Diagnosis of Liver Disease

Etsuko Hashimoto • Paul Y. Kwo
Arief A. Suriawinata • Wilson M. S. Tsui
Masaki Iwai

Editors

Diagnosis of Liver Disease

Second Edition

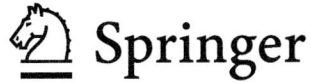 Springer

Editors
Etsuko Hashimoto
Department of Gastroenterology & Hepatology
Tokyo Women's Medical University
Shinjuku-ku
Tokyo
Japan

Arief A. Suriawinata
Department of Pathology and Laboratory
Medicine
Dartmouth–Hitchcock Medical Center
Lebanon, New Hampshire
USA

Masaki Iwai
Division of Gastroenterology, Hepatology &
Internal Medicine
Iwai Clinic
Kamigyo-ku
Kyoto
Japan

Paul Y. Kwo
Department of Gastroenterology/Hepatology
Stanford University School of Medicine
Palo Alto, CA
USA

Wilson M. S. Tsui
Department of Pathology
Caritas Medical Center
Kowloon
Hong Kong
China

Originally published by McGraw-Hill Education (Asia), Singapore, 2011
ISBN 978-981-13-6805-9   ISBN 978-981-13-6806-6 (eBook)
https://doi.org/10.1007/978-981-13-6806-6

This Springer imprint is published by the registered company Springer Nature Singapore Pte Ltd.
The registered company address is: 152 Beach Road, #21-01/04 Gateway East, Singapore 189721, Singapore

Preface

Our book is a primer that should guide practitioners, internists, gastroenterologists, and hepatologists in the assessment of patients with liver problems and is instructive for undergraduates and graduates in studying practical applications for diagnosis and treatment of liver diseases. Clinical manifestations, image analysis, and liver biopsy are essential for diagnosis and are combined throughout this book to assist clinicians in formulating differential diagnosis and treatment plan. Liver biopsy with or without peritoneoscopy is being replaced by noninvasive modalities for diagnosis. However, liver biopsy is still the "gold standard" for accurate diagnosis, and there is a significant emphasis on the role of macro- and microscopic pathology in elucidating pathogenesis as well as identifying confounding features of image findings in patients with liver disease that may lead to a more elaborate differential diagnosis. If appropriate, the role of light and electron microscopic examination—as well as the role of specific stains and molecular techniques—is illustrated.

Progress in diagnostic and therapeutic aspects of liver disease has been impressive, and our second book is edited by Professor Paul Y. Kwo, Professor Arief A. Suriawinata, Director Wilson M. S. Tsui, and Professor Etsuko Hashimoto as well as myself, and they also participate in authorship for their individual specialized chapters. We can also welcome Professor Takashi Kojima (anatomy and function), Associate Professor Yoshio Sumida (laboratory tests in liver disease), Associate Professor Yoshinori Harada (acute hepatitis), Professor Akio Ido (acute liver failure), Associate Professor Terumi Takahara (liver cirrhosis), Professor Mikio Zeniya (autoimmune liver diseases), Director Masahiko Koda (vascular and granulomatous liver diseases), Professor Toshinori Kamisako (hyperbilirubinemia), Associate Professor Naoshi Nishida (malignant liver tumors), and Professor Hironori Haga (liver pathology in transplantation) as authors. They describe essential and most current information for diagnosis of and therapy for liver diseases. Concepts related to each liver disease including the pathogenesis are summarized, and the diagnosis and therapy are presented in helpful tables. Concise, accurate, and up-to-date data on various diseases are provided in all chapters, and unresolved problems in diagnosis, treatment, and pathogenesis are clearly described. Thus, this book can be used as a textbook of clinical hepatology and can also be useful for gastroenterologists and hepatologists or researchers to explore topics and themes in the clinical field which should be scientifically investigated.

Practitioners, internists, gastroenterologists, and hepatologists encountering a patient with clinical manifestations of possible liver disease are often challenged when deciding how to reach a diagnosis for therapy by integrating clinical information, imaging studies, and potential liver biopsy. The latter may be accompanied simultaneously by peritoneoscopy showing macroscopic changes of the liver as well as image analysis to add accurate information for understanding the pathogenesis and generating a differential diagnosis. The findings should guide further management and assist in the final diagnosis of the liver disease and its treatment. The approach in this book is a practical one with a focus on the evaluation of representative cases, simultaneously illustrated with cross-sectional images (ultrasonography, computed tomography, magnetic resonance imaging, and angiography), pathological findings, and peritoneoscopic images. Our second book is cooperatively edited by specialists in hepatology and pathology and with the authors comprising experts from the United States, Europe, Asia, and Japan. This book should serve as a useful source of information for physicians, internists, hepatologists, gastroenterologists, radiologists, and pathologists worldwide.

Masaki Iwai, MD, PhD

Editors

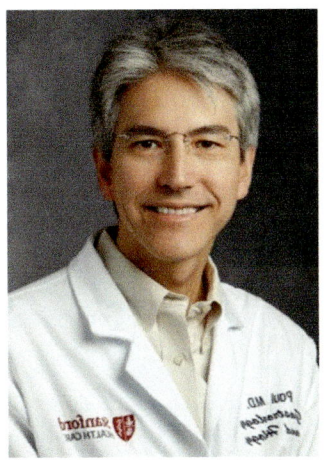

Professor Paul Y. Kwo, MD

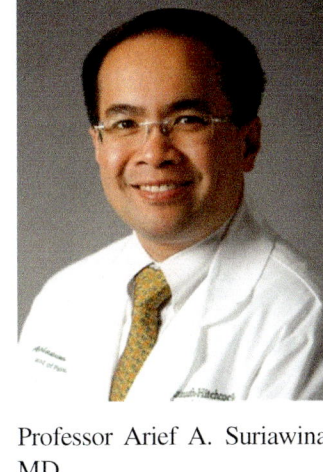

Professor Arief A. Suriawinata, MD

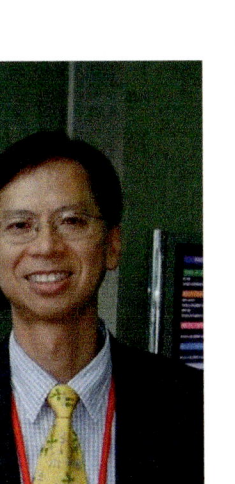

Director Masaki Iwai, MD, PhD

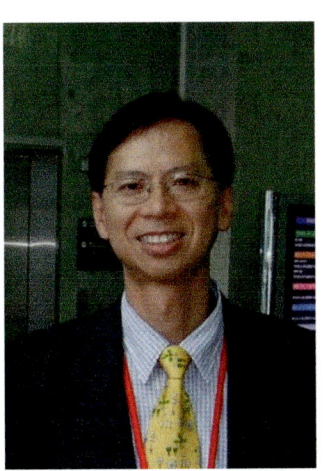

Director Wilson M. S. Tsui, MD, FRCPath

Professor Etsuko Hashimoto, MD, PhD

Acknowledgments I

The second edition of our book was supported by many doctors, whose contributions and warm assistance I hereby acknowledge: I am very happy to publish the second edition of Diagnosis of Liver Disease based upon the first edition for medical or graduate students, practitioners, hepatologists or gastroenterologists, radiologists, and clinical pathologists who want to study liver diseases. I expect that this book will be used for studying not only clinical manifestations, image analysis, and pathological features in liver diseases but also their pathogenesis. We were helped by contributions of Professors Alex Y. Chang, Dirk J. van Leeuwen, Paul Y. Kwo, Arief A. Suriawinata, and Director Wilson M. S. Tsui to the first edition preceding the second edition, and we acknowledge in the second edition all colleagues in the Department of Molecular Gastroenterology and Hepatology, Kyoto Prefectural University Graduate School of Medical Science, Otsu Municipal Hospital, Kyoto First Red Cross Hospital, North Medical Center Kyoto Prefectural University of Medicine, Kyoto Municipal Hospital, Kyoto Mitsubishi Hospital, Osaka Railway General Hospital, Kyoto Kizugawa Hospital, Kanagawa Prefectural Ashigarakami Hospital, Faculty of Medicine Tottori University, Tokyo Women's Medical University, and Caritas Medical Centre for presenting various kinds of liver diseases. I was much encouraged by editors and many authors to publish the second edition, and this textbook is dedicated not only to all colleagues working with us but also to medical students, internists, practitioners, gastroenterologists, hepatologists, radiologists, pathologists, and investigators who are studying liver diseases. I am also grateful to Springer Nature, Thieme Medical Publishers, Wiley, Wolters Kluwer, Japanese Society of Gastroenterology, Gastroenterological Endoscopy or Hepatology, and Kyoto Prefectural University of Medicine for kind permission to reproduce illustrations from their publications. Finally, I express my thanks to Subramaniam Vinodhini, a project manager and Sasirekka Nijanthan, a project coordinator in SPi Global, and Sachiko Hayakawa, an editor in Springer, for their continuous encouragement and kind support at all times in the publication of our second edition.

Masaki Iwai, MD, PhD

Acknowledgments II

We acknowledge Emeritus Professor Hisao Hayashi, Aichi-Gakuin University School of Pharmacy, Aichi; Dr. Akitoshi Douhara, Saiseikai Hospital, Sakurai; Dr. Yuji Eso, Kyoto University Graduate School of Medicine; Dr. Michiaki Ishii, Ayabe City Hospital; Dr. Hiroyuki Kimura, Kyoto First Red Cross Hospital; Dr. Hironori Mitsuyoshi, Kyoto Chubu Medical Center; Dr. Motoshige Nabeshima and Dr. Junya Tanaka, Mitsubishi Kyoto Hospital; Dr. Yorihisa Okada, Kameoka City Hospital; Dr. Hiroyuki Shintani, Kyoto Municipal Hospital; Dr. Kengo Takimoto, National Hospital Organization Kyoto Medical Center; Dr. Kazuhiro Tsuji, Kyoto Kizugawa Hospital, Kyoto, Japan, for their contributing to production of our book by its review and illustrating precious cases of liver diseases.

Editors

Contents

Contributors

Hironori Haga, MD, PhD Department of Clinical Pathology, Kyoto University Graduate School of Medicine, Kyoto, Japan

Yoshinori Harada, MD, PhD Department of Pathology and Cell Regulation, Graduate School of Medical Sciences, Kyoto Prefectural University of Medicine, Kyoto, Japan

Etsuko Hashimoto, MD, PhD Department of Gastroenterology and Hepatology, Tokyo Women's Medical University, Tokyo, Japan

Yutaka Horie, MD, PhD Division of Gastroinestinal Unit, Saiseikai Gotsu General Hospital, Shimane, Japan

Akio Ido, MD, PhD Digestive and Lifestyle Diseases, Department of Human and Environmental Sciences, Kagoshima University Graduate School of Medical and Dental Sciences, Kagoshima, Japan

Hajime Isomoto, MD, PhD Division of Medicine and Clinical Science, Department of Multidisciplinary Internal Medicine, Tottori University Faculty of Medicine, Tottori, Japan

Masaki Iwai, MD, PhD Division of Gastroenterology, Hepatology and Internal Medicine, Iwai Clinic, Kyoto, Japan

Nimy John, MD Department of Medicine, Gastroenterology and Hepatology, Stanford University School of Medicine, Palo Alto, CA, USA

Yoshihiro Kamada, MD, PhD Department of Molecular Biochemistry and Clinical Investigation, Osaka University, Graduate School of Medicine, Osaka, Japan

Department of Gastroenterology and Hepatology, Osaka University, Graduate School of Medicine, Osaka, Japan

Toshinori Kamisako, MD, PhD Department of Clinical Laboratory Medicine, Kindai University Faculty of Medicine, Osaka, Japan

Atsushi Kitamura, MD, PhD Division of Gastrointestinal Unit, Saiseikai Gotsu General Hospital, Shimane, Japan

Ryuichi Kita, MD, PhD Department of Gastroenterology and Hepatology, Osaka Red Cross Hospital, Osaka, Japan

Masahiko Koda, MD, PhD Hino Hospital, Tottori, Japan

Takashi Kojima, PhD Department of Cell Science, Research Institute for Frontier Medicine, Sapporo Medical University School of Medicine, Sapporo, Japan

Yosuke Kunishi, MD, PhD Department of Gastroenterology, Kanagawa Prefectural Ashigarakami Hospital, Tochigi, Japan

Paul Y. Kwo, MD Department of Medicine, Gastroenterology and Hepatology, Stanford University School of Medicine, Palo Alto, CA, USA

Tomomitsu Matono, MD, PhD Division of Medicine and Clinical Science, Department of Multidisciplinary Internal Medicine, Faculty of Medicine Tottori University, Tottori, Japan

Seiichi Mawatari, MD, PhD Digestive and Lifestyle Diseases, Department of Human and Environmental Sciences, Kagoshima University Graduate School of Medical and Dental Sciences, Kagoshima, Japan

Masako Mishima, MD Department of Gastroenterology and Hepatology, Kyoto University Graduate School of Medicine, Kyoto, Japan

Kenichi Miyoshi, MD, PhD Division of Medicine and Clinical Science, Department of Multidisciplinary Internal Medicine, Faculty of Medicine Tottori University, Tottori, Japan

Takahiro Mori, MD, PhD Division of Gastroenterology and Hepatology, Community Health Care Organization Kobe Central Hospital, Hyogo, Japan

Naoshi Nishida, MD, PhD Department of Gastroenterology and Hepatology, Kindai University Faculty of Medicine, Osaka, Japan

Bing Ren, MD, PhD Pathology and Laboratory Medicine, Department of Pathology and Laboratory Medicine, Dartmouth-Hitchcock Medical Center, Lebanon, NH, USA

Yoshio Sumida, MD, PhD, MBA Division of Gastroenterology and Hepatology, Department of Internal Medicine, Aichi Medical University, Aichi, Japan

Arief A. Suriawinata, MD Department of Pathology and Laboratory Medicine, Dartmouth-Hitchcock Medical Center, Lebanon, NH, USA

Terumi Takahara, MD, PhD Department of Gastroenterology and Hapatology, Toyama University Faculty of Medicine, Toyama, Japan

Makiko Taniai, MD, PhD Department of Gastroenterology and Hepatology, Tokyo Women's Medical University, Tokyo, Japan

Wilson M. S. Tsui, MD, FRCPath Department of Pathology, Caritas Medical Center, Kowloon, Hong Kong, China

Louis Vaickus, MD Department of Pathology and Laboratory Medicine, Dartmouth-Hitchcock Medical Center, Lebanon, NH, USA

Masashi Yoneda, MD, PhD Division of Hepatology and Pancreatology, Department of Internal Medicine, Aichi Medical University, Aichi, Japan

Mikio Zeniya, MD, PhD, FAASLD Sanno Medical Center, International University of Health and Welfare, Tokyo, Japan

Anatomy and Function

Masaki Iwai, Takashi Kojima, and Arief A. Suriawinata

Contents

1.1	Anatomy of the Liver	1
1.2	Anatomy of the Biliary Tract	3
1.3	Development of the Liver	3
1.4	Functional Heterogeneity of the Liver	6
1.5	Microanatomy of the Liver	7
1.6	Junctional Complex Between Hepatocytes	9
1.7	Regeneration	14
References		16

Abbreviations

AFP	Alpha fetoprotein
cAMP	cyclic adenosine $3',5'$-monophosphate
cGMP	cyclic guanosine $3',5'$-monophosphate
Cx	Connexin
EGFR	Epidermal growth factor receptor
GVHD	Graft-versus-host disease
HCV	Hepatitis C virus
IL-6	Interleukin-6
JAMs	Junctional adhesion molecules
PDZ	Postsynaptic density 95; Discs large, zonula occludens
PKC	Protein kinase C
PSC	Primary sclerosing cholangitis
SR-BI	Scavenger receptor BI
TNF	Tumor necrosis factor
ZO	Zonula occludens

M. Iwai, MD, PhD (✉)
Kyoto, Japan
e-mail: masaiwai@koto.kpu-m.ac.jp

T. Kojima, PhD
Sapporo, Japan

A. A. Suriawinata, MD
New Hampshire, USA

1.1 Anatomy of the Liver

The liver weighing 1200–1500 g is the largest organ in the human adult and occupies about 2% of body weight. There are two anatomical lobes in the liver, right and left, with the right lobe six times in volume than the left lobe. The right and left lobes are separated anteriorly by the falciform ligament, posteriorly by ligamentum venosum, and inferiorly by ligamentum teres. The Couinaud classification [1] defines eight segments of the liver, and the Bismuth classification [2] divides it into four sectors; they are subdivided into right anterior (V and VIII), right posterior (VI and VII), left medial (IV), or left lateral (II and III) segment and caudate lobe (I) (Fig. 1.1).

The liver receives double blood supply from the portal vein and hepatic artery. The portal vein brings about 65% of hepatic blood flow to the liver from the intestine and spleen, while the hepatic artery brings the remainder 35% from the celiac axis. These vessels enter the liver through the porta hepatis. Inside

© Springer Nature Singapore Pte Ltd. 2019
E. Hashimoto et al. (eds.), *Diagnosis of Liver Disease*, https://doi.org/10.1007/978-981-13-6806-6_1

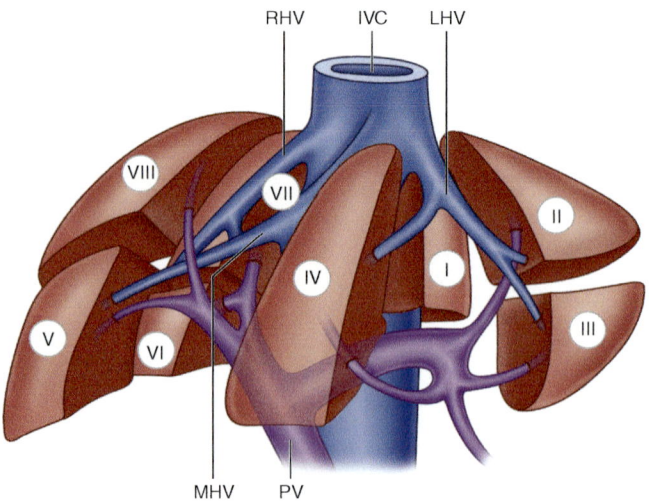

Fig. 1.1 Schematic demonstration of the vascular relations with the segments of the liver (Bismuth classification). The right anterior sector contains segments V and VIII; right posterior sector, segments VI and VII; left medial sector, segment IV; left lateral sector, segments II and III; caudate lobe, segment I. *IVC* inferior vena cava, *LHV* left hepatic vein, *MHV* middle hepatic vein, *RHV* right hepatic vein, *PV* portal vein

the porta hepatis, the portal vein and hepatic artery branch into the right and left lobes. Venous blood from the liver drains into the right and left hepatic veins and enters the inferior vena cava very near to the entry of the right atrium. Lymphatic channels are divided into deep and superficial networks. The former runs parallel to the branches of the portal vessels and hepatic veins, while the latter is found in the capsule, with numerous anastomoses among these networks. The right and left hepatic bile ducts join to form the common hepatic duct. The hepatic nerve plexus contains fiber from the synaptic ganglia, and it accompanies the hepatic artery and bile ducts in the portal tracts. A few fibers enter at the porta hepatis, and arteries are innervated by sympathetic fibers. The bile ducts are innervated by both sympathetic and parasympathetic fibers (Fig. 1.2a). Nerve fibers are present in the portal tract (Fig. 1.2b), and these unmyelinated sympathetic fibers innervate the hepatic parenchyma. Most hepatic nerve fibers are aminergic or peptidergic. Vasoactive intestinal peptide, neuropeptide Y, glucagon, somatostatin, neurotensin, and calcitonin gene-related peptide are present in hepatic nerve fibers (Fig. 1.2c) [3].

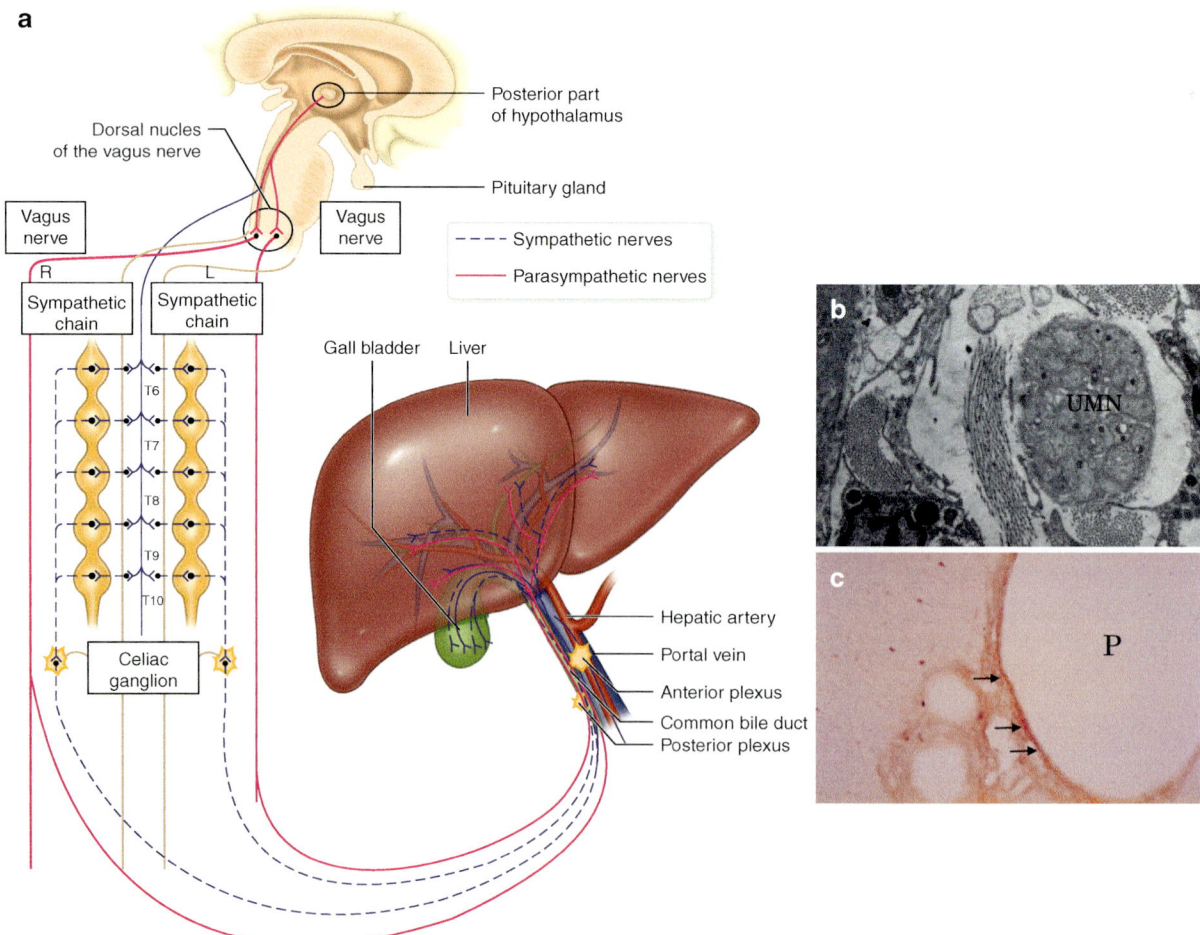

Fig. 1.2 Hepatic nerves. (**a**) Parasympathetic nerve fibers are derived from the dorsal nucleus of vagus nerve, while sympathetic nerve fibers are derived from spinal segments of T6 or 7–T10. They form intercommunicating plexuses around the hepatic artery and portal vein. (**b**) Unmyelinated nerve (UMN) bundle is seen in portal tract of rat liver. (**c**) Glucagon-immunoreactivity (arrow) is seen on nerve fibers in the wall of rat portal vein (P). (**b**, **c**); reuse of Iwai M, et al. Immunoreactive glucagon in rats with normal or regenerative livers induced by galactosamine. Biomedical Res. 1988;9:85–92, with permission of its chief editor

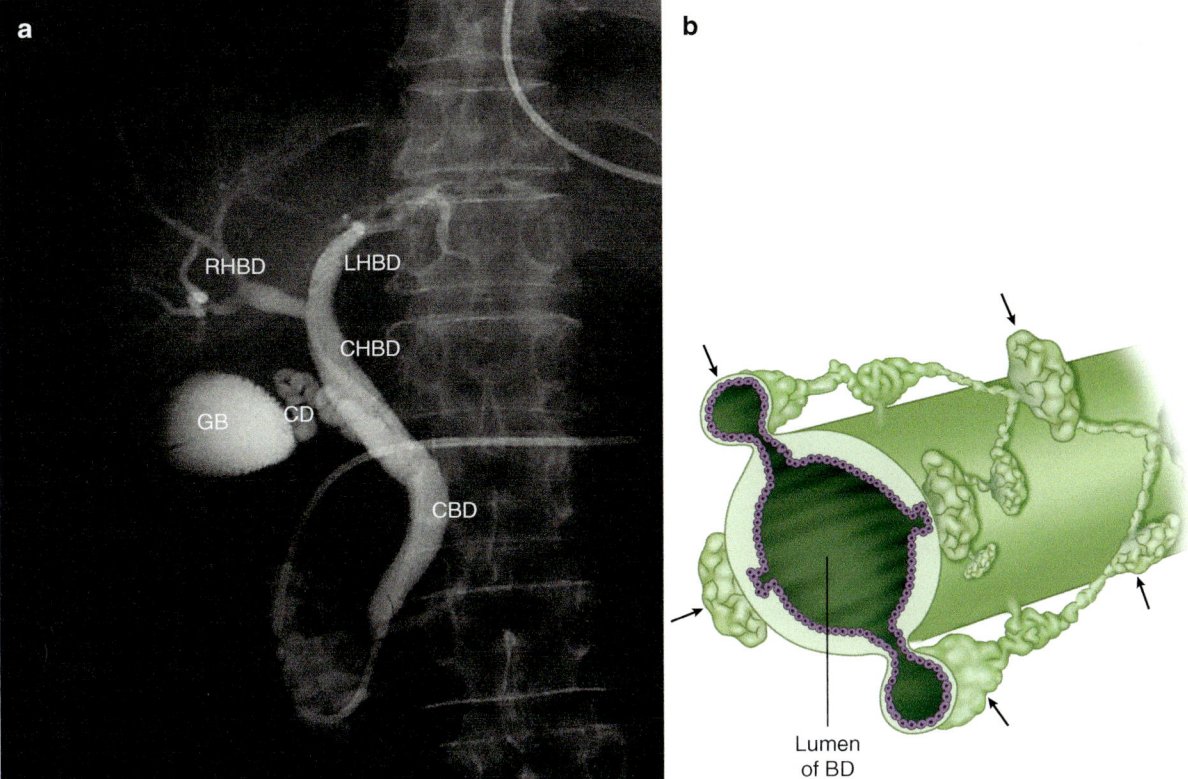

Fig. 1.3 Anatomy of bile duct (BD) and peribiliary gland. (**a**) Cholangiography under therapy of endoscopic biliary drainage shows common bile duct (CBD), common hepatic bile duct (CHBD), right or left hepatic bile duct (RHBD or LHBD), and gall bladder (GB) with cystic duct (CD). (**b**) Peribiliary glands (arrow) are communicating with large bile ducts

The liver takes important roles for metabolism of amino acid/protein, carbohydrate, lipid/lipoprotein, bile acid, bilirubin, hormones, vitamins, and porphyrin. Biotransformation and detoxification of trace elements, acid-base balance, and alcohol degradation also occur in the liver. The morphological and functional integrity of the liver is vital to the health of body, and disturbance of their integrity is closely associated with pathogenesis of liver diseases.

1.2 Anatomy of the Biliary Tract

The right and left hepatic bile ducts (diameter: >800 μm) emerge from the liver and unite at the porta hepatis to form the common hepatic duct (diameter: 0.4 mm–1.3 cm). They are joined by the cystic duct from the gall bladder to form the common bile duct (Fig. 1.3a). Large bile ducts are lined by columnar epithelium with thicker fibrous walls. In primary sclerosing cholangitis (PSC) and IgG4-related cholangitis, the large bile ducts or extrahepatic bile duct is stenotic.

Small intrahepatic bile ducts are classified into septal (diameter >100 μm) and interlobular bile ducts (diameter 40–100 μm). The interlobular bile ducts are connected to the bile canalicular network by ductules and the canals of Hering (diameter: <15 μm). Small bile ducts less than 100 μm are the focus of examination in chronic allograft rejection, GVHD, and Alagille syndrome and are severely damaged in primary biliary cholangitis.

Peribiliary glands are seen within the walls of extrahepatic bile ducts and along the large intrahepatic bile ducts and drain secretory component into the bile duct lumen via their own conduit [4] (Fig. 1.3b). They are thought to have absorptive and secretory activities and may be a site of biliary epithelial regeneration. Cystic lesion, hyperplasia, adenoma, and adenocarcinoma can arise from peribiliary glands.

1.3 Development of the Liver

The human liver arises from hepatic diverticulum of the foregut during the third or fourth week of gestation (Fig. 1.4a). The left and right vitelline veins around the foregut communicate to each other and form sinusoids [5]. The umbilical veins pass on each side of the liver and connect to the hepatic sinusoids (Fig. 1.4b). As the embryo develops, blood, supplying this region, delivers nutrients from the yolk sac, placenta, and gut [6]. Hepatocyte precursors, hepatoblasts, arise from endodermal cells at the front of the diverticulum and invade the mesoderm of septum transversum. The confluence of endodermal cells from the hepatic diverticulum that grows

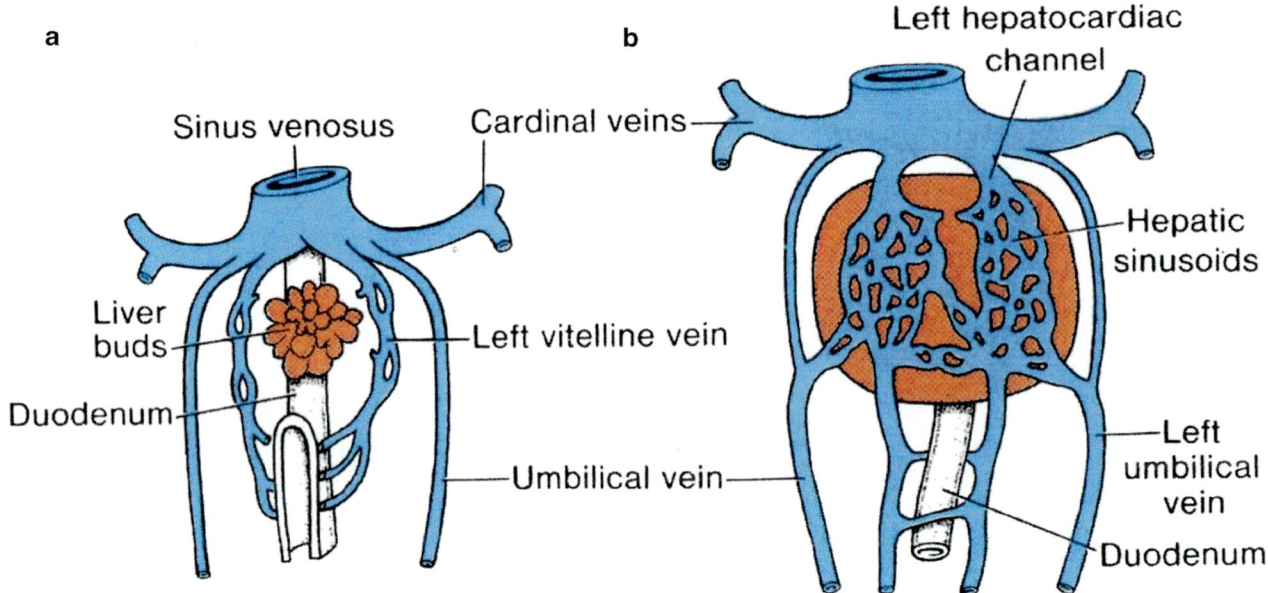

a

Sinus venosus **Cardinal veins**

Liver buds **Left vitelline vein**

Duodenum

Umbilical vein

b

Left hepatocardiac channel

Hepatic sinusoids

Left umbilical vein

Duodenum

Fig. 1.4 Development of the vitelline and umbilical veins during the fourth (**a**) and fifth (**b**) week. Note the plexus around the duodenum, formation of the hepatic sinusoids, and initiation of left-to-right shunts between the vitelline veins. (**a**) Liver buds arise from the ventral wall of the future duodenum. (**b**) Blood from umbilical veins drains to the sinusoidal plexus and passes through symmetrical right and left hepato-cardiac channels, to enter the sinus venous. (Reproduced from Sadler's, Langman's Medical Embryology, tenth edition with permission from Wolters Kluwer)

Fig. 1.5 Sagittal section of a human embryo at approximately 32 days of development. The confluence of endodermal cells from hepatic diverticulum invades septum transversum

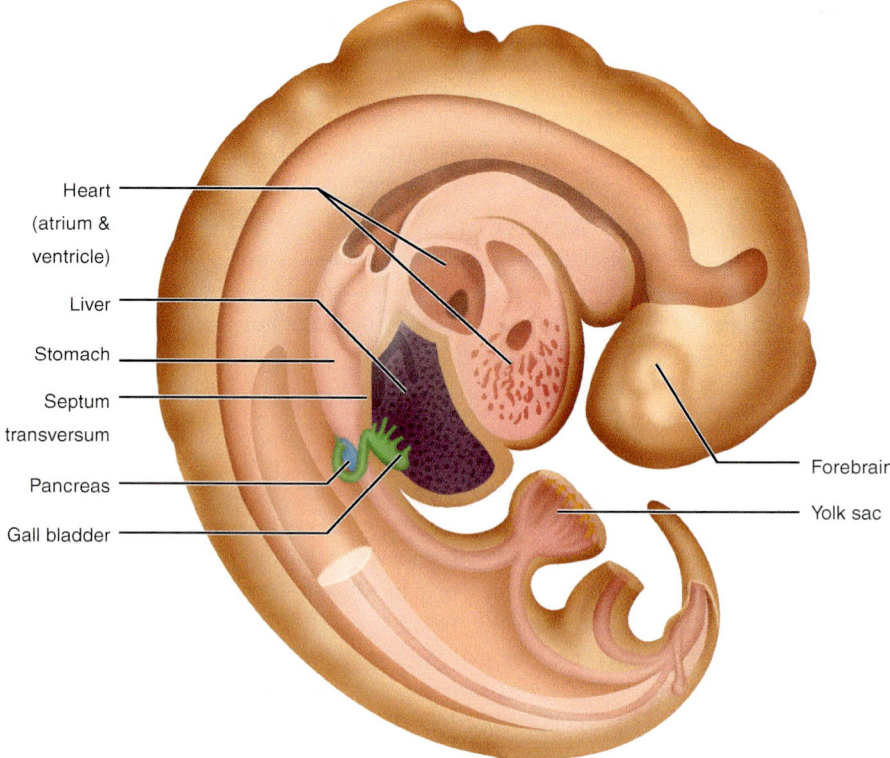

Heart (atrium & ventricle)

Liver

Stomach

Septum transversum

Pancreas

Gall bladder

Forebrain

Yolk sac

into host mesenchyme creates the solid organ destined to be liver, while hepatoblasts form trabecular structures (Fig. 1.5). The vitelline veins traverse the region, bridging blood from the yolk sac and digestive tube to the heart. As hepatoblasts invade the mesenchyme, they disrupt the vitelline veins of which segments become the portal veins. The hepatic bud is subdivided into cords by new capillaries of sinusoids, and the sinusoidal flow coalesces into three major hepatic veins.

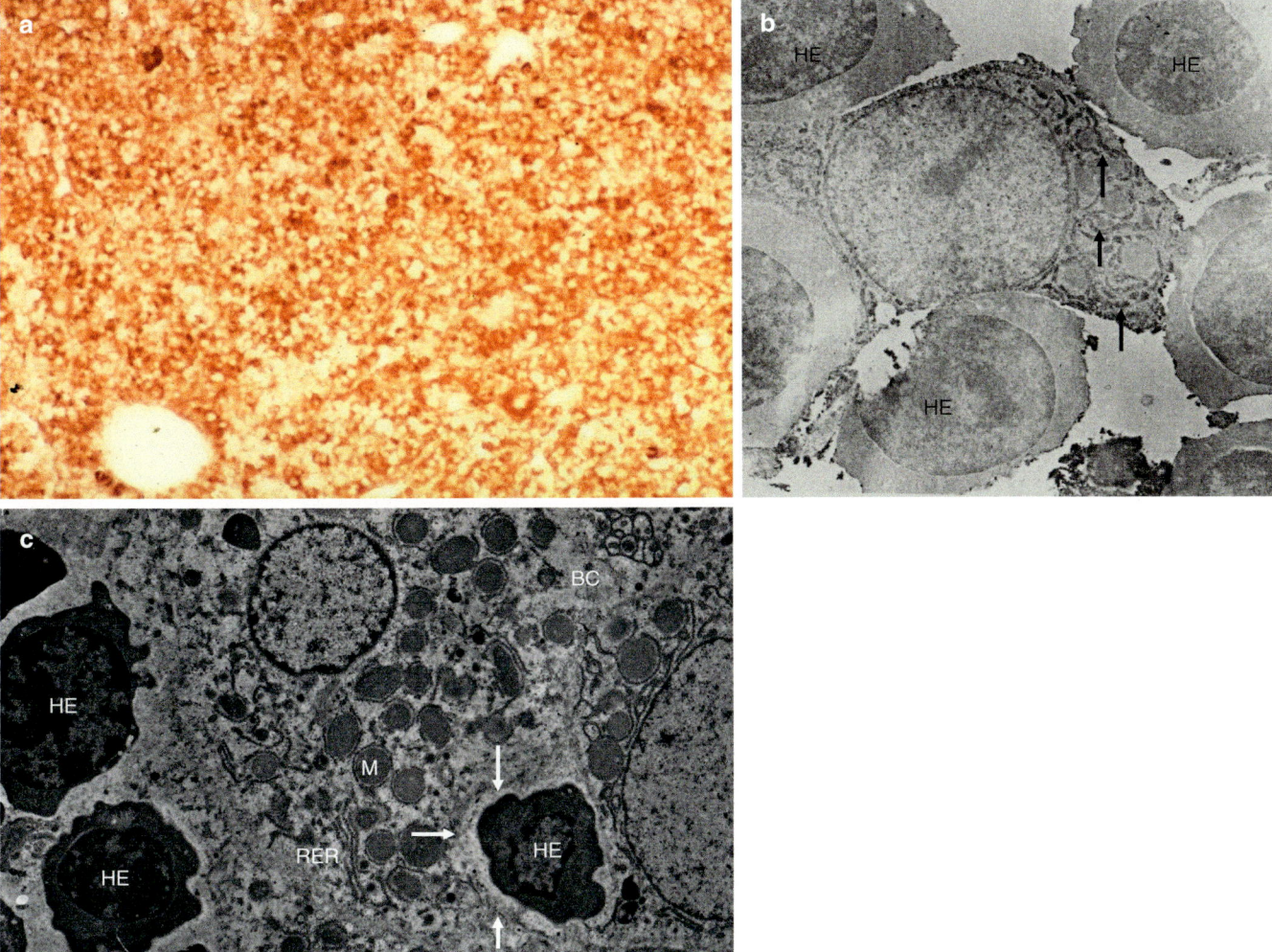

Fig. 1.6 AFP-positive hepatocytes in prenatal liver of rat an Immunohistochemistry for AFP in the liver of prenatal period. (**a**) AFP immunoreactivity is present in all hepatocytes. (**b**) Immunoelectron microscopy of AFP. AFP immunoreactivity (arrow) is detected in poor lamellar structure of rough endoplasmic reticulum. AFP-positive cell is in contact with hematopoietic cells (HE) and is oppressed by HE. (**c**) Electron microscopy shows hepatocytes surrounded by HE, and they have poorly structured rough endoplasmic reticulum (RER) and mitochondria (M), and microvilli (arrow) and bile canaliculi (BC) are visible

Hepatoblast cords develop into anastomosing tubular structures with central bile canaliculi that eventually communicate with the bile ducts. Most hepatoblasts produce AFP (Fig. 1.6a, b) and differentiate into hepatocytes. Numerous hematopoietic cells are found in the sinusoids even at birth and surround immature hepatocytes (Fig. 1.6c), but they are largely gone from the liver by 4 weeks of age.

Hepatoblasts adjacent to the portal mesenchyme differentiate into a layer of duct progenitors called the ductal plate [7]. The ductal plate gradually becomes bilayer and forms ductal segments with lumina. These ductal segments migrate away from the limiting plate to a more central location in the portal tracts near the portal veins. Portion of the ductal plate is resorbed, leaving a complex anastomosing network of ducts which continues to simplify in the weeks after birth. Abnormal remodeling of the embryonic ductal plate causes neonatal biliary atresia [8], congenital hepatic fibrosis, Caroli's disease, microhamartoma, choledochal cyst, and polycystic disease in which there is a genetic abnormality in cholangiocytic cilia leading to disruption of fluid transport and cholangiocyte proliferation [9]. The common bile duct, left and right hepatic ducts, and gallbladder develop in the stalk region of the hepatic diverticulum. These ducts are connected with the ductal plate at the cranial end of the diverticulum.

The liver occupies most of the abdominal cavity in the third month of gestation, in part because of large masses of sinusoidal hematopoietic cells. Thereafter, the right lobe grows faster than the left lobe but less than the growth rate of the rest of the body. The liver cell cords remain tubular until birth when they begin to remodel into double-cell plates and eventually into single-cell plates by 5 years of age.

1.4   Functional Heterogeneity of the Liver

Rappaport advocates a series of functional acini, each centered on the portal tract with its terminal branch of portal vein, hepatic artery and bile duct (Fig. 1.7a), [10] and fibrous tissue supports the structure of the portal tract and central vein (Fig. 1.7b). Hepatocytes show different structural and functional characteristics depending on their acinar location. The relative functions of cells in acini area adjacent to terminal hepatic veins (zone 3) are different from those in the area of zone 1. The zonation is related to the lobular/

acinar oxygen gradient and to signaling via Wnt/beta-catenin pathway [11]. Glycogenesis, fatty acid metabolism, and protein, albumin, or fibrinogen synthesis are more active in zone 1 than in zone 3 hepatocytes (Fig. 1.8a, b). Urea synthesis and glutaminase are found in the highest concentration in zone 1, whereas glutamine synthetase is more active at perivenular zone 3. The drug-metabolizing P450 enzymes are present in greater amounts in zone 3, which is the site of detoxification and biotransformation of drugs. The cells in zone 3 receive their oxygen supply last and are particularly prone to anoxic liver injury. Sharply defined

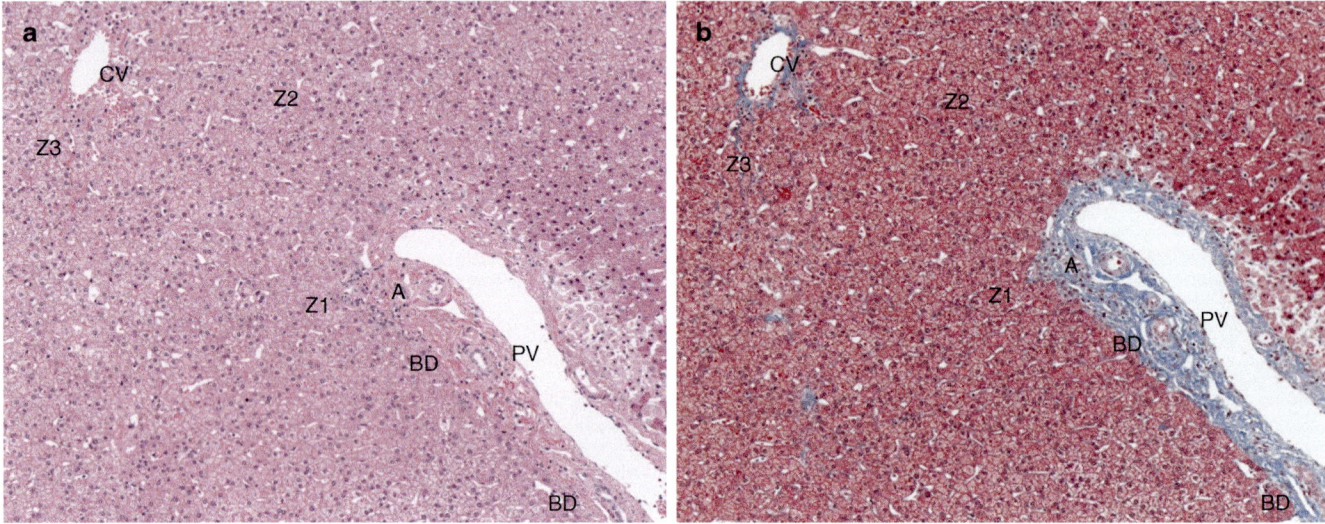

Fig. 1.7 Normal architecture of hepatic acini in adult liver. (**a**) Cords of liver cells are radiating from a central vein (CV) and interlaced in ordered fashion by sinusoids, and at the periphery a portal tract contains arteriole (A), bile duct (BD), and portal vein (PV). Z1, 2, and 3; zone 1,

zone 2, and zone 3. H&E staining. (**b**) Portal tract and central vein are supported by fibrous tissue, which is scarcely seen along hepatocytes. Masson trichrome staining. (Courtesy of Dr. Y Harada)

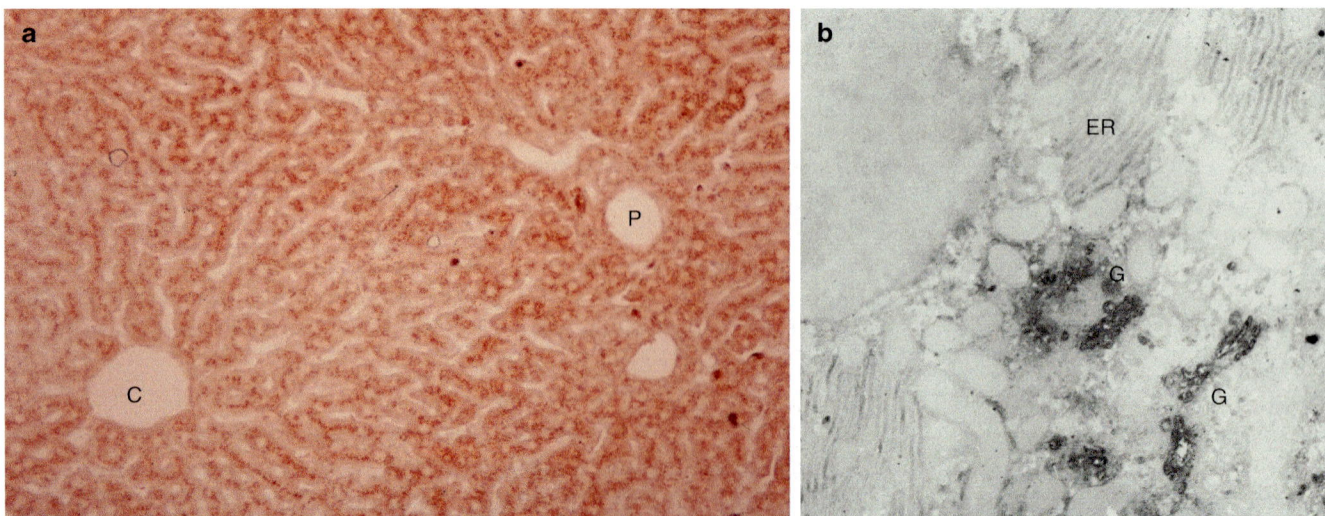

Fig. 1.8 Immunohistochemistry of albumin-positive hepatocytes in a lobule of adult rat and ultrastructural finding of albumin immunoreactivity. (**a**) All hepatocytes contain albumin immunoreactivity, and its

intensity is stronger in periportal area than in pericentral one (C). *P* portal vein; *C* central vein. (**b**) Albumin immunoreactivity is visible in rough endoplasmic reticulum (ER) and Golgi (G) apparatus

Table 1.1 Functional and ultrastructural heterogeneity of hepatocytes in acini

	Zone 1	Zone 3
Organelle	Golgi complex; rich Mitochondria; numerous, larger, more inner membranes	Smooth ER; rich Mitochondria; smaller, less inner membranes
Protein synthesis (albumin fibrinogen)	3+	1+
Carbohydrate	Gluconeogenesis	Glycolysis
Glutathione	2+	1+
Ammonia metabolism	1+	2+
Cytochrome 450	+	3+
Oxygen supply	3+	+
Bile formation		
Bile salt dependent	2+	1+
Non-bile salt dependent	1+	2+

zone 3 necrosis is characteristic of toxicity from acetaminophen, pyrrolizidine alkaloids, and various hydrocarbons such as halothane and carbon tetrachloride. Zone 1 necrosis has been found with allyl alcohol, phosphorus, and high-dose iron ingestion (Table 1.1).

1.5   Microanatomy of the Liver (Fig. 1.9)

Hepatocytes: The life span of liver cells is about 150 days in experimental animals, and hepatocytes comprise about 65% of the liver. They are arranged in plates of one cell in thickness and polygonal in shape, ranging from 30 to 40 μm in diameter. Microvilli project into the perisinusoidal space, providing active secretion or absorption of nutrients from the space of Disse. Hepatocytes are attached to one another by tight junctions, gap junctions, and desmosomes. There are

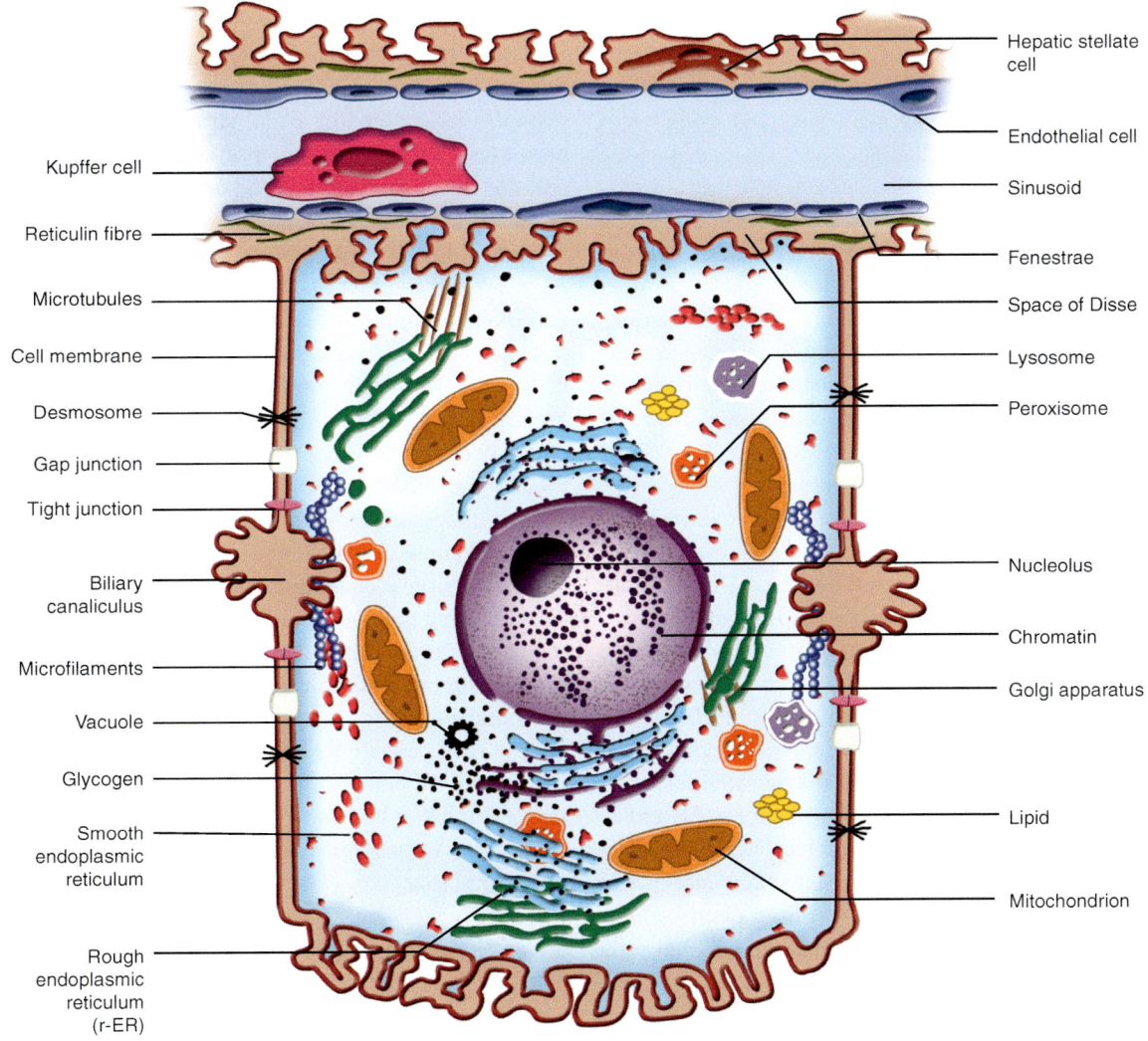

Fig. 1.9 Ultrastructural scheme of hepatocyte and mesenchymal cells within the lobule. Hepatocytes are attached to one another by junctional complex and they have abundant organellae, projecting microvilli in the perisinusoidal space. Sinusoids are composed of endothelial and stellate cells, and infiltrated by Kupffer cells

three surfaces: sinusoidal, basolateral, and canalicular surfaces. The polarity of the cell membrane is maintained by tight junctions [12].

The hepatocytes have single nucleus or, sometimes, multiple nuclei. The cytoplasm is rich in rough or smooth endoplasmic reticulum, mitochondria, peroxisomes, and lysosomes. Cell functions associated with the endoplasmic reticulum include protein synthesis, metabolism of fatty acids, production of cholesterol or triglyceride and bile acids, xenobiotic metabolism, and heme degradation. Golgi complex, lying near the canaliculus, has a role not only for secretion of proteins but also for glycosylation of secretory proteins. Production of energy and oxidative phosphorylation take place in mitochondria. The mitochondria also contain various enzymes useful for cycle of citric acid, beta-oxidation of fatty acid, and heme synthesis. Lysosomes located adjacent to the bile canaliculi contain many hydrolytic enzymes which can destroy the cell. The lysosomes are the site of deposition of ferritin, copper, bile pigment, lipofuscin, and senescent organelles. The peroxisomes are enzyme-rich and oxidative-reactive structures. The enzymes include simple oxidases and those involved in beta-oxidation cycles, glyoxylate cycle, lipid synthesis, and cholesterol biosynthesis.

The cytoskeleton supporting the hepatic structure consists of microtubules, microfilaments, and intermediate filaments [13]. Microtubules that contain tubulin control subcellular motility, vesicle movement, and secretion of plasma protein or glycoprotein. Microfilaments made up of actin are contractile and are important for the motility of bile canaliculus and for the bile flow. Intermediate filaments consisting of cytokeratins are essential for the stability and special organization of hepatocytes.

Endothelial cells: The sinusoidal endothelial cells constitute 70% of sinusoidal cells, and they do not have intercellular junctions or a conventional basement membrane. They act as a sieve between sinusoid and space of Disse due to presence of fenestrations. The fenestrations are larger in zone 1, but smaller and more numerous in zone 3, filtering macromolecules of different sizes [14]. The fenestrations can change in size in response to stimuli of pressure, neural impulses, endotoxins, alcohol, serotonin, and nicotine. They also have specific and non-specific endocytic activities and a variety of receptors. Receptor-mediated endocytosis exists for several molecules including transferrin, ceruloplasmin, and high- or low-density lipoprotein. Sinusoidal endothelial cells can clear small particles (<0.1 μm) from circulation as well as denatured collagen. Unlike vascular endothelial cells elsewhere in the body, sinusoidal endothelial cells do not express CD34 or factor VIII-related antigen. However, in chronic liver disease or liver cirrhosis, they undergo a phenotypic shift to conventional vascular endothelium and are referred as capillarization of sinusoids [15].

Kupffer cells: Kupffer cells are the resident macrophages attached to the endothelial cell lining of the sinusoids and can be mobilized. They are derived from monocytes in bone marrow and are found in greater number in the periportal area. Their cytoplasm contains microvilli, intracytoplasmic-coated vesicles, and dense bodies made up by lysosomal apparatus. They are responsible for removing old blood cells, cellular debris, bacteria, viruses, parasites, and tumor cells by endocytosis through receptor- or non-receptor-mediated mechanisms [16]. They are activated by agents of endotoxin, sepsis, shock, interferon-gamma, arachidonic acid, and tumor necrosis factor. They produce cytokines; hydrogen peroxide; nitric oxide; tumor necrosis factor; interleukin 1, 6, or 10; interferon alpha; transforming growth factor; and prostanoids [17].

Hepatic stellate cells: They are known as fat-storing cells, stellate cells, Ito cells, or lipocytes. They lie within the subendothelial space of Disse. Cytoplasmic droplets contain abundant vitamin A in the form of retinol palmitate [18], which can be identified by their immunoreactivity to smooth muscle actin. When the droplets are scanty, they resemble fibroblasts, which contain actin and myosin and contract in response to endothelin-1 and substance P [19] to regulate blood flow and to influence portal pressure [20]. In hepatocellular injury, hepatic Kupffer cells are activated, releasing many cytokines. Stellate cells transform to myofibroblast-like phenotype, producing collagen types 1, 3, and 4 and laminin. They also release matrix proteinases and their inhibitory molecules. In normal condition or liver injury, hepatic stellate cells play a role in regeneration, induced by hepatic growth factor in response to insulin-like growth factor 2 [21].

Pit cells: Pit cells are natural killer-lymphocytes attached to the sinusoidal surface of the endothelium [22] and are numerous in sinusoids of zone 1. They are short-lived cells that are renewed from circulating large granular lymphocytes. They have characteristic granules which contain perforin injuring cell membrane [22] and have a role for killing tumor cells and virus-infected hepatocytes.

Bile duct epithelial cells: Biliary epithelial cells that are columnar in shape, lining intrahepatic and extrahepatic bile duct system, constitute 3.0–5.0% of all hepatic cells [23]. Compared to hepatocytes, biliary epithelial cells contain fewer mitochondria and less endoplasmic reticulum. They are rich in cytoskeleton and contain prominent Golgi apparatus, numerous vesicles, and short luminal microvilli. Cholangiocytes lining small ducts transport water and organic solutes under hormonal control (secretin and somatostatin). IgA and IgM are secreted through cholangiocytes [24]. Bile acids are absorbed by biliary epithelium and are recirculated by a cholehepatic shunt pathway via the peribiliary plexus, [25] which promotes bile acid-dependent bile flow in the ducts [26].

1.6 Junctional Complex Between Hepatocytes

Hepatocytes are attached to each other by tight junctions, gap junctions, and desmosomes. There are three surfaces of hepatocytes: sinusoidal, basolateral, and canalicular domains. The polarity of cell membrane is maintained by tight junctions [12].

Tight junctions constitute the permeability barrier to macromolecules between the bile canaliculus and the rest of the intercellular space, preventing passage of the bile out of the canaliculus. The most apically located intercellular junctional complexes inhibit solute and water flow through the paracellular space (termed the "barrier" function) [27, 28], and they also separate the apical from the basolateral cell surface domains to establish cell polarity (termed the "fence" function)) [29, 30] (Fig. 1.10a). Recent evidence suggests that tight junctions also participate in signal transduction mechanisms that regulate epithelial cell proliferation, gene expression, differentiation, and morphogenesis [31]. The tight junctions are formed by not only the integral membrane proteins claudins, occludins, and JAMs (Fig. 1.10b) but also many peripheral membrane proteins, including the scaffold PDZ-expression proteins, cell polarity molecules, and non-PDZ-expressing proteins (Fig. 1.10c) [32–34]. Tricellulin was identified at tricellular contacts where there are three epithelial cells and has shown to have a barrier function (Fig. 1.10b) [35].

In the human liver, occludin, JAM-A, ZO-1, ZO-2, claudin-1, claudin-2, claudin-3, claudin-7, claudin-8, claudin-12, claudin-14, and tricellulin are detected together in well-developed tight junction structures (Fig. 1.11a, c). Claudin-2 shows a lobular gradient increasing from periportal to pericentral hepatocytes as in the livers of rat and mouse, whereas claudin-1 is expressed in the whole liver lobule (Fig. 1.11b). Tricellulin is detected in the regions of bile canaliculi where tight junctions can be identified as a set of branching intramembranous strands in freeze-fracture replicas (Fig. 1.12a, b) [36]. Claudin-1 and claudin-2 in hepatocytes are regulated by various cytokines and growth factors via distinct signal transduction pathways (Fig. 1.13a, b) [37, 38].

As a genetic disease of human tight junction protein, missense mutations in ZO-2 have been identified in patients with familial hypercholanemia [39]. In neonatal ichthyosis-sclerosing cholangitis (NISCH) syndrome, mutations of claudin-1 may lead to increased paracellular permeability between bile duct epithelial cells [40].

HCV is an enveloped positive-stranded RNA hepatotropic virus. Three host cell molecules are important entry factors or receptors for HCV internalization: scavenger receptor BI (SR-BI), tetraspanin CD81, and claudin-1 [41]. CD81 and claudin-1 act as co-receptors during late stages in the HCV

Fig. 1.10 Structure of tight junction. (**a**) Fence or barrier function of tight junction and its signal transduction. (**b**) Molecular structure of tight junction. (**c**) Tight junctional formation in cell membrane in association with actin filament

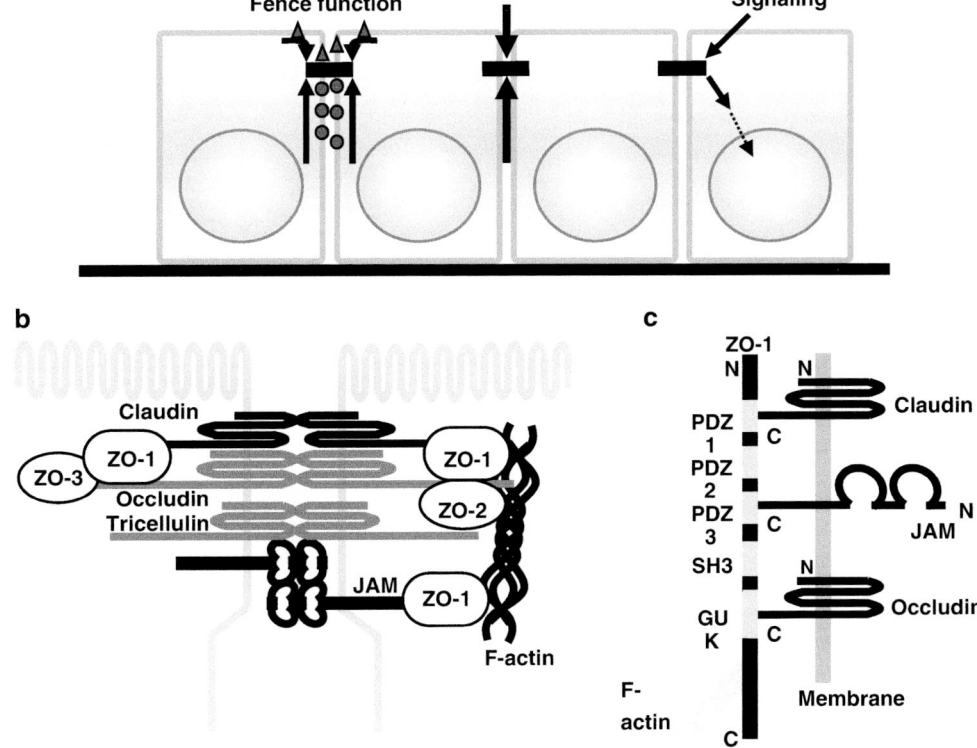

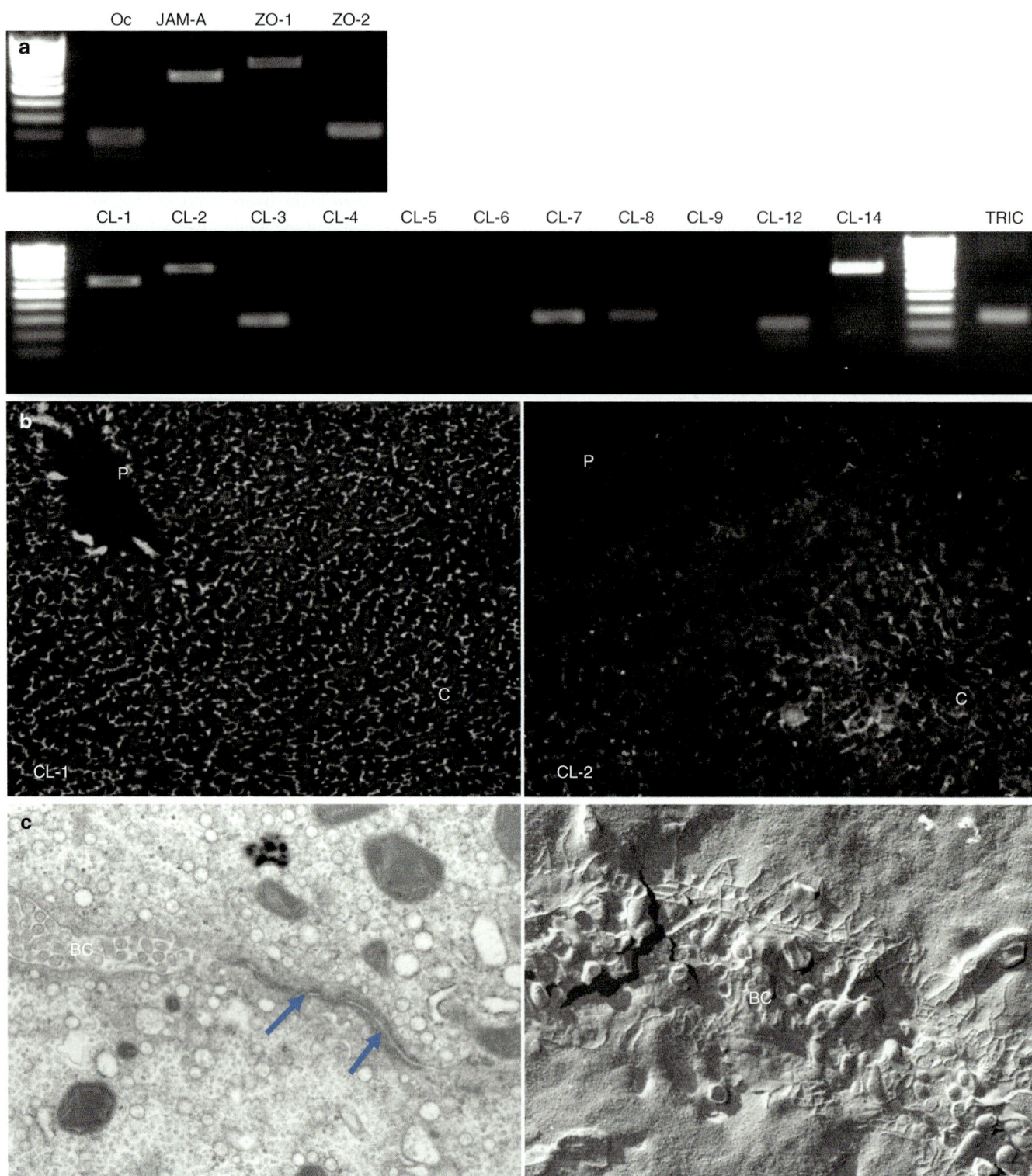

Fig. 1.11 Molecular structure of tight junction. (**a**) Western blot shows expression of JAM, Z-1, ZO-2, CL-1, CL-2, CL3, CL-7, CL-8, CL-12, and CL-14 in human liver. (**b**) Immunohistochemistry of CL-1 and CL-2. CL-1-immunoreactivity is seen diffusely on bile canaliculus of all hepatocytes, and CL-2 is detected on bile canaliculus of hepatocytes in pericentral area. (**c**) TEM and freeze fracture show tight junctional structure (arrow). *BC* bile canaliculus

human liver

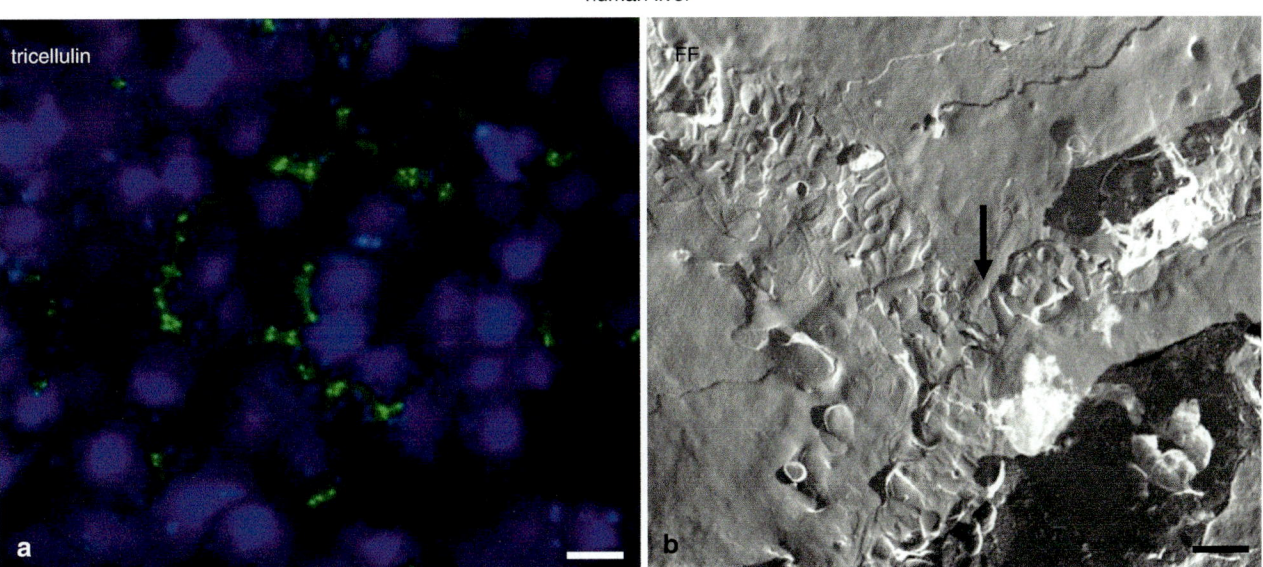

Fig. 1.12 Immunohistochemistry of tricellulin and its observation by freeze-fracture method. (**a**) Tricellulin-positive immunofluorescence is seen on bile canaliculi. (**b**) Freeze-fracture replicas show branched intramembranous strands in tight junction

Fig. 1.13 Relation between tight junction and various cytokines. (**a**) Association of tight junction and oncostatin, IL-1beta, TNF alpha, IL-6, EGF, HGF, and TGF beta produced by non-parenchymal cells. (**b**) Oncostatin, EGF, and TGF beta suppress Claudin-1 expression in hepatocytes. Oncostatin, IL-1 beta, EGF, HGF, and TGF beta can induce expression of Claudin-2

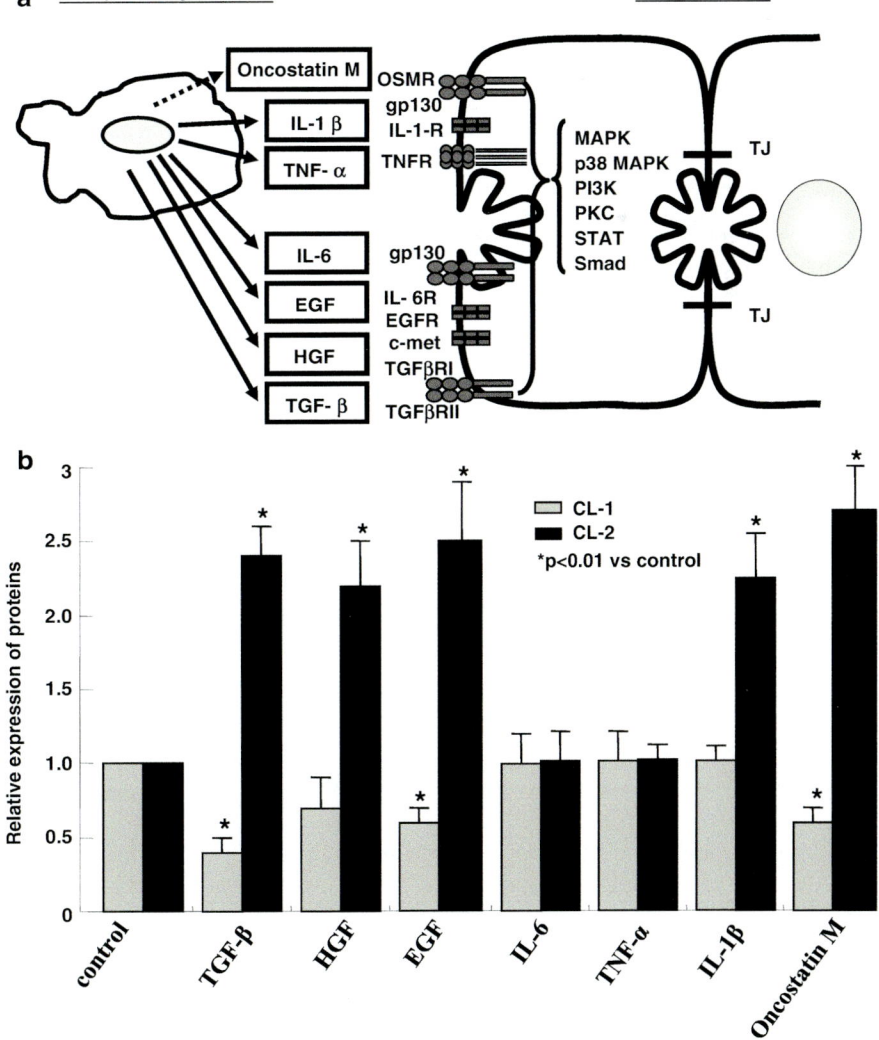

entry process. The first extracellular loop of claudin-1 in the liver is critical for the entry [42]. Occludin is also reported to be required for HCV entry [43, 44]. The tight junction proteins, claudin and occludin, are novel key factors for HCV infection. Both are potential targets for antiviral drugs.

Gap junctions are composed of 12 subunits (connexin) (Fig. 1.14a, b), six of which are contributed by each neighboring cell; the six-subunit assembly contributed by each cell is called a connexon or hemichannel (Fig. 1.14a, c) [45]. Intercellular communications occur at the gap junctions, involving calcium ion, second messenger RNA, and nerve impulses from zone 1–3. Connexin (Cx) 32 are permeable to both cAMP and cGMP, whereas heteromeric connexons composed of Cx32 and Cx26 lose permeability to cAMP but not to cGMP (Fig. 1.14d) [46]. The gap junctions also play an important role in liver homeostasis, [47] liver development [48], cancer, [49–52] and non-tumor liver diseases (hepatitis, liver fibrosis, cirrhosis, cholestasis, hepatic ischemia, and reperfusion injury) [47]. Hemichannels of

connexon are made up of Cx32 in pericentral area of adult liver (Fig. 1.15a), and they are mixed with Cx32 and Cx26 in periportal area (Fig. 1.15b, c) [53]. The cells of the liver capsule, Ito (fat-storing) cells, cholangiocytes, and endothelial cells express Cx43 as a major gap junction protein (Fig. 1.15d) [46].

In freeze-fracture images, hepatic gap junctions are recognizable as plaques of approximately 8- to 9-nm intramembranous particles present in the P fracture face in vertebrate tissues; complementary pits appear on the E fracture face (Fig. 1.16a). These plaques are generally round or oval and can be quite large in hepatocytes. Furthermore, small gap junction plaques are associated with tight junction strands in some cell types including hepatocytes (Fig. 1.16b), and Cx32 is partly colocalized with occludin and claudin-1 forming tight junction structures [54]. In Cx32-transfectanted immortalized mouse hepatocytes, which lack endogenous Cx32 and Cx26, induction of tight junction strands, and the integral tight junction proteins, occludins and claudins are observed,

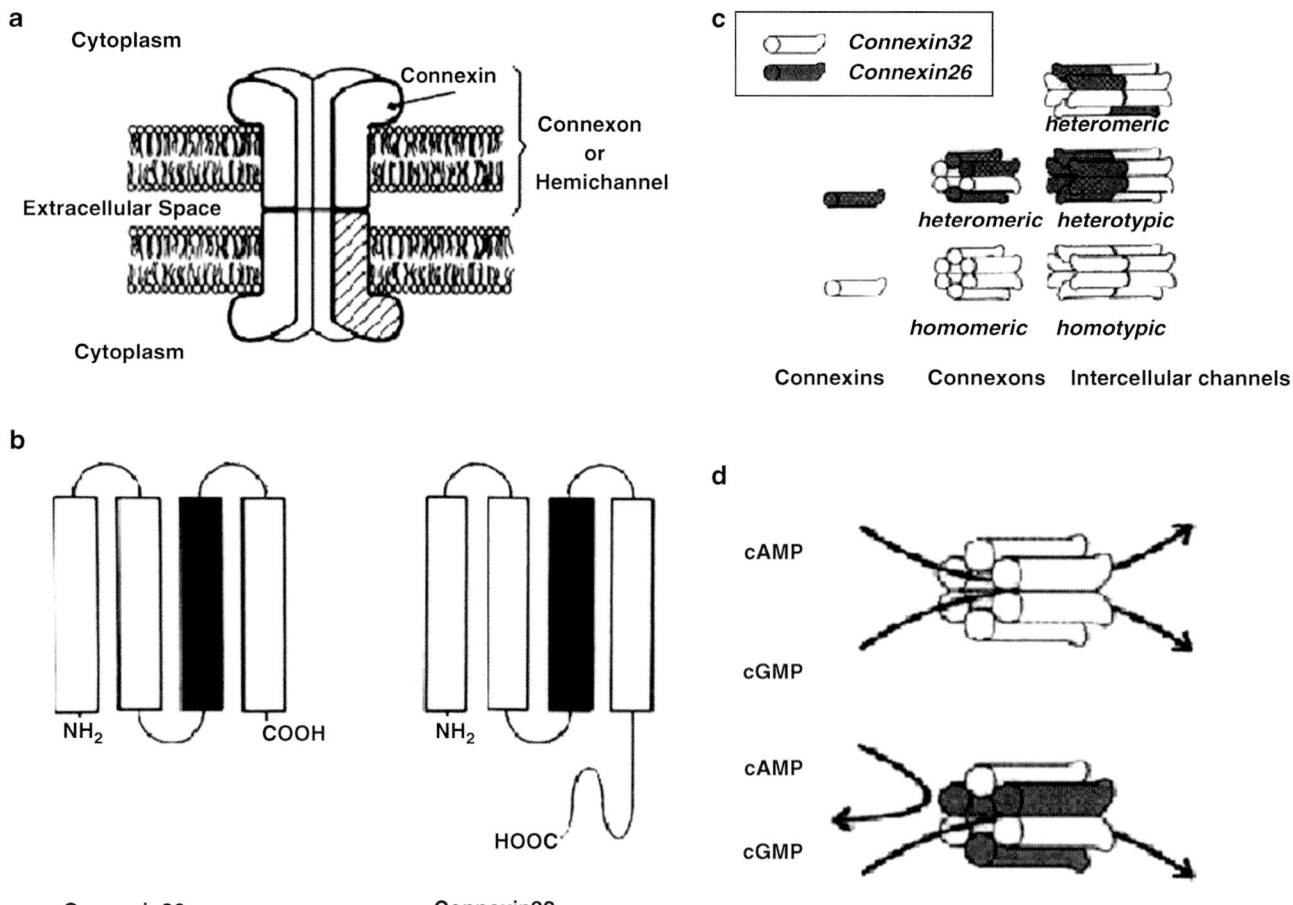

Fig. 1.14 Structure of gap junctions. (**a**) Connexon or hemichannel of gap junction is composed of six subunits of connexin. (**b**) There are two types of connexin in hepatocytes, and connexin 26 or 32 is a penetrating protein in cell membrane. (**c**) There are homomeric or heteromeric

hemichannels, and there are homotypic or heterotypic intercellular channels. (**d**) Homomeric channels of Cx32 are permeable to both cAMP and cGMP, whereas heteromeric connexons lose permeability to cAMP but not to cGMP

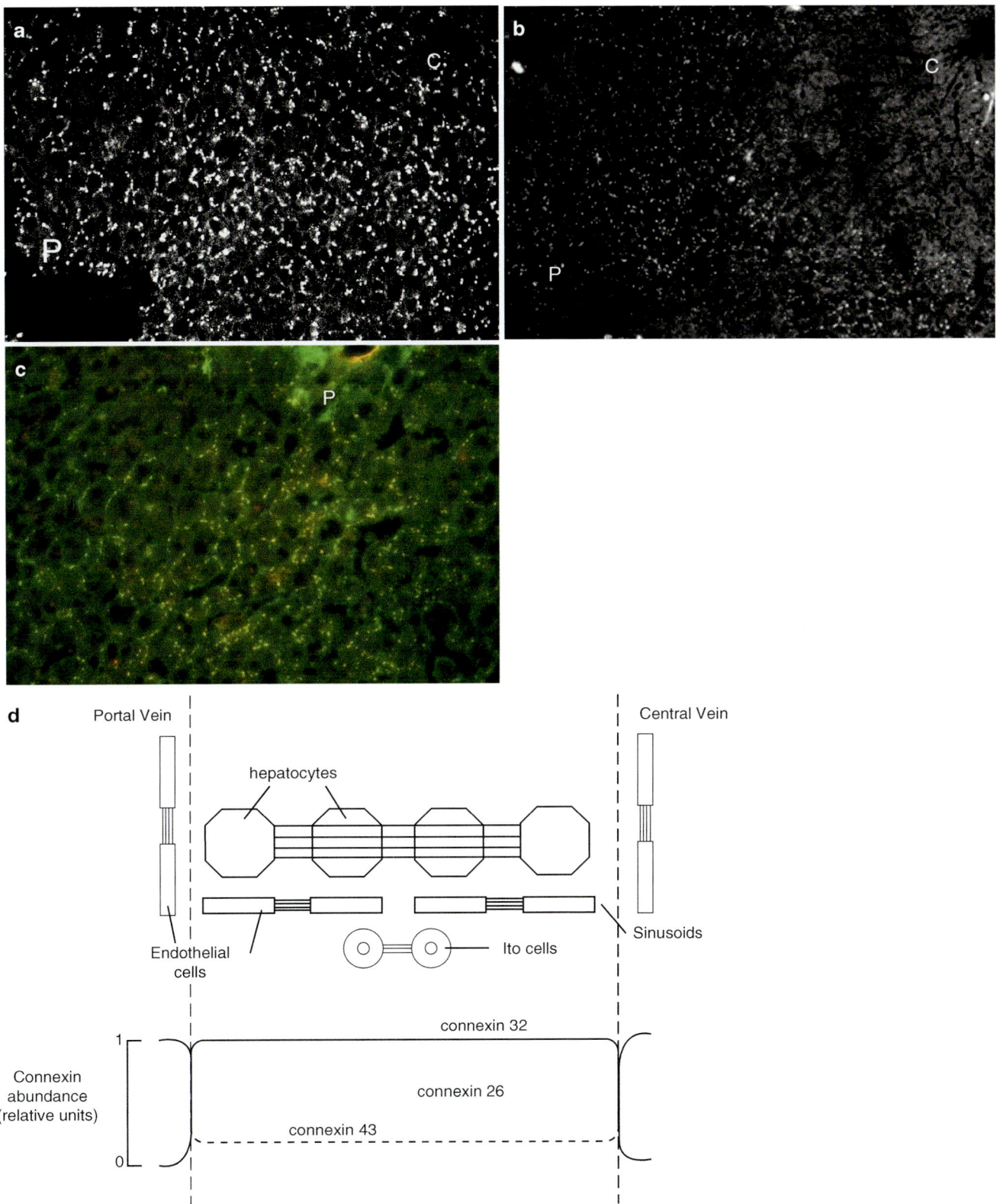

Fig. 1.15 Expression of connexin 26, 32, and 43. (**a**) Immunofluorescence of connexin 32. Connexin 32-positive fluorescence is seen on cell membrane of all hepatocytes. (**b**) Immunofluorescence of connexin 26. Connexin 26-positive fluorescence is present on the cell membrane of periportal hepatocytes. (**c**) Double immunocytochemistry of Cx32 and Cx26. Cx32 labeled with fluorescence and Cx26 labeled with rhodamine are seen in simultane- ous dots on cytoplasmic membrane of periportal area (orange color), and fluorescence-positive dots of Cx32 are seen in pericentral area (green color) (rat liver). (**d**) Cx43 are expressed in endothelial cells or Ito cells, and Cx26 expression is gradually decreased in zone 2 to zone 3, and Cx32 are diffusely expressed in a lobule. *P* portal tract, *C* pericentral area

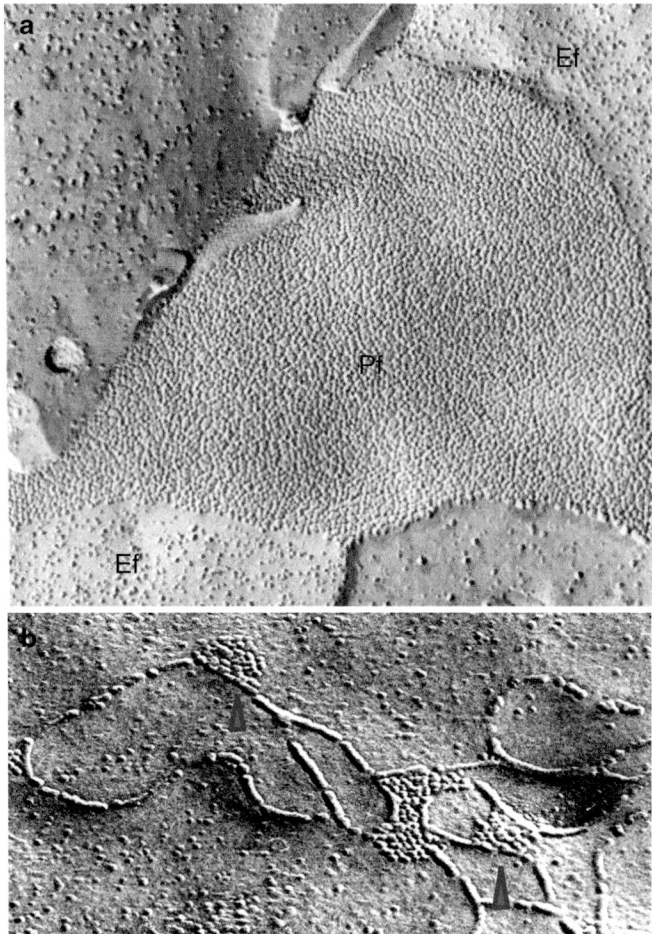

Fig. 1.16 Freeze-fracture images. (**a**) Hepatic gap junctions are recognizable as plaques of approximately 8- to 9-nm intramembranous particles present in the P fracture face (Pf), and complementary pits appear on the E fracture (Ef) face. (**b**) Small gap junction plaques are associated with tight junctional strands (arrow head)

and the induced endogenous occludin protein in the transfectants is found to bind to the exogenously expressed Cx32 protein [55, 56]. Gap junction and tight junction expression are closely correlated in hepatocytes, and gap junction expression may play a crucial role in the establishment of cell polarity via regulation of tight junction proteins. Studies of protein-protein interactions and coordinate/subordinate regulation of gene families are soon expected to disclose the intricacies of inter- and intracellular signaling and growth control at gap junctions and the regulatory mechanisms of the "blood-biliary barrier" formed by tight junctions [57].

1.7   Regeneration

Normal liver structure and function depend upon a balance between cell death and proliferation, [58] and the liver converts to a proliferative organ after surgical resection or massive injury and recovers its mass slowly and can store three-quarters of its mass within 6 months after surgical resection, but it has not been clearly understood from where or how parenchymal cell proliferate in partial hepatectomized liver and injured liver.

Protein kinase C (PKC) alpha type is reported to take an important role in early event of liver regeneration, not only phosphorylating Raf and mitogens but also activating proto-oncogene [59]. Our experimental study using combined technique of immunocytochemistry for PKC alpha and autoradiography with^{3}H-thymidine reveals that it is expressed in periportal area 6 h after 2/3 hepatectomy and that proliferating hepatocytes appear around portal tract at the same time and PKC alpha expression and proliferating hepatocytes reach a peak 12 and 48 h (Fig. 1.17a, c), then PKC alpha may take a role for early event of liver regeneration after hepatectomy, and DNA synthesis begins in hepatocytes of periportal area after stimulation of PKC alpha. Progenitor cells or proliferating hepatocytes around a portal tract spread to central area in the hepatectomized liver (Fig. 1.17b).

Liver structure is restored by regeneration of parenchymal and mesenchymal cells after liver injury. AFP, which is considered to be a regenerating marker, [60–63] is elevated in serum just after a peak of s-GOT in rat with acute liver injury (Fig. 1.18a), and AFP-positive cells are detected in surrounding area of central necrosis (Fig. 1.18b, c). Proliferating parenchymal cells labeled with ^{3}H-thymidine are found not only in surrounding area of central necrosis but also in periportal area (Fig. 1.19), and then restoration of parenchymal cells after liver injury occurs not only in vicinity of necrosis but also in periportal tract.

Polypeptide growth factors like hepatocyte growth factor [64], epidermal growth factor [65], transforming growth factor [66], heparin-binding EGR-like growth factor, [67] and insulin-like growth factor [68] are known to be capable of inducing hepatocyte replication at the beginning of regenerative process. Regenerating liver requires nutrition and various hormones of insulin, glucagon, thyroid and adrenal cortical, parathyroid, prolactin, vasopressin, prostaglandin, or catecholamines, and sex hormones[69].

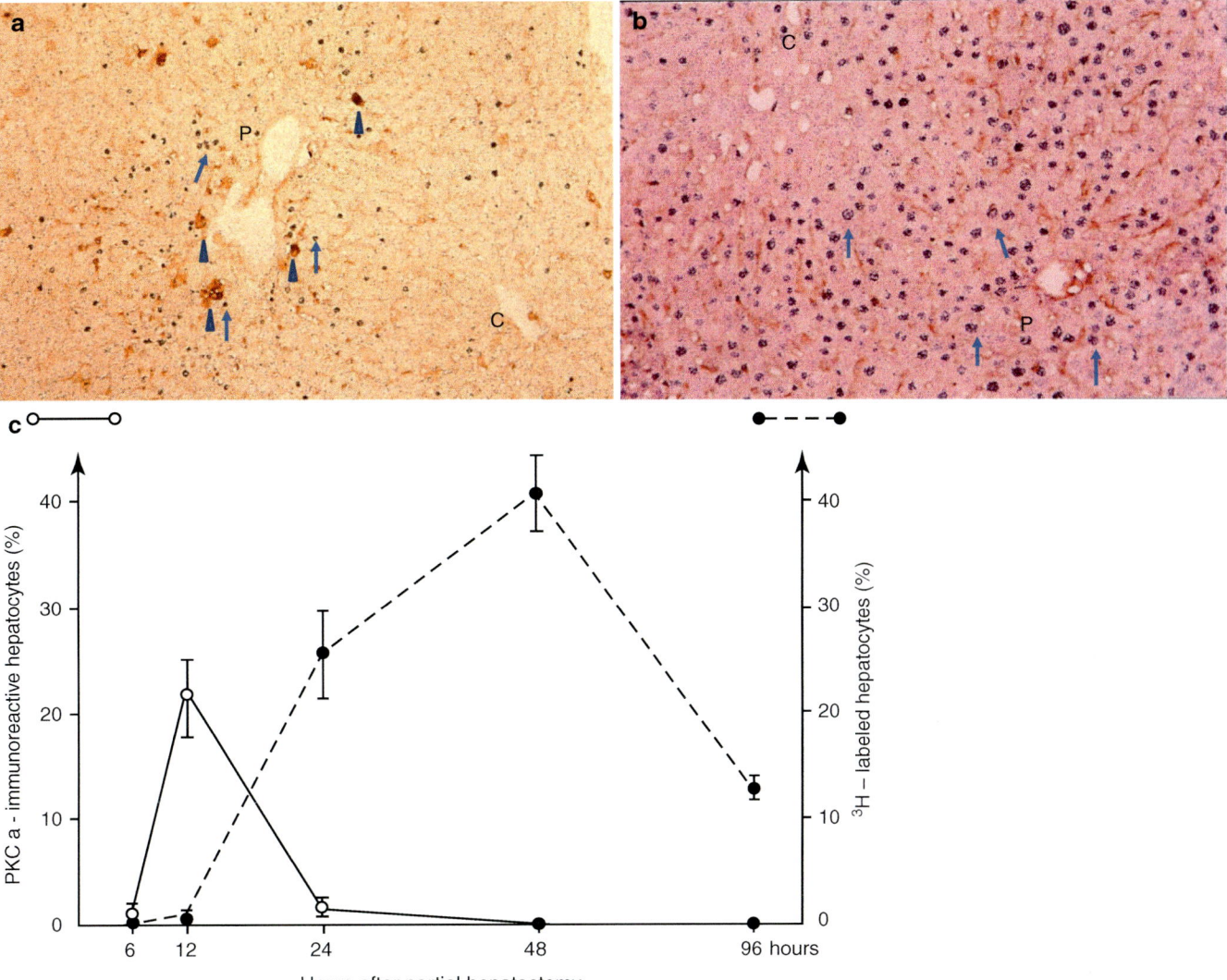

Fig. 1.17 Relation between expression of PKC alpha and presence of ^{3}H-thymidine-labeled hepatocytes in rat liver after 2/3 partial hepatectomy. (**a**) Combined technique of immunohistochemistry for PKC alpha and autoradiography with ^{3}H-thymidine. PKC alpha (arrow head) is expressed from periportal area 9 h after hepatectomy, and ^{3}H-thymidine-labeled hepatocytes (arrow) are first seen in periportal area. (**b**) Combined technique of immunohistochemistry and autoradiography. PKC alpha-immunoreactivity is invisible in 48 h, and ^{3}H-labeled hepatocytes are spread from periportal tract to pericentral area. (**c**) Expression of PKC alpha and ^{3}H-labeled hepatocytes after hepatectomy Expression of PKC alpha reaches a peak in 12 h, and labeled hepatocytes are in a peak in 48 h. *P* portal tract, *C* central vein. (Redrawn from Ishii Y. Expression and significance of PKC alpha in regenerating liver of rats after partial hepatectomy and CCL$_4$ administration. Jpn J Gastroenterol. 1996;93:717–24, with permission of Japanese Society of Gastroenterology)

Cytokines of IL-6 and TNF alpha play a critical role in the regulation of liver regeneration. Further studies are required to answer remaining questions on liver regeneration [70–72] so that we may treat patients with acute or chronic liver failure effectively. What cells are involved in the liver regeneration after its injury or partial hepatectomy? How are the architecture and function of the liver retained during its regeneration? Which signals are responsible for the turning off of the growth response once the mass of the liver is reconstituted?

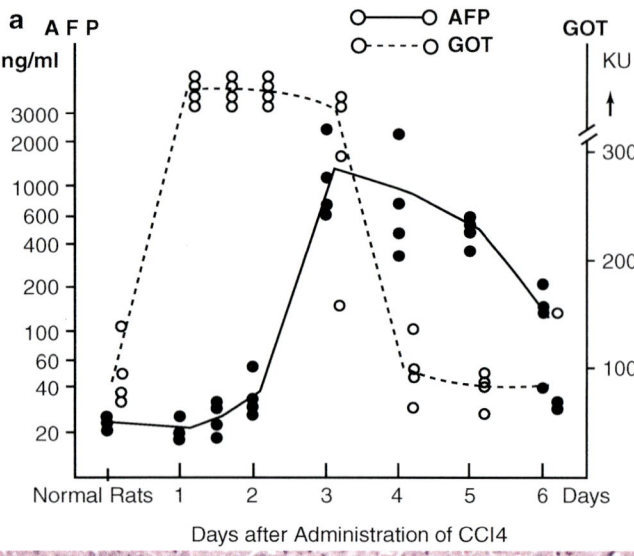

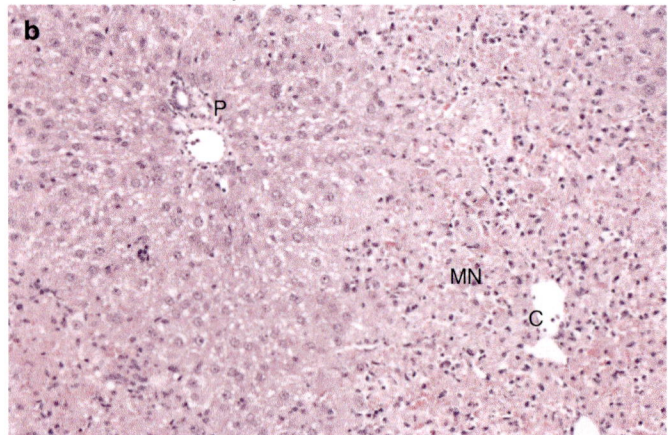

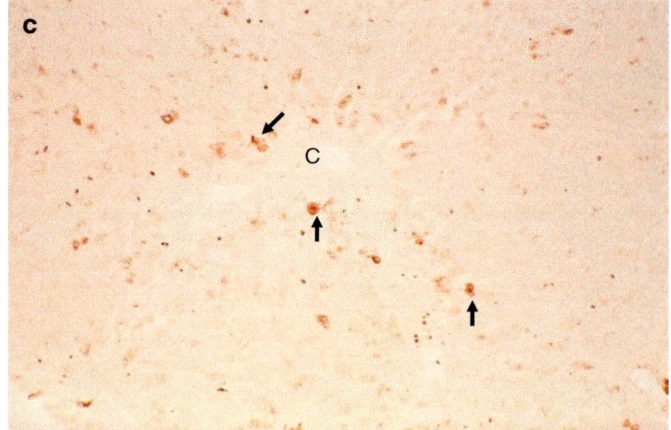

Fig. 1.18 Acute liver injury of rat induced by CCL₄. (**a**) Change of serum GOT and AFP after administration of CCL₄. Serum value of GOT is highest day 1 or 2 and AFP is highest day 3. (Reuse of a printed figure in Shoukakibyo-Gakkai Zasshi 93: p720 with permission of the Japanese Society of Gastroenterology). (**b**) Massive necrosis (MN) is seen around central vein day 1. (**c**) AFP-positive cells (arrow) are distributed in vicinity of central necrosis day 3. *P* portal tract, *C* central vein

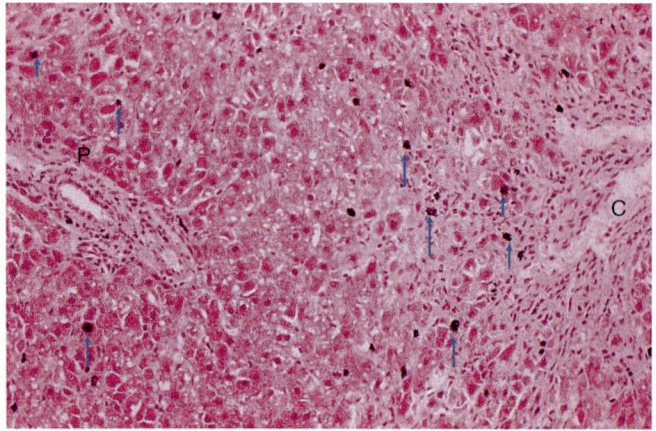

Fig. 1.19 Autoradiographic study of proliferating hepatocytes in acute liver injury induced by CCL₄, using ³H-thymidine ³H-thymidine-labeled hepatocytes (arrow) are seen not only in vicinity of central necrosis day 1 but also in periportal area. *P* portal tract, *C* central vein

References

1. Le Foie CC. Etudes anatomiques et chirurgicales. Paris: Masson; 1957.
2. Bismuth H. Surgical anatomy and anatomical surgery of the liver. World J Surg. 1982;6:3–9.
3. Timmermans JP, Geerts A. Nerves in liver: superfluous structures? A special issue of the anatomical record updating our reviews on hepatic innervation. Anat Rec B New Anat. 2005;282:4.
4. Nakanuma Y, Katayanagi K, Terada T, Saito K. Intrahepatic peribiliary glands of humans. I. Anatomy, development and presumed functions. J Gastroenterol Hepatol. 1994;9:75–9.
5. Severn CB. A morphological study of the development of the human liver. 1. Development of the hepatic diverticulum. Am J Anat. 1971;13:133–58.
6. Strasberg SM. Terminology of liver anatomy and liver resections: coming to grips with hepatic babel. J Am Coll Surg. 1997;184:413–34.
7. Haruna Y, Saito K, Spaulding S, et al. Identification of bipotential progenitor cells in human liver development. Hepatology. 1996;23:476–81.

8. Desmet VJ. Congenital diseases of intrahepatic bile ducts: variations on the theme "ductal plate malformation". Hepatology. 1992;16:1069–83.

9. Masyuk T, Masyuk A, LaRusso N. Cholangiociliopathies: genetics, molecular mechanisms and potential therapies. Curr Opin Gastroenterol. 2009;25:265–71.

10. Rappaport AM. The of normal and pathologic hepatic structure. Beitr Pathol. 1976;157:215–43.

11. Torre C, Perret C, Colnot S. Transcription dynamics in a physiological process: beta-catenin signaling directs liver metabolic zonation. Int J Biochem Cell Biol. 2011;43:271–8.

12. Mitic L, Anderson JM. Molecular architecture of tight junctions. Annu Rev Physiol. 1998;60:121–41.

13. Feldmann G. The cytoskeleton of the hepatocyte. Structure and functions. J Hepatol. 1989;8:380–6.

14. Wisse E, Braet F, Luo D, et al. Structure and function of sinusoidal lining cells in the liver. Toxicol Pathol. 1996;24:100–11.

15. Schaffner F, Papper H. Capillarization of hepatic sinusoids in man. Gastroenterology. 1963;44:239–42.

16. Toth CA, Thomas P. Liver endocytosis and kupffer cells. Hepatology. 1992;24:255–66.

17. Smedsrod B, LeCouteur D, Ikejima K, et al. Hepatic sinusoidal cells in health and disease: update from the 14th international symposium. Liver Int. 2009;29:490–9.

18. Mathew J, Geerts A, Burt AD. Pathobiology of hepatic stellate cells. Hepato-Gastroenterology. 1996;43:72–91.

19. Sakamoto M, Ueno T, Kin M, et al. Ito cell contraction in response to endothelin-1 and substance P. Hepatology. 1993;18:973–83.

20. Rockey DC, Weisiger RA. Endothelin induced contractility of stellate cells from normal and cirrhotic rat liver: implications for regulation of portal pressure and resistance. Hepatology. 1996;24:233–40.

21. Skirtic S, Wallenius V, Ekberg S, et al. Insulin-like growth factors stimulate expression of hepatocyte growth factor but not transforming growth factors beta 1 in cultured hepatic stellate cells. Endocrinology. 1997;138:4683–9.

22. Wisse E, Luo D, Vermijlen D, et al. On the function of pit cells, the liver specific natural killer cells. Semin Liver Dis. 1997;17:265–86.

23. Alpini G, Prall RT, LaRusso NF. The pathobiology of biliary epithelia. In: Arias IM, Boyer JL, Chisari FV, et al., editors. The liver biology and pathobiology. 4th ed. London: Lippincott Williams & Wilkins; 2001. p. 421–35.

24. Sugiura H, Nakanuma Y. Secretory components and immunoglobulins in the intrahepatic biliary tree and peribiliary glands in normal livers and hepatolithiasis. Gastroenterol Jpn. 1989;24:308–14.

25. Ishida F, Terada T, Nakanuma Y. Histologic and scanning electron microscopic observations of intrahepatic peribiliary glands in normal human livers. Lab Investig. 1989;60:260–5.

26. Hofmann AF, Yeh H-Z, Schteingart CD, et al. The cholehepatic circulation of organic anions: a decade of progress. In: Alvaro D, Benedeti A, Strazzabosco M, editors. Vanishing bile duct syndrome-pathophysiology and treatment. Dordrecht: Kluwer Academic; 1997. p. 90–103.

27. Gumbiner BM. Breaking through the tight junction barrier. J Cell Biol. 1993;123:1631–3.

28. Schneeberger EE, Lynch RD. Structure, function, and regulation of cellular tight junctions. Am J Phys. 1992;262:L647–L661.100.

29. van Meer G, Simon K. The function of tight junctions in maintaining differences in lipid composition between the apical and basolateral cell surface domains of MDCK cells. EMBO J. 1986;5:1455–64.

30. Cereijido M, Valdés J, Shoshani L, et al. Role of tight junctions in establishing and maintaining cell polarity. Annu Rev Physiol. 1998;60:161–77.

31. Matter K, Balda MS. Signalling to and from tight junctions. Nat Rev Mol Cell Biol. 2003;4:225–36.

32. Schneeberger EE, Lynch RD. The tight junction: a multifunctional complex. Am J Physiol Cell Physiol. 2004;286:C1213–28.

33. Tsukita S, Furuse M, Itoh M. Multifunctional strands in tight junctions. Nat Rev Mol Cell Biol. 2001;4:285–93.

34. Sawada N, Murata M, Kikuchi K, Osanai M, Tobioka H, Kojima T, Chiba H. Tight junctions and human diseases. Med Electron Microsc. 2003;36:147–56.

35. Ikenouchi J, Furuse M, Furuse K, Sasaki H, Tsukita S, Tsukita S. Tricellulin constitutes a novel barrier at tricellular contacts of epithelial cells. J Cell Biol. 2005;171:939–45.

36. Kojima T, Ninomiya T, Konno T, Kohno T, Taniguchi M, Sawada N. Expression of tricellulin in epithelial cells and non-epithelial cells. Histol Histopathol. 2013;28:1383–92.

37. Kojima T, Sawada N, Yamaguchi H, Fort AG, Spray DC. Gap and tight junctions in liver: composition, regulation, and function. In: Arias IM, et al., editors. The liver: biology and pathobiology. 5th ed. Philadelphia: Lippincott Williams & Wilkins; 2009a. p. 201–20.

38. Kojima T, Murata M, Yamamoto T, Lan M, Imamura M, Son S, Takano K, Yamaguchi H, Ito T, Tanaka S, Chiba H, Hirata K, Sawada N. Tight junction proteins and signal transduction pathways in hepatocytes. Histol Histopathol. 2009b;24:1463–72.

39. Carlton VE, Harris BZ, Puffenberger EG, Batta AK, Knisely AS, Robinson DL, Strauss KA, Shneider BL, Lim WA, Salen G, Morton DH, Bull LN. Complex inheritance of familial hypercholanemia with associated mutations in TJP2 and BAAT. Nat Genet. 2003;34:91–6.

40. Hadj-Rabia S, Baala L, Vabres P, Hamel-Teillac D, Jacquemin E, Fabre M, Lyonnet S, De Prost Y, Munnich A, Hadchouel M, Smahi A. Claudin-1 gene mutations in neonatal sclerosing cholangitis associated with ichthyosis: a tight junction disease. Gastroenterology. 2004;127:1386–90.

41. Helle F, Dubuisson J. Hepatitis C virus entry into host cells. Cell Mol Life Sci. 2008;65:100–12.

42. Evans MJ, von Hahn T, Tscherne DM, Syder AJ, Panis M, Wölk B, Hatziioannou T, McKeating JA, Bieniasz PD, Rice CM. Claudin-1 is a hepatitis C virus co-receptor required for a late step in entry. Nature. 2007;446:801–5.

43. Benedicto I, Molina-Jiménez F, Barreiro O, Maldonado-Rodríguez A, Prieto J, Moreno-Otero R, Aldabe R, López-Cabrera M, Majano PL. Hepatitis C virus envelope components alter localization of hepatocyte tight junction-associated proteins and promote occludin retention in the endoplasmic reticulum. Hepatology. 2008;48:1044–53.

44. Liu S, Yang W, Shen L, Turner JR, Coyne CB, Wang T. Tight junction proteins claudin-1 and occludin control hepatitis C virus entry and are downregulated during infection to prevent superinfection. J Virol. 2009;83:2011–4.

45. Kumar NM, Gilula NB. The gap junction communication channel. Cell. 1996;84:381–8.

46. Ayad WA, Locke D, Koreen IV, Harris AL. Heteromeric, but not homomeric, connexin channels are selectively permeable to inositol phosphates. J Biol Chem. 2006;281:16727–39.

47. Maes M, Cogliati B, Crespo Yanguas S, Willebrords J, Vinken M. Roles of connexin and pannexin in digestive homeostasis. Cell Mol Life Sci. 2015;72:2809–21.

48. Iwai M, Harada Y, Muramatsu A, Tanaka S, Mori T, Okanoue T, Katoh F, Ohkusa T, Kashima K. Development of gap junctional channels and intercellular communication in rat liver during ontogenesis. J Hepatol. 2000;32:11–8.

49. Temme A, Buchmann A, Gabriel HD, Nelles E, Schwarz M, Willecke K. High incidence of spontaneous and chemically induced liver tumors in mice deficient for connexin32. Curr Biol. 1997;7:713–6.

50. Vinken M, De Kock J, Oliveira AG, Menezes GB, Cogliati B, Dagli ML, Vanhaecke T, Rogiers V. Modifications in connexin expression in liver development and cancer. Cell Commun Adhes. 2012;19:55–62.

51. Caro JF, Poulos J, Ittoop O, et al. Insulin-like growth factor 1 binding in hepatocytes from human liver, human hepatoma, and normal regenerating and fetal rat liver. J Clin Invest. 1988;81:976–81.

52. Muramatsu A, Iwai M, Morikawa T, Tanaka S, Mori T, Harada Y, Okanoue T. Influence of transfection with connexin 26 gene on malignant potential of human hepatoma cells. Carcinogenesis. 2002;23:351–8.

53. Maes M, Decrock E, Cogliati B, Oliveira AG, Marques PE, Dagli ML, Menezes GB, Mennecier G, Leybaert L, Vanhaecke T, Rogiers V, Vinken M. Connexin and pannexin (hemi) channels in the liver. Front Physiol. 2014;4:405.

54. Kojima T, Kokai Y, Chiba H, Yamamoto M, Mochizuki Y, Sawada N. Cx32 but not Cx26 is associated with tight junctions in primary cultures of rat hepatocytes. Exp Cell Res. 2001;263(2):193–201.

55. Kojima T, Sawada N, Chiba H, Kokai Y, Yamamoto M, Urban M, Lee GH, Hertzberg EL, Mochizuki Y, Spray DC. Induction of tight junctions in human connexin 32 (hCx32)-transfected mouse hepatocytes: connexin 32 interacts with occludin. Biochem Biophys Res Commun. 1999;266:222–9.

56. Kojima T, Spray DC, Kokai Y, Chiba H, Mochizuki Y, Sawada N. Cx32 formation and/or Cx32-mediated intercellular communication induces expression and function of tight junctions in hepatocytic cell line. Exp Cell Res. 2002;276:40–51.

57. Kojima T, Yamamoto T, Murata M, Chiba H, Kokai Y, Sawada N. Regulation of the blood-biliary barrier: interaction between gap and tight junctions in hepatocytes. Med Electron Microsc. 2003;36:157–64.

58. Fausto N. Liver regeneration and repair: hepatocytes, progenitor cells, and stem cells. Hepatology. 2004;39:1477–87.

59. Angel P, Karin M. The role of Jun, Fos and the AP-1 complex in cell-proliferation and transformation. Biochim Biophys Acta. 1991;1072:129–57.

60. Kuhlmann WD, Peschke P. Hepatic progenitor cells, stem cells, and AFP expression in models of liver injury. Int J Exp Pathol. 2006;87:343–59.

61. Kakisaka K, Kataoka K, Onodera M, Suzuki A, Endo K, Tatemichi Y, Kuroda H, Ishida K, Takikawa Y. Alpha-fetoprotein: a biomarker for the recruitment of progenitor cells in the liver in patients with acute liver injury or failure. Hepatol Res. 2015;45:E12–20.

62. Tournier I, Legrès L, Schoevaert D, Feldmann G, Bernuau D. Cellular analysis of alpha-fetoprotein gene activation during carbon tetrachloride and D-galactosamine-induced acute liver injury in rats. Lab Investig. 1988;59:657–65.

63. Seo SI, Kim SS, Choi BY, Lee SH, Kim SJ, Park HW, Kim HS, Shin WG, Kim KH, Lee JH, Kim HY, Jang MK. Clinical significance of elevated serum alpha-fetoprotein (AFP) level in acute viral hepatitis a (AHA). Hepato-Gastroenterology. 2013;60:1592–6.

64. Ueki T, Kaneda Y, Tsutsui H, et al. Hepatocyte growth factor gene therapy of liver cirrhosis in rats. Nat Med. 1999;5:226–30.

65. Marti U, Burwen SJ, Jones AL. Hepatic sequestration and biliary secretion of epidermal growth factors: evidence for a high-capacity uptake system. Proc Natl Acad Sci U S A. 1983;80:3797–801.

66. Mead JE, Fausto N. Transforming growth factor alpha may be a physiological regulator of liver regeneration by means of an autocrine mechanism. Proc Natl Acad Sci U S A. 1989;86:4–13.

67. Kan M, Huang J, Mansson PE, et al. Heparin-binding growth factor type 1(acidic fibroblast growth factor): a potential biphasic autocrine and paracrine regulator of hepatocyte regeneration. Proc Natl Acad Sci U S A. 1989;86:7432–6.

68. Caro JE, Poulos J, Ittoop O, et al. Insulin-like growth factor 1 binding in hepatocytes from human liver, human hepatoma, and normal regenerating, and fetal rat liver. J Clin Invest. 1988;81:976–81.

69. Bucher NLR, Strain AJ. Regulatory mechanisms in hepatic regeneration. In: Millward-Sadler GH, Wright R, Arthur MJP, editors. Wright's liver and biliary disease. London: Saunders; 1992. p. 258–74.

70. Riehle KJ, Dan YY, Campbell JS, Fausto N. New concepts in liver regeneration. J Gastroenterol Hepatol. 2011;26(Suppl 1):203–12.

71. Michalpoulos GK. Liver regeneration after partial hepatectomy. Am J Pathol. 2010;176:2–13.

72. Duncan AW, Dorrell C, Grompe M. Stem cells and liver regeneration. Gastroenterology. 2009;137:466–81.

Laboratory Tests in Liver Diseases

2

Yoshio Sumida, Yoshihiro Kamada, Masaki Iwai,
Paul Y. Kwo, and Masashi Yoneda

Contents

Y. Sumida, MD, PhD (✉) · M. Yoneda, MD, PhD
Aichi, Japan
e-mail: sumida.yoshio.500@mail.aichi-med-u.ac.jp

Y. Kamada, MD, PhD
Osaka, Japan

M. Iwai, MD, PhD
Kyoto, Japan

P. Y. Kwo, MD
California, CA, USA

© Springer Nature Singapore Pte Ltd. 2019
E. Hashimoto et al. (eds.), *Diagnosis of Liver Disease*, https://doi.org/10.1007/978-981-13-6806-6_2

Abbreviations

AA	Aromatic amino acid
AASLD	American Association for the Study of Liver Diseases
ACA	Anti-centromere antibodies
ACG	American College of Gastroenterology
AFP	α-fetoprotein
AFP-L3	Fucosylated AFP
AIH	Autoimmune hepatitis
ALBI	Albumin-bilirubin
ALD	Alcoholic liver disease
ALP	Alkaline phosphatase
ALT	Alanine aminotransferase
ANA	Antinuclear antibodies
anti-LKM	Antibodies to liver/kidney microsome
APASL	Asian Pacific Association for the Study of the Liver
APRI	AST to platelet ratio index
ARFI	Acoustic radiation force impulse
ASMA	Anti-smooth muscle antibodies
AST	Aspartate aminotransferase
AAR	AST to ALT ratio
BCAA	Branched-chain amino acid
BTR	BCAA/tyrosine ratio
CHB	Chronic hepatitis B
CHC	Chronic hepatitis C
CK	Creatine kinase
CLD	Chronic liver disease
DCP	Des-γ-carboxyprothrombin
DIC	Disseminated intravascular coagulation
DILI	Drug-induced liver injury
EASL	European Association for the Study of the Liver
ECM	Extracellular matrix
ELF score	Enhanced liver fibrosis score
FIB4 index	Fibrosis-4 index
GGT	γ-glutamyl transferase
GPC3	Glypican-3
GPI	Glycosylphosphatidylinositol
HBV	Hepatitis B virus
HCC	Hepatocellular carcinoma
HCV	Hepatitis C virus
HIV	Human immunodeficiency virus
HPLC	High-performance liquid chromatography
HSC	Hepatic stellate cell
HSPG	Heparan sulfate proteoglycan
ICG	Indocyanine green
ICP	Intrahepatic cholestasis of pregnancy
IFN-γ	Interferon-γ
IgA	Immunoglobulin A
IgE	Immunoglobulin E
IgG	Immunoglobulin G
IgM	Immunoglobulin M
INR	International normalized ratio
IL-6	Interleukin-6
JSH	Japanese Society of Hepatology
LCA	*Lens culinaris* agglutinin A
LDH	Lactate dehydrogenase
LSEC	Liver sinusoidal endothelial cell
M2BP	Mac-2 binding protein
M2BPGi	Mac-2-binding protein glycosylation isomer
MELD	Model for end-stage liver disease
MRE	Magnetic resonance elastography
MRI	Magnetic resonance imaging
NAFLD	Nonalcoholic fatty liver disease
PIIINP	Procollagen type III N-terminal peptide
PBC	Primary biliary cholangitis
PDD	Pulse dye densitometer
Pro-C3	N-terminal propeptide of type III collagen
PSC	Primary sclerosing cholangitis
PT	Prothrombin time
SRCR	Scavenger receptor cysteine-rich domain
SVR	Sustained virological response
T4C7S	Type 4 collagen 7S
TIMP-1	Tissue inhibitor of matrix metalloprotease-1
TIPS	Transjugular intrahepatic portosystemic shunt
TNF-α	Tumor necrosis factor-α
UDP	Uridine diphosphate
WFA	*Wisteria floribunda* agglutinin

2.1 Biochemistry

2.1.1 Transaminases

Aspartate aminotransferase (AST) and alanine aminotransferase (ALT) are enzymes present in hepatocytes and are released into the bloodstream in response to hepatocyte injury or death (hepatitis). Elevations in either of these enzymes are the most common abnormality seen on liver blood test profiles. Both enzymes are present in many differing types of tissue, but ALT is considered more liver-specific since it is present in low concentrations in non-hepatic tissue, and non-liver-related elevations are uncommon. However, AST is abundantly present in skeletal, cardiac, and smooth muscle and so may be elevated in patients with myocardial infarction or myositis. Although ALT is considered a more specific indicator of liver disease, the concentration of AST may be a more sensitive indicator of liver injury in conditions such as alcoholic liver disease (ALD), congestive liver due to heart failure, and in some cases of autoimmune hepatitis (AIH). Creatine kinase (CK) measurement may help to determine whether an isolated rise in AST is due to an underlying muscle disorders, such as myocardial infarction, myositis, and various muscular dystrophies. AST is increased also in patients with hemolysis. Globally normal values of ALT are up to ~30 IU/L in men and up to ~19 IU/L in women [1]. The practice guideline of the American College of Gastroenterology (ACG) defined true healthy normal ALT value ranging from 29 to 33 IU/L for males and 19 to 25 IU/L for females based on an increased risk of liver-related mortality at ALT levels that were higher than these [2]. The degree of ALT elevation may correlate with the extent of hepatic injury but is generally not of prognostic importance. AST and ALT are not markers of liver function and should be referred to as liver chemistry or liver tests. Amino transaminase levels may be higher than 3000 IU/L in acute viral hepatitis, drug-induced liver injury (DILI), acute liver failure, or ischemic hepatitis (shock liver) though very high ALT levels are generally more common in acetaminophen overdose and ischemic injury to the liver. In ALD patients, the serum AST is usually no more than two to ten times the upper limit of normal with a AST/ALT ratio (AAR) >2. In contrast, in nonalcoholic fatty liver disease (NAFLD), ALT is typically higher than AST until cirrhosis develops. Mild to moderate elevations of aminotransferase levels are typical of chronic viral hepatitis, AIH, NAFLD, hemochromatosis, and Wilson disease. Abnormally low amino transaminase levels may be associated with uremia and chronic dialysis; chronic viral hepatitis in this population may not result in aminotransferase elevation. Rarely, isolated AST elevation without concurrent elevation in other liver enzymes is noted, and this is a result of the presence of macro-AST enzyme [3], because AST can exist as a macroenzyme by forming a complex with an immunoglobulin G (IgG). This is of no clinical consequence.

2.1.2 Biliary Enzymes

Alkaline phosphatase (ALP) [4] is produced mainly in the liver (from the hepatocyte canalicular membrane with a significantly lesser contribution from the biliary epithelium) but is also found in abundance in the bone and in smaller quantities in the intestines, kidneys, and white blood cells. Levels are physiologically higher in childhood, associated with bone growth, and in pregnancy due to placental production. Pathologically increased levels occur mainly in bone disease (e.g., metastatic bone disease and bone fractures) and cholestatic liver disease—for example, primary biliary cholangitis (PBC), primary sclerosing cholangitis (PSC), common bile duct obstruction, intrahepatic duct obstruction (metastases), and drug-induced cholestasis. Furthermore, hepatic congestion secondary to right-sided heart failure can also lead to cholestasis (elevated ALP levels and/or bilirubin). When ALP is elevated in isolation, the measurement of γ-glutamyltransferase (GGT) can indicate whether the ALP is of hepatic or non-hepatic origin. While there are no data on the most likely causes of an isolated raised ALP in an asymptomatic population, the most common cause is likely to be vitamin D deficiency or normal increase seen in childhood

due to rapid growth. Other causes include Paget's disease and bony metastases. If doubt still exists, the use of electrophoresis to separate the isoenzymes of ALP can differentiate hepatic from non-hepatic causes of increased ALP. In subjects with blood types B and O, serum ALP may increase after a fatty meal due to influx of intestinal ALP [5]. There are also reports of a benign familial occurrence of elevated serum ALP due to intestinal ALP. GGT is abundant in the liver and also present in the kidney, intestine, prostate, and pancreas but not in the bone; therefore it can be useful in confirming that an elevated ALP is of liver and not bony origin. GGT is most commonly elevated as a result of obesity and excess alcohol consumption or may be induced by drugs such as phenytoin or barbiturates. Although an elevated GGT has a low specificity for liver disease, it is one of the best predictors of liver mortality. It is particularly useful in children to establish the likelihood of biliary disease when ALP is not a reliable indicator. Predominant causes of cholestasis in children include congenital abnormalities of the biliary tract and genetic disorders affecting bile synthesis and excretion. We should be aware that GGT level is usually normal in intrahepatic cholestasis of pregnancy (ICP).

2.1.3 Hepatic Synthetic Function

Albumin is a protein that is produced only in the liver and has multiple biological actions, including maintenance of oncotic pressure and binding of other substances (such as fatty acids, bilirubin, thyroid hormone and drugs, metabolism of compounds, including lipids, and antioxidant properties). As albumin is only produced by the liver, the serum albumin concentration is often considered as a marker of the synthetic function of the liver. However, overinterpretation of the measured concentrations of albumin as a marker of the severity of liver disease is not always merited. Albumin concentrations are reduced in many clinical situations, including sepsis, systemic inflammatory disorders, nephrotic syndrome, malabsorption, and gastrointestinal protein loss. Albumin has a plasma half-life of 3 weeks, resulting slow change in serum concentration in response to acute alteration in hepatic function.

Prothrombin time (PT) and international normalized ratio (INR) are assessments of blood clotting, which are used to measure liver function, as the underlying protein clotting factors (II, V, VII, IX, and X) are made in the liver. If there is significant liver injury (usually loss of >70% of synthetic function), this results in a reduction in clotting factor production and subsequent coagulopathy, as confirmed by a prolonged PT or INR. While a prolonged PT/INR can indicate either acute or chronic liver dysfunction, it can also be caused by vitamin K deficiency as seen in fat malabsorption and chronic cholestasis. It should be noted that PT can be elevated with warfarin, heparin bolus, disseminated intravascular coagulation (DIC), and hypothermia.

2.1.4 Severity of Liver Disease

Bilirubin is a breakdown product of hemoglobin and, to a lesser extent, heme-containing enzymes; 95% of bilirubin is derived from senescent red blood cells. After red cell breakdown in the reticuloendothelial system, heme is degraded by the enzyme heme oxygenase in the endoplasmic reticulum. The daily formation of bilirubin is 250–350 mg. Bilirubin from this process passes into the blood, where it is bound to albumin to form unconjugated bilirubin. Unconjugated bilirubin is lipid soluble, is not filtered by the glomerulus, and does not appear in the urine. It is rapidly cleared from the blood in less than 5 min by hepatocytes and then conjugated with glucuronic acid by uridine diphosphate (UDP)-glucuronyl transferase to form a more water-soluble compound that can be excreted in bile. Conjugated bilirubin and unconjugated bilirubin are also referred to as direct and indirect bilirubin, respectively, based on their reaction with diazo dyes. In clinical practice, most clinical laboratories today measure total and direct bilirubin and calculate in indirect bilirubin. However, because direct bilirubin detected by this method also measures delta bilirubin (δ-bilirubin), it is not an accurate measurement of conjugated bilirubin. Delta bilirubin (δ-bilirubin) is covalently conjugated to albumin during times of liver injury and cholestasis. Accordingly, δ-bilirubin has a half-life similar to albumin (17–20 days). Recovery of icterus after removing biliary obstruction is often late because of elevation in δ-bilirubin (Table 2.1). Gilbert syndrome commonly causes unconjugated hyperbilirubinemia and is not associated with liver injury. Unconjugated hyperbilirubinemia is also seen in patients with hemolysis (elevated lactate dehydrogenase [LDH], low haptoglobin). Conjugated hyperbilirubinemia is usually seen in liver diseases, both obstructive and hepatocellular.

Blood ammonia is often measured in cirrhotic patients and known or suspected hepatic encephalopathy with altered mental status or coma. However, blood ammonia levels do not always accurately correlate with metal status of patients with liver disease, and increased levels are not required to make the diagnosis of hepatic encephalopathy though a recent guideline [6] has suggested that if the ammonia level is normal in a patient with cirrhosis, other causes of mental status changes should be investigated. Thus, the primary clinical utility of blood ammonia levels is to monitor treatments in patients with encephalopathy.

2.1.4.1 BTR (Branched-Chain Amino Acids/Tyrosine Ratio)

Fischer's ratio (a molar ratio of branched-chain amino acids [BCAA] to aromatic amino acids [AA] (tyrosine + phenylalanine]) was measured by conventional high-performance liquid chromatography (HPLC). A molar ratio of free BCAAs to tyrosine (BTR) was determined in the plasma of patients with liver diseases using a new enzymatic method. Significant correlation was also found between enzymatically determined BTR and Fischer's ratio obtained by HPLC. Changes of BTR in clinical courses were found to be in parallel with those of Fischer's ratio. BTR is a quite simple method and is also considered to be a very useful parameter of the clinical conditions of patients with liver diseases.

Indocyanine green (ICG) is a nontoxic water-soluble dye that can be absorbed by the liver stromal cells and almost completely discharged through excreted bile rather than extrahepatic removal or enterohepatic circulation. Minimally invasive pulse dye densitometry (PDD), as the primary approach for ICG detection test, has been commonly used for quantitative evaluation of liver function before hepatectomy [5]. PDD has been proven to be a safe, sensitive, and accurate method for early prediction and diagnosis of postoperative liver failure [7, 8]. Previous investigations have demonstrated that the ICG detection rate is of significance for predicting the survival rates of both grafts and patients [2, 5, 9]. Dynamic detection of ICG is able to identify early liver dysfunction and hepatic insufficiency [10, 11].

2.2 Peripheral Blood Cell Count

2.2.1 Platelets

A reduction in platelets, termed thrombocytopenia, is the most common hematological abnormality found in patients with chronic liver disease and is an indicator of advanced disease. Multiple factors culminate in a low platelet count: decreased production, splenic sequestration, and increased destruction. Decreased production is a consequence of bone marrow suppression, as caused by alcohol, iron overload, drugs, and viridae and also by a reduction in thrombopoietin levels in chronic liver injury. Splenic sequestration results from hypersplenism, which is a consequence of portal hypertension seen in advanced liver fibrosis. Platelet

Table 2.1 Under HPLC, bilirubin separates into four peaks (α, β, γ, and δ)

	Bilirubin peaks on HPLC			
	α	β	γ	δ
Bilirubin species	Unconjugated	Singly conjugated	Doubly conjugated	Conjugated to albumin
	Total—bilirubin			
Commonly performed laboratory test	Indirect bilirubin (calculated)	Direct bilirubin		
On request	Unconjugated	Conjugated		Delta (calculated)

destruction is also increased nonspecifically in liver cirrhosis owing to shear stress, fibrinolysis, and bacterial translocation, whereas in specific causes of autoimmune liver disease, immunologically mediated destruction of platelets occurs owing to antiplatelet immunoglobulin. Several scoring systems such as AST to platelet ratio index (APRI), Forns test, and fibrosis-4 (FIB4) index use platelet count in their scoring algorithm to predict stages of hepatic fibrosis.

2.3 Immunological Tests

Immunoglobulins are often increased nonspecifically in chronic liver disease (CLD), especially in cirrhosis. Elevated IgG, IgA, and IgM suggest AIH, ALD, and PBC, respectively. IgA is also elevated in some cases of NASH with advanced fibrosis [12]. In cases with DILI, serum IgE levels are occasionally abnormal. In patients with elevated IgG4 levels, IgG4-related hepatobiliary diseases should be considered. IgG4-related hepatobiliary diseases are part of a multi-organ fibroinflammatory condition termed IgG4-related disease and include IgG4-related sclerosing cholangitis (IgG4-SC), IgG4-related AIH, and IgG4-related hepatopathy. The traditional markers of AIH include antinuclear antibodies (ANA), anti-smooth muscle antibodies (ASMA), and antibodies to liver/kidney microsome 1 (anti-LKM1). The characteristic serologic hallmark of PBC is the AMA, a highly disease-specific autoantibody found in 90–95% of patients and less than 1% of normal control. Fewer than 5% of patients with PBC are AMA-negative [13]. Nearly all of AMA-negative patients have ANA, ASMA, and/or anti-centromere antibodies (ACA).

2.4 Other Blood Tests

Serum copper levels are increased in cholestatic diseases and decreased in Wilson disease.

Serum ceruloplasmin levels are decreased in patients with Wilson disease (<20 mg/dL). Serum ferritin is increased in a variety of liver diseases, such as hemochromatosis, ALD, chronic hepatitis C (CHC), and NASH. Ferritin, however, is also an acute-phase reactive protein and may be elevated in inflammatory conditions. Transferrin saturation (serum iron/total iron-binding capacity × 100) should be evaluated to differentiate hemochromatosis from other diseases.

2.5 Hepatic Fibrosis Markers

Chronic damage to the liver induces liver fibrosis resulting from wound-healing process and subsequent development of liver cirrhosis. Liver fibrosis comprises the excessive deposition of extracellular matrix (ECM) in the liver [14]. Excessive accumulation of ECM in the liver triggers the various complications of end-stage liver diseases, such as ascites, varices, and liver failure (including encephalopathy, synthetic dysfunction, and impaired metabolic capacity) [15–17]. Liver biopsy remains the definitive test, but liver biopsy has significant limitations such as pain, risk of severe complications, sampling error, cost, and patient unwillingness to undergo invasive testing [18, 19]. Therefore, reliable, accurate, disease-specific, and noninvasive biomarkers of fibrosis are critically needed to assess the degree of liver fibrosis accurately.

Novel noninvasive approaches [e.g., transient elastography (FibroScan), acoustic radiation force impulse (ARFI), and magnetic resonance elastography (MRE)] and various scoring systems can be used to measure the severity of fibrosis in patients with chronic liver diseases [20–26]. Ultrasound elastography is very useful for excluding advanced liver fibrosis and cirrhosis. However, there are some problems in elastography approach. For example, transient elastography is technically difficult in patients with early-stage fibrosis, moderate to severe steatosis, ascites, or increased body mass index. MRE is useful for the assessment of liver fibrosis even in early stage and obese people.

A variety of cells are associated with liver fibrosis pathophysiology, including hepatocytes, Kupffer cells, liver sinusoidal endothelial cells (LSECs), and hepatic stellate cells (HSCs). Among these cells, HSC is thought to play central roles in liver fibrosis progression and produces various kinds of ECM protein [14, 27]. HSC is located in the perisinusoidal space and is the predominant hepatic vitamin A storage cell in quiescent state [28]. When HSC is activated by inflammatory cytokines and/or fibrogenic cytokines, HSC migrates and accumulates at the liver injury site and secretes large amount of ECM [14]. Serum levels of ECM proteins directly relate to liver fibrosis progression, and used as liver fibrosis biomarkers, including hyaluronic acid, type 4 collagen 7S (T4C7S), procollagen type III N-terminal peptide (PIIINP), and N-terminal propeptide of type III collagen (Pro-C3). In addition, recent development in glycobiology could establish a novel liver fibrosis biomarker, M2BPGi (Mac-2-binding protein glycosylation isomer), which is clinically used in Japan since 2015 [29].

2.5.1 Hyaluronic Acid

Hyaluronic acid (hyaluronan) is a high molecular weight glycosaminoglycan and is highly present in the ECM in the liver [30]. The liver is the most important organ involved in the synthesis of hyaluronic acid. HSC synthesizes hyaluronic acid, and LSECs are involved in its degradation [31]. Degradation of hyaluronic acid occurs rapidly, and its half-life in the blood is very short (about 2–5 min) [32]. Serum hyaluronic acid levels may be dependent on the clearance via receptor-mediated uptake to the liver and sinusoidal endothelial cell function, and serum hyaluronic acid levels in healthy people are typically low due to the rapid clearance [33]. As the liver fibrosis progresses, hyaluronic acid clearance decreases, and serum hyaluronic acid levels can be used as a liver fibrosis biomarker in various chronic liver diseases. As we see later in this book, hyaluronic acid is included in enhanced liver fibrosis (ELF) score [34].

In injured liver, inflammatory cytokines, such as interleukin-6 (IL-6) and tumor necrosis factor-α (TNF-α), stimulate HSC to produce hyaluronic acid [33, 35]. Serum hyaluronic acid concentration significantly correlated with fibrosis stage in cCHC patients, and treatment of HCV with interferon and ribavirin decreased serum hyaluronic acid levels in sustained virological response (SVR) patients [36–38]. In patients with chronic hepatitis B (CHB), hyaluronic acid levels also correlated with liver fibrosis stage [39, 40]. Treatment of hepatitis B virus (HBV) with entecavir decreased serum hyaluronic acid levels in CHB patients [41]. In nonviral chronic liver diseases, such as PBC, PSC, ALD, and NAFLD, serum hyaluronic acid levels also increased with the liver fibrosis progression [33, 42–45].

2.5.2 Type 4 Collagen 7S

Type 4 collagen (T4C) is widely distributed and found exclusively in the basement membranes [46, 47]. T4C is a non-fibrillar collagen and is categorized into network-forming collagen [48]. T4C chains (α1-α6) are encoded by *COL4A1-COL4A* genes, and all chains have similar domain structures. The α-chain can be separated into three domains: an N-terminal non-collagenous 7S domain, a middle triple-helical collagenous domain, and a C-terminal globular non-collagenous (NC)-1 domain [49]. In the liver, LSEC, HSC, biliary epithelial cells, and fibroblasts secrete T4C as one of the basement membrane components [50, 51].

With the liver fibrosis progression, T4C is highly upregulated, and its relative increase is highest among all collagen types [52]. Antigen related to the 7S domain of T4C (T4C7S) has been evaluated as biomarkers of chronic liver diseases, such as CHC [53], CHB [54, 55], ALD [56, 57], and NAFLD [25, 58]. These indicate that increase in serum T4C7S levels reflects perisinusoidal basement membrane metabolism caused by chronic liver diseases. Serum T4C7S would be derived from the degradation of basement membrane associated with ECM remodeling during fibrogenesis. Circulating T4C7S levels decreased after interferon therapy in CHC patients [59].

2.5.3 Pro-C3

Procollagen type III N-terminal peptide (PIIINP) represents collagen turnover, and serum levels of PIIINP are used as a liver fibrosis biomarker [60]. PIIINP levels increases in hepatitis and correlate with serum levels of aminotransferase [61].

PIIINP levels are associated with advanced fibrosis in chronic liver diseases and used as one of the ELF score factors [62, 63]. However, PIIINP is not specific for liver fibrosis and can reflect fibrosis and inflammation in other organs as a consequence of tissue repair [64]. N-terminal propeptide of type III collagen (Pro-C3) is cleaved by N-proteases and is exclusively derived from type III procollagen cleavage during collagen deposition. The measurement of Pro-C3 was developed to assess true formation of type III collagen [65]. A conventional PIIINP is a marker of both fibrogenesis and fibrolysis, and a novel Pro-C3 is a pure synthesis marker of collagen type III. Serum levels of PIIINP and Pro-C3 showed no correlation in healthy human [65]. Serum Pro-C3 levels correlated to fibrosis scores in CHC patients, and it can predict fibrosis changes in clinical course [66]. Pro-C3 measurement is also useful for liver fibrosis assessment in NAFLD patients [67]. Pro-C3 not only can identify liver fibrosis degree but also can respond to a potential anti-fibrotic therapy [68].

2.5.4 M2BPGi (Mac-2-Binding Protein Glycosylation Isomer)

Mac-2-binding protein (Mac-2 bp) is a highly glycosylated secreted glycoprotein that was firstly identified from breast cancer patient in 1986 [69]. Mac-2bp specifically bounds galectin-3 (Mac-2) via a carbohydrate-specific interaction [70]. It is identical to a previously described tumor-associated antigen (90K, named after its molecular mass) released in the culture media of human breast cancer cells [71]. Mac-2bp belongs to the scavenger receptor cysteine-rich domain (SRCR) superfamily of proteins and is involved in immune defense and regulation [72]. Mac-2bp is expressed in many tissues, and its expression in macrophages can be upregulated by adherence and the inflammatory cytokines TNF-α and interferon-γ (IFN-γ) in mice [73]. In addition, Mac-2bp may regulate cell adhesion by binding to cellular matrix proteins including β1-integrin, collagens, and fibronectins [74]. Thus, Mac-2bp is a widely known glycoprotein, but its physiological functions are not fully understood. Serum levels of Mac-2bp are elevated as liver fibrosis stage progression in NAFLD patients [75].

Recently, Kuno et al. reported that WFA⁺-M2BP [*Wisteria floribunda* agglutinin (WFA)-positive Mac-2bp] is a novel liver fibrosis biomarker for CHC [29]. They developed an automatic measurement system that can detect M2BPGi (Mac-2-binding protein glycosylation isomer) within 20 min. WFA⁺-M2BP has a characteristic glycan structure that is recognized by WFA. WFA recognizes terminal *N*-acetylgalactosaminides and specifically binds with the disaccharide LacdiNAc (β-D-GalNAc-[1 → 4]-D-GlcNAc; GalNAc *N*-acetylgalactosamine, GlcNAC *N*-acetylglucosamine) [76].

M2BPGi quantification is based on a lectin-antibody sandwich immunoassay performed using a fully automatic immunoanalyzer (HISCL-2000i, Sysmex Co., Hyogo, Japan) [29]. The measured values of WFA$^+$-M2BP conjugated to WFA were indexed with the obtained values using the following calculating formula:

$$\text{Cutoff index}\left(\text{C.O.I.}\right) = \left(\left[\text{WFA}^+\text{-M2BP}\right]_{\text{sample}} - \left[\text{WFA}^+\text{-M2BP}\right]_{\text{NC}}\right) / \left(\left[\text{WFA}^+\text{-M2BP}\right]_{\text{PC}} - \left[\text{WFA}^+\text{-M2BP}\right]_{\text{NC}}\right)$$

[WFA$^+$-M2BP]$_{\text{sample}}$ was the WFA$^+$-M2BP count for the serum sample, PC was the positive control, and NC was the negative control. The positive control was supplied as a calibration solution preliminarily standardized to yield a C.O.I. value of 1.0 [77].

M2BPGi is very useful as a liver fibrosis biomarker for CHC and for predicting HCC development in CHC patients [78]. In Japan, M2BPGi has been used clinically as a novel liver fibrosis biomarker since 2015. M2BPGi can be also used for the other chronic liver diseases (e.g., NAFLD, CHB, PBC, and AIH) [29, 79–82]

2.5.5 Scoring Systems

Many serum biomarkers in routine laboratory tests are not specific for the liver fibrosis and can elevate on inflammation of other organs. Recently, combinations of several biomarkers (scoring systems) have been established for liver fibrosis assessment. Among these scoring systems, ELF score [based on the serum levels of hyaluronic acid, PIIINP, and tissue inhibitor of matrix metalloprotease-1 (TIMP-1)] [60], FIB4 index (based on the age, platelet count, serum AST and ALT levels) [83], AAR [84], APRI [85], and BARD score [based on the body mass index (BMI), AAR,

Table 2.2 Effective scoring system for detection of liver fibrosis in chronic liver diseases

Name	Calculation formula
ELF score	$2.278 + 0.851 \times \ln[\text{hyaluronic acid}] + 0.751 \times \ln[\text{PIIINP}] + 0.394 \times \ln[\text{TIMP-1}]$
AST to ALT ratio (AAR)	AST/ALT
AST to platelet ratio index (APRI)	[AST/upper limit of normal range (U/L)]/platelet count (10^9/L) × 100
FIB4 index	Age × AST (U/L)/platelet count (× 10^9/L)/$\sqrt{\text{ALT}}$ (U/L)

and diabetes] [23] are often used for the assessment of liver fibrosis in chronic liver diseases (Table 2.2). These scoring systems are especially useful for the exclusion of advanced liver fibrosis and cirrhosis but less useful for early-stage liver fibrosis [86, 87].

2.5.5.1 Enhanced Liver Fibrosis (ELF) Score

ELF score contains serum concentration of three direct markers of fibrosis including hyaluronic acid, PIIINP, and TIMP-1 [60]. The ELF score is calculated by the instrument employing the following equation [88]:

$$\text{ELF score} = 2.278 + 0.851 \times \ln\left[\text{hyaluronic acid}\right] + 0.751 \times \ln\left[\text{PIIINP}\right] + 0.394 \times \ln\left[\text{TIMP-1}\right]$$

The concentration of these three biomarkers is used to calculate ELF score. ELF score well-correlates with the histological stage of liver fibrosis [89] and is superior to liver biopsy for predicting clinical outcomes in patients with chronic liver diseases [90]. ELF score has been shown to have good performance for liver fibrosis diagnosis in CHC [91], CHB [92], NAFLD [93], and ALD patients [60]. However, ELF score can be influenced by gender and age [94]. Therefore, results need to be adjusted appropriately by these influence factors [95].

2.5.5.2 AAR (AST to ALT Ratio)

Serum AST and ALT are transaminases, which are released from damaged hepatocytes, and are used as liver damage tests. In 1988, the AAR was reported to be less than 1.0 in the majority of chronic hepatitis patients, but there was a significant correlation between AAR and the presence of liver cirrhosis [94]. AAR in the patients without cirrhosis is often smaller than 0.8 but greater than 1.0 in those with liver cirrhosis in virus and non-virus-associated liver diseases [95].

2.5.5.3 APRI (AST to Platelet Ratio Index)

APRI was firstly proposed as a noninvasive diagnostic method for CHC patients [85]. APRI is one of the simplest scoring systems that can diagnose advanced fibrosis and cirrhosis with acceptable accuracy. APRI is calculated by the following simple equation:

$$\left[\text{AST} / \text{upper limit of normal range} \left(\text{U} / \text{L}\right)\right] / \text{platelet count} \left(10^9 / \text{L}\right) \times 100$$

APRI can diagnose significant liver fibrosis and cirrhosis in various CLDs, including CHC [85], CHB [98, 99], ALD [100], and NAFLD [10, 101].

2.5.5.4 FIB4 Index

The FIB4 index was developed as a noninvasive scoring system to assess liver fibrosis stage in patients with human immunodeficiency virus (HIV) and hepatitis C virus (HCV) coinfection [83]. FIB4 index is calculated with the following formula:

$$\text{FIB4 index} = \text{age} \times \text{AST}\ (\text{U}/\text{L})/\text{platelet count}\ \left(\times 10^{9}/\text{L}\right)/\sqrt{\text{ALT}}\ (\text{U}/\text{L})$$

Age, AST, ALT, and platelet count are routinely measured in clinical use. FIB4 index is useful for the diagnosis of advanced fibrosis in CHC [7], CHB [8], and NAFLD patients [102]. FIB4 index has better performance characteristics for the diagnosis of advanced fibrosis in Caucasian [102] and Japanese NAFLD patients [101].

2.6   Approach to Evaluation of Liver Injury Pattern

The initial evaluation of a patient with abnormal liver tests includes obtaining a history to identify potential risk factors for liver disease and performing a physical examination to look for clues to the etiology and for signs of chronic liver disease. A thorough medical history is central to the evaluation of a patient with abnormal liver tests. The history should determine if the patient has had exposure to any potential hepatotoxins (including alcohol and medications), is at risk for viral hepatitis, has other disorders that are associated with liver disease, or has symptoms that may be related to the liver disease or a possible predisposing condition. Alcohol consumption is a common cause of liver disease, although obtaining an accurate history can be difficult. The American Association for the Study of Liver Diseases (AASLD) defines significant alcohol consumption as an average consumption of >210 grams of alcohol per week in men or >140 grams of alcohol per week in women over at least a 2-year period. Questioning about drug use should seek to identify all drugs used, the amounts ingested, and the durations of use. Drug use is not limited to prescription medications but also includes over-the-counter medications, herbal and dietary supplements, and illicit drug use. Features that suggest drug toxicity include lack of illness prior to ingesting the drug, clinical illness or biochemical abnormalities developing after beginning the drug, and improvement after the drug is withdrawn. Risk factors for viral hepatitis include potential parenteral exposures (e.g., intravenous drug use, blood transfusion prior to 1992), travel to areas endemic for hepatitis, and exposure to patients with jaundice. Hepatitis B and C are transmitted parenterally, whereas hepatitis A and E are transmitted from person to person via a fecal-oral route (often via contaminated food). It should be considered in patients who live in or have travelled to Asia, Africa, the Middle East, or Central America and has been seen increasingly in Europe as a result of consumption of contaminated swine and game meat. Patients should be asked about conditions that are associated with hepatobiliary disease, such as right-sided heart failure (congestive hepatopathy), diabetes mellitus, skin pigmentation, arthritis, hypogonadism and dilated cardiomyopathy (hemochromatosis), and obesity (nonalcoholic fatty liver disease), pregnancy (gallstones), inflammatory bowel disease (primary sclerosing cholangitis, gallstones), early-onset emphysema (alpha-1 antitrypsin deficiency), celiac disease, and thyroid disease. Finally, patients should be questioned about occupational or recreational exposure to hepatotoxins (e.g., mushroom picking). Examples of hepatitis due to exposures to hepatotoxins include industrial chemicals such as vinyl chloride and the mushrooms *Amanita phalloides* and *Amanita verna*, which contain a potent hepatotoxin (amatoxin). A variety of liver examinations are listed to examine the etiology of liver test abnormality (Table 2.3).

Pattern recognition of liver enzyme abnormalities is the most frequent cognitive mechanism used by physicians in the evaluation of liver disease. An R ratio defined as (ALT/ULN) ÷ (ALP/ULN) is often used to determine the pattern of injury; this is labeled "cholestatic "when R less than is 2, "mixed" when R is between 2 and 5, and "hepatocellular" when R greater than is 5 [10].

Table 2.3 Laboratory tests performed in the evaluation of acute and chronic liver injury

Etiology		Tests
Viral hepatitis	HAV	Anti-IgM-HA
	HBV	HBsAg, Anti-IgM-HBc
	HCV	Anti HCV, HCV RNA
	HEV	IgA-HEV
	Other virus	IgM-CMV, EBV VCA IgM, IgM-HSV
Autoimmune	AIH	IgG, ANA, ASMA, anti-LKM1
	PBC	IgM, AMA (anti-M2)
	PSC	pANCA
	IgG4-related diseases	IgG4
Metabolic disease	Wilson	Serum copper, ceruloplasmin, 24-hr urine copper
	Hemochromatosis	Serum ferritin, transferrin saturation, HFE mutation
	ALD	IgA, mAST
	NAFLD/NASH	HOMA-IR Hepatic fibrosis markers (FIB4 index, type 4 collagen 7s, Mac2-bp, Pro-C3)

2.6.1   Evaluation of Acute Liver Injury

Acute liver injury/acute liver disease is defined as the presence of abnormal liver tests for less than 6 months in a patient without preexisting liver diseases. Algorithm for evaluation of acute liver injury was shown in Fig. 2.1.

2.6.2   Evaluation of Chronic Liver Injury/ Chronic Liver Disease

The term of chronic liver injury/*chronic liver disease* is used when abnormal ALT levels persist for more than 6 months

or if there is evidence of chronic liver injury on liver histology. Algorithm for evaluation of chronic liver injury/CLD was shown in Fig. 2.2. If NAFLD is diagnosed, algorithm is shown in Fig. 2.3. Accumulating evidences suggest that FIB4 index is the most reliable and simple index to exclude severe fibrosis in NAFLD. FIB4 index is of use for predicting mortality and carcinogenesis in NAFLD patients. NAFLD patients with low FIB4 index (<1.3) who are unlikely to have severe fibrosis can be followed up, whereas those with inderminate or high FIB4 index cannot be excluded to have severe fibrosis. General physicians refer these patients to refer to hepatologists. Hepatologists should perform to examine liver fibrosis markers (type 4 collagen

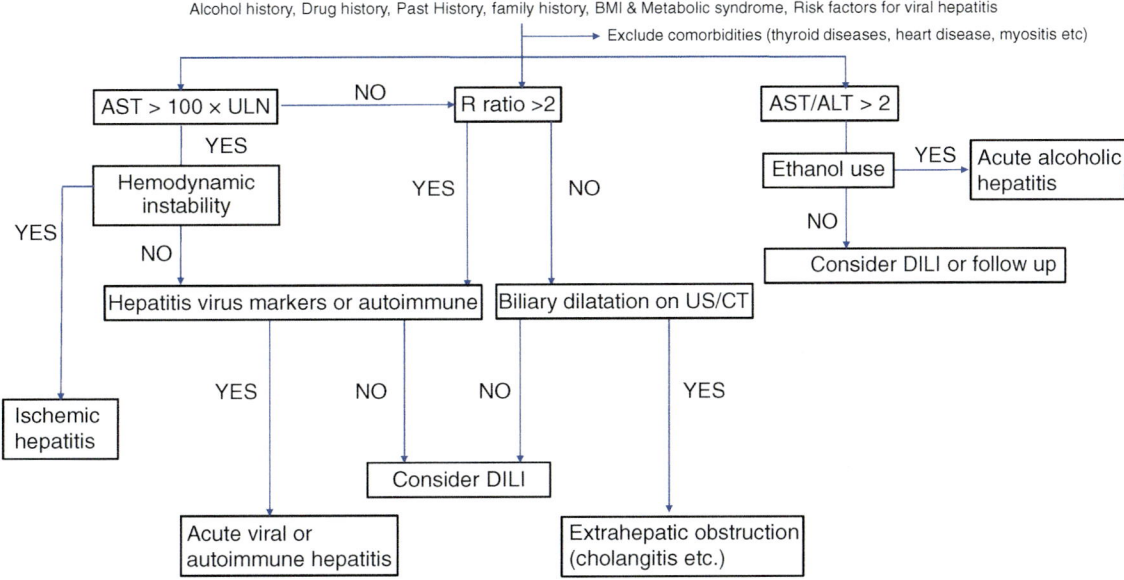

Fig. 2.1   Hepatobiliary enzyme elevation (acute)

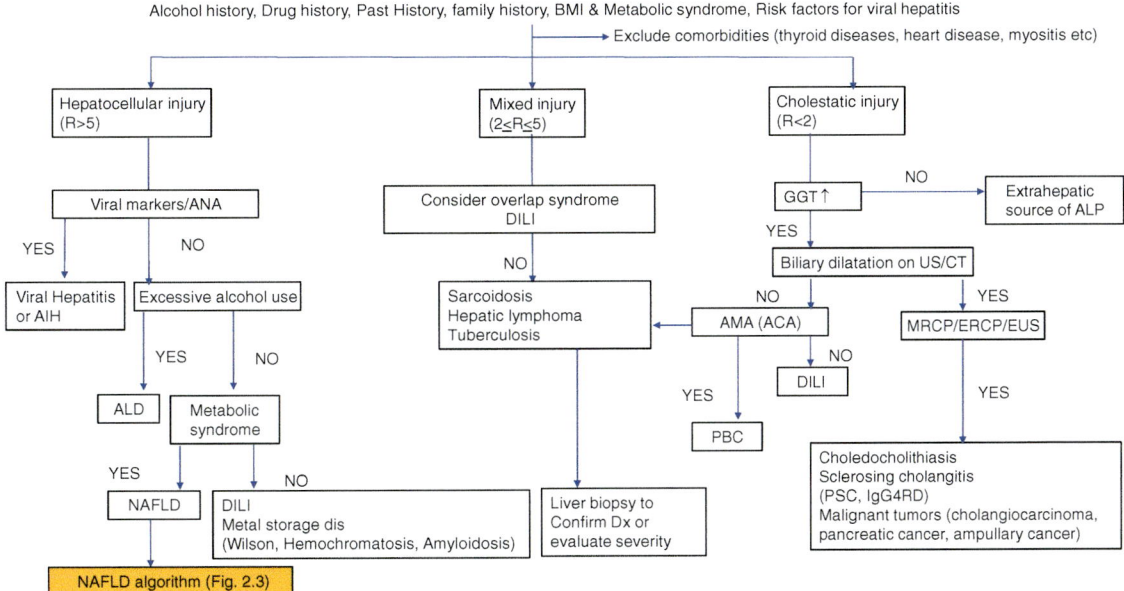

Fig. 2.2   Hepatobiliary enzyme elevation (chronic)

7S, M2bp, and Pro-C3) and elastography (FibroScan, MRE). NAFLD patients who are likely to have severe fibrosis should be considered performing liver biopsies and screening hepatocellular carcinoma (HCC)/esophageal varices (Fig. 2.3).

2.7 Assessing the Severity of Cirrhosis

2.7.1 Child-Pugh Score (Table 2.4)

The Child-Pugh score, initially derived to predict survival after portacaval shunt surgery, is the most widely used. The score divides patients into class A, B, and C based on three laboratory tests (prothrombin time, bilirubin, and albumin) and two clinical features (ascites, hepatic encephalopathy). Two-year survival for patients in class A is 85%, compared 60% and 35% for patients in class B and C, respectively.

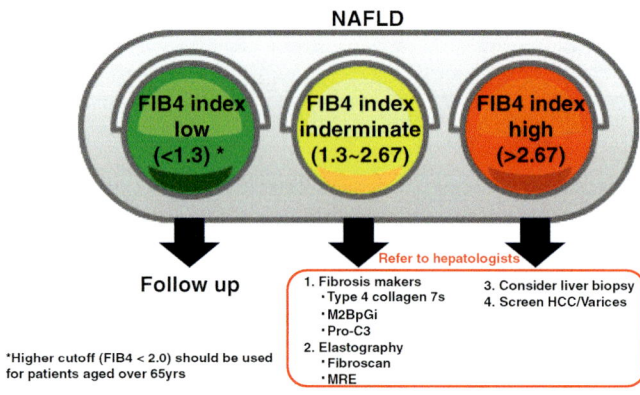

Fig. 2.3 NAFLD algorithm

Table 2.4 Child-Pugh score

Measure	1 point	2 points	3 points
Total bilirubin (mg/dL)	<2.0	2.1–3.0	>3.0
Serum albumin, g/dL	>3.5	2.8–3.5	<2.8
Prothrombin time, prolongation, or INR	<4.0 <1.7	4.0–6.0 1.7–2.3	> 6.0 >2.3
Ascites	None	Mild (or suppressed with medication)	Moderate to severe (or refractory)
Hepatic encephalopathy	None	Grades I–II	Grades III–IV

Scores: class A, 5–6; class B, 7–9; class C, 10–15

Table 2.5 Model for end-stage liver disease (MELD) score

Score	3-month mortality
<10	2–8%
10–19	6–29%
20–29	50–76%
30–39	62–83%
>40	100%

2.7.2 The Model for End-Stage Liver Disease (MELD) Score (Table 2.5)

The MELD score (Table 2.3) was originally developed to predict 3-month mortality following transjugular intrahepatic portosystemic shunt (TIPS) placement [7]. Now, the MELD scale is a reliable measure of mortality risk in patients with end-stage liver disease and suitable for use as a disease severity index to determine organ allocation priorities [8]. Several online tools are available for calculating the MELD score (https://www.mayoclinic.org/medical-professionals/model-end-stage-liver-disease/meld-model). MELD = $3.8*\log_e$(serum bilirubin [mg/dL]) + $11.2*\log_e$(INR) + $9.6*\log_e$(serum creatinine [mg/dL]) + 6.4. The MELD score is based entirely on objective data. Serum sodium has recently been added to the MELD score as the MELD-Na score to improve its performance [102, 103].

2.7.3 ALBI (Albumin-Bilirubin) Grade

The Child-Pugh classification has some nonobjective factors (ascites, hepatic encephalopathy). Recently, albumin-bilirubin (ALBI) scoring/grading, consisting of only albumin and total bilirubin, has been proposed to evaluate hepatic function. ALBI grade = ($\log_{10}$ bilirubin × 0.66) + (albumin × −0.085), where bilirubin is in μmol/L and albumin in g/L. ALBI score used for grading; ≤−2.60 = grade 1, greater than −2.60 to ≤−1.39 = grade 2, greater than −1.39 = grade 3 [9]. ALBI grade is a simple, evidence-based, objective, and discriminatory method of assessing liver function. This new model eliminates the need for subjective variables such as ascites and encephalopathy, a requirement in the conventional Child-Pugh classification. ALBI grade provided better prognostic performance than Child-Pugh score [11].

2.8 Tumor Markers

As major tumor biomarkers for HCC, α-fetoprotein (AFP), fucosylated AFP (AFP-L3), and des-γ-carboxyprothrombin (DCP) are used during clinical follow-up [104]. These bio-

Table 2.6 High-risk populations and risk factors for the development of HCC

1. High-risk population
• Patients with chronic hepatitis type B (including cirrhosis)
• Patients with chronic hepatitis type C (including cirrhosis)
• Liver cirrhosis patients caused by other than HBV or HCV
2. Risk factors
• HBV infection
• HCV infection
• Obesity
• Diabetes mellitus
• Older age
• Male gender
• Heavy alcohol drinker

markers can be used not only for the detection of HCC but also for the recurrence detection markers in the follow-up of HCC patients. However, approximately 30% of HCC are negative for AFP and DCP. Therefore, combination of these biomarkers is clinically used, and many researchers still have tried to establish novel HCC biomarkers. High-risk populations and risk factors for the development of HCC are proposed in Table 2.6. Among various risk factors for HCC development, HBV and HCV are most important [105–108]. Especially, HBV-/HCV-induced liver cirrhosis patients are super high-risk group for HCC. About 10% of virus-associated CLDs develop liver cirrhosis, and 5–10% of these cirrhosis patients develop HCC per year. Among patients with HCC, the prevalence of liver cirrhosis has been estimated to be 85–95% [109]. However, the ratio of cirrhosis patients in NAFLD-related HCC is about 50–60% [110–112]. In Japanese male NAFLD patients, more than half of HCC is developed from F0 to F3 stage patients [112, 113]. This finding is very important in the clinical surveillance of HCC for NAFLD patients.

Recently, the number of NAFLD-induced HCC is increasing around the world. CLD patients with virus (HBV, HCV) positive, obesity, diabetes mellitus, older age, male gender, and heavy alcohol drink are at high risk for the development of HCC. Outpatients with these risk factors should receive HCC surveillance. According to the guidelines for HCC treatment, the Asian Pacific Association for the Study of the Liver (APASL) and the *European Association for the Study of the Liver* (EASL) recommend HCC surveillance using tumor biomarker and abdominal ultrasonography (US) [106, 107]. These guidelines recommend AFP measurements every 6 months with abdominal US in high-risk patients for HCC development, especially in virus-associated liver cirrhosis patients. However, surveillance with AFP alone is not recommended as a confirmatory test in small HCC [106–108]. Combination of two or more tumor biomarkers would contribute to increase sensitivity without decreasing specificity [104]. In Japan, three HCC biomarkers (AFP, DCP, AFP-L3) are cov-

ered by the national health insurance in clinical settings for HCC surveillance. The Japanese Society of Hepatology (JSH) recommends the measurements of AFP, DCP, and/or AFP-L3 with imaging screening (US, dynamic CT, dynamic MRI) [105]. In contrast, AASLD practice guidelines recommend that US examination as the primary modality (without AFP) should be part of HCC surveillance [108]. However, cases with a very rough background liver parenchyma (e.g., cirrhosis, obesity) have difficulty for US evaluation; periodic imaging screening using dynamic CT and/or dynamic MRI every 6–12 months is proposed [105]. Imaging screening needs each testing equipment and involves significant cost, while measurements of tumor biomarkers are convenient and relatively low less expensive for HCC screening. Therefore, reliable biomarkers are needed for HCC surveillance.

2.8.1 α-Fetoprotein (AFP)

AFP is the most common and classical tumor marker for HCC. AFP was first identified in the sera of patients with HCC [114]. The serum levels of AFP higher than 500 ng/mL were diagnostic in the 1970s when most patients with HCC were diagnosed at advanced stage [115]. The usefulness of AFP is limited in small HCC diagnosis. The human AFP gene is mapped to chromosome 4 (4q11–q13) and is part of the albuminoid gene superfamily that encodes several proteins, including albumin in addition to AFP [116, 117]. AFP is synthesized by the yolk sac in early fetal life and later by the fetal liver. In adults the serum AFP concentration is approximately 5–10 μg/L under normal conditions [118]. APASL and EASL recommend AFP cutoff value of 200 ng/mL in a surveillance [106, 107]. It is to be noted that AFP levels increase in patients with active hepatitis, cirrhosis, AFP producing digestive tract tumor, and yolk sac tumor. An increase in the serum level of AFP is mainly used as a tumor marker for HCC.

2.8.2 AFP-L3 (Fucosylated AFP)

Recent findings in glycobiology include direct evidence of the involvement of oligosaccharide changes in human diseases [119]. Glycoproteomics has been in focus as a postgenomic research field for the identification of diagnostic markers [120, 121]. In particular, fucosylation, characterized by the addition of fucose to the glycans, is one of the most important models of glycosylation involved in hepatocarcinogenesis [122]. Various fucosylated proteins are reported to be biomarkers for human diseases including HCC [123–125].

AFP-L3 is a fucosylated variant of AFP that reacts with LCA (*Lens culinaris* agglutinin A) which recognizes α1-6 fucosylation. AFP-L3 is synthesized through the reaction of α1-6 fucosyltransferase (Fut8) in the presence of GDP-fucose as a donor substrate. While the enzymatic activity of Fut8 was not higher in HCC tissues than in the surrounding non-tumor tissues, the level of GDP-fucose, a donor substrate for Fut8, was dramatically increased in HCC tissues [126]. The lectin-dependent fractionation of AFP was originally described by Breborowicz [127] and Taketa [128].

The AFP concentration often increases in patients with active chronic liver diseases, and the low specificity of AFP for a diagnosis for HCC is a clinical problem. In contrast, AFP-L3 is a more specific marker for HCC than AFP alone [129–131]. The specificity of AFP-L3 for a differential diagnosis of HCC from chronic liver diseases is quite high [129]. Certain cases of benign liver diseases with high levels of AFP-L3 include those with severe acute hepatitis or fulminant hepatitis. A high level of AFP-L3 in HCC indicates a poor prognosis [132]. Therefore, AFP-L3 is considered to be much more useful than AFP as a tumor biomarker for HCC. AFP-L3 (%) is usually described as ratio to total AFP concentration, and it could not be measured when total AFP levels were less than 10 ng/mL. Recently, a highly sensitive measurement system was developed which enables AFP-L3 measurement even in the range of AFP less than 10 ng/mL [133].

2.8.3 Des-Gamma-Carboxyprothrombin (DCP)

DCP is also known as prothrombin induced by vitamin K absence or antagonist II (PIVKA-II). DCP is an abnormal product of liver carboxylation during the formation of thrombogen that acts as an autologous mitogen for HCC cell lines [134]. DCP is an abnormal prothrombin that was identified as an HCC biomarker in 1984 [135], and elevated DCP is most notably found in advanced cases with portal vein invasion [136, 137]. DCP has been recognized as a highly specific HCC biomarker and as a useful prognostic biomarker, for HCC [138, 139]. In NAFLD-associated HCC, DCP is reported to have a higher positive rate than AFP [112, 113].

Serum DCP levels are not correlated with the AFP, and about 30% of AFP-negative HCC is DCP-positive [140]. In small HCC cases, measurement of AFP and DCP is recommended. A high level of DCP indicates poor prognosis, and an increase in the DCP level after HCC therapy could be a marker of HCC recurrence [138, 139]. Interestingly, DCP is reported to have a biologic function in the growth of HCC. DCP acts as a growth factor in both autocrine and paracrine manners [134]. DCP also induces cell proliferation and migration of human umbilical vein endothelial cells [141]. DCP cannot be used in patients on vitamin K antagonists such as warfarin.

2.8.4 Glypican-3 (GPC3)

Glypican-3 (GPC3) is a family of the heparan sulfate proteoglycans (HSPGs) that are linked to the cell surface by a glycosylphosphatidylinositol (GPI) anchor [142]. GPC3 was identified as a gene developmentally expressed in rat intestine [143]. GPC3 has pivotal roles in cell growth, differentiation, and migration [144, 145]. GPC3 is highly expressed in fetal organs but is scarcely expressed in adult tissues [146]. In most HCCs, GPC3 mRNA levels and protein expression are significantly increased compared with benign liver lesions of the normal liver [146, 147]. In addition, serum levels of GPC3 also increased in HCC patients [146]. Thus, GPC3 is considered as a good candidate for HCC biomarker. The combination of GPC3 and AFP could significantly increase the sensitivity for the diagnosis of HCC [146]. Although GPC3 is expressed even in early small HCC, it is difficult to detect serum GPC3 in the patients with small HCC in such low serum levels. Diagnostic accuracy of serum GPC3 for early HCC is still unsatisfactory mainly due to unestablished assay system [148]. At this moment, GPC3 is of some help for the diagnosis of HCC.

References

1. Prati D, Taioli E, Zanella A, et al. Updated definitions of healthy ranges for serum alanine aminotransferase levels. Ann Intern Med. 2002;137:1–10.
2. Kwo PY, Cohen SM, Lim JK. ACG Clinical Guideline: evaluation of abnormal liver chemistries. Am J Gastroenterol. 2017;112:18–35.
3. Litin SC, O'Brien JF, Pruett S, et al. Macroenzyme as a cause of unexplained elevation of aspartate aminotransferase. Mayo Clin Proc. 1987;62:681–7.
4. Poupon R. Liver alkaline phosphatase: a missing link between choleresis and biliary inflammation. Hepatology. 2015;61(6):2080–90.
5. Matsushita M, Komoda T. Relationship between the effects of a high-fat meal and blood group in determination of alkaline phosphatase activity. Rinsho Byori. 2011;59:923–9.
6. Vilstrup H, Amodio P, Bajaj J, et al. Hepatic encephalopathy in chronic liver disease: 2014 Practice Guideline by the American Association for the Study of Liver Diseases and the European Association for the Study of the Liver. Hepatology. 2014;60:715–35.
7. Kamath PS, Wiesner RH, Malinchoc M, et al. A model to predict survival in patients with end-stage liver disease. Hepatology. 2001;33:464–70.
8. Wiesner R, Edwards E, Freeman R, et al. Model for end-stage liver disease (MELD) and allocation of donor livers. Gastroenterology. 2003;124:91–6.
9. Johnson PJ, Berhane S, Kagebayashi C, et al. Assessment of liver function in patients with hepatocellular carcinoma: a new evidence-based approach-the ALBI grade. J Clin Oncol. 2015;33:550–8.
10. Chalasani NP, Hayashi PH, Bonkovsky HL, et al. ACG Clinical Guideline: the diagnosis and management of idiosyncratic drug-induced liver injury. Am J Gastroenterol. 2014;109:950–66.
11. Hiraoka A, Kumada T, Michitaka K, et al. Usefulness of albumin-bilirubin grade for evaluation of prognosis of 2584 Japanese

patients with hepatocellular carcinoma. J Gastroenterol Hepatol. 2016;31:1031–6.

12. Maleki I, Aminafshari MR, Taghvaei T, et al. Serum immunoglobulin A concentration is a reliable biomarker for liver fibrosis in non-alcoholic fatty liver disease. World J Gastroenterol. 2014;20:12566–73.

13. Oertelt S, Rieger R, Selmi C, et al. A sensitive bead assay for antimitochondrial antibodies: chipping away at AMA-negative primary biliary cirrhosis. Hepatology. 2007;45:659–65.

14. Bataller R, Brenner DA. Liver fibrosis. J Clin Invest. 2005;115:209–18.

15. Svegliati-Baroni G, De Minicis S, Marzioni M. Hepatic fibrogenesis in response to chronic liver injury: novel insights on the role of cell-to-cell interaction and transition. Liver Int. 2008;28:1052–64.

16. Moller S, Henriksen JH. Cardiovascular complications of cirrhosis. Postgrad Med J. 2009;85:44–54.

17. Mas VR, Fisher RA, Archer KJ, et al. Proteomics and liver fibrosis: identifying markers of fibrogenesis. Expert Rev Proteomics. 2009;6:421–31.

18. Piccinino F, Sagnelli E, Pasquale G, et al. Complications following percutaneous liver biopsy. A multicentre retrospective study on 68,276 biopsies. J Hepatol. 1986;2:165–73.

19. Ratziu V, Charlotte F, Heurtier A, et al. Sampling variability of liver biopsy in nonalcoholic fatty liver disease. Gastroenterology. 2005;128:1898–906.

20. Yoneda M, Yoneda M, Fujita K, et al. Transient elastography in patients with non-alcoholic fatty liver disease (NAFLD). Gut. 2007;56:1330–1.

21. Yoneda M, Suzuki K, Kato S, et al. Nonalcoholic fatty liver disease: US-based acoustic radiation force impulse elastography. Radiology. 2010;256:640–7.

22. Castera L, Forns X, Alberti A. Non-invasive evaluation of liver fibrosis using transient elastography. J Hepatol. 2008;48:835–47.

23. Harrison SA, Oliver D, Arnold HL, et al. Development and validation of a simple NAFLD clinical scoring system for identifying patients without advanced disease. Gut. 2008;57:1441–7.

24. Angulo P, Hui JM, Marchesini G, et al. The NAFLD fibrosis score: a noninvasive system that identifies liver fibrosis in patients with NAFLD. Hepatology. 2007;45:846–54.

25. Sumida Y, Yoneda M, Hyogo H, et al. A simple clinical scoring system using ferritin, fasting insulin, and type IV collagen 7S for predicting steatohepatitis in nonalcoholic fatty liver disease. J Gastroenterol. 2011;46:257–68.

26. Imajo K, Kessoku T, Honda Y, et al. Magnetic resonance imaging more accurately classifies steatosis and fibrosis in patients with onalcoholic fatty liver disease than transient elastography. Gastroenterology. 2016;150:626–37.

27. Friedman SL. Molecular regulation of hepatic fibrosis, an integrated cellular response to tissue injury. J Biol Chem. 2000;275:2247–50.

28. Wake K. Perisinusoidal stellate cells (fat-storing cells, interstitial cells, lipocytes), their related structure in and around the liver sinusoids, and vitamin A-storing cells in extrahepatic organs. Int Rev Cytol. 1980;66:303–53.

29. Kuno A, Ikehara Y, Tanaka Y, et al. A serum "sweet-doughnut" protein facilitates fibrosis evaluation and therapy assessment in patients with viral hepatitis. Sci Rep. 2013;3:1065.

30. Neuman MG, Cohen LB, Nanau RM. Hyaluronic acid as a non-invasive biomarker of liver fibrosis. Clin Biochem. 2016;49:302–15.

31. Guéchot J, Laudat A, Loria A, et al. Diagnostic accuracy of hyaluronan and type III procollagen amino-terminal peptide serum assays as markers of liver fibrosis in chronic viral hepatitis C evaluated by ROC curve analysis. Clin Chem. 1996;42:558–63.

32. Schanté CE, Zuber G, Herlin C, et al. Chemical modifications of hyaluronic acid for the synthesis of derivatives for a broad range of biomedical applications. Carbohydr Polym. 2011;85:469–89.

33. Stickel F, Poeschl G, Schuppan D, et al. Serum hyaluronate correlates with histological progression in alcoholic liver disease. Eur J Gastroenterol Hepatol. 2003;15:945–50.

34. Rosenberg WMC, Voelker M, Thiel R, et al. Serum markers detect the presence of liver fibrosis: a cohort study. Gastroenterology. 2014;127:1704–13.

35. Toda K, Kumagai N, Kaneko F, et al. Pentoxifylline prevents pig serum-induced rat liver fibrosis by inhibiting interleukin-6 production. J Gastroenterol Hepatol. 2009;24:860–5.

36. Fontana RJ, Dienstag JL, Bonkovsky HL, et al. Serum fibrosis markers are associated with liver disease progression in non-responder patients with chronic hepatitis C. Gut. 2010;59:1401–9.

37. Arima Y, Kawabe N, Hashimoto S, et al. Reduction of liver stiffness by interferon treatment in the patients with chronic hepatitis C. Hepatol Res. 2010;40:383–92.

38. Andersen ES, Moessner BK, Christensen PB, et al. Lower liver stiffness in patients with sustained virological response 4 years after treatment for chronic hepatitis C. Eur J Gastroenterol Hepatol. 2011;23:41–4.

39. Park SH, Kim CH, Kim DJ, et al. Usefulness of multiple biomarkers for the prediction of significant fibrosis in chronic hepatitis B. J Clin Gastroenterol. 2011;45:361–5.

40. Chen J, Liu C, Chen H, et al. Study on noninvasive laboratory tests for fibrosis in chronic HBV infection and their evaluation. J Clin Lab Anal. 2013;27:5–11.

41. Koo JH, Lee MH, Kim SS, et al. Changes in serum histologic surrogate markers and procollagen III N-terminal peptide as independent predictors of HBeAg loss in patients with chronic hepatitis B during entecavir therapy. Clin Biochem. 2012;45:31–6.

42. Corpechot C, Carrat F, Poujol-Robert A, et al. Noninvasive elastography-based assessment of liver fibrosis progression and prognosis in primary biliary cirrhosis. Hepatology. 2012;56:198–208.

43. Corpechot C, Gaouar F, El Naggar A, et al. Baseline values and changes in liver stiffness measured by transient elastography are associated with severity of fibrosis and outcomes of patients with primary sclerosing cholangitis. Gastroenterology. 2014;146:970–9.

44. Alkhouri N, Carter–Kent C, Lopez R, et al. A combination of the pediatric NAFLD fibrosis index and enhanced liver fibrosis test identifies children with fibrosis. Clin Gastroenterol Hepatol. 2011;9:150–5.

45. Tomita K, Teratani T, Yokoyama H, et al. Serum immunoglobulin a concentration is an independent predictor of liver fibrosis in nonalcoholic steatohepatitis before the cirrhotic stage. Dig Dis Sci. 2011;56:3648–54.

46. Martinez-Hernandez A, Amenta PS. The hepatic extracellular matrix. I. Components and distribution in normal liver. Virchows Arch A Pathol Anat Histopathol. 1993;423:1–11.

47. Kefalides NA, Borel JP. Structural macromolecules: laminins, entactin/nidogen, and proteoglycans (Perlecan, Agrin). Curr Top Membr. 2005;56:147–97.

48. Birk DE, Brückner P. Collagens, suprastructures, and collagen fibril assembly. In: The extracellular matrix: an overview. Berlin: Springer; 2011. p. 77–115.

49. Kalluri R. Angiogenesis: basement membranes: structure, assembly and role in tumour angiogenesis. Nat Rev Cancer. 2003;3:422.

50. Wells RG. Cellular sources of extracellular matrix in hepatic fibrosis. Clin Liver Dis. 2008;12:759–68.

51. Mak KM, Mei R. Basement membrane type IV collagen and laminin: an overview of their biology and value as fibrosis biomarkers of liver disease. Anat Rec (Hoboken). 2017;300:1371–90.

52. Rojkind M, Ponce-Noyola P. The extracellular matrix of the liver. Coll Relat Res. 1982;2:151–75.

53. Murawaki Y, Ikuta Y, Koda M, et al. Comparison of serum 7S fragment of type IV collagen and serum central triple-helix of type IV collagen for assessment of liver fibrosis in patients with chronic viral liver disease. J Hepatol. 1996;24:148–54.

54. Murawaki Y, Ikuta Y, Nishimura Y, et al. Serum markers for connective tissue turnover in patients with chronic hepatitis B and chronic hepatitis C: a comparative analysis. J Hepatol. 1995;23:145–52.

55. Shimamura T, Nakajima Y, Une Y, et al. Serum levels of the type IV collagen 7s domain in patients with chronic viral liver diseases. Int J Oncol. 1996;8:153–7.

56. Niemela O, Risteli J, Blake JE, et al. Markers of fibrogenesis and basement membrane formation in alcoholic liver disease. Relation to severity, presence of hepatitis, and alcohol intake. Gastroenterology. 1990;98:1612–9.

57. Hirayama C, Suzuki H, Takada A, et al. Serum type IV collagen in various liver diseases in comparison with serum 7S collagen, laminin, and type III procollagen peptide. J Gastroenterol. 1996;31:242–8.

58. Yoneda M, Mawatari H, Fujita K, et al. Type IV collagen 7s domain is an independent clinical marker of the severity of fibrosis in patients with nonalcoholic steatohepatitis before the cirrhotic stage. J Gastroenterol. 2007;42:375–81.

59. Kojima H, Hongo Y, Harada H, et al. Long-term histological prognosis and serum fibrosis markers in chronic hepatitis C patients treated with interferon. J Gastroenterol Hepatol. 2001;16:1015–21.

60. Rosenberg WM, Voelker M, Thiel R, et al. Serum markers detect the presence of liver fibrosis: a cohort study. Gastroenterology. 2004;127:1704–13.

61. Montalto G, Soresi M, Aragona F, et al. Procollagen III and laminin in chronic viral hepatopathies. Presse medicale (Paris, France: 1983). 1996;25:59–62.

62. Hayasaka A, Schuppan D, Ohnishi K, et al. Serum concentrations of the carboxy terminal cross-linking domain of procollagen type IV (NC1) and the aminoterminal propeptide of procollagen type III (PIIIP) in chronic liver disease. J Hepatol. 1990;10:17–22.

63. Tanwar S, Trembling PM, Guha IN, et al. Validation of terminal peptide of procollagen III for the detection and assessment of nonalcoholic steatohepatitis in patients with nonalcoholic fatty liver disease. Hepatology. 2013;57:103–11.

64. Gluba A, Bielecka-Dabrowa A, Mikhailidis DP, et al. An update on biomarkers of heart failure in hypertensive patients. J Hypertens. 2012;30:1681–9.

65. Nielsen MJ, Nedergaard AF, Sun S, et al. The neo-epitope specific PRO-C3 ELISA measures true formation of type III collagen associated with liver and muscle parameters. Am J Transl Res. 2013;5:303.

66. Nielsen MJ, Veidal SS, Karsdal MA, et al. Plasma Pro-C3 (N-terminal type III collagen propeptide) predicts fibrosis progression in patients with chronic hepatitis C. Liver Int. 2015;35:429–37.

67. Daniels S, Nielsen M, Krag A, et al. Serum Pro-C3 combined with clinical parameters is superior to established serological fibrosis tests at identifying patients with advanced fibrosis among patients with non-alcoholic fatty liver disease. J Hepatol. 2017;66:S671.

68. Karsdal MA, Henriksen K, Nielsen MJ, et al. Fibrogenesis assessed by serological type III collagen formation identifies patients with progressive liver fibrosis and responders to a potential antifibrotic therapy. Am J Physiol Gastrointest Liver Physiol. 2016;311:G1009–17.

69. Iacobelli S, Arno E, D'Orazio A, et al. Detection of antigens recognized by a novel monoclonal antibody in tissue and serum from patients with breast cancer. Cancer Res. 1986;46:3005–10.

70. Koths K, Taylor E, Halenbeck R, et al. Cloning and characterization of a human Mac-2-binding protein, a new member of the superfamily defined by the macrophage scavenger receptor cysteine-rich domain. J Biol Chem. 1993;268:14245–9.

71. Tinari N, Kuwabara I, Huflejt ME, et al. Glycoprotein 90K/MAC-2BP interacts with galectin-1 and mediates galectin-1-induced cell aggregation. Int J Cancer. 2001;91:167–72.

72. Resnick D, Pearson A, Krieger M. The SRCR superfamily: a family reminiscent of the Ig superfamily. Trends Biochem Sci. 1994;19:5–8.

73. Trahey M, Weissman IL. Cyclophilin C-associated protein: a normal secreted glycoprotein that down-modulates endotoxin and proinflammatory responses in vivo. Proc Natl Acad Sci U S A. 1999;96:3006–11.

74. Ochieng J, Leite-Browning ML, Warfield P. Regulation of cellular adhesion to extracellular matrix proteins by galectin-3. Biochem Biophys Res Commun. 1998;246:788–91.

75. Kamada Y, Ono M, Hyogo H, et al. A novel noninvasive diagnostic method for nonalcoholic steatohepatitis using two glycobiomarkers. Hepatology. 2015;62:1433–43.

76. Haji-Ghassemi O, Gilbert M, Spence J, et al. Molecular basis for recognition of the cancer glycobiomarker, LacdiNAc (GalNAc[beta1-->4]GlcNAc), by *Wisteria floribunda* Agglutinin. J Biol Chem. 2016;291:24085–95.

77. Kuno A, Sato T, Shimazaki H, et al. Reconstruction of a robust glycodiagnostic agent supported by multiple lectin-assisted glycan profiling. Proteomics Clin Appl. 2013;7:642–7.

78. Yamasaki K, Tateyama M, Abiru S, et al. Elevated serum levels of *Wisteria floribunda* agglutinin-positive human Mac-2 binding protein predict the development of hepatocellular carcinoma in hepatitis C patients. Hepatology. 2014;60:1563–70.

79. Abe M, Miyake T, Kuno A, et al. Association between *Wisteria floribunda* agglutinin-positive Mac-2 binding protein and the fibrosis stage of non-alcoholic fatty liver disease. J Gastroenterol. 2015;50:776–84.

80. Zou X, Zhu MY, Yu DM, et al. Serum WFA+ -M2BP levels for evaluation of early stages of liver fibrosis in patients with chronic hepatitis B virus infection. Liver Int. 2017;37:35–44.

81. Nishikawa H, Enomoto H, Iwata Y, et al. Impact of serum *Wisteria floribunda* agglutinin positive Mac-2-binding protein and serum interferon-gamma-inducible protein-10 in primary biliary cirrhosis. Hepatol Res. 2016;46:575–83.

82. Nishikawa H, Enomoto H, Iwata Y, et al. Clinical significance of serum *Wisteria floribunda* agglutinin positive Mac-2-binding protein level and high-sensitivity C-reactive protein concentration in autoimmune hepatitis. Hepatol Res. 2016;46:613–21.

83. Sterling RK, Lissen E, Clumeck N, et al. Development of a simple noninvasive index to predict significant fibrosis in patients with HIV/HCV coinfection. Hepatology. 2006;43:1317–25.

84. Imperiale TF, Said AT, Cummings OW, et al. Need for validation of clinical decision aids: use of the AST/ALT ratio in predicting cirrhosis in chronic hepatitis C. Am J Gastroenterol. 2000;95:2328–32.

85. Wai CT, Greenson JK, Fontana RJ, et al. A simple noninvasive index can predict both significant fibrosis and cirrhosis in patients with chronic hepatitis C. Hepatology. 2003;38:518–26.

86. Bedossa P, Carrat F. Liver biopsy: the best, not the gold standard. J Hepatology. 2009;50:1–3.

87. Castera L, Pinzani M. Biopsy and non-invasive methods for the diagnosis of liver fibrosis: does it take two to tango? Gut. 2010;59(7):861–6. BMJ Publishing Group.

88. Kennedy OJ, Parkes J, Tanwar S, et al. The enhanced liver fibrosis (ELF) panel: analyte stability under common sample storage conditions used in clinical practice. J Appl Lab Med. 2017;1:720–8.

89. Nobili V, Parkes J, Bottazzo G, et al. Performance of ELF serum markers in predicting fibrosis stage in pediatric non-alcoholic fatty liver disease. Gastroenterology. 2009;136:160–7.

90. Parkes J, Roderick P, Harris S, et al. Enhanced liver fibrosis test can predict clinical outcomes in patients with chronic liver disease. Gut. 2010;59:1245–51.

91. Sands CJ, Guha IN, Kyriakides M, et al. Metabolic phenotyping for enhanced mechanistic stratification of chronic hepatitis C-induced liver fibrosis. Am J Gastroenterol. 2015;110:159–69.

92. Gumusay O, Ozenirler S, Atak A, et al. Diagnostic potential of serum direct markers and non-invasive fibrosis models in patients with chronic hepatitis B. Hepatol Res. 2013;43:228–37.

93. Karlas T, Dietrich A, Peter V, et al. Evaluation of transient elastography, acoustic radiation force impulse imaging (ARFI), and enhanced liver function (ELF) score for detection of fibrosis in morbidly obese patients. PLoS One. 2015;10:e0141649.

94. Fagan KJ, Pretorius CJ, Horsfall LU, et al. ELF score >/=9.8 indicates advanced hepatic fibrosis and is influenced by age, steatosis and histological activity. Liver Int. 2015;35:1673–81.

95. Lichtinghagen R, Pietsch D, Bantel H, et al. The enhanced liver fibrosis (ELF) score: normal values, influence factors and proposed cut-off values. J Hepatol. 2013;59:236–42.

96. Williams AL, Hoofnagle JH. Ratio of serum aspartate to alanine aminotransferase in chronic hepatitis relationship to cirrhosis. Gastroenterology. 1988;95:734–9.

97. Lurie Y, Webb M, Cytter-Kuint R, et al. Non-invasive diagnosis of liver fibrosis and cirrhosis. World J Gastroenterol. 2015;21:11567.

98. Zhu X, Wang L-C, Chen E-Q, et al. Prospective evaluation of FibroScan for the diagnosis of hepatic fibrosis compared with liver biopsy/AST platelet ratio index and FIB-4 in patients with chronic HBV infection. Dig Dis Sci. 2001;56:2742–9.

99. Shin W, Park S, Jang M, et al. Aspartate aminotransferase to platelet ratio index (APRI) can predict liver fibrosis in chronic hepatitis B. Dig Liver Dis. 2008;40:267–74.

100. Naveau S, Gaudé G, Asnacios A, et al. Diagnostic and prognostic values of noninvasive biomarkers of fibrosis in patients with alcoholic liver disease. Hepatology. 2009;49:97–105.

101. Sumida Y, Yoneda M, Hyogo H, et al. Validation of the FIB4 index in a Japanese nonalcoholic fatty liver disease population. BMC Gastroenterol. 2012;12:2.

102. Biggins SW, Rodriguez HJ, Bacchetti P, et al. Serum sodium predicts mortality in patients listed for liver transplantation. Hepatology. 2005;41:32–9.

103. Kim WR, Biggins SW, Kremers WK, et al. Hyponatremia and mortality among patients on the liver-transplant waiting list. N Engl J Med. 2008;359:1018–26.

104. Tateishi R, Yoshida H, Matsuyama Y, et al. Diagnostic accuracy of tumor markers for hepatocellular carcinoma: a systematic review. Hepatol Int. 2018;2:17–30.

105. Kudo M, Izumi N, Kokudo N, et al. Management of hepatocellular carcinoma in Japan: Consensus-Based Clinical Practice Guidelines proposed by the Japan Society of Hepatology (JSH) 2010 updated version. Dig Dis. 2011;29:339–64.

106. Omata M, Cheng AL, Kokudo N, et al. Asia-Pacific clinical practice guidelines on the management of hepatocellular carcinoma: a 2017 update. Hepatol Int. 2017;11:317–70.

107. de Lope CR, Tremosini S, Forner A, et al. Management of HCC. J Hepatol. 2012;56(Suppl 1):S75–87.

108. Heimbach JK, Kulik LM, Finn RS, et al. AASLD guidelines for the treatment of hepatocellular carcinoma. Hepatology. 2018;67:358–80.

109. Kanwal F, Hoang T, Kramer JR, et al. Increasing prevalence of HCC and cirrhosis in patients with chronic hepatitis C virus infection. Gastroenterology. 2011;140:1182–1188.e1.

110. Mittal S, Sada YH, El-Serag HB, et al. Temporal trends of nonalcoholic fatty liver disease-related hepatocellular carcinoma in the veteran affairs population. Clin Gastroenterol Hepatol. 2015;13:594–601.e1.

111. Ertle J, Dechene A, Sowa JP, et al. Non-alcoholic fatty liver disease progresses to hepatocellular carcinoma in the absence of apparent cirrhosis. Int J Cancer. 2011;128:2436–43.

112. Tokushige K, Hyogo H, Nakajima T, et al. Hepatocellular carcinoma in Japanese patients with nonalcoholic fatty liver disease and alcoholic liver disease: multicenter survey. J Gastroenterol. 2016;51:586–96.

113. Yasui K, Hashimoto E, Komorizono Y, et al. Characteristics of patients with nonalcoholic steatohepatitis who develop hepatocellular carcinoma. Clin Gastroenterol Hepatol. 2011;9:428–33.

114. IuS T. Detection of embryo-specific alpha-globulin in the blood serum of a patient with primary liver cancer. Vopr Med Khim. 1964;10:90–1.

115. Kew M. Alpha-fetoprotein. In: Modern trends in gastroenterology, vol. 5; 1975. p. 91.

116. Koteish A, Thuluvath PJ. Screening for hepatocellular carcinoma. J Vasc Interv Radiol. 2002;13:S185–90.

117. McLeod JF, Cooke NE. The vitamin D-binding protein, alpha-fetoprotein, albumin multigene family: detection of transcripts in multiple tissues. J Biol Chem. 1989;264:21760–9.

118. Ruoslahti E, Seppala M. Studies of carcino-fetal proteins. 3. Development of a radioimmunoassay for -fetoprotein. Demonstration of -fetoprotein in serum of healthy human adults. Int J Cancer. 1971;8:374–833.

119. Ohtsubo K, Marth JD. Glycosylation in cellular mechanisms of health and disease. Cell. 2006;126:855–67.

120. Callewaert N, Van Vlierberghe H, Van Hecke A, et al. Noninvasive diagnosis of liver cirrhosis using DNA sequencer-based total serum protein glycomics. Nat Med. 2004;10:429–34.

121. Ito K, Kuno A, Ikehara Y, et al. LecT-hepa, a glyco-marker derived from multiple lectins, as a predictor of liver fibrosis in chronic hepatitis C patients. Hepatology. 2012;56:1448–56.

122. Miyoshi E, Moriwaki K, Nakagawa T. Biological function of fucosylation in cancer biology. J Biochem. 2008;143:725–9.

123. Hashimoto S, Asao T, Takahashi J, et al. alpha1-acid glycoprotein fucosylation as a marker of carcinoma progression and prognosis. Cancer. 2004;101:2825–36.

124. Wang M, Long RE, Comunale MA, et al. Novel fucosylated biomarkers for the early detection of hepatocellular carcinoma. Cancer Epidemiol Biomark Prev. 2009;18:1914–21.

125. Okuyama N, Ide Y, Nakano M, et al. Fucosylated haptoglobin is a novel marker for pancreatic cancer: a detailed analysis of the oligosaccharide structure and a possible mechanism for fucosylation. Int J Cancer. 2006;118:2803–8.

126. Noda K, Miyoshi E, Gu J, et al. Relationship between elevated FX expression and increased production of GDP-L-fucose, a common donor substrate for fucosylation in human hepatocellular carcinoma and hepatoma cell lines. Cancer Res. 2003;63:6282–9.

127. Breborowicz J, Mackiewicz A, Breborowicz D. Microheterogeneity of alpha-fetoprotein in patient serum as demonstrated by lectin affino-electrophoresis. Scand J Immunol. 1981;14:15–20.

128. Taketa K, Izumi M, Ichikawa E. Distinct molecular species of human alpha-fetoprotein due to differential affinities to lectins. Ann N Y Acad Sci. 1983;417:61–8.

129. Aoyagi Y. Carbohydrate-based measurements on alpha-fetoprotein in the early diagnosis of hepatocellular carcinoma. Glycoconj J. 1995;12:194–9.

130. Sato Y, Nakata K, Kato Y, et al. Early recognition of hepatocellular carcinoma based on altered profiles of alpha-fetoprotein. N Engl J Med. 1993;328:1802–6.

131. Taketa K, Endo Y, Sekiya C, et al. A collaborative study for the evaluation of lectin-reactive alpha-fetoproteins in early detection of hepatocellular carcinoma. Cancer Res. 1993;53:5419–23.

132. Yamashita F, Tanaka M, Satomura S, et al. Prognostic significance of *Lens culinaris* agglutinin A-reactive alpha-fetoprotein in small hepatocellular carcinomas. Gastroenterology. 1996;111:996–1001.

133. Kagebayashi C, Yamaguchi I, Akinaga A, et al. Automated immunoassay system for AFP-L3% using on-chip electrokinetic reaction and separation by affinity electrophoresis. Anal Biochem. 2009;388:306–11.

134. Suzuki M, Shiraha H, Fujikawa T, et al. Des-gamma-carboxy prothrombin is a potential autologous growth factor for hepatocellular carcinoma. J Biol Chem. 2005;280:6409–15.

135. Liebman HA, Furie BC, Tong MJ, et al. Des-γ-carboxy (abnormal) prothrombin as a serum marker of primary hepatocellular carcinoma. N Engl J Med. 1984;310:1427–31.

136. Koike Y, Shiratori Y, Sato S, et al. Des-γ-carboxy prothrombin as a useful predisposing factor for the development of portal venous invasion in patients with hepatocellular carcinoma. Cancer. 2001;91:561–9.

137. Hagiwara S, Kudo M, Kawasaki T, et al. Prognostic factors for portal venous invasion in patients with hepatocellular carcinoma. J Gastroenterol. 2006;41:1214–9.

138. Suehiro T, Sugimachi K, Matsumata T, et al. Protein induced by vitamin K absence or antagonist II as a prognostic marker in hepatocellular carcinoma. Comparison with alpha-fetoprotein. Cancer. 1994;73:2464–71.

139. Imamura H, Matsuyama Y, Miyagawa Y, et al. Prognostic significance of anatomical resection and des-γ-carboxy prothrombin in patients with hepatocellular carcinoma. Br J Surg. 1999;86:1032–8.

140. Toyoda H, Kumada T, Kiriyama S, et al. Prognostic significance of simultaneous measurement of three tumor markers in patients with hepatocellular carcinoma. Clin Gastroenterol Hepatol. 2006;4:111–7.

141. Fujikawa T, Shiraha H, Ueda N, et al. Des-gamma-carboxyl prothrombin-promoted vascular endothelial cell proliferation and migration. J Biol Chem. 2007;282:8741–8.

142. Filmus J, Selleck SB. Glypicans: proteoglycans with a surprise. J Clin Invest. 2001;108:497–501.

143. Filmus J, Church JG, Buick RN. Isolation of a cDNA corresponding to a developmentally regulated transcript in rat intestine. Mol Cell Biol. 1988;8:4243–9.

144. Li M, Choo B, Wong ZM, et al. Expression of OCI-5/glypican 3 during intestinal morphogenesis: regulation by cell shape in intestinal epithelial cells. Exp Cell Res. 1997;235:3–12.

145. Farooq M, Hwang SY, Park MK, et al. Blocking endogenous glypican-3 expression releases Hep 3B cells from G1 arrest. Mol Cells. 2003;15:356–60.

146. Capurro M, Wanless IR, Sherman M, et al. Glypican-3: a novel serum and histochemical marker for hepatocellular carcinoma. Gastroenterology. 2003;125:89–97.

147. Zhu Z, Friess H, Wang L, et al. Enhanced glypican-3 expression differentiates the majority of hepatocellular carcinomas from benign hepatic disorders. Gut. 2001;48:558–64.

148. Jia X, Liu J, Gao Y, et al. Diagnosis accuracy of serum glypican-3 in patients with hepatocellular carcinoma: a systematic review with meta-analysis. Arch Med Res. 2014;45:580–8.

Acute Hepatitis

3

Yoshinori Harada and Masaki Iwai

Contents

Abbreviations

CMV	Cytomegalovirus
DIC	Disseminated intravascular coagulation
EBNA	EBV nuclear antigen
EBV	Epstein-Barr virus
HAV	Hepatitis A virus
HBV	Hepatitis B virus
HCV	Hepatitis C virus
HDV	Hepatitis D virus
HEV	Hepatitis E virus
HSV	Herpes simplex virus
IgM-HA	Anti-HAV IgM antibody
VCA	Viral-capsid antigen

Y. Harada, MD, PhD (✉)
Kyoto, Japan
e-mail: yoharada@koto.kpu-m.ac.jp

M. Iwai, MD, PhD
Kyoto, Japan

Acute viral hepatitis is sporadic or endemic mainly due to hepatitis virus. It is spread by the oral-fecal route or parenterally by blood transfusion, intravenous drug abuse, and sexual intercourse. The hepatitis virus is defined as a virus that has a greater affinity for the liver and produces a characteristic inflammatory reaction in the liver. The virus includes types A, B, C, D, and E. Types A is transmitted via the oral-fecal route, whereas types B, C, and D are transmitted by parenteral route. Type E is mostly transmitted through the fecal-oral route, but it can be transmitted via blood transfusions (Table 3.1). Systemic infections of Epstein-Barr virus (EBV), cytomegalovirus, herpesvirus, adenovirus, and rubella rarely produce acute concomitant hepatitis. EBV causes hepatitis in the acute phase of systemic infection; and acute hepatitis due to herpesvirus, cytomegalovirus, adenovirus, or rubella occurs in immunosuppressed patients and young children.

Acute attacks of hepatitis virus are frequently subclinical or anicteric. If symptoms are present, they may be either characteristic or nonspecific. Typical symptoms include anorexia and nausea in the early stages, followed in the icteric form by dark urine and jaundice. In the anicteric form, jaundice is absent or unnoticed, and portal hypertension and ascites develop in some patients with acute hepatitis. These complications are partly the

© Springer Nature Singapore Pte Ltd. 2019
E. Hashimoto et al. (eds.), *Diagnosis of Liver Disease*, https://doi.org/10.1007/978-981-13-6806-6_3

result of liver cell injury and consequent collapse of the sinusoidal network. Biochemical changes in acute hepatitis are associated with hepatocellular damage, and serum aminotransferase activities are high, showing a peak preceding the onset of jaundice. Prothrombin time provides good information regarding liver failure, and serum bilirubin levels correlate with the severity of liver injury. In addition, polymorphonuclear leukocytes may be a secondary response to epithelial injury and are often seen with bile ductular proliferation.

Peritoneoscopy in acute viral hepatitis shows an enlarged liver with a red surface, whereas a green surface is seen in acute hepatitis with jaundice (Fig. 3.1).

In approximately 1–2% of patients with acute hepatitis, it is fulminant, and once fulminant, the death rate increases. Therefore, when diagnosing a patient with acute hepatitis, it is necessary for clinicians to clarify the cause and to determine whether inflammation has passed the acme phase. If there is an indication of severity or fulminant signs, one should consult a specialized medical institution promptly. It is also necessary to track until the virus is eliminated in order not to overlook chronicity.

Table 3.1 Hepatitis viruses

Virus	Type	Spread and disease
Hepatitis A	RNA hepatovirus	Fecal-oral, acute, and fulminant
Hepatitis B	DNA hepadnavirus	Parenteral, acute, fulminant, and chronic, hepatocellular carcinoma
Hepatitis C	RNA hepacivirus	Parenteral or sporadic, acute, more often chronic and rarely fulminant, hepatocellular carcinoma
Hepatitis D	RNA delta virus	Pathogenic when combined with hepatitis B virus
Hepatitis E	RNA hepevirus	Fecal-oral and parenteral, epidemic or sporadic
		Acute and fulminant
		Chronic in immunocompromised hosts

3.1 Hepatitis A Virus

Hepatitis A virus (HAV) is a common cause of acute hepatitis. It rarely causes fulminant hepatitis and is not associated with chronic hepatitis. The rate of lethality in acute hepatitis A is exceptionally low. HAV infections generally occur via the oral-fecal route and are related to shedding of the virus in the stool for 2–3 weeks before and 1 week after the onset of jaundice [1, 2]. Sporadic HAV infection can occur after ingestion of contaminated shellfish. HAV can cause epidemic hepatitis in countries with poor public hygiene.

HAV, 27 nm in diameter, is a nonenveloped, positive-strand RNA virus [3]. The virus itself is considered not to have direct toxic effects on hepatocytes. T cell-mediated immune response appears to cause hepatocyte injury. A representative course of acute hepatitis A is shown in Fig. 3.2 [1, 2]. Anti-HAV IgM antibody (IgM-HA) emerges in the serum at the symptomatic onset. Detection of IgM-HA is a good serological indicator for acute hepatitis A. A large amount of virus is discharged into the feces of the patient before onset. Therefore, infection expands even during the incubation period. Emission of virus is greatest at onset. After infection with HAV, a high-titer defensive antibody is produced, resulting in acquisition of permanent immunity.

There are two histopathological features in acute hepatitis A [4, 5]. The first is a periportal pattern of inflammation and necrosis with little or no perivenular necrosis. In severe hepatitis A, the virus may cause virus-associated hemophagocytic syndrome [6], and hepatocytes in the periportal area become swollen and develop a microvesicular formation. The second feature is perivenular cholestasis with little or no associated hepatocellular necrosis.

Case 3.1

A 44-year-old male complained of a common cold, and laboratory tests showed TBIL 3.7 mg/dL, ALT 7070 IU/L, AST

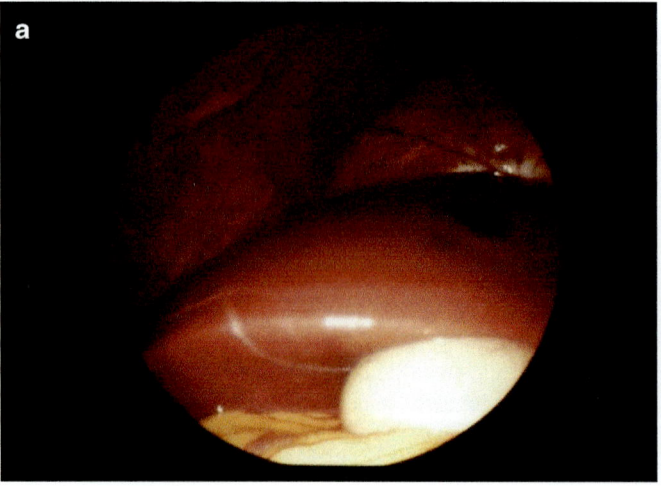
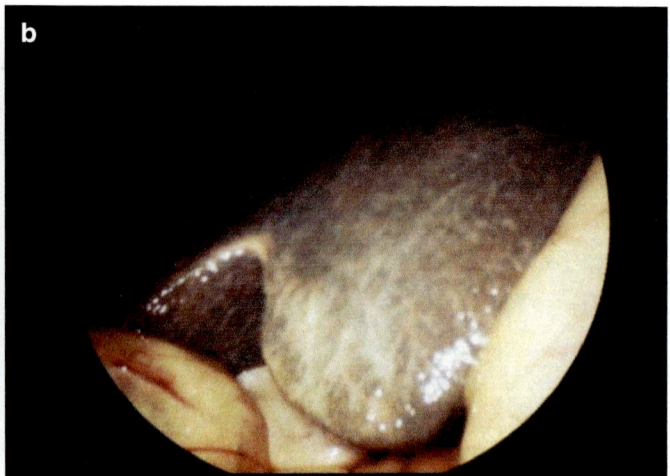

Fig. 3.1 Peritoneoscopic findings in acute hepatitis. (**a**) Liver is diffusely swollen, with a red surface. (**b**) Liver is enlarged, with a smooth surface and green color

5800 IU/L, LDH 4400 IU/L, ALP 515 IU/L, GGT 365 IU/L, PT 17.9 s, and IgM-HA positive. Liver biopsy 10 days after onset showed disarrayed trabecular structure and infiltration of mononuclear cells, neutrophils, and histiocytes in the portal tract (Fig. 3.3).

Case 3.2

A 40-year-old-female complained of fever for several days and epigastric pain with nausea. She was icteric and had dark urine. Liver function test 1 week after onset showed TBIL 3.29 mg/dL, ALT 1018 IU/L, AST 702 IU/L, ALP 16.6 KAU, LAP 280 IU/L, GGT 62 IU/L, TTT 7.8 U, and IgM-HA posi-

tive. Liver biopsy 3 weeks after onset showed bridging necrosis from portal tracts with infiltration of mononuclear cells and dilated sinusoids; the magnified view of the portal tracts showed a cluster of phagocytosing histiocytes and lymphocytes with an abnormal configuration of bile ducts (Fig. 3.4).

Acute viral hepatitis A is caused by an enterally transmitted RNA virus, and with good hygienic living standards, infection shifts to adulthood. A fulminant course is rare, and there is no causative relation with development of hepatocellular carcinoma. Transition to chronic hepatitis need not be feared. It is easy to make a diagnosis of acute hepatitis A serologically. HAV IgM rises in the serum during the first week of the disease, and it persists for 2 or 3 months.

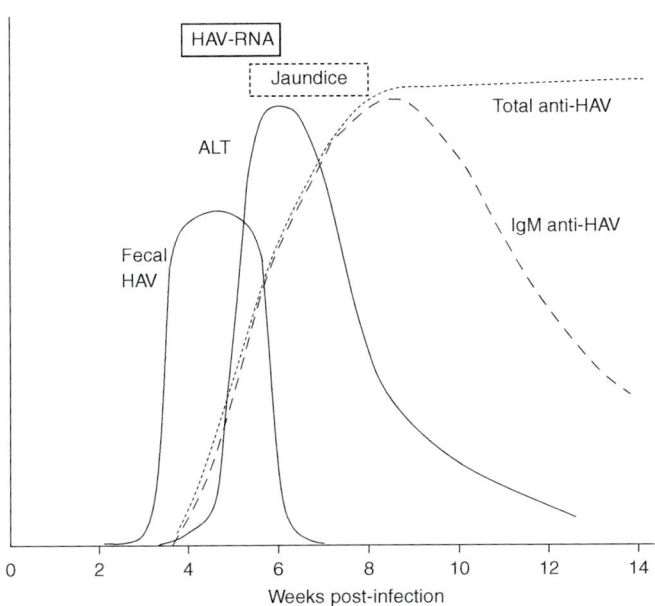

Fig. 3.2 Clinical course of acute hepatitis A. The mean incubation period for hepatitis A is 2–4 weeks

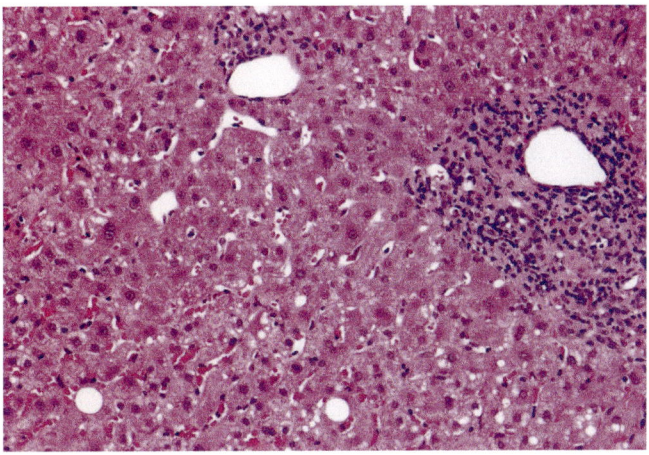

Fig. 3.3 Acute hepatitis A. Trabecular structure is disarrayed, and mononuclear cells, neutrophils, and histiocytes are seen in the portal tract

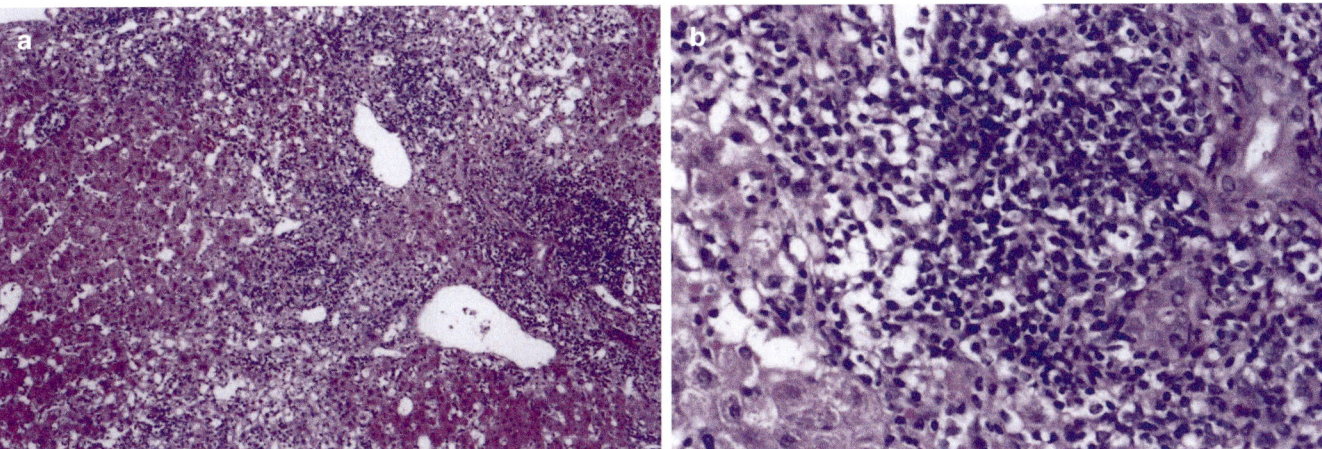

Fig. 3.4 Acute hepatitis A. (**a**) Submassive necrosis in the portal tract, with disarray of the lobular structure and dilated sinusoids. (**b**) Infiltration of mononuclear, neutrophilic, and histiocytic cells, with destruction of the bile ducts in the portal tract

3.2   Hepatitis B Virus

Hepatitis B virus (HBV) is a partially double-stranded DNA virus of the *Hepadnaviridae* family, and HBV is subdivided into ten different genotypes of A (HBV/A) to J (HBV/J), on the basis of sequence comparison [7–10]. The distribution of each HBV genotype is known to vary geographically [11]. Acute HBV infection in adults causes acute hepatitis, fulminant hepatitis, chronic hepatitis, and an asymptomatic carrier state. Sixty percent to 65% of adult infections with HBV result in subclinical disease, but 20–25% of HBV-infected patients develop acute hepatitis, and <1% of them progress to fulminant hepatitis. Five percent to 10% of adult HBV infections develop into chronic hepatitis [2]. Persistence of HBV is reported to be associated with genotype HBV/A [12]. When a stop codon mutation occurs in the precore/core promoter region, HBe antigen is not produced, which increases the risk of severity. That is, detection of the stop codon mutation is necessary to select therapeutic agents when acute hepatitis B is suspected of causing fulminant hepatitis [12].

HBV is transmitted via blood or body fluids; the principal routes of infection are sexual contact, blood transfusion, medical accidents, and mother-to-child transmission. The typical course of acute hepatitis B is shown in Fig. 3.5 [2, 11]. Acute hepatitis B develops after an incubation period of 1–4 months, and HB antigen appears in the sera about 1 month before onset [2, 11]. Anti-HBc IgM antibody is of value in the diagnosis of acute hepatitis B: IgM-HBc antibody may be positive even with acute exacerbation in an

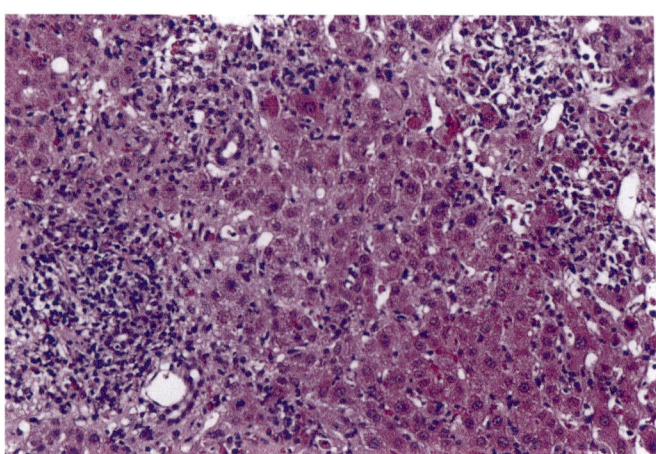

Fig. 3.6 Acute hepatitis B. Edematous portal tract with infiltration by inflammatory cells and scattered acidophilic bodies in the lobule and central necrosis showing infiltration of lymphocytes

HBV carrier, but generally its titer is low. It is possible to distinguish acute hepatitis B from acute exacerbation in an HBV carrier.

Histopathology in acute hepatitis B infection appears similar to that in other forms of viral hepatitis, demonstrating periportal hepatitis, perivenular confluent necrosis, acidophilic bodies, and parenchymal collapse.

Case 3.3

A 30-year-old male complained of general malaise, common cold-like symptoms, and was icteric. Liver chemistries demonstrated a peak 2 weeks after onset: TBIL 9.5 mg/dL, ALT 3245 IU/L, AST 1788 IU/L, ALP 396 IU/L, GGT 133 IU/L, and anti-HBcAb IgM 3.4. Liver biopsy 2 months after onset showed periportal hepatitis and intralobular necrosis; there was infiltration of mononuclear cells in portal tracts, and scattered acidophilic bodies were seen (Fig. 3.6).

3.3   Hepatitis C Virus

Hepatitis C virus (HCV), a family of *Flaviviridae* viruses, contains a positive-sense, single-stranded RNA molecule [13]. The HCV viral genome is translated into a single polyprotein of about 3000 amino acids. Clinical manifestations on acute infection of HCV are milder than in the case of HBV. Seventy-five percent of cases in acute HCV infection are asymptomatic [14, 15]. Only one in four cases develops symptomatic acute hepatitis C. The incubation period of HCV in acute symptomatic patients is usually 6–12 weeks [2]. HCV infection resolves spontaneously in 25% of patients, but about 75% of acute hepatitis C cases become chronic and persistent. Chronic hepatitis C is reported to result in the development of cirrhosis in about 20% of cases [2].

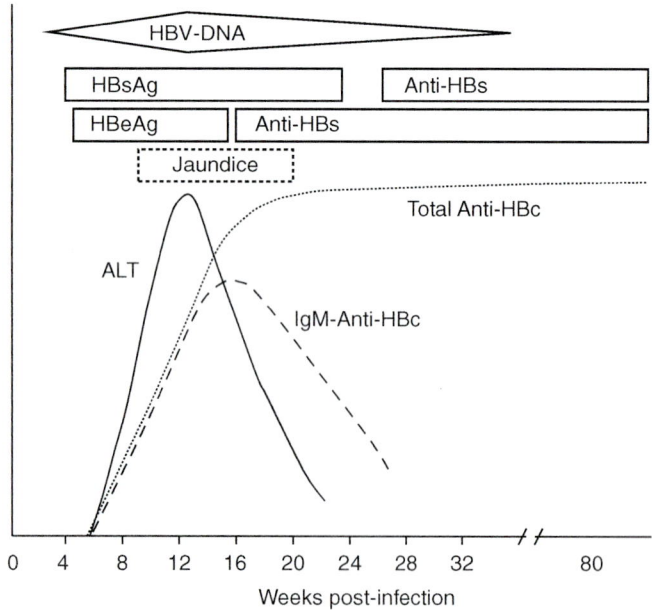

Fig. 3.5 Clinical course of acute hepatitis B with resolution. The mean incubation period for hepatitis B is 1–4 months

The clinical course of acute hepatitis C is shown in Figs. 3.7 and 3.8 [2, 16]. As mentioned above, acute hepatitis C most commonly becomes chronic and persistent. A diagnosis of acute hepatitis C is confirmed primarily by the presence of HCV RNA in the sera of a previously HCV-negative patient or seroconversion from anti-HCV antibody-negative to anti-HCV-positive [17]. Note that serum HCV RNA can be detected 1–3 weeks after exposure to HCV, whereas seroconversion may occur 4–10 weeks after exposure to HCV [18, 19].

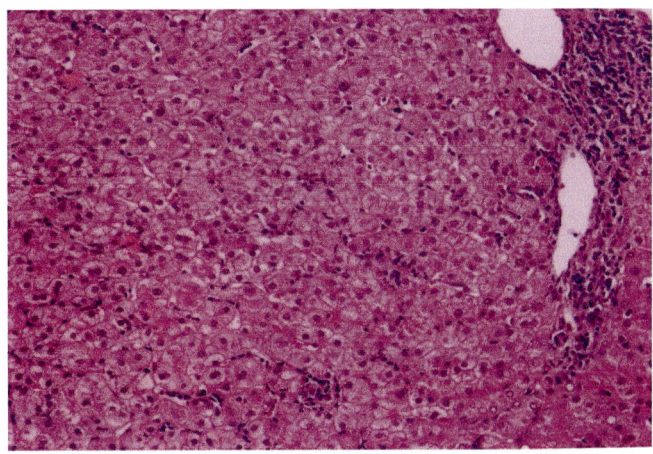

Fig. 3.9 Acute hepatitis C. Infiltration of the portal tract by inflammatory cells, along with scattered spotty necrosis and infiltration of the sinusoids by lymphocytes

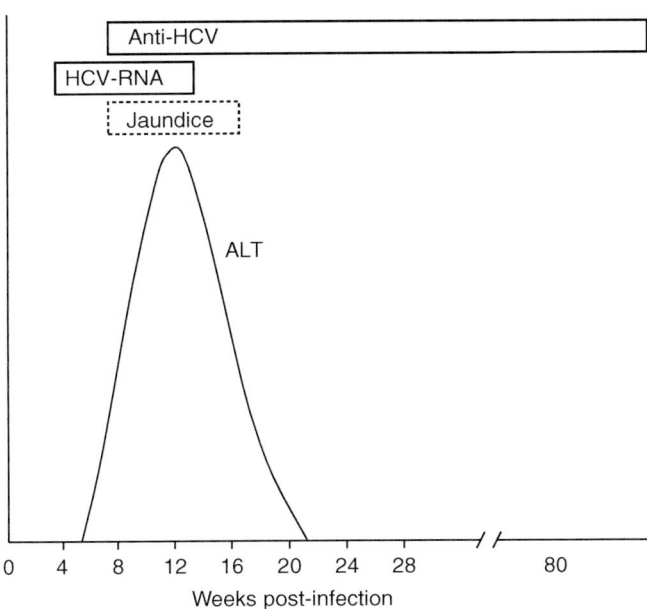

Fig. 3.7 Clinical course of acute hepatitis C with resolution

Histological features of infection by the hepatitis C virus are similar to those of acute hepatitis A and B, and infiltration of lymphocytes is distributed along the sinusoids in the absence of severe liver cell damage [20].

Case 3.4
Due to a fracture of the femoral bone, a 17-year-old female underwent surgery with blood transfusion. Ten weeks after transfusion, her liver function test showed ALT 260 IU/L and AST 150 IU/L. Liver biopsy 3 weeks after onset of hepatitis showed infiltration of lymphocytes in the portal tract and scattered spotty necrosis in a lobule. Lymphocytes infiltrated along the sinusoids (Fig. 3.9).

3.4 Hepatitis D Virus

Hepatitis D virus (HDV) infection is found only in coexistence with HBV infection: it is either HDV infection in an HBV carrier or coinfection with HBV and HDV as acute hepatitis. Both HDV antibody and HB antigen are positive. The chronicity rate after acute hepatitis is about 2–7%, and the fulminating rate is about 1–2%.

3.5 Hepatitis E Virus

Hepatitis E is caused by infection with hepatitis E virus (HEV) and usually develops into transient acute hepatitis. Acute hepatitis E causes epidemics in Asia and is found in Africa and North America. The incubation period is about 15–50 days. Clinical pictures are almost identical to those of acute hepatitis A, and clinical findings and symptoms regress within 2 or 3 weeks. Hepatitis E does not generally become chronic in patients with normal immunity; however, in the case of immunocompromised hosts, chronic hepatitis can develop due to HEV infection [21].

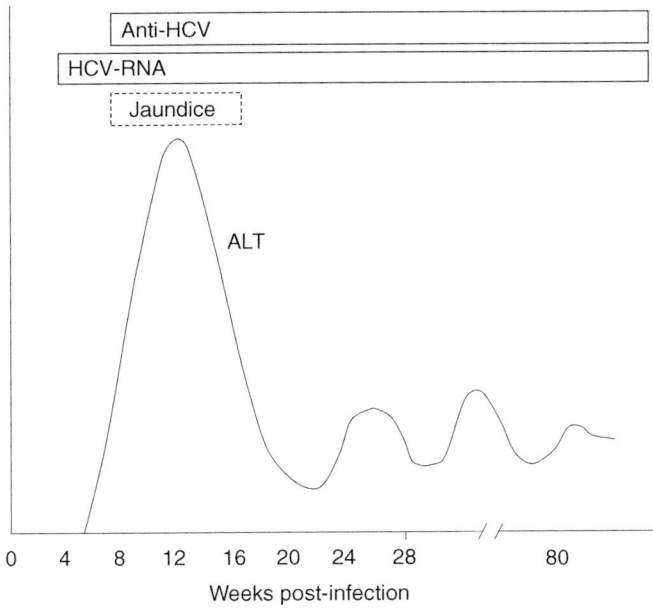

Fig. 3.8 Clinical course of acute hepatitis C with progression to chronicity

HEV is the sole member of the family *Hepeviridae* and includes four genotypes (genotypes 1–4) which cause hepatitis E [22]. Of these, genotype 1 and 2 HEVs infect only humans and are responsible for epidemic and sporadic hepatitis E due to fecal-oral infections in developing countries. On the other hand, genotype 3 and 4 HEVs are zoonotic viruses which are isolated from both humans and animals, such as pigs, wild boars, etc. Intake of undercooked contaminated meat causes sporadic hepatitis E [23]. Transfusion-borne hepatitis E is also increasingly recognized.

The typical course of acute hepatitis E is shown in Fig. 3.10. In individual cases, severe courses of acute hepatitis occur with transaminase values >2000 IU/L and a high value of total bilirubin [24], and fulminant hepatitis occurs in 2–3%. Pregnant women are susceptible, and mortality in the third trimester is high (10–25%) [25]. The histological appearance of the liver in HEV is similar to that of hepatitis A; cholestasis and portal or periportal inflammation can be observed [26]. For the diagnosis of acute hepatitis E, IgM anti-HEV antibody, IgA anti-HEV antibody, and/or HEV-RNA is used [27, 28]. IgM anti-HEV antibody and HEV-RNA are detected at onset and for a relatively short period. Since IgA anti-HEV antibody appears even after the recovery phase of hepatitis in addition to the acute phase, clinicians should try to detect HEV-RNA for the diagnosis of acute hepatitis E if IgA anti-HEV antibody is found in the early period of hepatitis. When acute hepatitis E is diagnosed, the genotype of HEV should also be determined. By assessing genotype of HEV, physicians can speculate as to the source of infection, infectious route, and possible prognosis of individual cases [29].

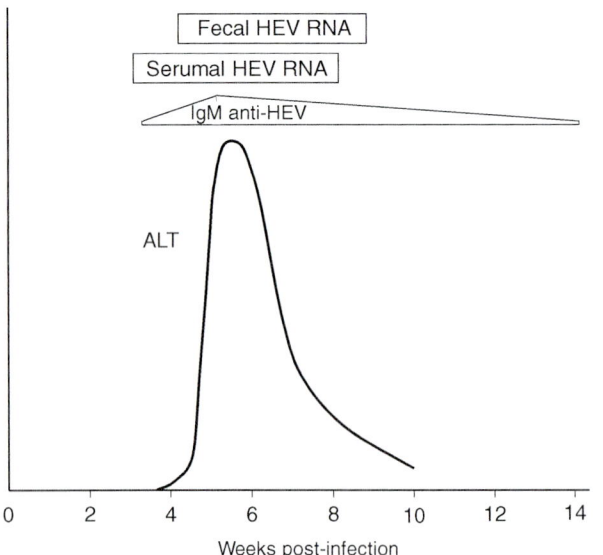

Fig. 3.10 Clinical course of acute hepatitis E. The incubation period is about 15–56 days

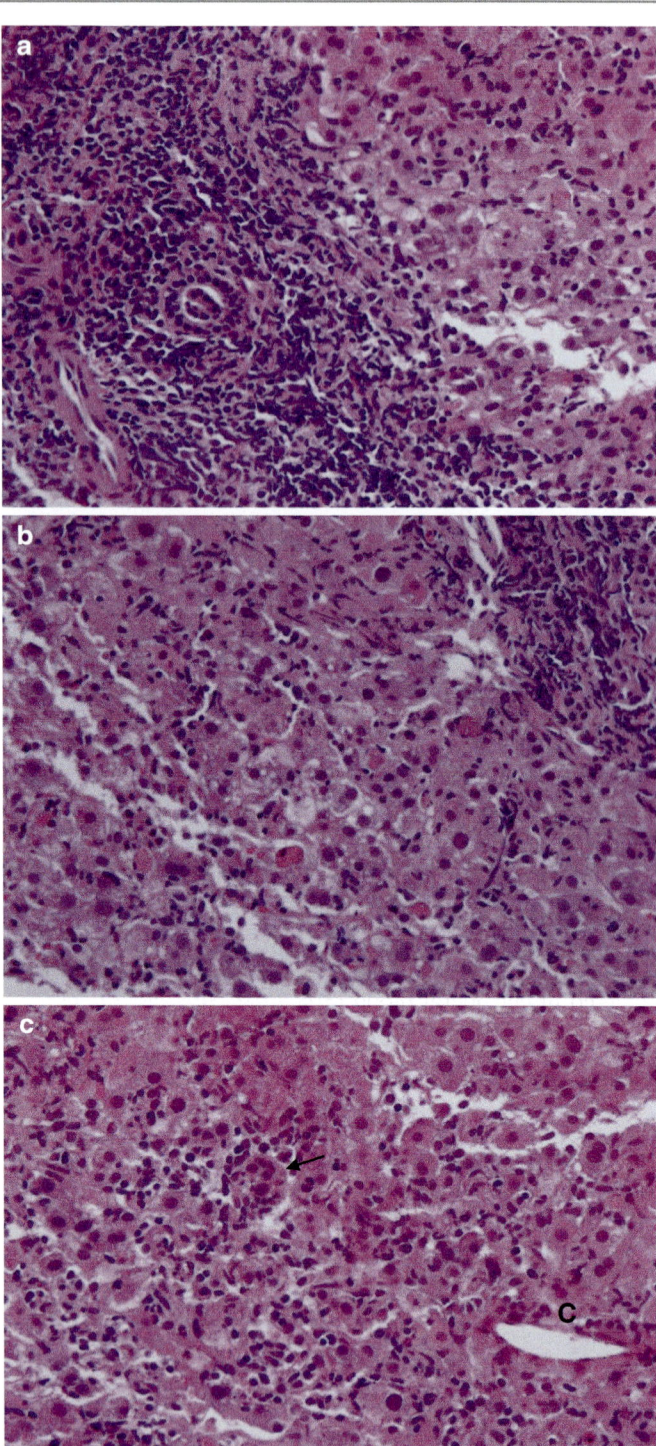

Fig. 3.11 Acute hepatitis E. (**a**) Lymphocytes, neutrophilic leukocytes, and plasma cells are infiltrated in the portal tract and periportal area. (**b**) Lobular architecture is disarrayed, vacuolated hepatocytes remain in the periportal area, and acidophilic bodies are seen. (**c**) There is focal necrosis, giant cells (arrow), and infiltration of many lymphocytes and neutrophilic leukocytes around phlebitis of the central vein. *C* central vein

Case 3.5

A 55-year-old Japanese male working in China complained of general malaise, icterus, and febrile sense. Acute hepatitis E was suspected. His liver chemistry in 2 weeks showed TBIL 9.7 mg/dL, AST 1227 IU/L, ALT 2003 IU/L, ALP 811 U/L, GGT 180 U/L, IgG 2012 mg/dL, IgM 261 mg/dL, PT 73.5%, and HEV-RNA positive. Liver biopsy showed disarray of lobular architecture and infiltration of many inflammatory cells in the portal tract and periportal area; acidophilic bodies or vacuolated hepatocytes were seen with infiltration of lymphocytes, neutrophilic leukocytes, and Kupffer cells in zone 1; and there were spotty necrosis, multinucleated cells, and many inflammatory cells around the central vein with phlebitis (Fig. 3.11). He gradually recovered from his liver disorder; the jaundice disappeared after 2 months, and his liver chemistry reverted to normal values after 3 months.

3.6 Hepatitis Associated with Epstein-Barr Virus

Epstein-Barr virus (EBV) is a DNA virus belonging to a member of the herpesvirus family and is transmitted through saliva. EBV infection is common among children in the tropics, and it is also seen in adolescents in developed countries. It causes infectious mononucleosis, which is a clinical syndrome. Pharyngeal pain, fever, splenomegaly, and lymph node swelling are present, and atypical lymphocytes are detected in peripheral blood [30]. Infectious mononucleosis is diagnosed by the early detection of IgM antibody against EBV viral-capsid antigen (EBV-VCA), and IgG antibody against EBV nuclear antigen (EBNA) is not detected (Fig. 3.12) [30]. There is hepatic involvement, but cholestasis is rare [31, 32], and fulminant hepatitis is infrequent [33]. The common histological feature of the liver in EBV infec-

tion is of a diffuse lymphocytic infiltrate in the sinusoids, and fatty change may occur [34]. At times, EBV infection causes virus-associated hemophagocytic syndrome [35].

Case 3.6

A 29-year-old female complained of persistent high fever and pharyngeal pain. Laboratory data showed TBIL 7.9 mg/dL, ALT 295 IU/L, AST 408 IU/L, LDH 1595 IU/L, ALP 4340 IU/L, WBC 26,700 with atypical lymphocytes, and VCA IgM positive. Liver biopsy 3 weeks after onset showed a cluster of inflammatory cells in the portal tract, and sinusoids were dilated and infiltrated with inflammatory cells; a magnified view of the portal tracts showed infiltration of lymphocytes, plasma cells, histiocytic cells, eosinophils, and neutrophilic leukocytes, while the bile ducts were infiltrated by lymphocytes, and the nuclei of cholangiocytes were vacuolated (Fig. 3.13).

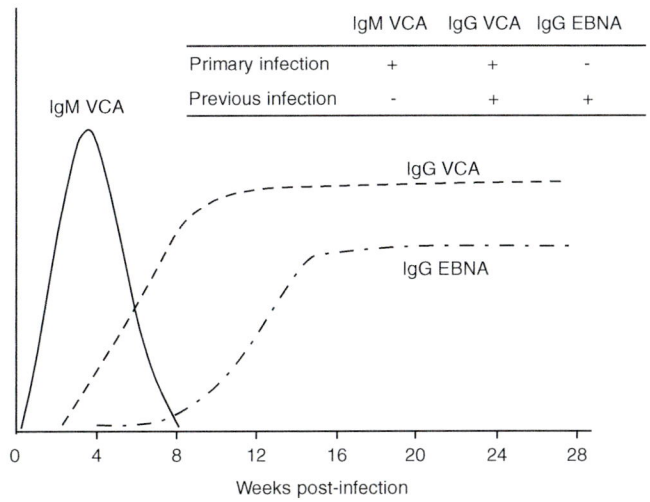

	IgM VCA	IgG VCA	IgG EBNA
Primary infection	+	+	-
Previous infection	-	+	+

Fig. 3.12 Sequence of antibody responses in infectious mononucleosis. *VCA* viral-capsid antigen. *EBNA* EBV nuclear antigen

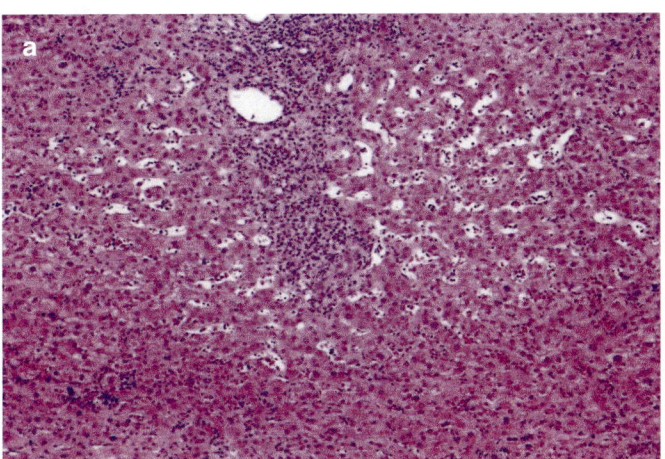

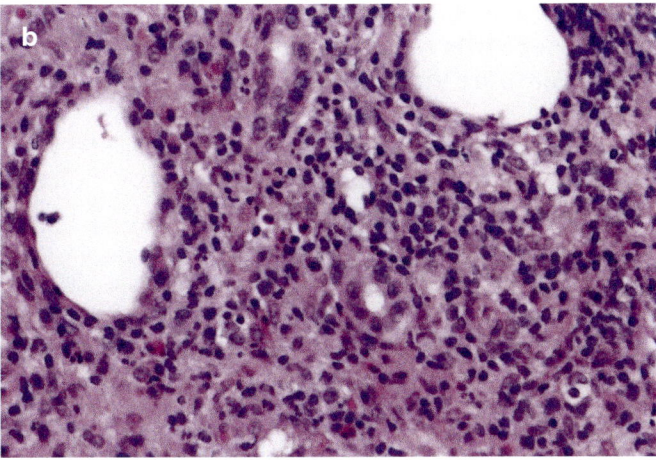

Fig. 3.13 Acute liver injury with Epstein-Barr virus. (**a**) Preserved lobular architecture with infiltration of the portal tract by numerous inflammatory cells and dilated sinusoids showing infiltration by mononuclear cells.

(**b**) Infiltration of the portal tract by lymphocytes, polymorphonuclear or eosinophilic leukocytes, and histiocytic cells surrounding the bile ducts, and the nuclei of cholangiocytes showing vacuolation

3.7 Hepatitis Associated with Cytomegalovirus (CMV)

CMV has broad organotropism and persistently infects multiple organs, such as the salivary glands and kidneys. It is excreted in breast milk, saliva, etc., and these become sources of infection. The frequency of infection of the liver is high. CMV infections include congenital CMV infection transmitted across the placenta; acquired infection transmitted via saliva, lactation, or blood; and opportunistic infection transmitted by organ transplantation [36, 37].

The most acquired infections with CMV among healthy subjects appear as occult infections, but occasionally infectious mononucleosis symptoms are seen [38, 39]. Fever, liver dysfunction, cervical lymphadenopathy, and hepatosplenomegaly are the main symptoms. Liver dysfunctions are usually mild, resolving in 2–3 weeks, and there is no chronicity, but there are reports of cholestatic jaundice and fulminant hepatitis. Opportunistic infections tend to cause systemic CMV infection and cause death.

The CMV antigenemia method for detecting CMV antigen and the PCR method for the detection of CMV DNA are suitable for diagnosis of CMV infection and determination of therapeutic effect. In C7HRP, one of the CMV antigenemia methods, the number of CMV antigen-positive cells in peripheral leukocytes is measured. IgM-CMV antibody detection is also used for acute infection with CMV [40, 41].

The histological findings for CMV hepatitis are similar to those for EBV hepatitis. Hepatocellular damage and necrosis are mild, but infiltration of mononuclear cells into sinusoids is conspicuous. Mononuclear cell infiltration into the portal region is moderate. Granulomatoid changes may also be observed. Opportunistic infections tend to result in extensive hepatocellular necrosis, but there are few immune cell reactions. Intranuclear inclusion in bile duct epithelia and hepatocytes is seen [42, 43].

3.8 Hepatitis Associated with Herpes Simplex Virus (HSV)

Herpes simplex virus (HSV) consists of HSV-1 and HSV-2. Originally, HSV-1 affects the oral mucosa, and HSV-2 affects the genitals. HSV hepatitis is caused by both HSV-1 and HSV-2. HSV infects newborns, HSV infection occurs frequently in children aged 1–3 years, and more than 80% of adults have HSV antibodies.

Systemic infections with HSV are rare in healthy adults but are seen in patients with opportunistic infection. It is reported that HSV hepatitis has a high mortality rate [44]. In HSV hepatitis, fever, mild jaundice, transaminase elevation, coagulation abnormalities, and thrombocytopenia are seen. Even when transaminase values are very elevated in the serum, values of bilirubin tract enzyme often show only mild elevation. If pyrogenic severe hepatitis with disseminated intravascular coagulation (DIC) is found, especially in immunocompromised individuals, consider HSV hepatitis. IgM-HSV is of diagnostic value for HSV hepatitis. Fulminant liver failure accompanied by DIC is often observed in HSV hepatitis: it is critical to make an early diagnosis for improvement of prognosis [45, 46]. Pathologically, HSV hepatitis presents random areas of coagulation necrosis of hepatocytes and bleeding of liver parenchyma. Inflammatory response is commonly weak. Ground-glass intranuclear inclusions are found.

As other viruses causing hepatitis, varicella zoster virus (VZV), adenovirus, measles virus, rubella virus, human parvovirus, paramyxovirus, coxsackie virus, ECHO virus, yellow fever virus, and others are described.

Acknowledgments Prof. Paul Y. Kwo was a coauthor of the first edition of this chapter.

References

1. Martin A, Lemon SM. Hepatitis A virus: from discovery to vaccines. Hepatology. 2006;43(S1):S164–72.
2. Kumar V, Abbas AK, Aster JC. Robbins basic pathology E-book. New York: Elsevier Health Sciences; 2017.
3. Feinstone SM, Kapikian AZ, Purceli RH. Hepatitis A: detection by immune electron microscopy of a viruslike antigen associated with acute illness. Science. 1973;182(4116):1026–8.
4. Abe H, et al. Light microscopic findings of liver biopsy specimens from patients with hepatitis type A and comparison with type B. Gastroenterology. 1982;82(5 Pt 1):938–47.
5. Teixeira MR, et al. The pathology of hepatitis A in man. Liver. 1982;2(1):53–60.
6. Watanabe M, et al. Hepatitis A virus infection associated with hemophagocytic syndrome: report of two cases. Intern Med. 2002;41(12):1188–92.
7. Yuen MF, Lai CL. Hepatitis B virus genotypes: natural history and implications for treatment. Expert Rev Gastroenterol Hepatol. 2007;1(2):321–8.
8. Kramvis A, Kew M, Francois G. Hepatitis B virus genotypes. Vaccine. 2005;23(19):2409–23.
9. Yu H, et al. Molecular and phylogenetic analyses suggest an additional hepatitis B virus genotype "I". PLoS One. 2010;5(2):e9297.
10. Tatematsu K, et al. A genetic variant of hepatitis B virus divergent from known human and ape genotypes isolated from a Japanese patient and provisionally assigned to new genotype J. J Virol. 2009;83(20):10538–47.
11. Jake LT. Hepatitis B: the virus and disease. Hepatology. 2009;49(S5):S13–21.
12. Atsushi O, et al. Influence of genotypes and precore mutations on fulminant or chronic outcome of acute hepatitis B virus infection. Hepatology. 2006;44(2):326–34.
13. De Francesco R. Molecular virology of the hepatitis C virus. J Hepatol. 1999;31:47–53.
14. Orland JR, Wright TL, Cooper S. Acute hepatitis C. Hepatology. 2001;33(2):321–7.
15. Blackard JT, et al. Acute hepatitis C virus infection: a chronic problem. Hepatology (Baltimore, MD). 2008;47(1):321–31.

16. Maheshwari A, Ray S, Thuluvath PJ. Acute hepatitis C. Lancet. 2008;372(9635):321–32.

17. Santantonio T, Wiegand J, Tilman Gerlach J. Acute hepatitis C: current status and remaining challenges. J Hepatol. 2008;49(4):625–33.

18. Mondelli MU, Cerino A, Cividini A. Acute hepatitis C: diagnosis and management. J Hepatol. 2005;42(Suppl 1):S108–14.

19. Jean-Michel P. Use and interpretation of virological tests for hepatitis C. Hepatology. 2002;36(5B):s65–73.

20. Bamber M, et al. Short incubation non-A, non-B hepatitis transmitted by factor VIII concentrates in patients with congenital coagulation disorders. Gut. 1981;22(10):854–9.

21. Kamar N, et al. Hepatitis E virus and chronic hepatitis in organ-transplant recipients. N Engl J Med. 2008;358(8):811–7.

22. Smith DB, et al. Consensus proposals for classification of the family Hepeviridae. J Gen Virol. 2014;95(Pt 10):2223–32.

23. Tei S, et al. Zoonotic transmission of hepatitis E virus from deer to human beings. Lancet. 2003;362(9381):371–3.

24. Rakesh A, Krzysztof K. Hepatitis E: an overview and recent advances in clinical and laboratory research. J Gastroenterol Hepatol. 2000;15(1):9–20.

25. Nanda SK, et al. Etiological role of hepatitis E virus in sporadic fulminant hepatitis. J Med Virol. 1994;42(2):133–7.

26. Dienes HP, et al. Hepatitis A-like non-A, non-B hepatitis: light and electron microscopic observations of three cases. Virchows Arch A Pathol Anat Histopathol. 1986;409(5):657–67.

27. Takahashi M, et al. Simultaneous detection of immunoglobulin A (IgA) and IgM antibodies against hepatitis E virus (HEV) is highly specific for diagnosis of acute HEV infection. J Clin Microbiol. 2005;43(1):49–56.

28. Davern TJ, et al. Acute hepatitis E infection accounts for some cases of suspected drug-induced liver injury. Gastroenterology. 2011;141(5):1665–72.e1-9.

29. Ankcorn MJ, Tedder RS. Hepatitis E: the current state of play. Transfus Med. 2017;27(2):84–95.

30. Luzuriaga K, Sullivan JL. Infectious mononucleosis. N Engl J Med. 2010;362(21):1993–2000.

31. Hinedi TB, Koff RS. Cholestatic hepatitis induced by Epstein-Barr virus infection in an adult. Dig Dis Sci. 2003;48(3):539–41.

32. Edoute Y, et al. Severe cholestatic jaundice induced by Epstein-Barr virus infection in the elderly. J Gastroenterol Hepatol. 1998;13(8):821–4.

33. Papatheodoridis GV, et al. Fulminant hepatitis due to Epstein-Barr virus infection. J Hepatol. 1995;23(3):348–50.

34. Purtilo DT, Sakamoto K. Epstein-Barr virus and human disease: immune responses determine the clinical and pathologic expression. Hum Pathol. 1981;12(8):677–9.

35. Ohshima K, et al. Clinicopathological findings of virus-associated hemophagocytic syndrome in bone marrow: association with Epstein-Barr virus and apoptosis. Pathol Int. 1999;49(6):533–40.

36. Marcelin JR, Beam E, Razonable RR. Cytomegalovirus infection in liver transplant recipients: updates on clinical management. World J Gastroenterol. 2014;20(31):10658–67.

37. Fowler KB, Boppana SB. Congenital cytomegalovirus infection. Semin Perinatol. 2018;42(3):149–54.

38. Cohen JI, Corey GR. Cytomegalovirus infection in the normal host. Medicine (Baltimore). 1985;64(2):100–14.

39. Evans AS. Infectious mononucleosis and related syndromes. Am J Med Sci. 1978;276(3):325–39.

40. Rowshani AT, et al. Clinical and immunologic aspects of cytomegalovirus infection in solid organ transplant recipients. Transplantation. 2005;79(4):381–6.

41. Revello MG, Gerna G. Diagnosis and management of human cytomegalovirus infection in the mother, fetus, and newborn infant. Clin Microbiol Rev. 2002;15(4):680–715.

42. Demetris AJ, et al. Pathology of hepatic transplantation: a review of 62 adult allograft recipients immunosuppressed with a cyclosporine/steroid regimen. Am J Pathol. 1985;118(1):151–61.

43. Colina F, et al. Histological diagnosis of cytomegalovirus hepatitis in liver allografts. J Clin Pathol. 1995;48(4):351–7.

44. Kaufman B, et al. Herpes simplex virus hepatitis: case report and review. Clin Infect Dis. 1997;24(3):334–8.

45. Norvell JP, et al. Herpes simplex virus hepatitis: an analysis of the published literature and institutional cases. Liver Transpl. 2007;13(10):1428–34.

46. Natu A, Iuppa G, Packer CD. Herpes simplex virus hepatitis: a presentation of multi-institutional cases to promote early diagnosis and management of the disease. Case Rep Hepatol. 2017;2017:3180984.

Acute Liver Failure

4

Seiichi Mawatari, Yoshinori Harada, Masaki Iwai,
Paul Y. Kwo, and Akio Ido

Contents

Abbreviations

ALF	Acute liver failure
EGF	Epidermal growth factor
HAV	Hepatitis A virus
HBV	Hepatitis B virus
HEV	Hepatitis E virus
HGF	Hepatocyte growth factor
HVP	High-volume plasmapheresis
IL	Interleukin
MARS	Molecular adsorbent recirculating system
OLT	Orthotopic liver transplantation
TGF-α	Transforming growth factor α
TNF	Tumor necrosis factor

S. Mawatari, MD, PhD · A. Ido, MD, PhD (✉)
Kagoshima, Japan
e-mail: ido-akio@m2.kufm.kagoshima-u.ac.jp

Y. Harada, MD, PhD
Kyoto, Japan

M. Iwai, MD, PhD
Kyoto, Japan

P. Y. Kwo, MD
California, USA

4.1 General Consideration and Classification

Acute liver failure (ALF) is defined as severe liver dysfunction characterized by an elevated prothrombin time with encephalopathy occurring within 8 weeks after onset of the first symptom without a history of chronic liver disease. The first symptom develops as jaundice [1]. Depending on the interval between jaundice and encephalopathy, liver failure can be classified into hyperacute, acute, and subacute types. The patient outcome is reported to be different in all three [2]. Hyperacute type develops encephalopathy within 7 days of onset, and the spontaneous survival rate is 80–90%. Common etiologies of hyperacute type are hepatitis A, acetaminophen overdose, and ischemia. Acute type indicates a jaundice-to-encephalopathy interval of 7–28 days, and the spontaneous survival rate is 50–60%. In subacute type, the interval from onset to encephalopathy ranges from 28 days to 2–3 months [3, 4], and the prognosis is worse than in hyperacute and acute type: the spontaneous survival rate is 15–20%. Acute or subacute type may be caused by viral hepatitis, drugs, herbal therapies, autoimmune hepatitis, hypoperfusion or ischemia, inherited diseases, malignant

© Springer Nature Singapore Pte Ltd. 2019
E. Hashimoto et al. (eds.), *Diagnosis of Liver Disease*, https://doi.org/10.1007/978-981-13-6806-6_4

Table 4.1 Etiologic factors in fulminant hepatic failure [6]

Viral	Hepatitis A, B, D, C, and E, CMV, HSV, EBV, VZV, HHV 6, parvovirus B19, parainfluenza, yellow fever, etc.
Toxic dose-dependent	Acetaminophen (paracetamol), *Amanita phalloides*, isoniazid, tetracycline, methotrexate, carbon tetrachloride, amphetamine
Idiosyncratic	Coumarins, carbamazepine, valproic acid, chinolones, halogenated hydrocarbons, methyldopa, phenytoin, rifampicin, penicillin, sulfonamides, etc.
Toxic synergistic	Ethanol + acetaminophen, barbiturate + acetaminophen, isoniazid + rifampicin
Metabolic	Wilson's disease, alpha-1 antitrypsin deficiency, galactosemia, tyrosinemia, Reye's syndrome, nonalcoholic steatohepatitis
Associated with pregnancy	Acute fatty liver of pregnancy, HELLP syndrome
Vascular	Budd-Chiari syndrome, veno-occlusive disease, shock, heart failure
Miscellaneous	Autoimmune hepatitis, malignant infiltration, sepsis, hyperthermia

infiltration of the liver, and mitochondrial defects in the liver [5]. The underlying causes of ALF are shown in Table 4.1 [6].

4.2 Pathogenesis of ALF and Regeneration Failure

ALF is characterized by a massive cell death and the suppression of the regenerative capacity of the liver [7]. Immune dysregulation leads to the large production of inflammatory cytokines such as TNF-α, IL-1, and IL-6. Apoptosis can be triggered by activating death receptors such as Fas and tumor necrosis factor (TNF) receptor, which are activated by inflammatory cytokines [8]. Oxidative stress of mitochondria and endoplasmic reticulum induces apoptosis [8]. Additionally, activation of Kupffer cells by intestinal-derived endotoxin causes local hypercoagulability [9], resulting in hepatocellular death. As viral factors that cause poor prognosis, 5′ non-translated region (5′NTR) of the HAV genome [10], pre-core or core promoter mutation in HBV [11], and genotype 4 in HEV [12] have been assumed.

Liver regeneration failure is caused when hepatocyte death exceeds hepatocyte proliferation or when hepatocyte proliferation itself is suppressed or insufficient. Generally TNF-α and IL-6 contribute to the initiation of the cell cycle (G0 to G1) by binding to their receptors [13]. Several growth factors such as hepatocyte growth factor (HGF), epidermal growth factor (EGF), and transforming growth factor α (TGF-α) are thought to initiate the G1 to S transition [14, 15]. These factors stimulate DNA replication and mitosis by binding to their corresponding receptors [14]. In the patients with fulminant hepatitis, HGF and TGF-α level in serum are elevated [16, 17]. It is considered to be a biological reaction trying to regenerate liver against extensive liver cell death. In fulminant hepatitis, receptors for growth factors on hepatocytes and subsequent signal transduction change, and as a result, liver regeneration is impaired [18, 19].

On the other hand, expression of strong inhibitors of hepatocyte proliferation such as TGF-β and IL-1β is also enhanced [20, 21]. In acute liver failure, proliferation of not only mature hepatocytes but also progenitor cells called oval cells is observed. Wnt/Notch signal is related to control of this cell [22]. In liver regeneration deficiency, liver stem cells and progenitor cells are suspected to have maturation and differentiation disorders, but details are unknown.

4.3 Symptoms

Symptoms of ALF are similar to those of acute hepatitis: general malaise, appetite loss, and jaundice. However, the severity of symptoms varies. Symptoms of acute hepatitis are improved after the onset of jaundice; however, patients with ALF worsen after the onset of jaundice. Severe general malaise and vomiting develop, and encephalopathy and coma are noted.

4.4 Hepatic Encephalopathy

The mechanism of hepatic encephalopathy in ALF has not been fully elucidated. Hyperammonemia is considered a fatal factor related to cerebral edema and hernia development [23, 24]. Alpha-ketoglutarate dehydrogenase is inhibited by ammonia, resulting in inhibition of tricarboxylic cycle, suppression of glucose metabolism, accumulation of lactic acid, reduction of adenosine triphosphate biosynthesis, and swelling of astrocytes [25].

Encephalopathy is classified into four grades [26]. The prognosis in ALF depends on the extent to which encephalopathy develops. Patients with grade 3 or 4 encephalopathy are at risk of developing cerebral edema and multiple organ failure [26, 27]. ALF occurs with complications of infection, hepatorenal syndrome, gastrointestinal hemorrhage, and disseminated intravascular coagulation. Infection is a common complication of ALF, and bacterial and fungal infections should be carefully watched for in the beginning.

4.5 Clinical Findings

The serum value of AST and ALT is generally >3000 IU/mL. As acute liver atrophy progresses, ascites and jaundice develop, ammonia in the serum is elevated, albumin is reduced, prothrombin time is prolonged, and triphasic waves are seen in electroencephalography.

4.6 Treatment

The most important prognostic indicators for predicting the outcome in ALF are the etiology of the disorder, the degree of encephalopathy, and the patient's age. Orthotopic liver transplantation (OLT) is the most effective treatment for patients with ALF, in addition to conservative medical management treating specific causes and supporting multiple organ system failure [27]. The European Liver and Intestine Transplant Association database showed 1-, 5- and 10-year patient and graft survival rates were 74%, 68%, and 63% and 63%, 57%, and 50%, respectively [28]. It follows that patients with ALF should be promptly referred to transplant centers for the management of variable medical conditions. The determination for OLT depends on the probability of hepatic recovery, which is difficult to predict [29]. A commonly used method for selecting potential candidates for OLT is the King's College Hospital criteria (Table 4.2) [6, 29]. However, OLT is not universally available, has shortage in the cadaveric donor, and has the risk of coercion, complication and death in the living donor. Less than 10% of liver transplantations are performed in patients with acute liver failure [7, 28].

There are some liver assist therapies, which aim to compensate liver synthesis and detoxification and to maintain the body metabolic environment until the liver obtains sufficient regeneration or liver transplantation. However, none of the therapies compensates efficiently all of these functions. Two randomized controlled studies about liver assist therapies have reported in ALF. Molecular adsorbent recirculating system (MARS) is one of the liver assist therapies, which allows albumin-bound toxins to be removed [30]. A multicenter, randomized, controlled study about MARS in ALF showed no survival benefit, but 75% of enrolled patients had been

undergoing liver transplantation within 24 h [31]. High-flow dialysate continuous hemodiafiltration had higher recovery late of encephalopathy than non-high-flow group; however, there was no difference about survival rate between high-flow and non-high-flow groups [32].

High-volume plasmapheresis (HVP) is also one of the therapies. In a recent study, HVP has been shown to significantly improve hospital survival, especially for patients with contraindications for liver transplantation [33]. However, the incidence of severe adverse events was similar in the control group [33].

Liver regeneration medicine is a field expected to be clinically applied to acute liver failure. Induced pluripotent stem cells (iPSc), mesenchymal stem cells (MSC), hepatic progenitor cells (HPC), human amniotic epithelial cells (hAEC), fibroblasts, and so on are potential alternative cell sources which can be used to generate hepatocytes [34]. In addition, among the potential therapies, anti-apoptotic or cell protective drugs are expected to become clinically available. Emricasan, a pan-caspase inhibitor [35]; ALF-5755, recombinanthepatocarcinoma-intestine-pancreas/pancreatitis-associated protein [36]; and recombinant human hepatocyte growth factor (rh-HGF) [37] are candidates that are currently being investigated in clinical trials.

4.7 Case Presentation

4.7.1 HBV carrier with Crohn's disease

A 29-year-old male complained of high fever, nausea, and general malaise 2 months after ileocecal resection and ileocolostomy for perforation of the ileum due to Crohn's disease. Liver chemistries showed TBIL 17.0 mg/dL, ALT 5400 IU/L, AST 5000 IU/L, PT 54%, and HBsAg and HBeAg positive. The high fever persisted, and he died of hepatic failure within 1 week. Necropsy showed massive necrosis with hemorrhage in the lobules, reticulin fibers were diffusely distributed, and bile ductular proliferation was observed around the portal tract; few viable hepatocytes were noted, and infiltration of polymorphonuclear leukocytes, small lymphocytes, and macrophage were seen around the portal tract with ductular proliferation or "oval cells" (Fig. 4.1). In another case, most hepatocytes were lost, hemorrhage was detected, and sinusoids were dilated although viable ductular structures remained (Fig. 4.2).

4.7.2 Anti-pyretic drug-induced liver injury

An 18-year-old girl with anorexia nervosa had taken a combination of drugs in a suicide attempt and was referred to our hospital several hours after stomach lavage. Liver tests 2 days after drug intake showed ALT 7162 IU/L, AST 6388 IU/L, and TBIL 3.54 mg/dL, and PT was unmeasur-

Table 4.2 King's College Hospital criteria for liver transplantation in fulminant hepatic failure [6, 29]

Acetaminophen	Arterial pH < 7.30 (irrespective of grade of encephalopathy) *OR* Prothrombin time > 100 s and serum creatinine > 300 μmol/L in patients with grade 3 or 4 encephalopathy
Nonacetaminophen patients	Prothrombin time > 100 s (irrespective of grade of encephalopathy) *OR* Any three of the following variables (irrespective of grade of encephalopathy):
	• Age < 10 years or >40 years
	• Etiology: non-A, non-B hepatitis, halothane hepatitis, idiosyncratic drug reactions
	• Duration of jaundice before onset of encephalopathy > 7 days
	• Prothrombin time > 50 s
	• Serum bilirubin > 300 μmol/L

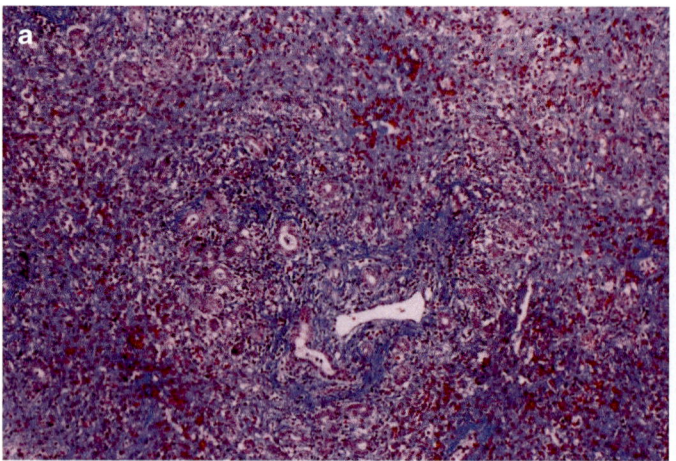

Fig. 4.1 Fulminant hepatitis. (**a**) Submassive necrosis of hepatocytes and collapse of the normal architecture with fine fibrosis are seen. Scattered hemorrhage and ductular proliferation are observed around the portal tracts. (**b**) Bile ductular structures are seen around the portal tracts, and matured bile ducts are absent. Lymphocytes and polymorphonuclear leukocytes infiltrate in the portal tracts with ductular proliferation

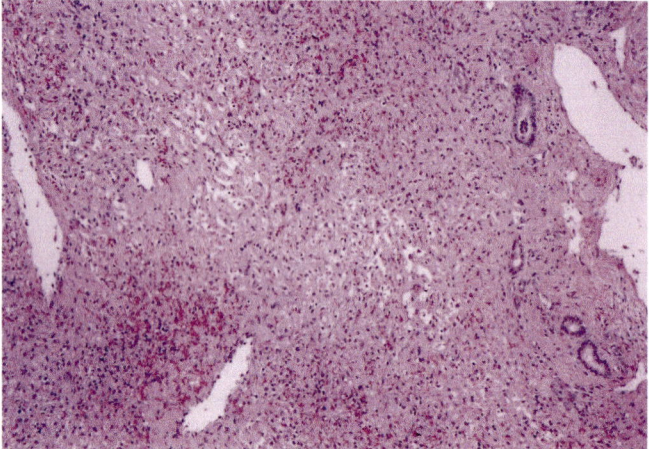

Fig. 4.2 Fulminant hepatitis. Most hepatocytes are absent, and dilatation of sinusoids and hemorrhage are seen, while bile ducts remain in the portal tracts

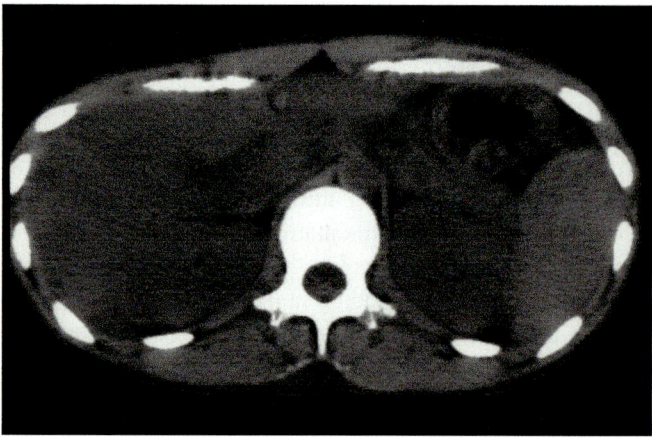

Fig. 4.3 CT in fulminant hepatitis due to toxic injury. CT without intravenous contrast medium shows heterogeneous density in the liver

able. She became comatose within 5 days and was scheduled for liver transplantation from a living donor. CT scan without contrast showed low or heterogeneous density in the liver (Fig. 4.3). The hepatectomized liver showed hemorrhagic necrosis around the central veins, pseudoglandular formations of immatured hepatocytes around the portal tracts, and infiltration of eosinophilic leukocytes, lymphocytes, plasma cells, and histiocytes in the portal tract (Fig. 4.4). Roxonin was positive on the drug lymphocyte stimulation test.

4.7.3 Autoimmune hepatitis

A 43-year-old female complained of general malaise and dark urine. Her liver function test showed AST 1015 IU/mL and ALT 925 IU/mL. One month later, her TBIL reached 26 mg/dL, and massive ascites were present. CT and ultrasonography demonstrated atrophic liver with nodular surface, and hepatic encephalopathy developed. Liver biopsy after onset of symptoms showed periportal necrosis and extensive cell loss with infiltration of neutrophilic leukocytes and small lymphocytes, as well as proliferation of bile ductules and rosette formations with abundant macrophages (Fig. 4.5a). The international autoimmune hepatitis score [38] was beyond that of the definite type, and the patient survived after plasma exchange and glucocorticoid administration. A second biopsy 4 months later demonstrated hepatic plates 2 or more cells thick, forming regenerative nodules consistent with cirrhosis, and stroma or inflammatory cells were decreased in number (Fig. 4.5b).

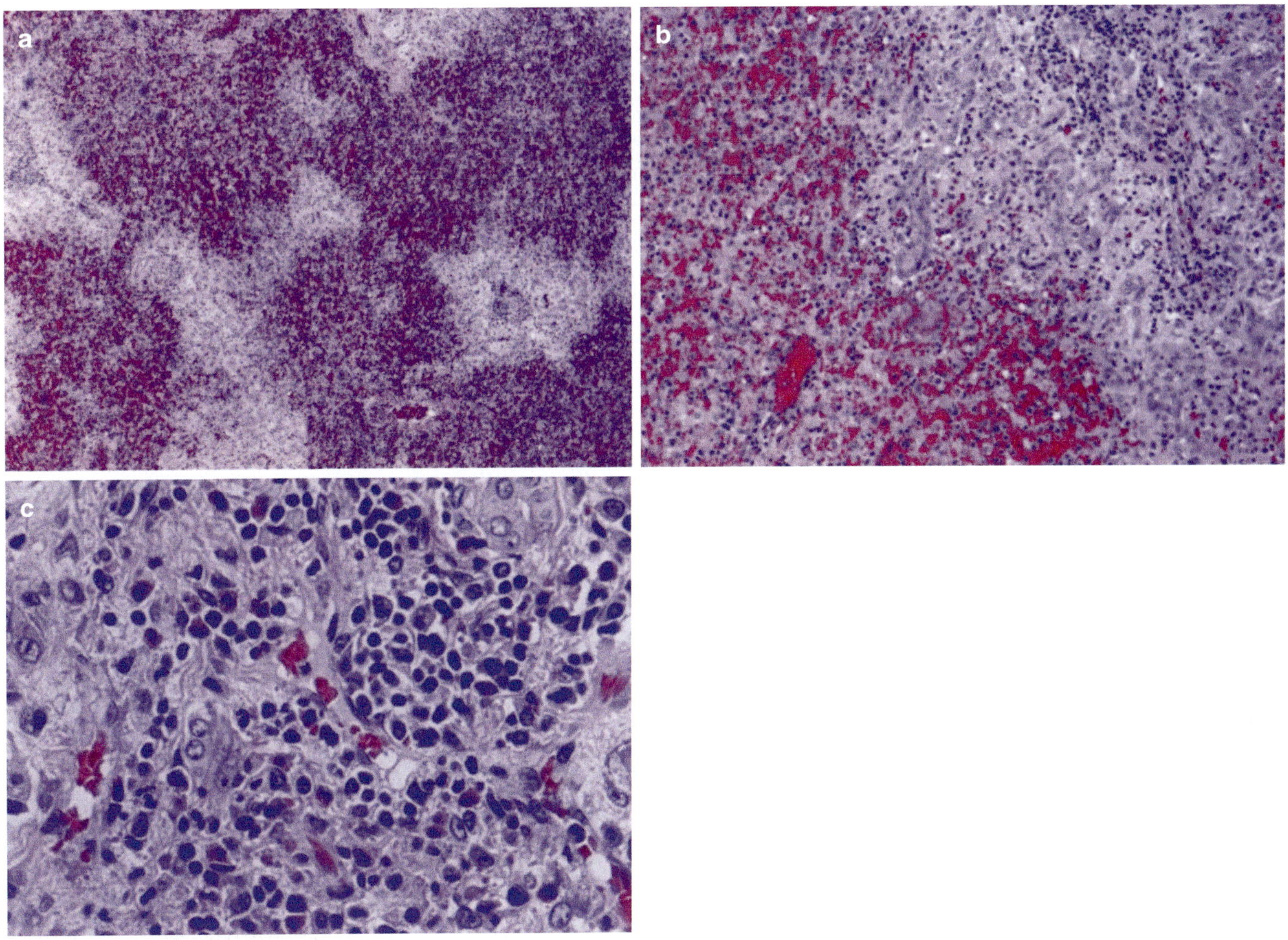

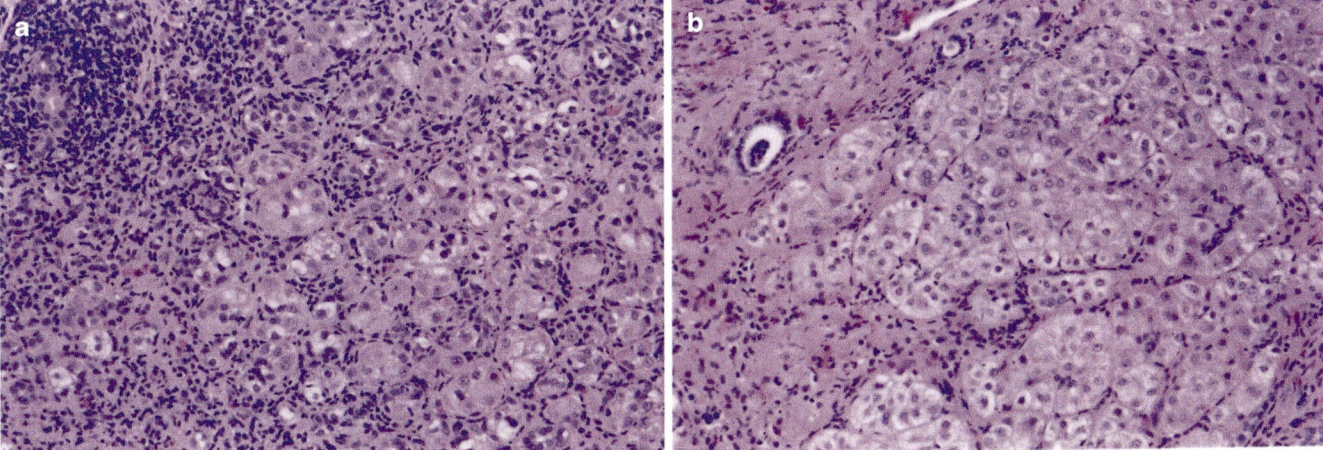

Fig. 4.4 Drug-induced liver injury. (**a**) Massive hemorrhagic necrosis is observed around the central veins. (**b**) Massive hemorrhagic necrosis is seen around the central vein, and the pseudoglandular structure of immature cells is noted around the portal tract as the liver attempts to regenerate. (**c**) The portal tract is infiltrated by eosinophilic leukocytes, plasma cells, and lymphocytes, and immature cells form pseudoglandular structures

Fig. 4.5 Severe liver injury in autoimmune hepatitis. (**a**) Many inflammatory cells and damaged cholangioles are seen in the portal tract. Residual hepatocytes show ballooning and rosette formations, which are surrounded by lymphocytes, plasma cells, and Kupffer cells. (**b**) Inflammatory cells are decreased after glucocorticoid therapy. Hepatocytes form plates that are two or three cells thick, and their cytoplasm becomes clear

References

1. Trey C, Davidson CS. The management of fulminant hepatic failure. Prog Liver Dis. 1970;3:282–98.
2. Stravitz RT. Critical management decisions in patients with acute liver failure. Chest. 2008;134:1092–102.
3. Bernuau J, Rueff B, Benhamou JP. Fulminant and subfulminant liver failure: definitions and causes. Semin Liver Dis. 1986;6:97–106.
4. Lee WM. Acute liver failure. N Engl J Med. 1993;329:1862–72.
5. Polson J, Lee WM. AASLD position paper: the management of acute liver failure. Hepatology. 2005;41:1179–97.
6. Gotthardt D, Riediger C, Weiss KH, Encke J, Schemmer P, Schmidt J, et al. Fulminant hepatic failure: etiology and indications for liver transplantation. Nephrol Dial Transplant. 2007;22(Suppl 8):viii5–8.
7. Bernal W, Wendon J. Acute liver failure. N Engl J Med. 2013;369:2525–34.
8. Kaplowitz N. Mechanisms of liver cell injury. J Hepatol. 2000;32:39–47.
9. Mochida S, Arai M, Ohno A, Yamanobe F, Ishikawa K, Matsui A, et al. Deranged blood coagulation equilibrium as a factor of massive liver necrosis following endotoxin administration in partially hepatectomized rats. Hepatology. 1999;29:1532–40.
10. Fujiwara K, Yokosuka O, Ehata T, Saisho H, Saotome N, Suzuki K, et al. Association between severity of type A hepatitis and nucleotide variations in the 5′ non-translated region of hepatitis A virus RNA: strains from fulminant hepatitis have fewer nucleotide substitutions. Gut. 2002;51:82–8.
11. Omata M, Ehata T, Yokosuka O, Hosoda K, Ohto M. Mutations in the precore region of hepatitis B virus DNA in patients with fulminant and severe hepatitis. N Engl J Med. 1991;324:1699–704.
12. Inoue J, Nishizawa T, Takahashi M, Aikawa T, Mizuo H, Suzuki K, et al. Analysis of the full-length genome of genotype 4 hepatitis E virus isolates from patients with fulminant or acute self-limited hepatitis E. J Med Virol. 2006;78:476–84.
13. Yamada Y, Kirillova I, Peschon JJ, Fausto N. Initiation of liver growth by tumor necrosis factor: deficient liver regeneration in mice lacking type I tumor necrosis factor receptor. Proc Natl Acad Sci. 1997;94:1441–6.
14. Michalopoulos GK, DeFrances MC. Liver regeneration. Science. 1997;276:60–6.
15. Pediaditakis P, Lopez-Talavera JC, Petersen B, Monga SP, Michalopoulos GK. The processing and utilization of hepatocyte growth factor/scatter factor following partial hepatectomy in the rat. Hepatology. 2001;34:688–93.
16. Tsubouchi H, Niitani Y, Hirono S, Nakayama H, Gohda E, Arakaki N, et al. Levels of the human hepatocyte growth factor in serum of patients with various liver diseases determined by an enzyme-linked immunosorbent assay. Hepatology. 1991;13:1–5.
17. Tomiya T, Fujiwara K. Liver regeneration in fulminant hepatitis as evaluated by serum transforming growth factor alpha levels. Hepatology. 1996;23:253–7.
18. Huh CG, Factor VM, Sanchez A, Uchida K, Conner EA, Thorgeirsson SS. Hepatocyte growth factor/c-met signaling pathway is required for efficient liver regeneration and repair. Proc Natl Acad Sci U S A. 2004;101:4477–82.
19. Nakamura K, Nonaka H, Saito H, Tanaka M, Miyajima A. Hepatocyte proliferation and tissue remodeling is impaired after liver injury in oncostatin M receptor knockout mice. Hepatology. 2004;39:635–44.
20. Miwa Y, Harrison PM, Farzaneh F, Langley PG, Williams R, Hughes RD. Plasma levels and hepatic mRNA expression of transforming growth factor-beta1 in patients with fulminant hepatic failure. J Hepatol. 1997;27:780–8.
21. Ogiso T, Nagaki M, Takai S, Tsukada Y, Mukai T, Kimura K, et al. Granulocyte colony-stimulating factor impairs liver regeneration in mice through the up-regulation of interleukin-1beta. J Hepatol. 2007;47:816–25.
22. Boulter L, Govaere O, Bird TG, Radulescu S, Ramachandran P, Pellicoro A, et al. Macrophage-derived Wnt opposes Notch signaling to specify hepatic progenitor cell fate in chronic liver disease. Nat Med. 2012;18:572–9.
23. Bernal W, Hall C, Karvellas CJ, Auzinger G, Sizer E, Wendon J. Arterial ammonia and clinical risk factors for encephalopathy and intracranial hypertension in acute liver failure. Hepatology. 2007;46:1844–52.
24. Clemmesen JO, Larsen FS, Kondrup J, Hansen BA, Ott P. Cerebral herniation in patients with acute liver failure is correlated with arterial ammonia concentration. Hepatology. 1999;29:648–53.
25. Haussinger D, Kircheis G, Fischer R, Schliess F, vom Dahl S. Hepatic encephalopathy in chronic liver disease: a clinical manifestation of astrocyte swelling and low-grade cerebral edema? J Hepatol. 2000;32:1035–8.
26. Caraceni P, Van Thiel DH. Acute liver failure. Lancet. 1995;345:163–9.
27. Munoz SJ, Robinson M, Northrup B, Bell R, Moritz M, Jarrell B, et al. Elevated intracranial pressure and computed tomography of the brain in fulminant hepatocellular failure. Hepatology. 1991;13:209–12.
28. Germani G, Theocharidou E, Adam R, Karam V, Wendon J, O'Grady J, et al. Liver transplantation for acute liver failure in Europe: outcomes over 20 years from the ELTR database. J Hepatol. 2012;57:288–96.
29. Cochran JB, Losek JD. Acute liver failure in children. Pediatr Emerg Care. 2007;23:129–35.
30. Stange J, Mitzner SR, Risler T, Erley CM, Lauchart W, Goehl H, et al. Molecular adsorbent recycling system (MARS): clinical results of a new membrane-based blood purification system for bioartificial liver support. Artif Organs. 1999;23:319–30.
31. Saliba F, Camus C, Durand F, Mathurin P, Letierce A, Delafosse B, et al. Albumin dialysis with a noncell artificial liver support device in patients with acute liver failure: a randomized, controlled trial. Ann Intern Med. 2013;159:522–31.
32. Yokoi T, Oda S, Shiga H, Matsuda K, Sadahiro T, Nakamura M, et al. Efficacy of high-flow dialysate continuous hemodiafiltration in the treatment of fulminant hepatic failure. Transfus Apher Sci. 2009;40:61–70.
33. Larsen FS, Schmidt LE, Bernsmeier C, Rasmussen A, Isoniemi H, Patel VC, et al. High-volume plasma exchange in patients with acute liver failure: an open randomised controlled trial. J Hepatol. 2016;64:69–78.
34. Lee CA. Hepatocyte transplantation and advancements in alternative cell sources for liver-based regenerative medicine. J Mol Med. 2018;96(6):469–81.
35. Baskin-Bey ES, Washburn K, Feng S, Oltersdorf T, Shapiro D, Huyghe M, et al. Clinical trial of the Pan-Caspase inhibitor, IDN-6556, in human liver preservation injury. Am J Transplant. 2007;7:218–25.
36. Nalpas B, Ichai P, Jamot L, Carbonell N, Rudler M, Mathurin P, et al. A proof of concept, phase II randomized European trial, on the efficacy of ALF-5755, a novel extracellular matrix-targeted antioxidant in patients with acute liver diseases. PLoS One. 2016;11:e0150733.
37. Ido A, Moriuchi A, Numata M, Murayama T, Teramukai S, Marusawa H, et al. Safety and pharmacokinetics of recombinant human hepatocyte growth factor (rh-HGF) in patients with fulminant hepatitis: a phase I/II clinical trial, following preclinical studies to ensure safety. J Transl Med. 2011;9:55.
38. Alvarez F, Berg PA, Bianchi FB, Bianchi L, Burroughs AK, Cancado EL, et al. International Autoimmune Hepatitis Group Report: review of criteria for diagnosis of autoimmune hepatitis. J Hepatol. 1999;31:929–38.

Chronic Hepatitis

5

Paul Y. Kwo and Nimy John

Contents

Abbreviations

AIH   Autoimmune hepatitis
ALT   Alanine aminotransferase
APRI   AST-to-platelet ratio index
DAAs   Direct-acting antiviral agents
DNA   Deoxyribonucleic acid
HBcAg   Hepatitis B core antigen
HBsAg   Hepatitis B surface antigen
HBV   Hepatitis B virus
HCC   Hepatocellular carcinoma
HCV   Hepatitis C virus
HDV   Hepatitis D virus
HIV   Human immunodeficiency virus
RNA   Ribonucleic acid
SVR   Sustained viral response

Chronic viral hepatitis is defined as persistent inflammation of the liver in an identifiable hepatotropic viral (most commonly hepatitis B or C virus) infection persisting for

P. Y. Kwo, MD (✉) · N. John, MD
California, USA
e-mail: pkwo@stanford.edu

6 months or longer after acute infection [1]. Patients with chronic viral hepatitis may be asymptomatic or may complain of general fatigue, mild right hypochondoralgia, loss of appetite, nausea, and weakness. Many patients are diagnosed as having chronic viral hepatitis during routine physical with biochemical examination revealing abnormal liver chemistries, typically mild elevation of serum aminotransferases. Occasionally, patients may have flares or exacerbation of necroinflammatory activity in the liver, particularly with hepatitis B [2]. Less common causes of chronic viral hepatitis include hepatitis B/D coinfection and rarely chronic hepatitis E in immunosuppressed patients [3, 4].

The recent advances in noninvasive tests in the management of patients with chronic viral hepatitis—including elastography, radiologic studies, and serologic markers for fibrosis—have reduced the immediate need for liver biopsy, though an assessment of fibrosis is essential as those with advanced fibrosis and viral hepatitis are at high risk for complications from portal hypertension as well as hepatocellular cancer. Elastography is a method of assessing liver stiffness as a surrogate for liver fibrosis that uses longitudinal sound waves (transient elastography) or acoustic radiation forces [5, 6]. Elastography may also be determined by magnetic resonance. Imaging of the liver may also reveal a cirrhotic liver with an enlarged portal vein diameter, nodular liver, and splenomegaly which may be seen on ultrasound, CT scan with contrast, or MR with contrast.

© Springer Nature Singapore Pte Ltd. 2019
E. Hashimoto et al. (eds.), *Diagnosis of Liver Disease*, https://doi.org/10.1007/978-981-13-6806-6_5

Clinicians may also use any number of serum tests to assess fibrosis such as AST to platelet ratio index (APRI) or FIB-4 index using commonly available laboratory tests including AST, ALT, and platelet count. Finally, a number of commercial assays are also available worldwide to assess fibrosis.

However, despite all of these advances, liver biopsy is still considered the gold standard by many physicians in guiding the treatment of patients with chronic viral hepatitis, particularly in patients with chronic hepatitis B. In addition to providing staging and grading of chronic viral hepatitis, liver biopsy can furnish histologic information that is not availed by other tests. This is often the case in patients with comorbidities such as fatty liver, alcoholic, and iron storage diseases. Screening for hepatocellular carcinoma (HCC) may lead to fine needle aspiration or core biopsy of suspicious space-occupying lesions, especially lesions with atypical enhancement patterns that are suspicious for hepatocellular carcinoma as a late complication of chronic viral hepatitis that do not meet standard radiologic criteria for hepatocellular cancer. Depending on the underlying disease, the risks of HCC development may vary considerably. For example, chronic hepatitis B virus (HBV) is associated with the development of HCC in both cirrhotic and non-cirrhotic livers, whereas HCC rarely occurs in non-cirrhotic hepatitis C virus (HCV) infection. Therapy nucleoside analogues (and much less commonly interferon) have been shown to be most effective in suppressing HBV DNA levels, preventing fibrosis and reducing the risk of HCC [7, 8]. Direct-acting antiviral agents (DAAs) have replaced the combination of interferon with ribavirin as the standard therapy for chronic hepatitis C with high rates of cure (>95%) with minimal side effects [9].

Peritoneoscopy of a patient with chronic hepatitis generally shows an irregular surface of the tan-white liver, with or without red markings (Fig. 5.1). In general, chronic hepatitis

is characterized by a combination of portal inflammation, interface hepatitis (previously referred to as piecemeal necrosis or periportal hepatitis), and mild lobular inflammation with scattered necroinflammatory foci. After years of continuous inflammation, fibrosis and cirrhosis may eventually develop.

Portal inflammation consists of lymphocytic infiltrate with a variable number of plasma cells. A mild degree of ductular reaction can be seen at the periphery of the portal tracts, which represents hepatic progenitor cell activation and correlates with the degree of interface hepatitis and fibrosis. Interface hepatitis is a common feature in chronic viral hepatitis, consisting of lymphocytic infiltrate at the limiting plate with associated necrosis or apoptosis of the periportal hepatocytes. This process results in the destruction of the periportal parenchyma, its replacement by fibrous tissue, stellate enlargement of the portal tracts, and portal-to-portal fibrous septum formation. The degree of interface hepatitis varies according to the activity of the disease; it is often focal or absent in mild disease activity. Focal ballooning degeneration of the periportal hepatocytes can be seen in severe interface hepatitis. Lobular inflammation in chronic viral hepatitis is typically variable in severity and spotty in distribution. Lymphocytes cluster around injured or apoptotic hepatocytes. In areas of hepatocyte necrosis, Kupffer cells may contain phagocytosed cellular debris. Lobular disarray, cholestasis, significant regeneration, and ballooning degeneration of the hepatocytes—similar to those seen in acute viral hepatitis—are uncommon in chronic viral hepatitis, unless there is severe exacerbation or injury due to other etiologies.

These histological features described above are not specific to chronic viral hepatitis; they are shared with other chronic liver diseases, most commonly autoimmune hepatitis (AIH), and drug-induced liver injury.

5.1 Hepatitis B Virus

Nearly 240 million people all over the world are chronic HBV surface antigen (HBsAg) carriers, with a large regional variation of HBsAg positive [10]. Chronic hepatitis B is characterized by various degrees of portal chronic inflammation, interface hepatitis, and lobular inflammation. The most distinctive histological feature of chronic hepatitis B is the presence of "ground-glass" hepatocytes (Fig. 5.2), which represents distended smooth endoplasmic reticulum containing abundant hepatitis B surface antigen (HBsAg). Ground-glass hepatocytes are seen in chronic hepatitis only and usually in biopsies that show minimal necroinflammatory activity and represent a marked increase of smooth endoplasmic reticulum which contains filamentous and spherical HBsAg particles. The accumulation of hepatitis B core antigen (HBcAg) within the hepatocyte nuclei produces the sanded nucleus appearance. Intrahepatic HBcAg positivity may correlate with a higher degree of necroinflammatory activity [11].

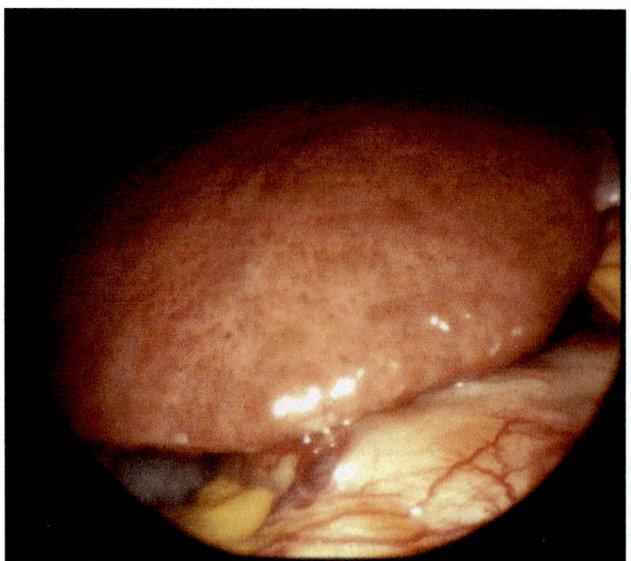

Fig. 5.1 Peritoneoscopic findings of liver with chronic hepatitis. Peritoneoscopy shows tan-white liver with red markings on the surface

The distribution of both HBV core and surface antigens and the subcellular localization of HBsAg in liver biopsy of patients with chronic hepatitis B and cirrhosis can be examined using immunohistochemistry and ultrastructural immunoperoxidase techniques. The distribution patterns of HBsAg in hepatocytes are membranous, cytoplasmic, festoon, and inclusion body types (Fig. 5.3). Both cytoplasmic and festoon types are seen more frequently than the membranous type. Extensive membranous staining for HBsAg is usually parallel to the staining of core antigen and associated with high viral replication. HBcAg is found predominantly in the nucleus and less prominently in the cytoplasm of hepatocytes, and electron microscopy shows clusters of HBV particles in the nucleus (Fig. 5.4). HBcAg immunoreactivity is detected in HBsAg-positive hepatocytes, and the staining pattern of HBsAg is the festoon and cytoplasmic type (Fig. 5.5). The inclusion body pattern of HBsAg is characteristic of liver cirrhosis with HCC, which suggests active syn-

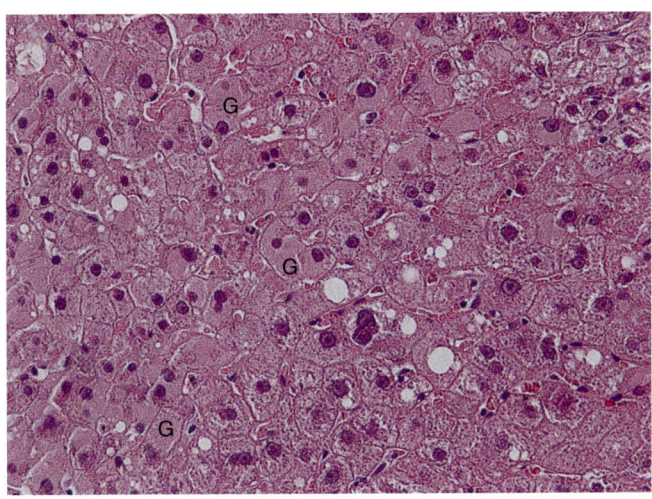

Fig. 5.2 Ground-glass hepatocytes (G) in chronic hepatitis B. Finely granular pink inclusions are identified in hepatocytes. Many ground-glass hepatocytes show a pale-staining halo in the cytoplasm

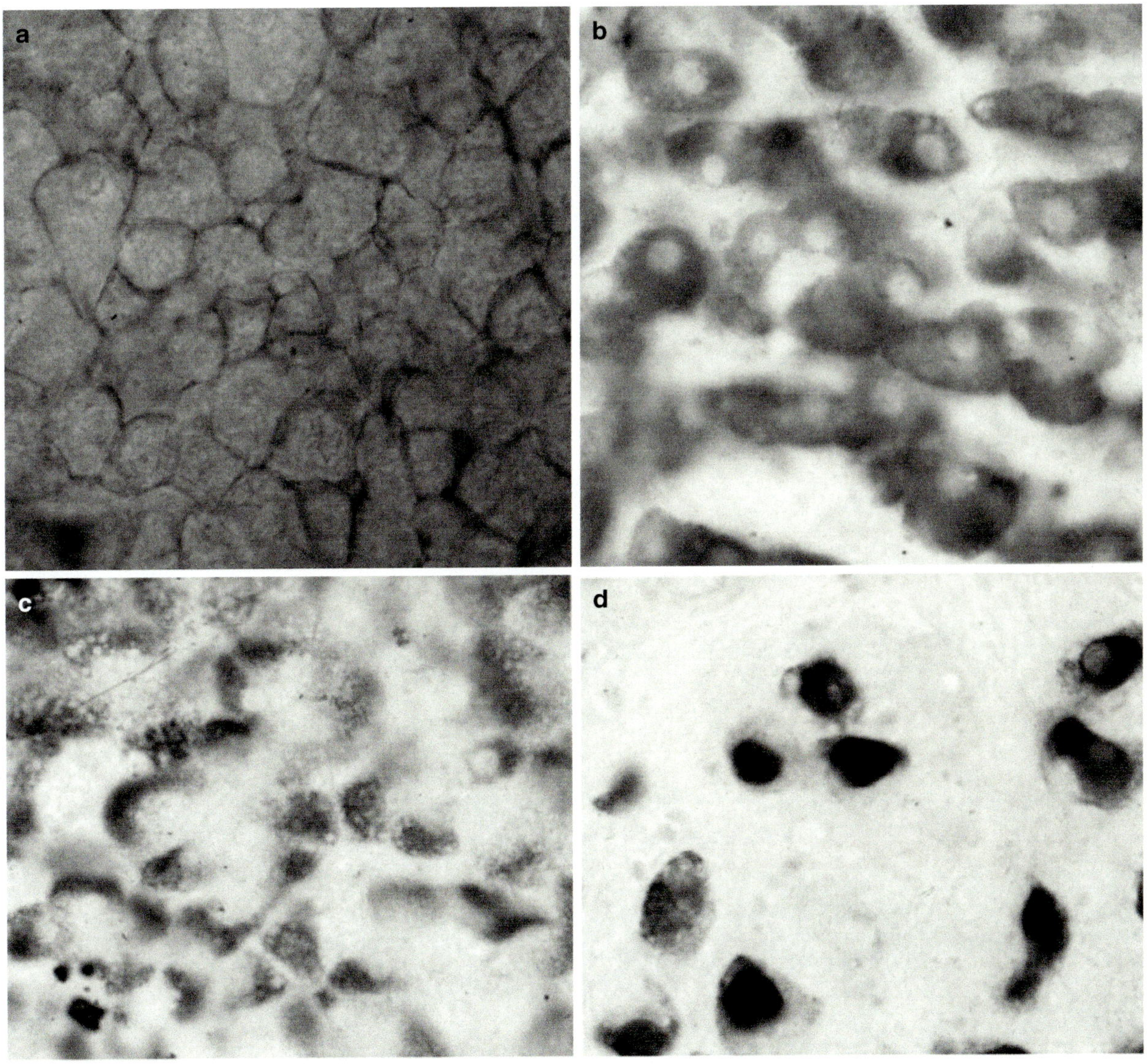

Fig. 5.3 HBsAg staining patterns. HBsAg localization reveals the membranous (**a**), cytoplasmic (**b**), festoon (**c**), and inclusion type (**d**)

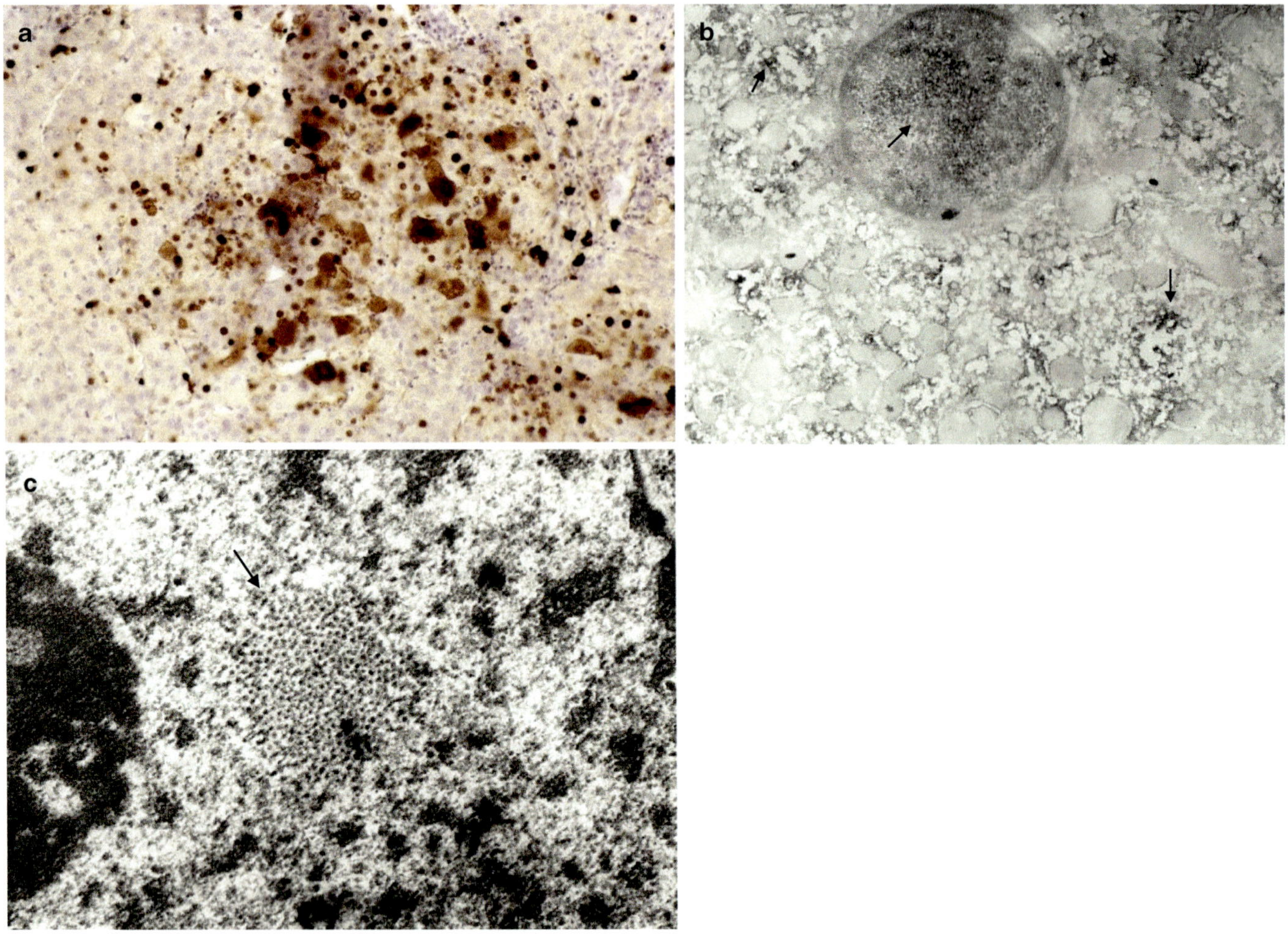

Fig. 5.4 HBcAg. (**a**) HBcAg immunoreactivity is seen not only in the nucleus of hepatocytes but also in the cytoplasm. (**b**) Immunoelectron microscopy shows the presence of HBcAg (arrow) in the nucleus and cytoplasm. (**c**) Electron microscopy shows a cluster of hepatitis B virus particles (arrow) in the nucleus

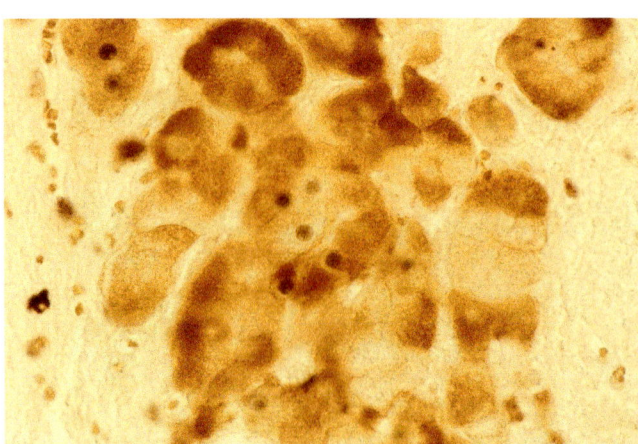

Fig. 5.5 Co-localization of HBsAg and HBcAg. Double staining shows the presence of HBcAg (purple) in the nucleus or cytoplasm of hepatocytes with cytoplasmic and festoon type of HBsAg (brown)

thesis of HBsAg in chronic hepatitis or cirrhosis, and that HBV is retained in the liver with HCC.

Hepatitis B treatments depend on E antigen status, extent of liver injury, HBV DNA level, and ALT level. For HBeAg-positive patients with elevated ALT (ALT more than twice the upper limit), the HBV threshold of treatment is 20,000 IU/L, and for HBeAg-negative patients with elevated ALT, HBV threshold of treatment is 2000 IU/L. In addition, AASLD suggests antiviral therapies to reduce the risk of perinatal transmission of hepatitis B in HBsAg-positive women with an HBV level >200,000 IU/mL. Approved agents for hepatitis B therapies include tenofovir disoproxil, tenofovir alafenamide, entecavir, telbivudine, adefovir, and lamivudine [2, 12, 13]. Interferon may also be given for a finite duration with lower rates of viral suppression but, in general, higher rates of HBeAg clearance and HBsAg clearance.

Hepatitis D virus (HDV, delta agent) superinfection requires HBsAg, and this phenomenon can be demonstrated using immunohistochemical stains. The clue to HDV infection is severe necroinflammatory activity in patients with HBV; therefore, HDV infection should be suspected in all patients with hepatitis B who develop severe exacerbation of disease activity or who have a severe clinical course. Diagnosis is confirmed via positivity for anti-HDV in a patient seropositive for HBsAg and/or quantitative/qualitative testing for serum HDV RNA. There are no approved therapies for hepatitis D though interferon has been used.

Fibrosing cholestatic hepatitis, an atypical form of chronic hepatitis B infection, may be encountered in patients with HIV infection or in immunosuppressed states, such as post-liver transplantation [14]. It is caused by the direct cytopathic effect of hepatitis B, seen in the high levels of HBV replication and massive HBcAg expression in the liver. The histological features include marked ductular reaction at the limiting plate, combined with cholangiolitis and extensive periportal sinusoidal fibrosis. With the advent of nucleoside/nucleotide analogues, fibrosing cholestatic hepatitis is readily treated.

5.2 Hepatitis C Virus

The total global HCV prevalence is estimated at 2.5% with an approximate 70 million of HCV RNA positive cases [15]. There are six main genotypes of hepatitis C; genotype 1b is the most common genotype worldwide followed by genotype 3 [16].

Most cases of chronic hepatitis C tend to show mild necroinflammatory activity on biopsies. The portal tract is infiltrated by dense aggregates of lymphocytes with follicle formation; the intralobular bile ducts are often found within the lymphocytic infiltrate and disrupted; and mild macro vesicular steatosis can be seen in the lobule, particularly in periportal hepatocytes (Fig. 5.6) [17, 18]. The lobular necroinflammatory activity is commonly represented by scattered acidophilic or apoptotic bodies in the lobules.

Steatosis in chronic hepatitis C can occur in the periportal or centrilobular region or both. Although steatosis tends to occur in hepatitis C genotype 3b infection [12], excessive centrilobular steatosis in genotype 3 or other genotypes may suggest concurrent steatohepatitis. Hepatitis C genotype 3

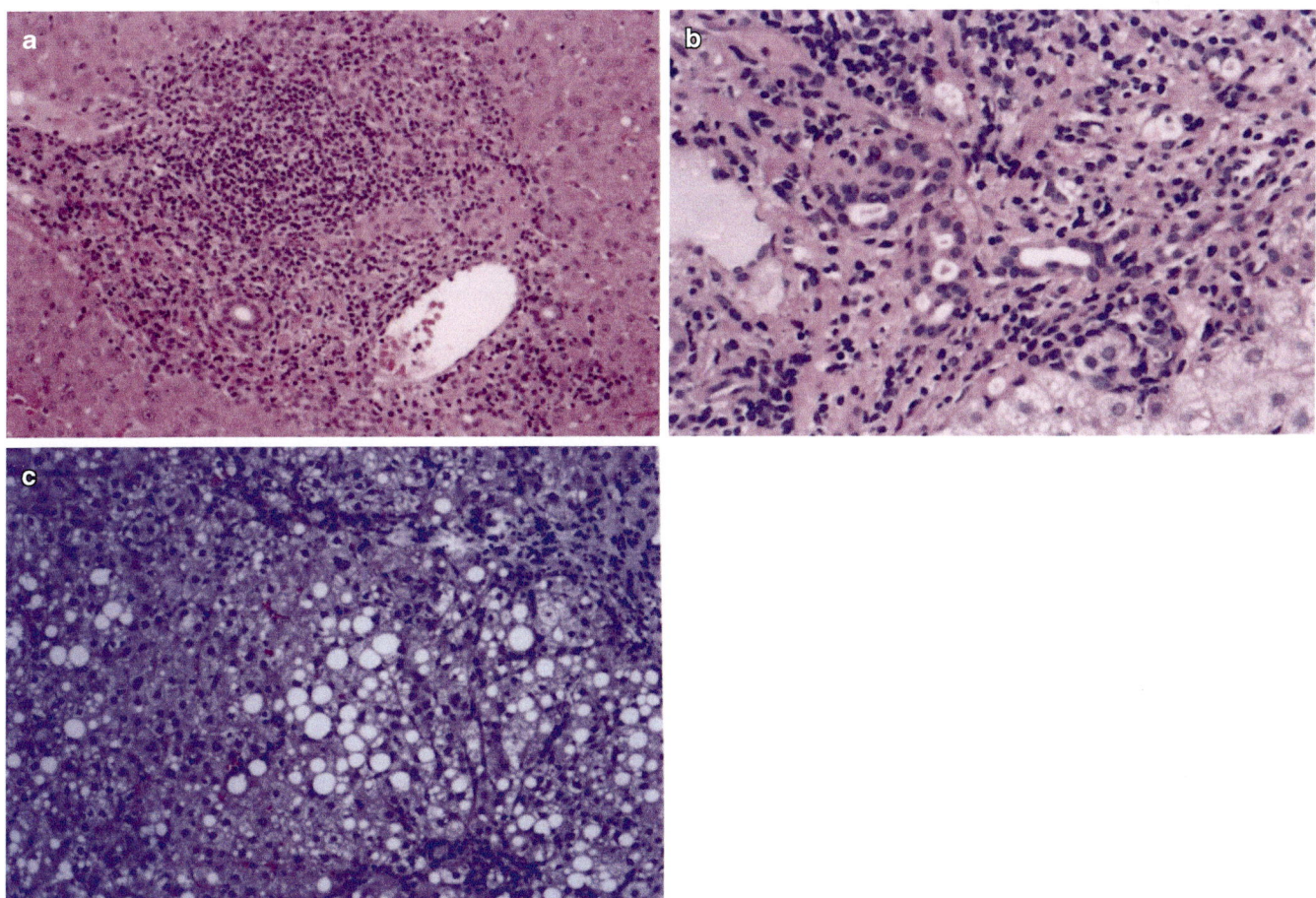

Fig. 5.6 Histological features of chronic hepatitis C. (**a**) The formation of lymphoid follicles is observed in the portal tract. (**b**) Bile duct damage is seen in the portal tract. (**c**) Steatosis is seen around the portal tract

also has the most aggressive natural history (fibrosis progression as well as HCC risk) [19].

Treatment for hepatitis C is recommended for all patients with chronic HCV infection, except those with short life expectancies owing to comorbid conditions. Agents currently used for hepatitis C treatment include ribavirin and direct-acting antiviral agents (DAAs) [20, 21]. The treatment regimen is selected based on the genotype, extent of liver damage, and response to previous treatment. There are multiple DAAs available for treatment. These agents belong to multiple classes and are combined to achieve high rates of cure: NS3 protease inhibitors, NS5A replication complex inhibitors, and NS5B polymerase inhibitors (sofosbuvir). DAAs have been proved very effective in multiple trials achieving a sustained viral response (SVR) or cure of greater than 95% of infected individuals even in genotype 3.

Hepatitis C may induce autoantibody formation, including antinuclear and anti-LKM type 1, but the titers are low. Clinically, these patients still resemble patients with chronic hepatitis C and not AIH. The presence of severe activity and a significant number of plasma cells—in the area of interface hepatitis in a liver biopsy specimen of a patient with chronic hepatitis C—suggest concurrent autoimmune features that are induced either by the HCV infection or by the interferon treatment. The overlap syndrome of AIH and chronic hepatitis C implies the coexistence of AIH with high titer of autoantibodies and high IgG level and detectable HCV RNA [22]. The diagnosis of AIH alone should not be rendered to patients who are known to harbor the virus, as corticosteroid therapy will enhance viral replication and disease progression. In the era of DAA therapy, it is now straightforward to treat hepatitis C patients with DAAs first to see if liver chemistries normalize and, if they do not, address the potential AIH.

In chronic hepatitis C, the rate of progression to cirrhosis correlates with serum HCV RNA levels, high-grade necroinflammatory activity, and advanced stage at initial biopsies [23, 24]. Other factors that may influence disease progression include viral genotype, sex, age, alcohol consumption, and iron overload. Genotype 3 is harder to treat in the era of DAAs though SVR rates still are excellent. Male and older individuals are more likely to show progressive fibrosis. Alcohol consumption increases viral replication and severity of disease. Iron overload may reduce the response to antiviral therapy.

Late complications of chronic hepatitis C infection include diabetes, cirrhosis with or without decompensation, lymphoma, hepatocellular cancer (HCC), and less commonly intrahepatic cholangiocarcinoma [25].

5.3 Hepatitis E Virus

There are 20 million HEV infections estimated worldwide, further leading to an estimated 3.3 million symptomatic cases of hepatitis E [26]. Hepatitis E is usually considered as a self-limiting illness lasting 1–3 months with spontaneous resolution. However, recent studies suggested that there is virus retention in posttransplant immunocompromised patients. HEV genotypes 3 and 4 can lead to chronic infection in transplant recipients and immunosuppressed subjects. Worsening of liver function, liver cirrhosis, and decompensation due to chronic HEV infection can occur as early as 2 years after infection with hepatitis E [27]. A 3-month course of ribavirin is recommended as treatment if an immunocompromised patient fails to clear the virus in 3 months after detection. If the patient has a detectable viral load after 3 months of ribavirin, a 6-month course of ribavirin is given. Pegylated interferon for 3 months has been used if ribavirin therapy fails.

5.4 Combined Viral Infection

Hepatitis B and C or hepatitis B/C and HIV coinfection is not uncommon due to shared modes of transmission [28]. In hepatitis B and C coinfection, the features of hepatitis C often predominate. If co-replication occurs, the disease is more likely to be severe and show faster progression of fibrosis.

HIV coinfection negatively impacts on the natural history of acute and chronic viral hepatitis, thereby increasing the risk of chronicity and progressive liver disease [29]. In addition, drug-induced liver injury related to antiretroviral therapy complicates the treatment of both diseases and should be considered in "exacerbation" or atypical presentation of chronic viral hepatitis. Treatment for coinfected patients is similar to monoinfected patients; drug-drug interactions must be accounted for, particularly with HIV/HCV coinfection with similar high rates of efficacy.

5.5 Non-viral Causes of Chronic Hepatitis

In most cases, chronic hepatitis is caused by hepatitis viruses B, C, and B/D; rare isolated cases are caused by non-hepatitis viruses (Epstein-Barr virus and cytomegalovirus), bacterial infection, and parasitic infestation [30–32]. Steatohepatitis due to metabolic syndrome is likely the most common form of non-viral chronic hepatitis worldwide [33]. Toxic substances such as alcohol, drugs, and chemicals also cause chronic hepatitis. Genetic and metabolic etiologies are relatively rare but should be taken into account. Chronic hepatic autoimmunopathies including AIH, primary biliary cirrhosis, primary sclerosing cholangitis, and overlap syndrome are more frequent than has hitherto been assumed.

AIH is reported to be due to disturbance of the immune system. Immunologically, it is classified into two types, of which type 1—with antinuclear antibody or anti-smooth muscle antibody-positive sera—is most frequent in AIH [34]. All AIH types are treated with administration of pred-

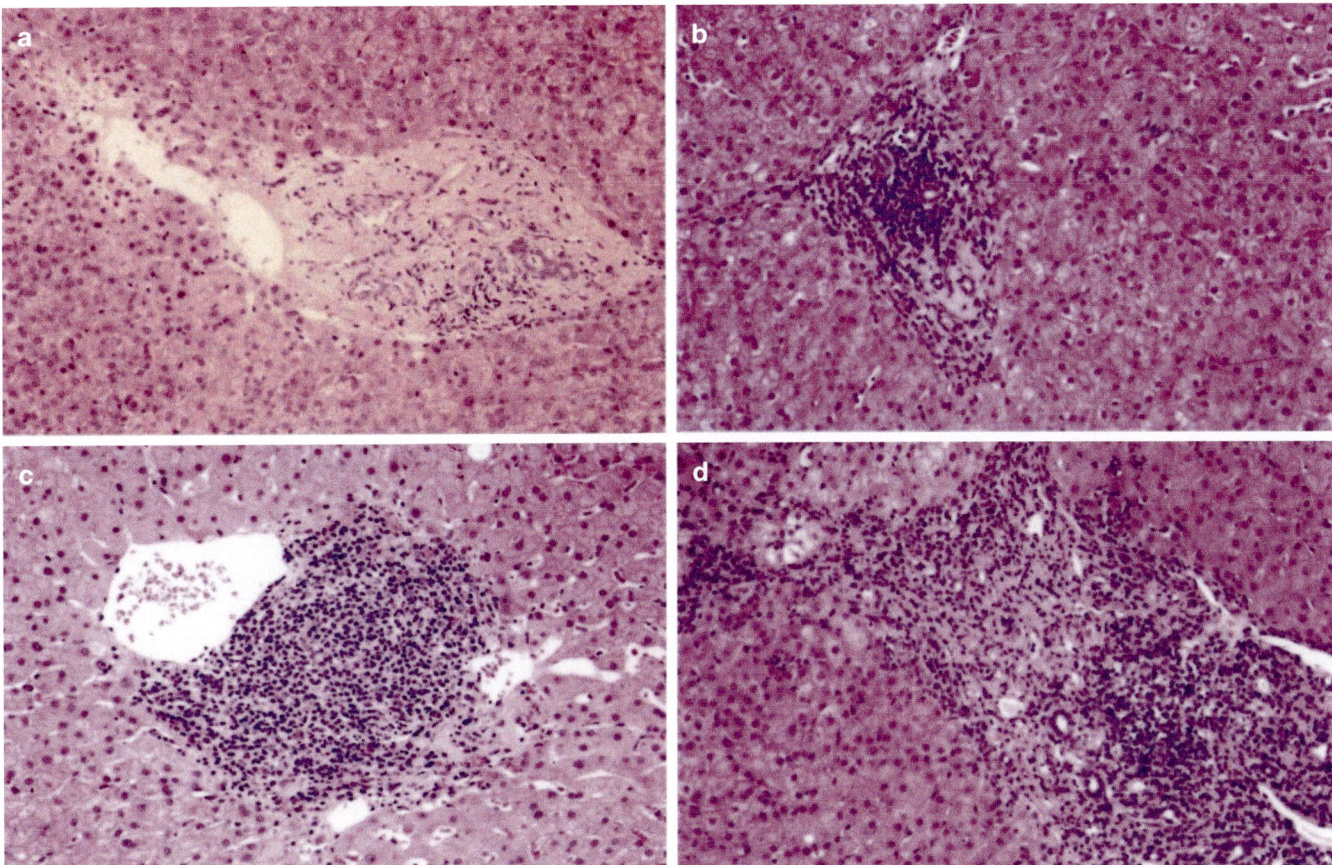

Fig. 5.7 Grading of inflammation in chronic hepatitis C. (**a**) No inflammation is observed in the portal tract, and necrosis is not seen in the lobule. (**b**) Mild inflammation is seen in the portal tract with mini- mal interface hepatitis. (**c**) Mild interface hepatitis with lymphoid follicle is seen in the portal tract. (**d**) Moderate interface hepatitis is seen, with the establishment of bridging fibrosis

nisolone with or without immunomodulators, and most individuals respond well. However, few cases that do not respond to prednisolone require high dosage or a combination with other immunomodulators. Cirrhosis may rapidly occur when the patient does not respond well to immunotherapy or when the diagnosis and therapy of AIH are delayed. Interface hepatitis with infiltration of lymphoplasmacytic cells is histologically characteristic of AIH, and lobular necrosis is frequently seen after acute onset, while bridging necrosis and fibrosis are observed in the chronic phase of AIH (Fig. 5.7). Cirrhotic change develops in asymptomatic patients when AIH is diagnosed.

5.6 Staging and Grading of Chronic Hepatitis

Several semiquantitative scoring systems were introduced over the years, including those of Knodell in 1981 [35], Scheuer in 1991 [36], Ishak in 1995 [1], Ludwig and Batts in 1995 [37], and METAVIR in 1996 [38]. Each system has its strengths and weaknesses in clinical practice or in investiga-

tive work. The Ishak system is often used in clinical trials, while the newer systems are simple to understand and allow greater reproducibility in everyday clinical practice.

Grading pertains to the intensity of inflammation. For example, according to the Ludwig and Batts system, a score of 0 indicates the absence of inflammation while 1 refers to minimal portal and lobular inflammation, 2 refers to mild or localized interface hepatitis and/or mild lobular inflammation, 3 refers to moderate or more extensive interface hepatitis and/or moderate lobular inflammation, and 4 indicates severe and widespread interface hepatitis (Fig. 5.8).

Staging refers to the degree of fibrosis and is also measured on a semiquantitative scale ranging from 0 to 4, with 0 indicating the lack of fibrosis while 1 refers to fibrosis confined to the portal tract, 2 refers to periportal or portal-to-portal septa, 3 refers to bridging fibrosis causing structural distortion (but without obvious cirrhosis), and 4 refers to cirrhosis (Fig. 5.9).

It is important to understand that the use of a scoring system for staging and grading is not meant to replace microscopic description and should include diagnosis of concurrent comorbidities, such as fatty liver and alcoholic and metabolic diseases, which may alter treatment decisions.

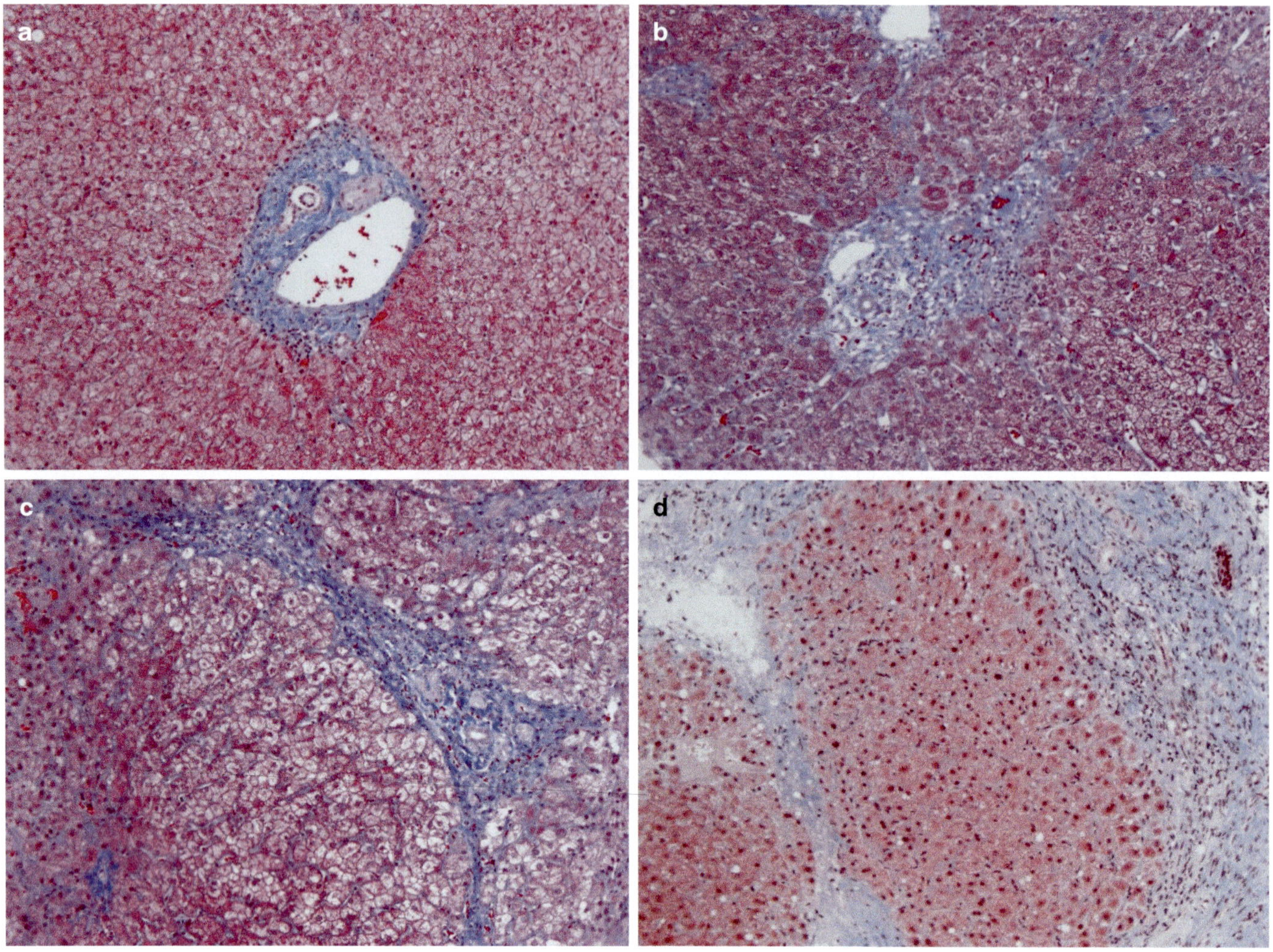

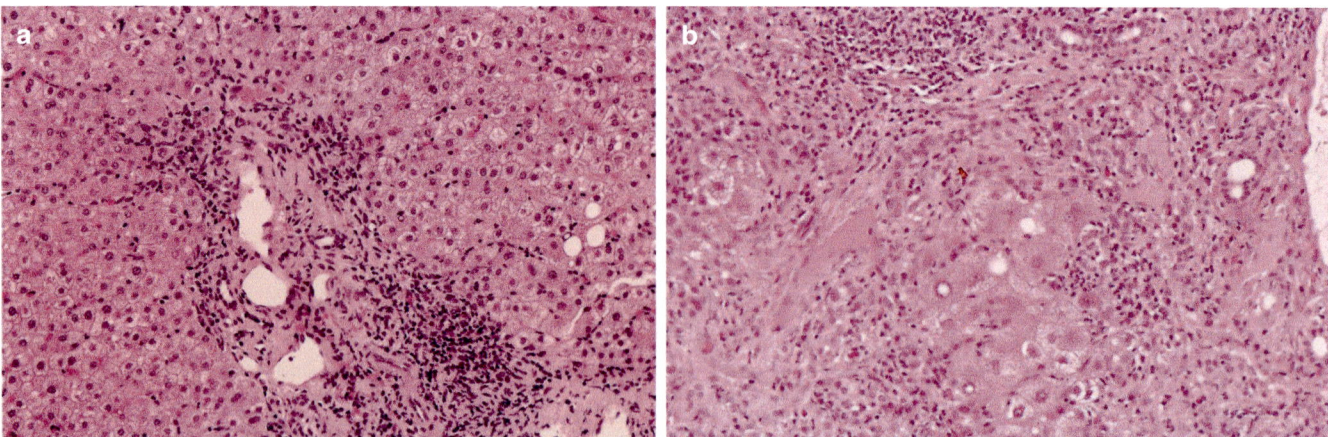

Fig. 5.8 Stages of chronic hepatitis C (Masson's trichrome stain). (**a**) Stage 1 = Localized fibrosis is seen in the portal tract. (**b**) Stage 2 = Portal fibrosis extends beyond the portal tract. (**c**) Stage 3 = Portal fibrosis extends beyond the portal tract, bridging fibrosis is seen, and the lobular structure is distorted. (**d**) Stage 4 = Pseudolobular formation is seen

Fig. 5.9 Autoimmune hepatitis (AIH) . (**a**) Interface hepatitis is seen, with infiltration of lymphoplasmacytic cells in AIH. (**b**) Bridging necrosis is observed in the chronic phase of AIH. (**c**) Intralobular necrosis is present with a cluster of lymphoplasmacytic cells, and rosette formation of hepatocytes is seen. (**d**) Bridging fibrosis develops simultaneously (Mallory-Azan stain)

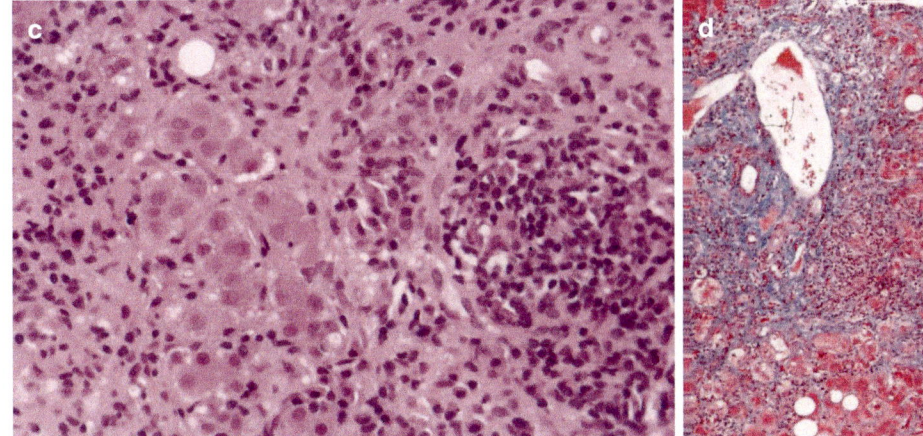
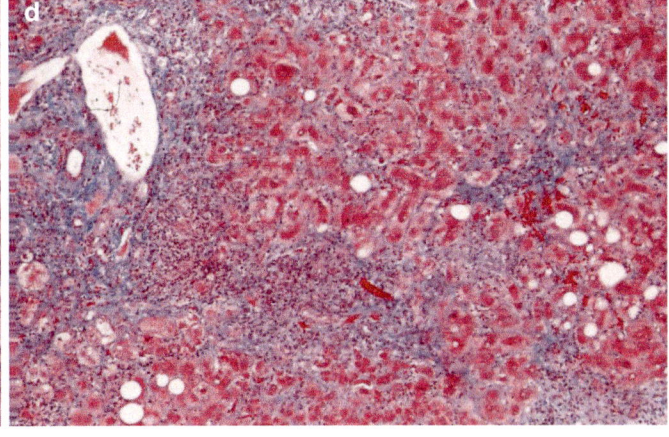

Fig. 5.9 (continued)

References

1. Ishak K, Baptista A, Bianchi L, et al. Histological grading and staging of chronic hepatitis. J Hepatol. 1995;22(6):696–9.
2. Terrault NA, Bzowej NH, Chang KM, et al. AASLD guidelines for treatment of chronic hepatitis B. Hepatology. 2016;63(1):261–83.
3. Jacobson IM, Dienstag JL, Werner BG, et al. Epidemiology and clinical impact of hepatitis D virus (delta) infection. Hepatology. 1985;5(2):188–91.
4. Kamar N, Selves J, Mansuy J-M, et al. Hepatitis E virus and chronic hepatitis in organ-transplant recipients. N Engl J Med. 2008;358(8):811–7.
5. Tamaki N, Kurosaki M, Matsuda S, et al. Prospective comparison of real-time tissue elastography and serum fibrosis markers for the estimation of liver fibrosis in chronic hepatitis C patients. Hepatol Res. 2014;44(7):720–7.
6. Afdhal NH, Bacon BR, Patel K, et al. Accuracy of fibroscan, compared with histology, in analysis of liver fibrosis in patients with hepatitis B or C: a United States multicenter study. Clin Gastroenterol Hepatol. 2015;13(4):772–9 e1-3.
7. Tong MJ, Kowdley KV, Pan C, et al. Improvement in liver histology among Asian patients with chronic hepatitis B after long-term treatment with entecavir. Liver Int. 2013;33(4):650–1.
8. Kuo YH, Lu SN, Chen CH, et al. The changes of liver stiffness and its associated factors for chronic hepatitis B patients with entecavir therapy. PLoS One. 2014;9(3):e93160.
9. Falade-Nwulia O, Suarez-Cuervo C, Nelson DR, et al. Oral direct-acting agent therapy for hepatitis C virus infection: a systematic review. Ann Intern Med. 2017;166(9):637–48.
10. Whitford K, Liu B, Micallef J, et al. Long-term impact of infant immunization on hepatitis B prevalence: a systematic review and meta-analysis. Bull World Health Organ. 2018;96(7):484.
11. Chisari FV, Ferrari C. Hepatitis B virus immunopathology. Semin Immunopathol. 1995;17(2-3):261–81.
12. Sarin S, Kumar M, Lau G, et al. Asian-Pacific clinical practice guidelines on the management of hepatitis B: a 2015 update. Hepatol Int. 2016;10(1):1–98.
13. Liver EAFTSOT. EASL 2017 clinical practice guidelines on the management of hepatitis B virus infection. J Hepatol. 2017;67(2):370–98.
14. Davies SE, Portmann BC, O'Grady JG, et al. Hepatic histological findings after transplantation for chronic hepatitis B virus infection, including a unique pattern of fibrosing cholestatic hepatitis. Hepatology. 1991;13(1):150–7.
15. Blach S, Zeuzem S, Manns M, et al. Global prevalence and genotype distribution of hepatitis C virus infection in 2015: a modelling study. Lancet Gastroenterol Hepatol. 2017;2(3):161–76.
16. Gower E, Estes C, Blach S, et al. Global epidemiology and genotype distribution of the hepatitis C virus infection. J Hepatol. 2014;61(1):S45–57.
17. Freni MA, Artuso D, Gerken G, et al. Focal lymphocytic aggregates in chronic hepatitis C: occurrence, immunohistochemical characterization, and relation to markers of autoimmunity. Hepatology. 1995;22(2):389–94.
18. Kaji K, Nakanuma Y, Sasaki M, et al. Hepatitic bile duct injuries in chronic hepatitis C: histopathologic and immunohistochemical studies. Mod Pathol. 1994;7(9):937–45.
19. Bochud PY, Cai T, Overbeck K, et al. Genotype 3 is associated with accelerated fibrosis progression in chronic hepatitis C. J Hepatol. 2009;51(4):655–66.
20. Panel AIHG, Chung RT, Davis GL, et al. Hepatitis C guidance: AASLD-IDSA recommendations for testing, managing, and treating adults infected with hepatitis C virus. Hepatology. 2015;62(3):932–54.
21. Pawlotsky J-M, Negro F, Aghemo A, et al. EASL recommendations on treatment of hepatitis C. J Hepatol. 2018.
22. Clifford BD, Donahue D, Smith L, et al. High prevalence of serological markers of autoimmunity in patients with chronic hepatitis C. Hepatology. 1995;21(3):613–9.
23. Kobayashi M, Tanaka E, Sodeyama T, et al. The natural course of chronic hepatitis C: a comparison between patients with genotypes 1 and 2 hepatitis C viruses. Hepatology. 1996;23(4):695–9.
24. Poynard T, Bedossa P, Opolon P. Natural history of liver fibrosis progression in patients with chronic hepatitis C. The OBSVIRC, METAVIR, CLINIVIR, and DOSVIRC groups. Lancet. 1997;349:825–32.
25. Davis GL, Albright JE, Cook SF, et al. Projecting future complications of chronic hepatitis C in the United States. Liver Transpl. 2003;9(4):331–8.
26. Kamar N, Dalton HR, Abravanel F, et al. Hepatitis E virus infection. Clin Microbiol Rev. 2014;27(1):116–38.
27. Sempoux C, Jibara G, Ward SC, et al. Intrahepatic cholangiocarcinoma: new insights in pathology. In: Seminars in liver disease. 20Thieme Medical; 2011.
28. Shepard CW, Finelli L, Alter MJ. Global epidemiology of hepatitis C virus infection. Lancet Infect Dis. 2005;5(9):558–67.
29. Di Martino V, Rufat P, Boyer N, et al. The influence of human immunodeficiency virus coinfection on chronic hepatitis C in injec-

tion drug users: a long-term retrospective cohort study. Hepatology. 2001;34(6):1193–9.

30. Drebber U, Kasper HU, Krupacz J, et al. The role of Epsteincohort studyction drug users: a longers: a. J Hepatol. 2006;44(5):879–85.

31. Tanaka S, Toh Y, Minagawa H, et al. Reactivation of cytomegalovirus in patients with cirrhosis: analysis of 122 cases. Hepatology. 1992;16(6):1409–14.

32. Larrey D. Bacterial hepatitis. Gastroenterol Clin Biol. 2003;27(5 Suppl):B27–31.

33. Bellentani S. The epidemiology of non-alcoholic fatty liver disease. Liver Int. 2017;37:81–4.

34. Vierling JM. Autoimmune hepatitis and overlap syndromes: diagnosis and management. Clin Gastroenterol Hepatol. 2015;13(12):2088–108.

35. Knodell RG, Ishak KG, Black WC, et al. Formulation and application of a numerical scoring system for assessing histological activity in asymptomatic chronic active hepatitis. Hepatology. 1981;1(5):431–5.

36. Scheuer PJ. Classification of chronic viral hepatitis: a need for reassessment. J Hepatol. 1991;13(3):372–4.

37. Batts KP, Ludwig J. Chronic hepatitis. An update on terminology and reporting. Am J Surg Pathol. 1995;19(12):1409–17.

38. Bedossa P, Poynard T. An algorithm for the grading of activity in chronic hepatitis C. The METAVIR Cooperative Study Group. Hepatology. 1996;24(2):289–93.

Liver Cirrhosis

6

Terumi Takahara, Masaki Iwai, and Wilson M. S. Tsui

Contents

Abbreviations

ARFI Acoustic radiation force impulse
DAA   Direct-acting antiviral
EVL   Endoscopic variceal band ligation
HBV   Hepatitis B virus
HCC   Hepatocellular carcinoma
HCV   Hepatitis C virus
HRS   Hepatorenal syndrome
HSC   Hepatic stellate cell

MELD The model for end-stage liver disease
MMP   Matrix metalloproteinase
MRE   Magnetic resonance elastography
NA   Nucleos(t)ide analogue
NASH Nonalcoholic steatohepatitis
SBP   Spontaneous bacterial peritonitis
SWE   Shear wave elastography
TE   Tissue elastography
TGF   Transforming growth factor
TIMP Tissue inhibitor of matrix metalloproteinase

T. Takahara, MD, PhD (✉)
Toyama, Japan
e-mail: taka@med.u-toyama.ac.jp

M. Iwai, MD, PhD
Kyoto, Japan

W. M. S. Tsui, MD, FRCPath
Hong Kong, China

Liver cirrhosis is anatomically defined as a diffuse disruption of the normal architecture of the liver with fibrosis and nodule formation. It is the end result of fibrogenesis caused by chronic liver injury. The anatomical architecture is the same with any etiology: continuous inflammation or hepatocyte damage causes fibrogenesis, and fibers extend from central or portal area, and finally fibrous septa is completely formed to

© Springer Nature Singapore Pte Ltd. 2019
E. Hashimoto et al. (eds.), *Diagnosis of Liver Disease*, https://doi.org/10.1007/978-981-13-6806-6_6

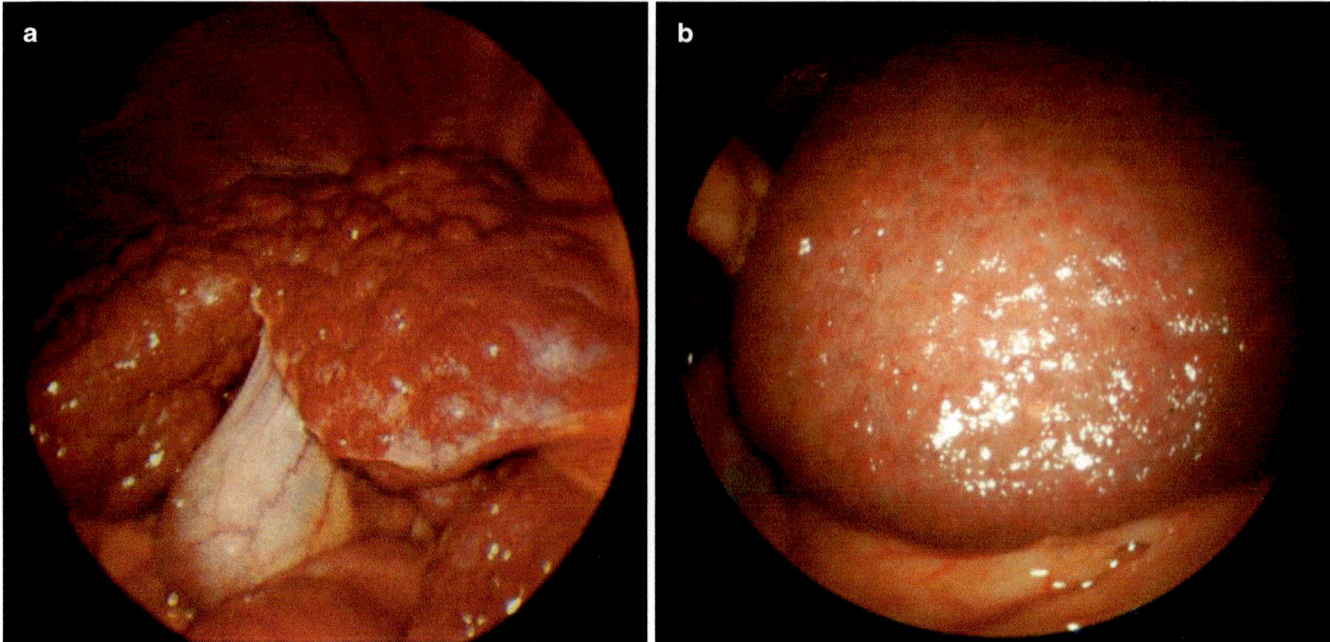

Fig. 6.1 Peritoneoscopic findings in liver cirrhosis. (**a**) Peritoneoscopic examination shows macronodules in the right lobe of liver cirrhosis with HBV infection. (**b**) Peritoneoscopic examination shows micronodules in left lobe of alcoholic liver cirrhosis

Table 6.1 Child-Pugh staging system and MELD score

Child-Pugh staging system			
Parameter	1 point	2 point	3 point
Total bilirubin			
μmol/L	<34	34–50	>50
mg/dL	<2	2–3	>3
Serum albumin			
g/L	>35	28–35	<28
INR	<1.7	1.71–2.3	>2.3
Ascites	None	Mild (controlled by diuretics)	Moderate to severe (refractory to diuretics)
Hepatic encephalopathy	None	Grades I–II (absent with medication)	Grades III–IV (recurrent)

Child A class is 5–6 points; B is 7–9 points; C is 10–15 points
MELD score
MELD = 3.78× [serum bilirubin (mg/dL)] + 11.2× [INR] + 9.57× [serum creatinine (mg/dL)] + 6.43

surround regenerative nodules. Thus liver cirrhosis is characterized with hepatocyte dysfunction and portal hypertension.

6.1 Classification

(a) Morphological classification

WHO classification of macropathology showed three nodular types, namely, macronodular (bigger than 3 mm nodule in diameter), micronodular (smaller than 3 mm nodule in diameter), and mixed. Micronodule is caused by alcohol, cholestasis, or hemochromatosis, and mac-

ronodule is caused by viral infection. However the dynamics is not specified, and micronodule can evolve to macronodule (Fig. 6.1) [1].

(b) Functional classification

Clinically cirrhosis is classified as compensated or decompensated stages. No significant symptoms are observed at compensated stage because protein synthesis and detoxification ability are reserved. However decompensation means one or more of the following: jaundice, ascites, bleeding varices, or hepatic encephalopathy.

Child-Pugh classification is used worldwide and is based on jaundice, ascites, encephalopathy, serum albumin concentration, and prothrombin time [2]. The total score classifies patients into grade A, B, or C (Table 6.1).

At the same time, MELD (the model for end-stage liver disease) score is used for prognostication of decompensated stage, which is derived from serum creatinine, prothrombin time (INR), and serum bilirubin. MELD score is applied to liver transplantation and found to predict the mortality in waiting list; thus it is now widely used as a criterion for organ allocation [3].

(c) Etiology

Liver cirrhosis is caused by several etiologies, and the incidence varies between different countries and genetic background. In Western countries the prevalence of alcoholic and nonalcoholic steatohepatitis (NASH) and viral cirrhosis, in particular hepatitis C, are all increasing. In developing countries, the predominant causes are hepatitis virus B and C. In Japan HCV is the cause in about 60%, alcohol 15%, and HBV 13% (Fig. 6.2) [4]. In China and Korea, HBV is the most predominant.

Recently, the incidence of NASH is increasing worldwide, especially in developing country.

6.1.1 Hepatitis C

HCV-mediated infection causes mild and persistent attacks in the liver. When degeneration and regenerative activity are mild, the excavations are small, and regenerative nodules are lower in height [5].

Case 6.1

A 65-year-old male suffering from persistent infection of HCV presented with serum HCV RNA 6.0 log copies/mL. Liver function test showed TBIL 1.04 mg/dL, AST 71 IU/L, ALT 48 IU/L, GGT 353 IU/L, PLT 7.8×10^4/μL, and hyaluronic acid 400 ng/mL. Peritoneoscopy showed white and wavy surface with dilated peripheral portal veins, and nodules were not apparent; histologically, pseudolobular formation was present, and the internodular space differed in

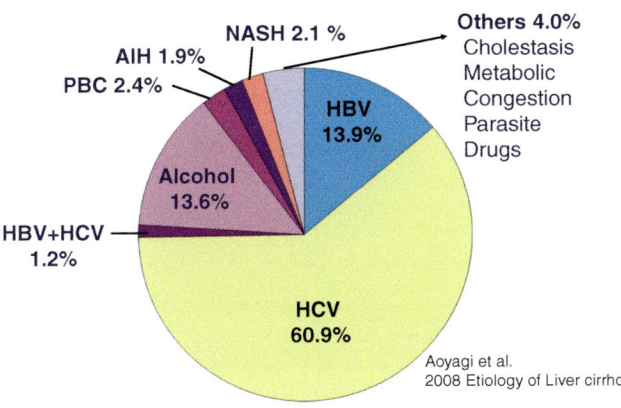

Etiology of liver cirrhosis in Japan (2008)

NASH 2.1 %
AIH 1.9%
PBC 2.4%
Others 4.0%
Cholestasis
Metabolic
Congestion
Parasite
Drugs
HBV 13.9%
Alcohol 13.6%
HBV+HCV 1.2%
HCV 60.9%
Aoyagi et al.
2008 Etiology of Liver cirrhosis

Fig. 6.2 Etiology of liver cirrhosis in Japan. HCV is the most predominant cause

each pseudolobule; and steatosis was seen in hepatocytes, and bile ducts were disorganized (Fig. 6.3).

6.1.2 Primary Biliary Cholangitis

In primary biliary cholangitis, interlobular bile ducts or septal bile ducts are initially destroyed, and their destruction is irregularly distributed. Therefore, excavation due to destruction of bile ducts is distributed irregularly, with liver surface becoming wavy or undulating. Nodules may become large and vary in size. Fibrosis spreads from the portal tracts, with destruction or disappearance of bile ducts [6], and proliferated fibrosis may cause the formation of pseudolobules.

Case 6.2

A 53-year-old female was suspected of having ascites and jaundice. Her liver function test showed TBIL 4.6 mg/dL, AST 93 IU/L, ALT 70 IU/L, ALP 1177 IU/L, GGT 331 IU/L, IgG 2350 mg/dL, IgM 645 mg/dL, anti-M2 antibody 2980 U/mL, ANA × 1280, and PLT 7.1×10^4/μL. Esophageal varices were detected by esophagogastroduodenoscope. Peritoneoscopy with liver biopsy showed formation of large nodules and presence of lymph follicles on wavy surface, while lobular architecture was microscopically destructed, pseudolobular formation was established, and bile ducts disappeared (Fig. 6.4). Ursodeoxycholic acid was administered, but serum value of TBIL and ALP gradually increased, and she died of hepatic failure after 3.5 years.

6.1.3 Wilson's Disease

In Wilson's disease, there is genetic disturbance of hepatobiliary copper discharge by copper-transporting ATPase [7], and copper is deposited in the liver and brain. Microscopically fatty metamorphosis, chronic active hepatitis, cirrhotic

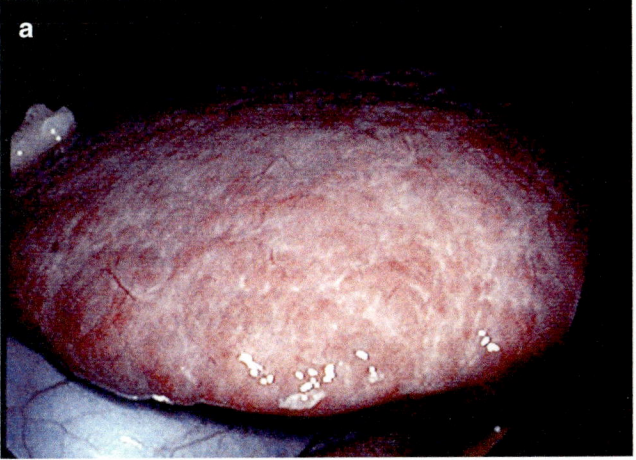
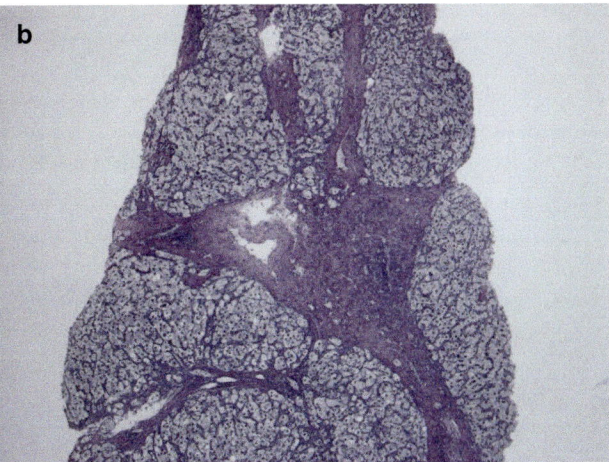

Fig. 6.3 Liver cirrhosis due to hepatitis C virus infection. (**a**) Peritoneoscopy shows nodules are regular in size and are low in height, and internodular space is narrow. (**b**) Pseudolobular formation is seen and nodules vary in size

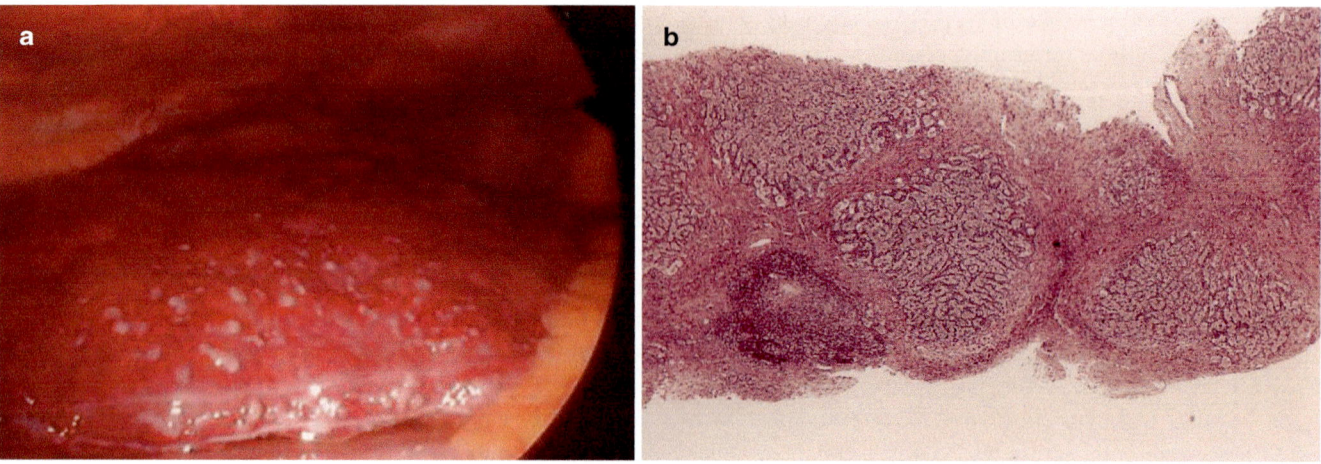

Fig. 6.4 Primary biliary cholangitis. (**a**) Peritoneoscopy shows nodules are irregular in size and are low in height, and lymph vesicles are seen on liver surface. (**b**) Pseudolobular formation with aggregate of lymphocytes is established. Pseudolobules vary in size, and septum fibrosis is wide

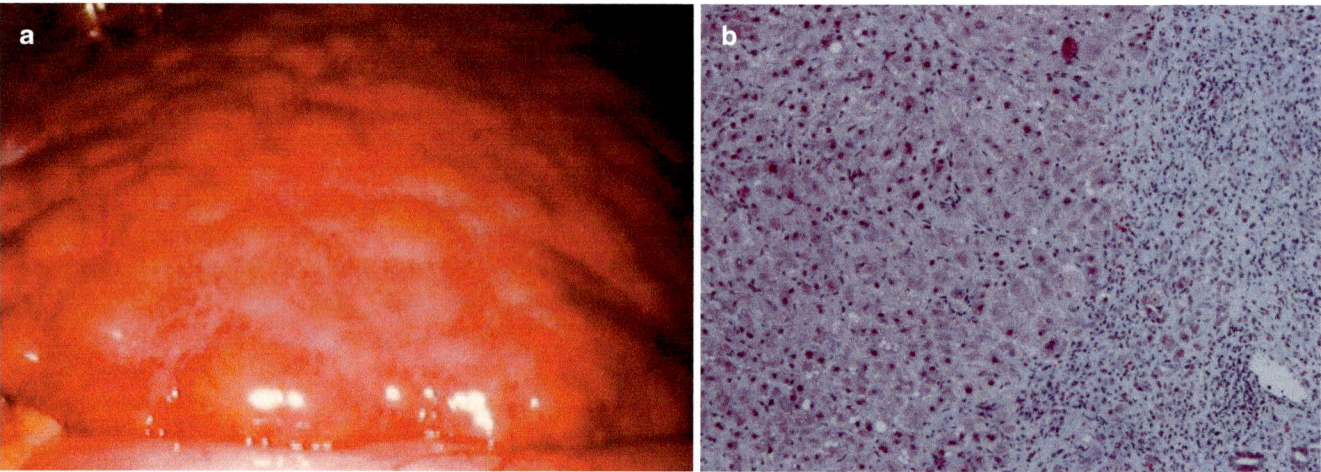

Fig. 6.5 Wilson's disease. (**a**) Peritoneoscopy shows nodular formation on yellow liver surface. Nodules are round and vary in size. (**b**) Masson trichrome stain shows pseudolobular formation, extension of fibrosis from portal tracts, and micro- and macrosteatosis

changes, and submassive necrosis occur in the liver of some patients with Wilson's disease. Cirrhotic change can develop with chronic hepatitis; therefore, the liver surface is typically yellow with red markings [8].

Case 6.3 (See Chap. 12)

Liver test performed on a 12-year-old boy showed abnormal values, including low ceruloplasmin in serum with high urinary copper. Wilson's disease was suspected. Peritoneoscopy showed round nodular formations on yellow liver surface, while pseudolobular formation with microvesicular or macrovesicular fatty change was observed under histology, and active inflammation was seen in portal tracts (Fig. 6.5).

6.1.4 Budd-Chiari Syndrome

Clinical manifestations in Budd-Chiari syndrome (BCS) vary from symptom-free to epigastric pain, hematemesis and hepatic encephalopathy, lower extremity edema, venous dilatation of abdominal wall, and ascites. BCS is classified into two types: with or without membranous obstruction of inferior vena cava (MOVC). Chronic obstruction leads to peliosis and hemorrhage between the parenchyma and portal area or subcapsular space. Hepatic capsule is thick and white in color, and necrosis of hepatocytes is persistent. Liver surface is darkly white, regenerative nodules are low in height, and subcapsular hemorrhage is seen on liver surface [9].

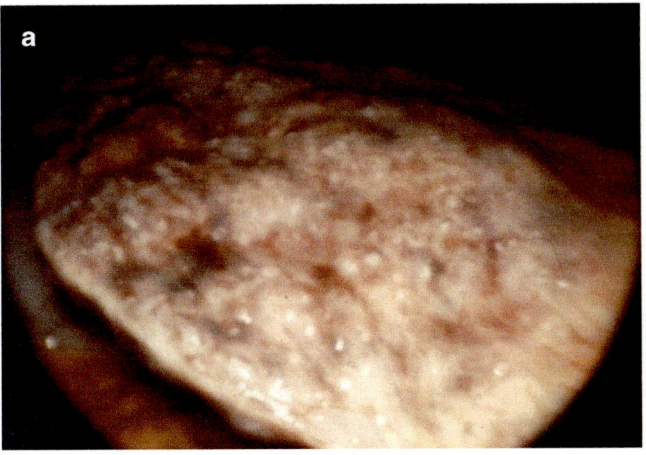
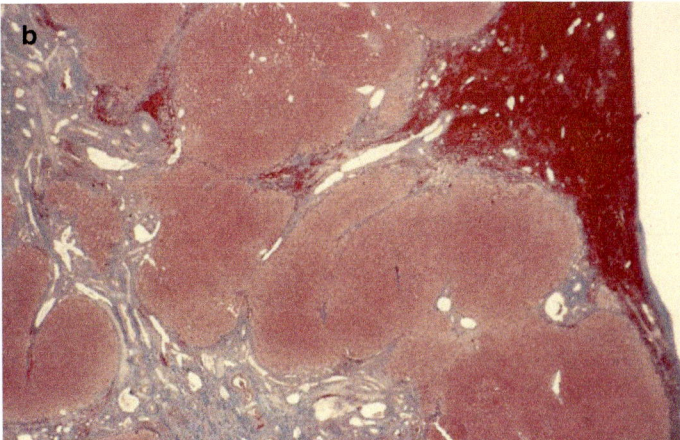

Fig. 6.6 Budd-Chiari syndrome. (**a**) Peritoneoscopy shows wavy and white-colored liver surface, and nodular formations are seen. Internodular space is wide, and subcapsular hemorrhage is observed (Redrawn from Iwai M, et al. Clinical features, image analysis, and laparoscopic and histological liver findings in Budd-Chiari syndrome. Hepato-Gastroenterol 1998; 45: 2359–68). (**b**) Subcapsular or periportal hemorrhage is seen, pseudolobular formation is established, and bridging fibrosis is observed between portal tracts

Case 6.4

A 66-year-old male had an esophagogastroduodenoscopic examination, and early gastric cancer was detected. Upper abdominal CT examination was performed prior to gastrectomy, and thrombus was detected in inferior vena cava (Chap. 11). Peritoneoscopy showed atrophic liver of left lobe with thick capsule, and subcapsular hemorrhage was seen on wavy surface of the liver; pseudolobular formation was established, and hemorrhage was seen in the subcapsular space. On histology, bridging fibrosis between portal tracts was noted, and central veins were not dilated (Fig. 6.6).

6.2 Pathology

Liver cirrhosis is caused by significant fibrosis due to the wound healing steps from continuous liver injuries together with structural changes of lobules and vessels.

In normal liver, low-density basement membrane composed of type IV collagen, glycoprotein (fibronectin and laminin), and proteoglycans is located in the space of Disse, which separates hepatocytes from sinusoidal endothelium. After hepatic injury there is a three- to eightfold increase of extracellular matrix, which is composed predominantly of interstitial fibril-forming collagens (types I and III) as well as other matrices. In addition, there are loss of endothelial cell fenestration and formation of basement membrane which is composed of high-density type IV collagen and laminin. This change is known as capillarization of sinusoid, which impedes the metabolic exchange between blood and hepatocytes.

The activated hepatic stellate cell (HSC) located in Disse's space is the principal cell involved in fibrogenesis. With liver injury, HSC undergoes phenotypic changes referred to as "activation" characterized as myofibroblastic changes. HSC activation can be divided into two phases such as initiation and perpetuation. Initiation is caused by different factors of liver injury depending on the disease etiology. Stimuli include oxidant stress signals, apoptotic bodies, lipopolysaccharide, and paracrine stimuli from neighboring cells such as Kupffer cells, sinusoidal endothelial cells, and hepatocytes which initiate HSC to respond to a host growth factor and cytokines. Perpetuation involves cellular events that amplify the activated phenotype through enhanced cytokine expression and responsiveness. Fibrosis is developing through enhanced HSC proliferation, contractility, chemotaxis, secretion of proinflammatory mediators, direct interaction between HSCs and the immune systems, and altered matrix degradation. Among cytokine, TGF-beta is the most potent fibrogenic cytokine (Fig. 6.7) [10].

Once the initiating injury signal is eliminated, HSCs either revert to the quiescent phenotype or are removed from the liver through programmed cell death or apoptosis.

Liver biopsy is the gold standard for diagnosis [11]. Interpretation may be limited by small size and sampling error. Specialist liver histopathology is essential. Even with small biopsies, the expert histopathologist may be able to make a diagnosis of cirrhosis by recognizing a rim of fibrosis at the periphery of the fragments and the lack of normally related portal tracts and hepatic venules in the parenchyma, often with a widened reticulin pattern or architectural disruption. Liver biopsy contributes to the determination of etiology by identifying features such as micronodule and pericellular fibrosis indicating alcoholic liver cirrhosis (Fig. 6.8), steatosis and ballooning indicating NASH, or plasma cell infiltration suggesting autoimmune hepatitis. Liver biopsy is not without risk. If there are contraindications such as ascites or prolonged coagulation time, the transjugular approach is suggested.

Fig. 6.7 Pathway of hepatic stellate cell (HSC) activation. HSC activation can be divided into two phases: initiation and perpetuation. Initiation is provoked by soluble stimuli including oxidative stress signals, cytokines from neighboring cells such as Kupffer cells, and apoptotic bodies. Perpetuation follows, characterized by a number of specific phenotype changes including proliferation, contractility, fibrogenesis, altered matrix degradation, chemotaxis, and inflammatory signaling

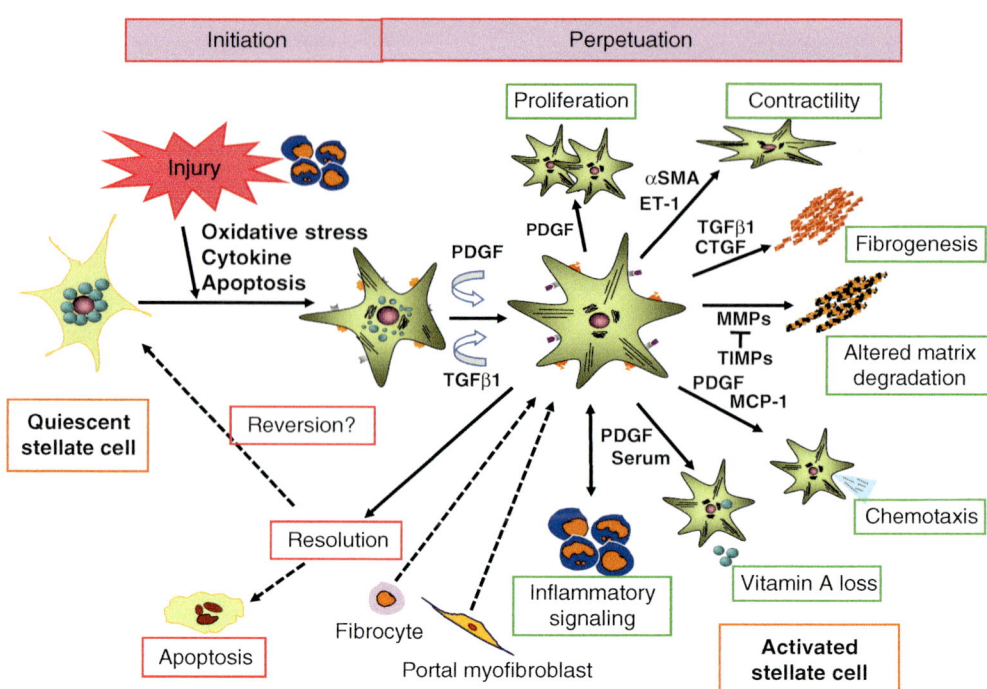

Fig. 6.8 Histology of alcoholic liver cirrhosis. Microscopy shows micronodule formation together with pericellular fibrosis

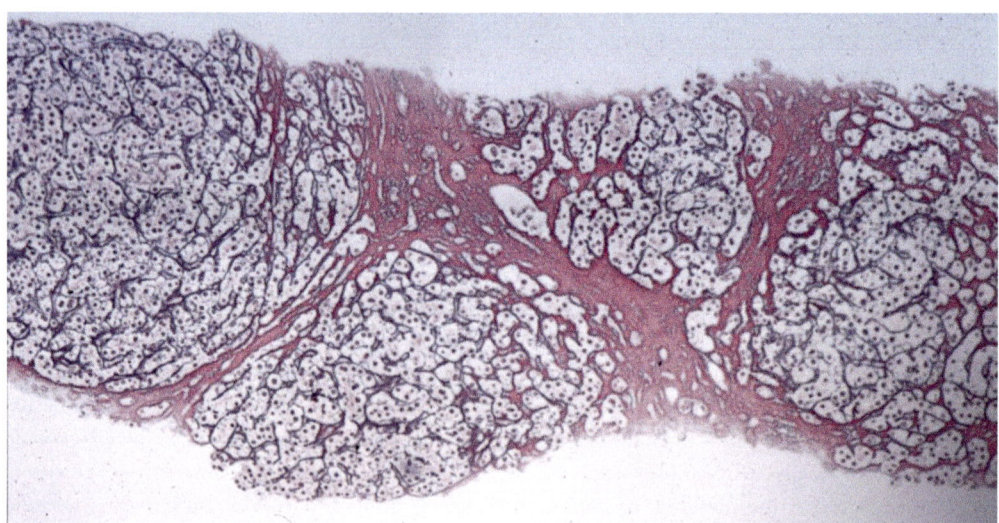

6.3   Clinical Symptoms

The symptoms are caused by both the loss of hepatocytes function and portal hypertension.

At the compensated stage, no significant symptoms are noted, and it is difficult to distinguish from chronic hepatitis. Non-specific symptom such as general fatigue, easy fatigability, anorexia, muscle cramp, itching, and loss of libido may be noted.

Vascular spider at the neck to forechest, palmar erythema, gynecomastia, asterixis, white nails, dark skin, malnutrition, and sarcopenia are also noticed. Right lobe of the liver becomes atrophic, and left lobe is hypertrophic; thus hard liver is palpable at epigastrium. Splenomegaly is also noted. Venous collaterals of abdominal wall from umbilical area, known as "caput medusa," are caused by portal hypertension (Fig. 6.9).

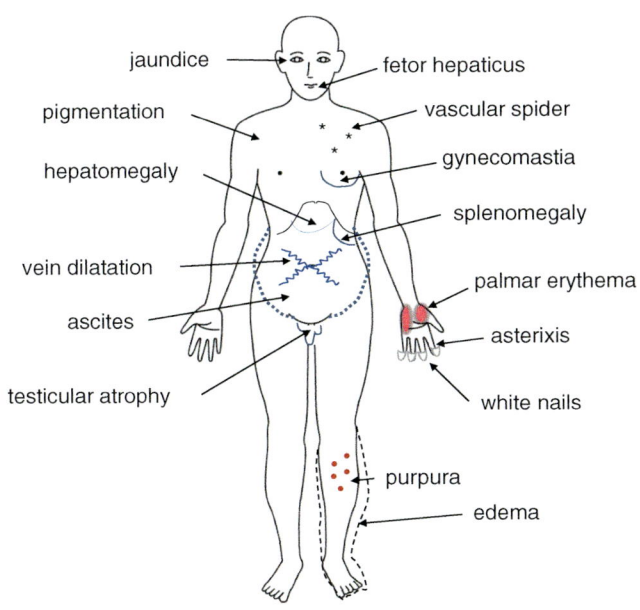

Fig. 6.9 Clinical symptoms of cirrhotic patient

Table 6.2 Laboratory investigations

Investigations			
Hematology	Red blood cell	↓	
	White blood cell	↓	
	Platelet	↓	
	Prothrombin time (INR)	↑	
Biochemistry	Albumin	↓	
	Cholinesterase	↓	
	Total cholesterol	↓	
	Bilirubin	↑	
	Transaminase	↑	
	AST/ALT>1		
	Ammonia	↑	
	ICG (R15)	↑	
	Fischer ratio	↓	
Protein fraction	g-globulin	↑	
	IgG	↑	
Fibrosis marker	P-III-P	↑	
	Type IV collagen	↑	
	Hyaluronic acid	↑	
	M2BPGi	↑	

At decompensated stage, leg edema and ascites, jaundice, consciousness disturbance due to hepatic coma, and hematemesis occur.

6.4   Laboratory Examination

(a) Biochemistry and blood cell count: Disturbance of hepatocyte function causes low level of synthesis, such as albumin, cholesterol, and cholinesterase, and elevated level of bilirubin and prothrombin time (INR) (Table 6.2). AST and ALT are rather low compared with that of chronic hepatitis, and AST is higher than ALT. Gamma globulin is elevated, and albumin/globulin ratio (A/G) is decreased. Hepatic fibrosis markers such as hyaluronic acid, type IV collagen, and Mac-2 binding protein glycan isomer (M2BPGi) are elevated together with fibrosis progression [12]. High level of ammonium suggests hepatic coma. Low level of Fisher ratio (BCAA/AAA) suggests the disturbance of protein metabolism. Indocyanine green tolerance test at 15 min (ICG R15) is more than 20% at cirrhotic stage. Alpha-fetoprotein is sometimes increased due to hepatocyte regeneration. Portal hypertension causes splenomegaly and pancytopenia, especially decrease in white blood cells and platelets.

(b) Image analyses: Many kinds of images are used because liver cirrhosis is highly associated with liver cancer. Ultrasonography is not reliable for the diagnosis of cir-

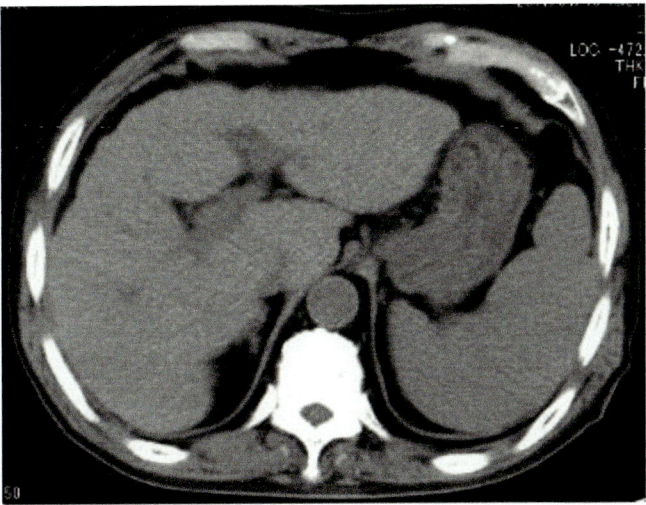

Fig. 6.10 CT scan in liver cirrhosis. CT shows the liver with irregular surface, enlargement of left lobe, and splenomegaly

rhosis but useful for screening for hepatocellular carcinoma. US shows the coarse echo pattern in the liver, irregular surface, dull edge, left lobe enlargement, splenomegaly, and sometimes ascites. CT scan can assess liver size and shape and identify liver nodules (Fig. 6.10). It provides an objective record for evaluating changes over time. Fatty change, focal liver lesions, ascites, collateral vessels, and splenomegaly can be identified. MRI is also useful for evaluating liver nodules.

(c) Noninvasive assessment of cirrhosis: Serum markers of fibrosis can be subclassified as direct and indirect markers. Direct markers such as serum hyaluronic acid, type IV collagen, procollagen type III amino-terminal peptide (PIIINP), matrix metalloproteinase-2 (MMP-2), tissue inhibitor of metalloproteinase-1 (TIMP-1), and TIMP-2 have been implicated in hepatic fibrosis. Indirect markers of fibrosis involve combinations of standard laboratory tests including AST/ALT, GGT, bilirubin, coagulation parameters, platelet count, and so on. APRI (AST to platelet ratio index) is a simple indirect marker that can be calculated from routine laboratory data. It has proven effective in predicting the presence of cirrhosis in HCV patients [13]. FIB-4 is another simple indirect marker that found to be a predictor of cirrhosis [14].

Liver stiffness measurement appears to have a better diagnostic accuracy compared with serum markers. Liver stiffness measurement has the advantage of being liver-specific and unaffected by extrahepatic inflammation and scarring. However, stiffness measurement has some disadvantages such as requiring a dedicated device and subjection to inter- and intraobserver variability unlike serum markers. Also it may not be measurable in certain patients, such as those with obesity or ascites [15]. Tissue elastography (TE) using FibroScan measures the velocity of a low-frequency (50 Hz) elastic shear wave propagating through the liver. The velocity is directly related to tissue stiffness, called the elastic modulus (expressed as $E = 3\,pv^2$, where v is the shear velocity and p is the density of tissue, assumed to be constant). The stiffer the tissue, the faster the shear wave propagates. The standard M probe is estimated to examine a liver volume 100 times larger than a standard biopsy. The results are expressed in kilopascals (kPa) and range from 1.5 to 75 kPa with normal values around 5 kPa. Result more than 17.0 kPa suggests liver cirrhosis (Fig. 6.11). TE takes only 5–10 min for the procedure and is simple, inexpensive, and reproducible. Acoustic radiation force impulse (ARFI) imaging, also called point shear wave elastography (pSWE), is an ultrasound-based elastography technique. Short acoustic pulse (~262 μs) generates shear waves causing microdisplacement of the hepatic parenchyma. The shear wave velocity is measured in m/sec. Liver stiffness measured by 2D shear wave elastography (2D-SWE) is another modality. The technique involves the real-time capture of transient shear waves induced in the hepatic parenchyma by focused ultrasonic beams. 2D-SWE has a lower failure rate than TE, and there has been a suggestion that 2D-SWE has better performance than both TE and ARFI/pSWE (Fig. 6.12). Magnetic resonance elastography (MRE) has not yet been adopted in routine clinical use due to its expense and time commitment. However, MRE provides excellent quantification of shear wave propagation using modified phase-contrast imaging.

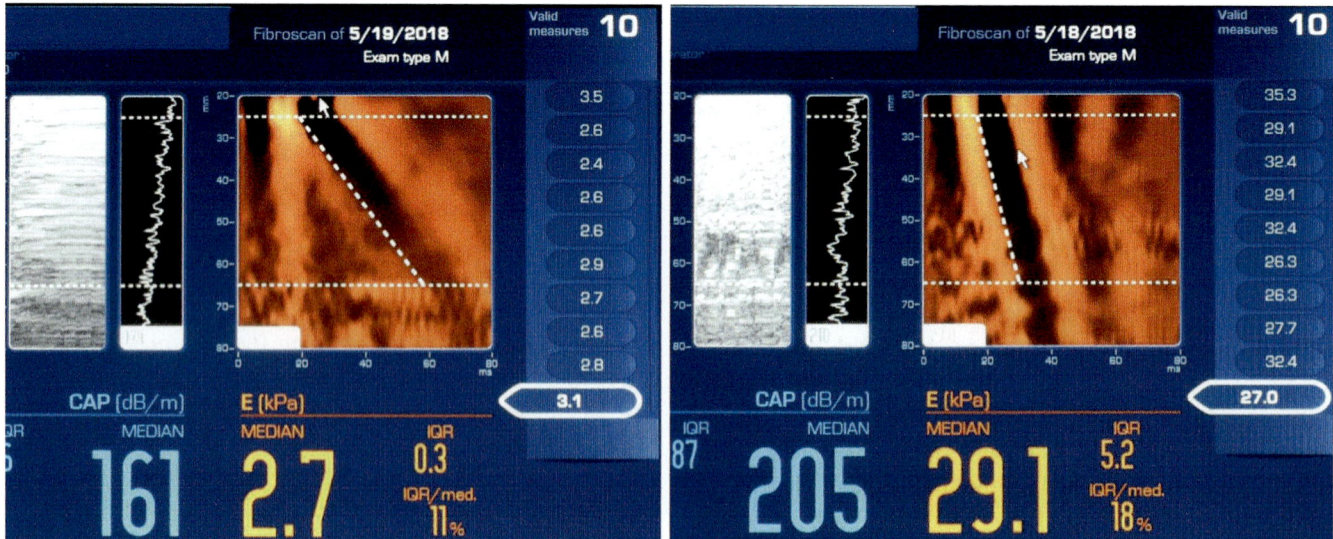

Fig. 6.11 Tissue elastography using FibroScan. Left: normal liver. The inclination is mild. Elasticity is 2.7 kPa. Right: liver cirrhosis. The inclination is steep. Elasticity is 29.1 kPa

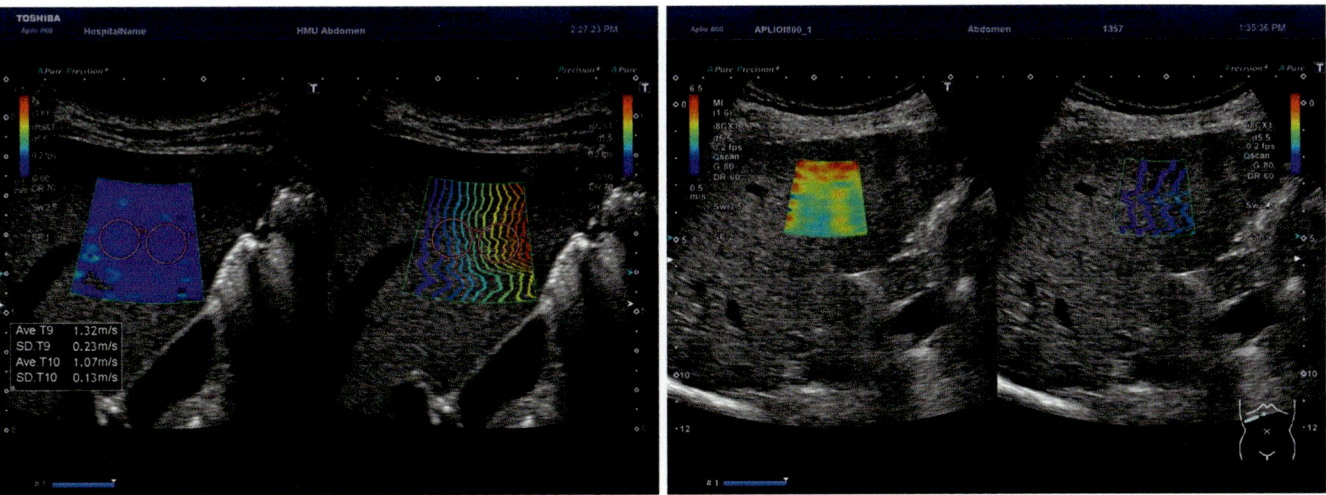

Fig. 6.12 2D-share wave elastography. Left: normal liver. Shear wave speed is slow (blue). The propagation is parallel and narrow. Right: liver cirrhosis. Shear wave speed is fast (red to yellow), and the propagation is wide

6.5   Complications

(a) Hepatocellular carcinoma (HCC): The most dreadful complication is HCC. The risk of HCC differs with the etiology of liver cirrhosis. The occurrence rate of HCC is reported at 7–8% per year in hepatitis C [16]. The guideline recommends regular imaging examination and tumor markers such as alpha-fetoprotein (AFP) and des-γ-carboxy prothrombin (DCP) in liver cirrhosis patients.

(b) Portal hypertension: Portal hypertension is noticed as gastroesophageal varices, portal hypertensive gastropathy, splenomegaly, and hepatic coma. Esophagogastroduodenoscopy is required to show gastroesophageal varices. Red color sign (RC sign), which is reddish area on the varices, is particularly important to evaluate the possibility of bleeding and to decide the preventive treatment (Fig. 6.13).

(c) Ascites: The ascites of liver cirrhosis is transudative with clear and yellowish fluid. The mechanisms of ascites formation are complicated, but portal (sinusoidal) hypertension and renal retention of sodium are universal. The natural history of cirrhotic ascites progresses from diuretic-responsive (uncomplicated) ascites to the development of dilutional hyponatremia, refractory ascites, and finally hepatorenal syndrome.

(d) Spontaneous bacterial peritonitis (SBP): One of the most common bacterial infections in cirrhosis is SBP. It is called spontaneous because it occurs in the absence of a contiguous source of infections and in the absence of an intra-abdominal inflammatory focus. The diagnostic puncture of ascites shows the increase of white blood cell more than 750/mm^3 or polymorphonuclear cells more than 250/mm^3 as an indication of SBP. Culture of bacteria is negative in approximately 50% of patients with clinical manifestations suggestive of SBP.

(e) Hepatorenal syndrome (HRS): HRS is a severe complication of cirrhosis that occurs in patients with ascites and hyponatremia and consists of the development of renal failure in the absence of any identifiable renal pathology. It is a functional disturbance, and the histology of the kidney is mostly normal. The syndrome involves intense splanchnic and peripheral vasodilation with consequent renal vasoconstriction.

(f) Hepatic encephalopathy: Hepatic encephalopathy in liver cirrhosis is characterized by neuropsychiatric abnormalities, ranging from indiscernible changes in cognition to obvious changes in intellect, behavior, motor function, and consciousness. This complication has detrimental effects on health-related quality of life, safety, and survival. Both hepatocellular failure and portal-systemic shunting are key to this development. Ammonia plays a key role in the pathogenesis of the syndrome via the induction of astrocyte swelling, and the development of low-grade cerebral edema, oxidative stress, disrupted glial-neuronal communication, and neuronal dysfunction follow. Asterixis (flapping tremor) is the best-known motor abnormality. Fetor hepaticus, a sour, musty, feculent smell, can be detected on the breath of some patients.

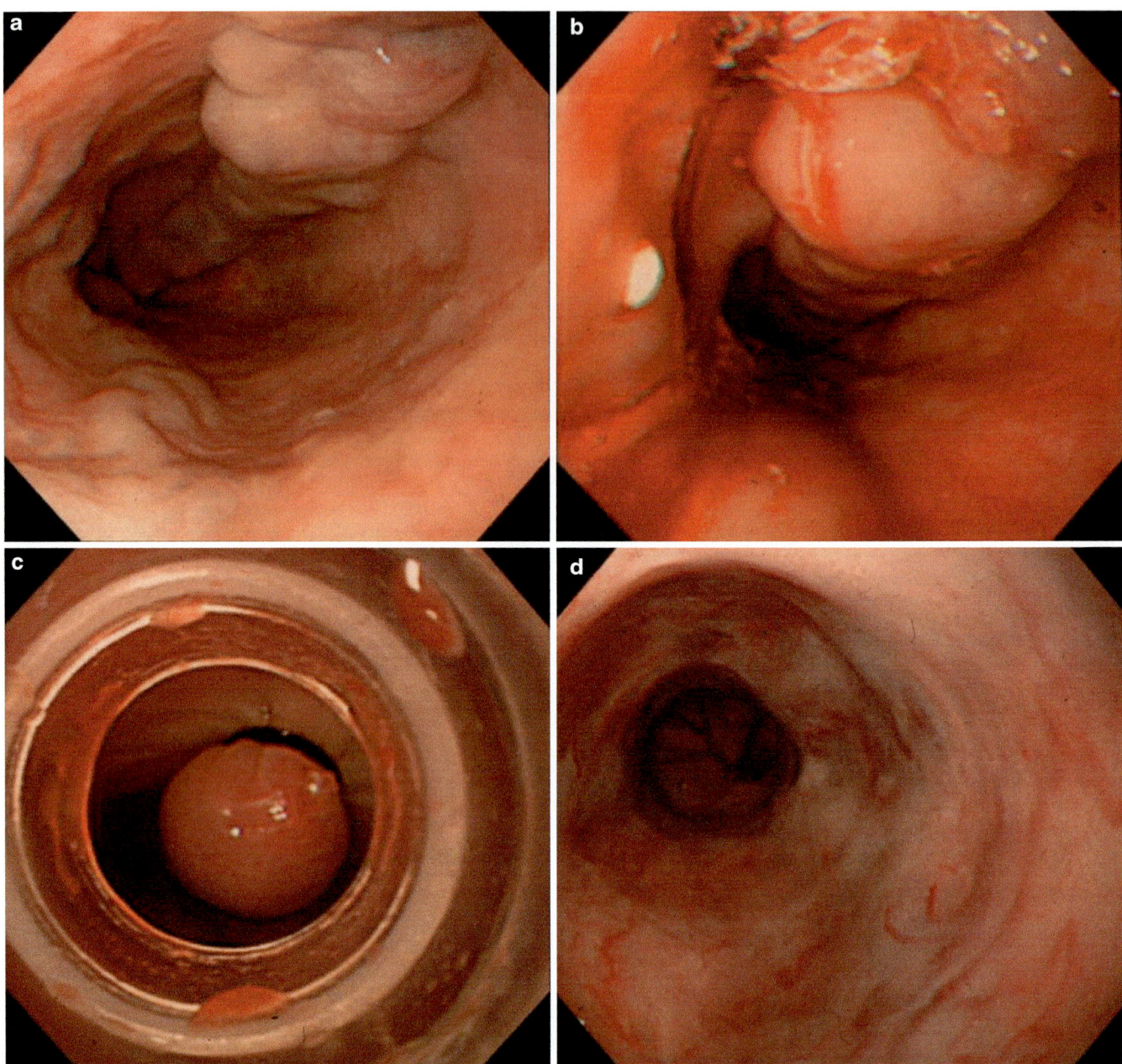

Fig. 6.13 Esophagogastroduodenoscopic findings. (**a**) Esophagogastroduodenoscopy shows meandered blue esophageal varices. (**b**) Bleeding from esophageal varices. (**c**) Endoscopic variceal band ligation is done to the ruptured varices. (**d**) Esophageal scaring is seen after EVL

6.6 Prognosis

Poor prognosis is associated with a prolonged prothrombin time, marked ascites, gastrointestinal bleeding, high serum bilirubin, low albumin values, and poor nutrition. If liver transplantation is done, the prognosis is getting better. The appearance of ascites is the most common first decompensating event, followed by variceal bleeding, encephalopathy, and jaundice.

6.7 Therapy

Treatment consists of two factors. One is the treatment for the cause of cirrhosis. The other is for treatment of its complications.

6.7.1 Etiology-Based Therapy

(a) Hepatitis B virus
    Liver cirrhosis with hepatitis B infection is treated with antiviral drug. Nucleos(t)ide analogue (NA) rather than interferon is used for the treatment of liver cirrhosis because interferon has many adverse events compared with NA. Tenofovir and entecavir are used as first-line drugs. Regression of fibrosis and reversal of cirrhosis can be observed in patients with maintained viral suppression after 3–5 years of continuous NA administration [17].

(b) Hepatitis C virus
    Treatment of hepatitis C has dramatically changed within recent several years. The efficacy of direct-acting antiviral (DAA) on hepatitis C is more than 95%. The sustained viral response will lead to resolution of the extended fibrosis, together with decreased incidence of HCC [18].

(c) Autoimmune hepatitis
    Autoimmune hepatitis can be treated with immunosuppressant reagents. Two general treatment strategies have developed: (1) prednisolone monotherapy and (2) combination therapy, either from the onset or with addition of azathioprine a few weeks later. Some may choose budesonide as first-line treatment instead of prednisolone.

(d) Primary biliary cholangitis
    The first-line licensed treatment is ursodeoxycholic acid (UDCA). Obeticholic acid (OCA) is now approved for use in both Europe and the USA in patients showing an inadequate response to or intolerant of UDCA. Liver transplantation remains the only effective treatment for patients with end-stage disease. Bilirubin level of >100 μmol/L (6 mg/dL) is a useful threshold at which transplant is actively considered.

(e) Alcoholic liver cirrhosis
    The most important measure is to ensure total and immediate abstinence from alcohol. Psychological and pharmacological treatments are available to help abstinence and prevent relapse.

(f) Wilson's disease
    Patients will require continuous treatment throughout their lifetime. The frontline agents are copper chelators such as D-penicillamine and trientine. After successful initial treatment, options for maintenance treatment include a reduction in the dose of chelator or its substitution by zinc.

(g) Hemochromatosis
    Venesections of 500 mL are carried out weekly and are continued until the serum ferritin level falls into low normal range. Other endpoints have been the development of anemia and a reduction in the mean cellular volume (MCV).

(h) NASH
    NASH has no approved pharmacotherapy yet. The mainstay of treatment remains diet and lifestyle change to promote weight loss. But this is either unattainable or not maintainable in some patients; thus pharmacotherapy is warranted. Exercise, calorie reduction, and weight loss are first recommended. Only vitamin E and thiazolidines have the beneficial evidence in treatment of NASH.

6.7.2 Complication Treatment

(a) Hepatocellular carcinoma (HCC): The strategy of HCC treatment is based on liver function and tumor status. Treatments can be divided into "curative" including liver resection, liver transplantation, and local ablation (mainly radiofrequency ablation) or "palliative" including hepatic artery embolization, chemoembolization, radiotherapy, various chemotherapy regimens, and recently targeted agents sorafenib, regorafenib, and lenvatinib.

(b) Portal hypertension: Pharmacological therapy aims at decreasing portal pressure. Traditional nonselective beta-blockers include propranolol and nadolol decrease portal pressure by reducing portal vein inflow. Carvedilol and terlipressin are also used. As an endoscopic treatment, endoscopic variceal band ligation (EVL) is more effective and safer than endoscopic variceal sclerotherapy (Fig. 6.13). As intervention procedure, transjugular intrahepatic portosystemic shunt (TIPS) and balloon-occluded retrograde transvenous obliteration (BRTO) are considered for constructing a shunt connecting the high-pressure portal vein with a low-pressure systemic vein.

(c) Ascites: Therapy of ascites reduces clinical symptoms and improves quality of life. The spectrum of therapeutic intervention ranges from sodium restriction alone to diuretic use, therapeutic paracentesis, and, for the most severe groups, TIPS and eventually liver transplantation. For diuretics, spironolactone is administered alone or in combination with furosemide in refractory case. Tolvaptan, a new vasopressin V2 receptor antagonist, may be considered to add if available. Recently long-term albumin administration was proved to prolong overall survival in uncomplicated ascites patients by decreasing the rate of spontaneous bacterial peritonitis and hepatorenal syndrome [19].

(d) Spontaneous bacterial peritonitis (SBP): When complicated with SBP, 10–33% of patients will die during the hospital admission. Main predictors of mortality are the development of renal dysfunction and lack of response to initial empirical antibiotic therapy. The most common infecting organisms are Escherichia coli and Klebsiella. Antibiotics should be started empirically, and first-line drugs are third-generation cephalosporins, usually cefotaxime, administered intravenously. Amoxicillin-clavulanic acid is as effective as cefotaxime. Lack of response can be due to resistant bacteria or secondary bacterial peritonitis. Then extended spectrum antibiotics (carbapenems, piperacillin/tazobactam) should be used as initial empirical therapy. In a randomized study, the administration of intravenous albumin to patients with SBP treated with cefotaxime significantly reduced the incidence of renal impairment [20].

(e) Hepatorenal syndrome: Liver transplantation is the only definitive therapy for HRS, resulting in improved survival, though the opportunity is limited. As pharmacological treatment, vasoconstrictors plus intravenous albumin constitute the current mainstay therapy. Administration of vasoconstrictors (ornipressin, terlipressin, noradrenaline) for periods greater than 3 days is associated with significant increases of mean arterial pressure and decreased serum creatinine. The best evidence supports the use of terlipressin, a synthetic analogue of vasopressin. Alternative vasoconstrictive therapy is the use of intravenous noradrenaline infusion, which has been shown to be as effective as terlipressin.

(f) Hepatic encephalopathy: Patients with cirrhosis are unable to effectively store glycogen. Patients should avoid fasting for longer than 3–6 h during the day time. Branched-chain amino acids have a beneficial effect on hepatic encephalopathy by promoting ammonia detoxification, correcting the plasma amino acid imbalance, and reducing the brain influx of aromatic amino acids. There are additional benefits associated with consumption of a late evening snack. The nonabsorbable disaccharide lactulose or lactitol is used widely as first-line treatment for hepatic encephalopa-

thy. This disaccharide has several beneficial effects: a laxative effect, bacterial uptake of ammonia, reduction of intestinal ammonia production, and improving gut microbiome. Antibiotics can be also used selectively to eliminate urease-producing organisms from the intestinal tract, thereby reducing the production of ammonia. Neomycin and rifaximin are poorly absorbed antibiotics and are used to treat hepatic encephalopathy. L-ornithine L-aspartate promotes hepatic removal of ammonia by stimulating residual hepatic urea cycle activity and by promoting glutamine synthesis, particularly in skeletal muscle.

6.8 Reversibility

It is widely believed that cirrhosis is an irreversible process that leads ultimately to liver failure. However, it has recently been reported that upon cessation of the injurious process, cirrhosis may reverse or at least improve histologically [17, 18]. Dense micronodular cirrhosis can undergo remodeling to a more attenuated, macronodular pattern, and fibrous septa is shown to become attenuated and then discontinued. Incomplete septal cirrhosis, a previously obscure entity, is now recognized as an indication of regression in fibrosis and a reversal of cirrhosis [21]. Histological clues of regression include delicate perforated septa, isolated thick collagen fibers, delicate periportal fibrosis spikes, portal tracts remnants, hepatic vein remnants, minute regenerative nodules, and aberrant parenchymal veins—so-called hepatic repair complex (Fig. 6.14). Despite the lack of significant fibrosis, patients with regressed cirrhosis may have portal hypertension. It has been advocated that the use of the word

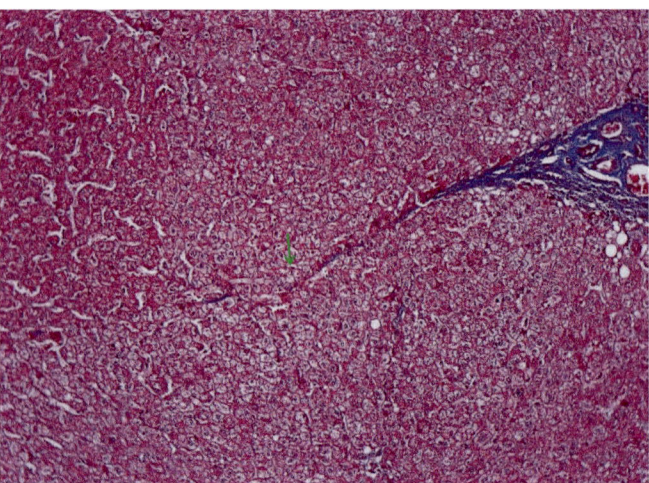

Fig. 6.14 Incomplete septal cirrhosis (cirrhosis with regressing fibrosis). Trichrome stain highlights a slender fibrous septum with perforation (arrow)

"cirrhosis" should be discontinued because of its connotation and that these patients labeled as having "chronic liver disease of advanced stage" should be provided treatment on the basis of clinicopathologic correlation of all available findings with the hope of disease regression [22].

Acknowledgment The authors thank Prof. Hiroko Iijima for her data of FibroScan and 2D shear wave elastography.

References

1. Goodman ZD. Chapter 6 Hepatic histopathology. In: Schiff ER, Maddrey WC, Reddy KR, editors. Shiff's disease of the liver. 12th ed. Hoboken: Wiley Balckwell; 2017. p. 135–99.
2. Infante-Rivard C, Esnaola S, Villeneuve JP. Clinical and statistical validity of conventional prognostic factors in predicting short-term survival among cirrhosis. Hepatology. 1987;7:660–4.
3. Kamath PS, Weisner RH, Malinchoc M, Kremers W, Therneau TM, Kosberg CL, et al. A model to predict survival in patients with end-stage liver disease. Hepatology. 2001;33:464–70.
4. Aoyagi Y, Nishiguchi S, Dougyou K, Tokumoto Y, Onji M. Etiology of liver cirrhosis in Japan. In: Onji M, editor. 2008 Etiology of liver cirrhosis. Tokyo: Chugai-igakusha; 2008.
5. Ohkawa K, Hayashi N, Yuki N, Kasahara A, Oshita M, Mochizuki K, et al. Disease stage of chronic hepatitis C assessed by both peritoneoscopic and histologic findings and its relationship with response to interferon therapy. Gastrointest Endosc. 1997;45:168–75.
6. Onji M, Yamashita Y, Kato T, Bandou H, Horiike N, Ohta Y. Laparoscopic histopathological analysis of "gentle undulation" findings observed in patients with primary biliary cirrhosis. Endoscopy. 1987;19:17–9.
7. Petrukhin K, Lutsenko S, Chemov I, Ross BM, Kaplan JH, Gillam TC. Characterization of the Wilson disease gene encoding a P-type copper transporting ATPase: genomic organization, alternative splicing, and structure/function predictions. Hum Mol Genet. 1994;3:1647–56.
8. Sakaida I, Kawaguchi K, Kimura T, Tamura F, Okita K. D-Penicillamine improved laparoscopic and histological findings of the liver in a patient with Wilson's disease: 3-year follow-up after diagnosis of Coombs-negative hemolytic anemia of Wilson's disease. J Gastroenterol. 2005;40:646–51.
9. Bhargawa DK, Arova A, Dasarathy AS. Laparoscopic features of the Budd-Chiari syndrome. Endoscopy. 1991;23:259–61.
10. Bansal MB, Friedman SL. Chapter6. Hepatic fibrogenesis. In: Dooley JS, Lok AS, Garcia-Tsao G, Pinzani M, editors. Sherlock's diseases of the liver and biliary system. 13th ed. Hoboken: Willey Blackwell; 2018. p. 82–92.
11. McCormick PA, Jalan R. Chapter 8. Hepatic cirrhosis. In: Dooley JS, Lok AS, Garcia-Tsao G, Pinzani M, editors. Sherlock's diseases of the liver and biliary system. 13th ed. Hoboken: Willey Blackwell; 2018. p. 107–26.
12. Shirabe K, Bekki Y, Gantumur D, Araki K, Ishii N, Kuno A, et al. Mac-2 binding protein glycan isomer (M2BPGi) is a new serum biomarker for assessing liver fibrosis: more than a biomarker of liver fibrosis. J Gastroenterol. 2018;53:819–26.
13. Wai CT, Greenson JK, Fontana RJ, et al. A simple noninvasive index can predict both significant fibrosis and cirrhosis in patients with chronic hepatitis C. Hepatology. 2003;38:518–26.
14. Sterling RK, Lissen E, Clumeck N, et al. Development of a simple noninvasive index to predict significant fibrosis in patients with HIV/HCV coinfection. Hepatology. 2006;43:1317–25.
15. European Association for the Study of the Liver. EASL-ALEH clinical practice guidelines: non-invasive tests for evaluation of liver disease severity and prognosis. J Hepatol. 2015;63:237–64.
16. Ikeda K, Saitoh S, Koida I, et al. A multivariate analysis of risk factors for hepatocellular carcinogenesis: a prospective observation of 795 patients with viral and alcoholic cirrhosis. Hepatology. 1993;18:47–53.
17. Marcellin P, Gane E, Buti M, et al. Regression of cirrhosis during treatment of with tenofovir disoproxil fumarate for chronic hepatitis B: a-5-year open label follow-up study. Lancet. 2013;381:468–75.
18. Akhtar E, Manne V, Saab S. Cirrhosis regression in hepatitis C patients with sustained virological response after antiviral therapy: a meta-analysis. Liver Int. 2015;35:30–6.
19. Caraceni P, Riggio O, Angeli P, Alessandria C, et al. Long-term albumin administration in decompensated cirrhosis (ANSWER): an open-label randomized trial. Lancet. 2018;391:2417–29.
20. Sort P, Navasa M, Arroyo, et al. Effect of intravenous albumin on renal impairment and mortality in patients with cirrhosis and spontaneous bacterial peritonitis. N Engl J Med. 1999;341:403–9.
21. Wanless I, Nakashima E, Sherman M. Regression of human cirrhosis. Morphologic features and the genesis of incomplete septal cirrhosis. Arch Pathol Lab Med. 2000;124:1599–607.
22. Hytiroglou P, Snover DC, Alves V, et al. Beyond "cirrhosis": a proposal from the International Liver Pathology Study Group. Am J Clin Pathol. 2012;137:5–9.

Alcoholic Liver Disease and Nonalcoholic Fatty Liver Disease/Nonalcoholic Steatohepatitis

7

Etsuko Hashimoto, Masaki Iwai, and Arief A. Suriawinata

Contents

7.1   Alcoholic Liver Disease (ALD)

Alcoholic liver disease (ALD) has been reported worldwide with a prevalence of 0–20% and remains one of the major causes of liver disease. The spectrum of ALD includes fatty liver, alcoholic hepatitis, alcoholic fibrosis, and cirrhosis. Hepatocellular carcinoma may also develop, especially in patients with cirrhosis. Histologically, ALD shows simple steatosis and steatohepatitis and eventually progresses to cirrhosis. These clinical and histological features overlap.

The diagnosis of ALD is based on a history of significant alcohol consumption and clinical evidence of liver disease, supported by laboratory abnormalities [1–3]. Significant total and daily ethanol intake is the most important risk factor for the development of ALD. Furthermore, the type of alcohol consumed and the drinking pattern (binge drinking), gender, ethnicity, and associated comorbidities, such as chronic viral hepatitis, obesity, and iron overload, may also have an influence. Epidemiological studies have shown that ALD can occur when the daily alcohol consumption exceeds 20 g in women and 30 g in men; fatty liver develops in about 90% of individuals who drink more than 60 g/day of alcohol. Risk of alcoholic fibrosis, cirrhosis, or alcoholic hepatitis increases markedly in patients with ALD who drink >40 g of alcohol/day for more than 5 years and even more so with >60 g/day.

There is no specific test for ALD. Laboratory data show elevation of aminotransferases, with the ratio of AST to ALT ≥ 2, and elevation of GGT induced by ethanol. Macrocytosis with a mean corpuscular volume (MCV) > 100 fL occurs due to the direct effect of alcohol on bone marrow or due to folate deficiency in malnutrition. Neutrophilic leukocytosis may result from elevation of cytokines in alcoholic hepatitis. Imaging modalities show fatty change and mild to severe enlargement of the liver, with or without evidence of cirrhosis. Liver biopsy is indicated if there are atypical clinical features and to rule out other chronic liver diseases. For patients with cirrhosis, α-fetoprotein and protein induced by vitamin K absence/antagonist-II (PIVKA-II) levels and liver ultrasonography should be done every 4 months to screen for hepatocellular carcinoma. The levels of PIVKA-II may increase in ALD patients without hepatocellular carcinoma, as a result of vitamin K deficiency in malnutrition or prolonged cholestasis.

Alcoholic fatty liver can result in an accumulation of triglyceride in the hepatocytes. Patients with alcoholic fatty liver are asymptomatic, and steatosis disappears after 2–6 weeks of abstinence. Continued significant alcohol consumption increases the risk of progression to alcoholic hepatitis, alcoholic fibrosis, and cirrhosis. Alcoholic

E. Hashimoto, MD, PhD (✉)
Tokyo, Japan
e-mail: drs-hashimoto@mti.biglobe.ne.jp

M. Iwai, MD, PhD
Kyoto, Japan

A. A. Suriawinata, MD
New Hampshire, USA

E. Hashimoto et al. (eds.), *Diagnosis of Liver Disease*, https://doi.org/10.1007/978-981-13-6806-6_7

hepatitis can occur in patients with ALD after several days of significant alcohol abuse. Severity of alcoholic hepatitis ranges from mild to life-threatening, and alcoholic hepatitis has a high risk of progression to cirrhosis. Symptoms may include fever, fatigue, right upper abdominal pain, abdominal distension, and jaundice. With abstinence, mild cases can be self-limited, but severe cases can progress to hepatic failure, disseminated intravascular coagulation, and sepsis, with a high risk of death. Severe cases should be treated aggressively with enteral nutritional therapy, and steroids or anticytokine therapy might be considered. Patients with decompensated cirrhosis have generalized fatigue, jaundice, encephalopathy, and features of portal hypertension, such as ascites, edema, or gastrointestinal varices.

The characteristic features of liver histology are macrovesicular steatosis, neutrophilic infiltrates, ballooning degeneration, giant mitochondria, Mallory-Denk bodies, perivenular fibrosis, pericellular fibrosis, central hyaline sclerosis, and stellate-shaped portal fibrosis [4–6]. The absence of steatosis, in the presence of other features, does not rule out the diagnosis of ALD.

Alcoholic foamy degeneration, which shows mainly microvesicular steatosis and minimal inflammation, has been previously described in severe liver injury. However, patients with benign prognosis have also been reported. There may be a purely degenerative process of steatosis. Mallory-Denk bodies or alcoholic hyaline are characteristic features of alcoholic hepatitis. Mallory-Denk bodies are clumps or strands of intermediate filaments of the hepatocyte cytoskeleton that are positive for cytokeratins 8 and 18, ubiquitin, and p62. Mallory-Denk bodies [4] are found in biopsies of heavy drinkers and disappear after abstinence. Neutrophils typically surround hepatocytes with Mallory-Denk bodies.

The pattern of early fibrosis in alcoholic liver disease is pericellular or perisinusoidal fibrosis, commonly referred to as "chicken wire" fibrosis, which begins in the centrilobular areas (zone 3). As the fibrosis progresses, occlusion of central hepatic venules occur, referred to as central hyaline sclerosis. Patients with central hyaline sclerosis can present with clinical features of portal hypertension in the absence of cirrhosis. Stellate-shaped portal and periportal fibrosis develops later in the progression of the disease, followed by central-to-central, central-to-portal, and portal-to-portal thin bridging fibrosis. Central hyaline sclerosis is not a histologic feature of nonalcoholic steatohepatitis. Cirrhosis in patients who are actively drinking is usually the micronodular type, and pericellular or perisinusoidal fibrosis can be gradually obscured by expansion of fibrosis and increasing parenchymal loss. Mild to moderate iron deposition is common in

ALD as a result of increased intestinal absorption, upregulation of transferrin receptor, hemolysis, or iron-containing alcoholic beverages.

Case 7.1

A 32-year-old housewife was admitted to our hospital due to abdominal distension. She denied alcoholism, but her family confirmed that she drank a half bottle of whisky (700 ml) daily for 3 years. Her laboratory data included T.Bil 2.0 mg/dL, D.Bil 1.2 mg/dl, AST 340 IU/L, ALT 99 IU/L, GGT 2415 IU/L, WBC 10,200/mm³, Plats 22.4 × 10⁴/μL prothrombin time (PT) 12.1 sec, and elevated CRP. Abdominal ultrasonography showed a large bright liver, increased hepatorenal contrast, deep attenuation, and vascular blurring (Fig. 7.1). Computed tomography (CT) with and without contrast enhancement showed enlargement of the liver, decrease of hepatic attenuation, and a decreased liver-to-spleen attenuation ratio (Fig. 7.2). Peritoneoscopy showed a smoothly enlarged, yellowish liver. Acinar markings were blurred, and the peripheral portal veins were dilated (Fig. 7.3). Liver biopsy revealed broad central fibrosis, central hyaline sclerosis, perisinusoidal fibrosis, and macrovesicular steatosis (Fig. 7.4). Electron microscopy revealed large fat droplets, a vesicular smooth-surfaced endoplasmic reticulum, distorted mitochondrial cristae, and nuclei com-

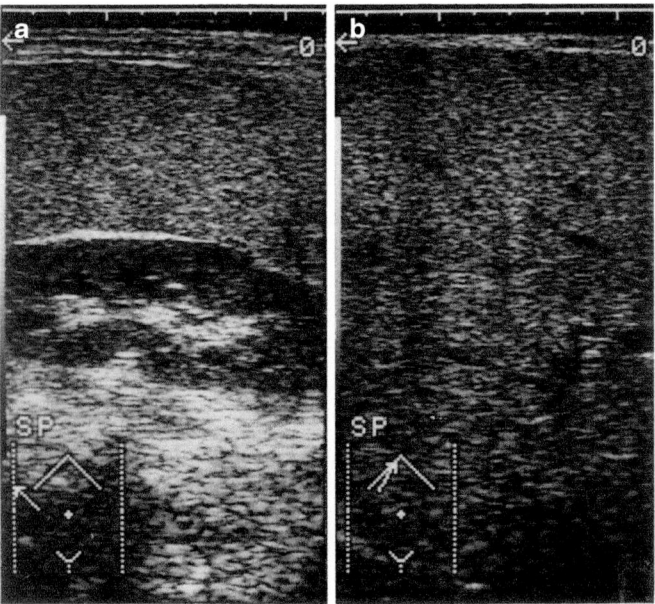

Fig. 7.1 Ultrasonographic features of the liver with alcoholic injury. (**a**) There is a different echo density between the liver and kidney, and the liver is bright. (**b**) Vision of intrahepatic vessels are blurred. (Reuse of Iwai M, et al. Alcoholic hepatitis in a kitchen drinker. J Kyoto Pref Univ Med 1991; 100: 149–157, with permission of its chief editor)

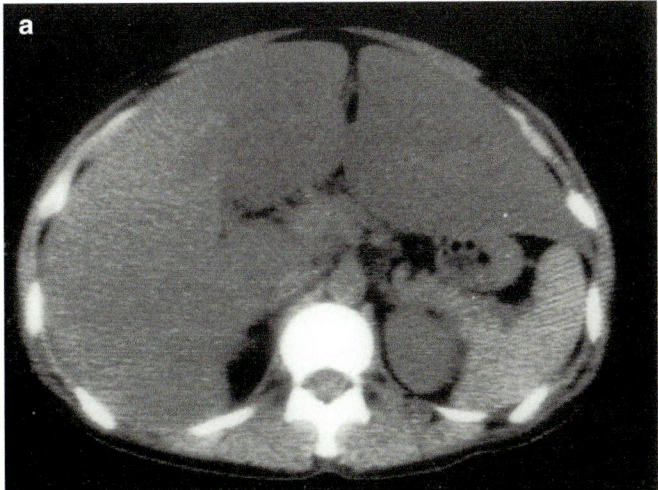

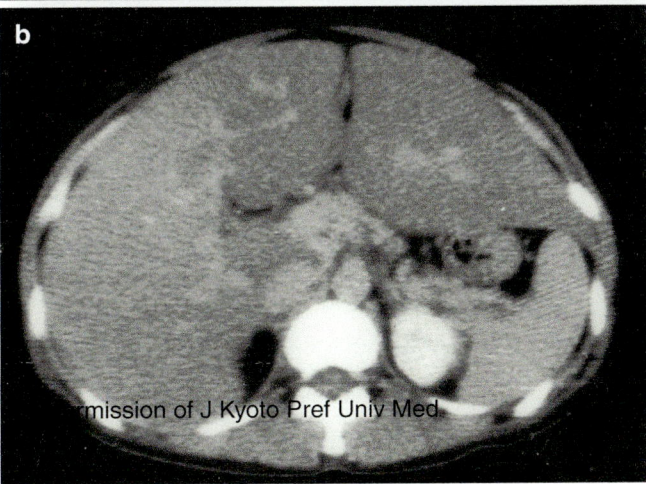

Fig. 7.2 CT in alcoholic liver injury. (**a**) CT without contrast medium shows heterogenous density in the liver, and density in the liver is lower than that in the spleen. (**b**) CT with contrast medium shows low density in the inner area of the right lobe and left lobe, and intrahepatic portal veins are enhanced (Reuse of Iwai M, et al. Alcoholic hepatitis in a kitchen drinker. J Kyoto Pref Univ Med 1991; 100: 149–157, with permission of its chief editor)

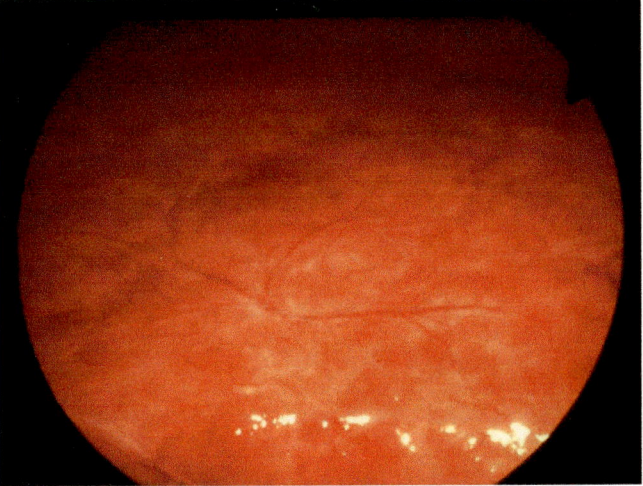

Fig. 7.3 Peritoneoscopic findings of the liver with alcoholic injury. Peritoneoscopy shows an enlarged yellow liver, and acinus markings are blurred on the liver surface with dilation of peripheral portal veins. (Reuse of Iwai M, et al. Alcoholic hepatitis in a kitchen drinker. J Kyoto Pref Univ Med 1991; 100: 149–157, with permission of its chief editor)

other alcoholic injury, such as depression, cardiomyopathy, chronic pancreatitis, and alcoholic neurotoxicity. Strict abstinence must be advised. Only abstinence improves the outcome of ALD.

Case 7.2

A 45-year-old man showed elevation of transaminases and GGT for 3 years. He had a history of heavy drinking for 25 years. He presented to our clinic complaining of abdominal fullness, jaundice, nausea, and diarrhea. His laboratory data showed TBIL 14.15 mg/dL, AST 234 IU/L, ALT 55 IU/L, ALP 295 IU/L, GGT 119 IU/L, WBC 13,000/mm^3, platelets (PLT) 6.2×10^4/μL, PT 19.1 s, and immunoglobulin A (IgA) 1139 mg/dL. Peritoneoscopy showed ascites and a green and yellow liver with fine nodule formation (Fig. 7.5). Liver biopsy specimens showed nodular formation with pericellular fibrosis and neutrophilic infiltrates. Residual hepatocytes showed ballooning degeneration. With abstinence and disappearance of ascites and jaundice, liver function tests gradually returned to normal over 6 months. However, 15 years later, he died of liver failure after bleeding from esophageal varices. In this patient, long-term alcohol intake from age of 20- to 45-year-old induced cirrhosis. Even though he stopped drinking after diagnosis of cirrhosis, and ALT and AST returned to normal, his portal hypertension gradually deteriorated accompanied by recurrent bleeding from esophageal varices, which eventually caused his death from liver failure.

pressed to the periphery of the hepatocytes by fat droplet; there were also giant mitochondria and a dilated smooth-surfaced endoplasmic reticulum, and neutrophilic infiltration was seen in the vicinity of damaged hepatocytes (Fig. 7.4). A repeat liver biopsy on the second admission within 6 months showed cirrhosis caused by central hyaline sclerosis. On the third admission after repeated drinking, the patient presented with hepatic failure. It is well known alcoholic hepatitis with histological hyaline sclerosis progresses rapidly to cirrhosis. Denial of alcohol abuse is very common, especially in female patients. It is also important for physicians to be aware of

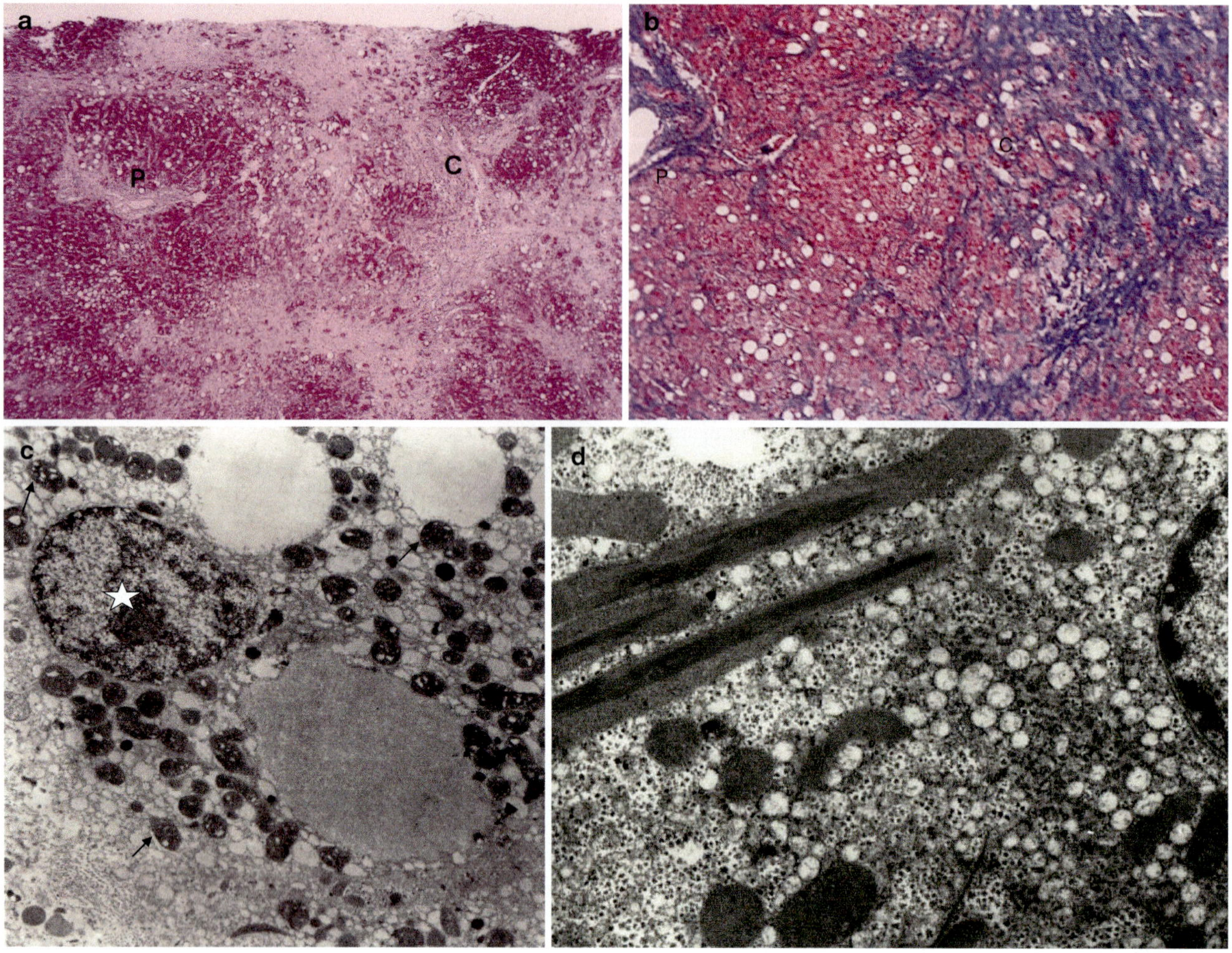

Fig. 7.4 Alcoholic liver injury. (**a**) PAS staining of the liver tissue shows a broad collapse in the central area, and there are residual hepatocytes containing macrovesicular droplets. *P* portal tract, *C* central vein. (Reuse of Iwai M, et al. Alcoholic hepatitis in a kitchen drinker. J Kyoto Pref Univ Med 1991; 100: 149–157, with permission of its chief editor). (**b**) Masson trichrome staining reveals broad fibrosis with occlusion of the central vein (central hyaline necrosis) and pericellular fibrosis, and the stellate fibrosis is seen in the portal tract. *P* portal tract, *C* central vein

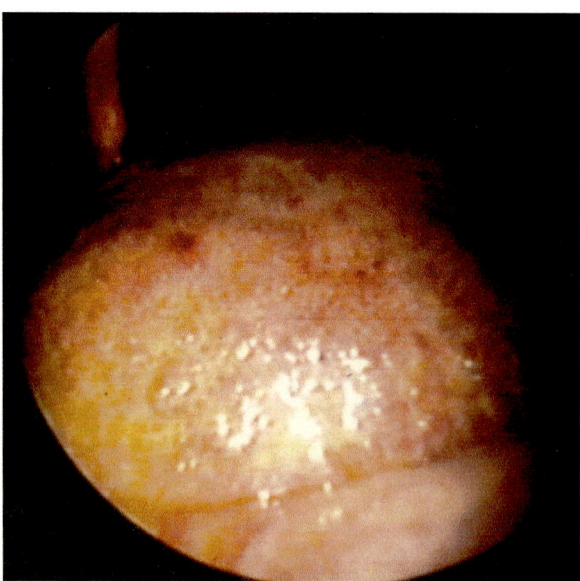

Fig. 7.5 Peritoneoscopic findings of the liver. Peritoneo-scopy shows a green and yellow liver with micronodular formation

Abstinence is the only therapeutic intervention for patients with ALD; however, when cirrhosis is established, it may be too late for complete recovery.

Case 7.3

A 52-year-old heavy drinker had edema and abdominal fullness, and his laboratory tests showed TBIL 5.3 mg/dL, AST 201 IU/L, ALT 91 IU/L, GGT 284 IU/L, CRP 10.8 mg/dL, and WBC 19,800/mm³. Peritoneoscopy showed an enlarged yellow liver, with dilated peripheral portal veins. Liver biopsy showed Mallory-Denk bodies in ballooned hepatocytes with pericellular fibrosis (Figs. 7.6 and 7.7). He stopped drinking for 6 months, but started drinking again, and later developed cirrhosis.

Abstinence is the only treatment for ALD patients. Appropriate treatment should be provided by physicians, psychologist, nurses, psychotherapists, and family members.

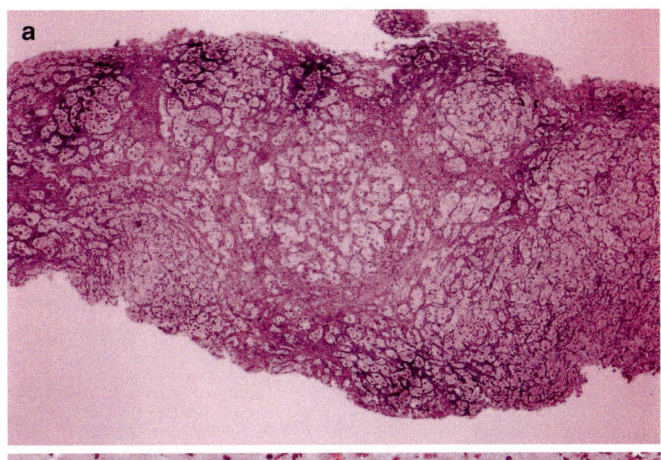

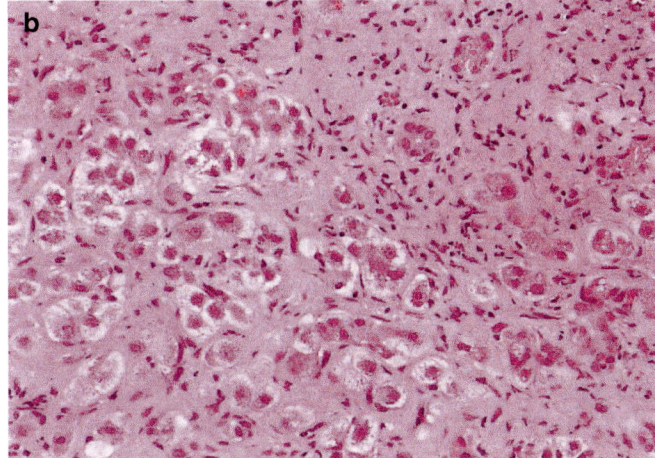

Fig. 7.6 Alcoholic liver injury. (**a**) Reticulum fiber staining shows pseudolobular formation with marked pericellular fibrosis. (**b**) Ballooning hepatocytes are surrounded by fibrosis and infiltration of neutrophils is noted. Hematoxylin-eosin staining

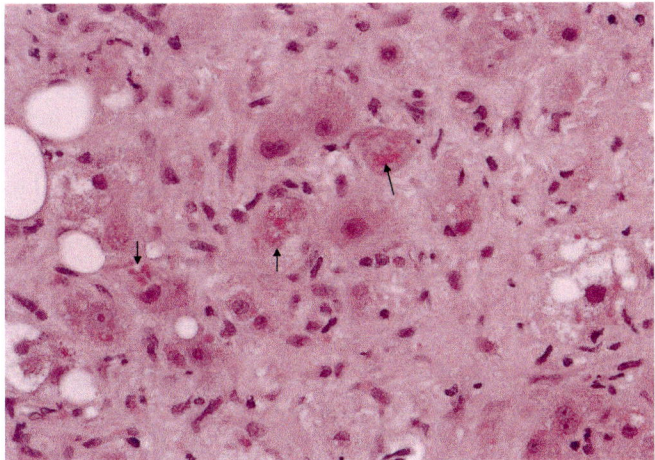

Fig. 7.7 Alcoholic liver injury. Ballooning hepatocytes contain Mallory Denk bodies (arrow) and some hepatocytes contain fat droplets and neutrophilic leukocytes are scatteredly seen. Hematoxylin-eosin staining

7.2 Nonalcoholic Fatty Liver Disease/Nonalcoholic Steatohepatitis

Changes in diet and lifestyle have resulted in a dramatic increase in obesity and metabolic syndrome worldwide. Nonalcoholic fatty liver disease (NAFLD) is a hepatic manifestation of metabolic syndrome, and it also has a causative role in it. Currently NAFLD is the most common chronic liver disease. A meta-analysis of a very large population (8,515,431 subjects from 22 countries) by Younossi et al. [7] showed that the global prevalence of NAFLD is 25.24% (95% confidence interval, 22.10–28.65), with the highest prevalence in the Middle East, followed by South America and Asia. The higher prevalence of NAFLD in these geographic areas can be explained by a higher prevalence of obesity and in addition to genetic factors. A single nucleotide polymorphism, patatin-like phospholipase 3 rs738409 (PNPLA3), is known to be the most important risk allele for the onset and progression of NAFLD; G allele is the risk factor [8]. This risk allele, of PNPLA3, is the most common in Hispanics, who are most susceptible to NAFLD, followed by Asians.

NAFLD consists of two clinical entities, which are known, i.e., nonalcoholic fatty liver (NAFL) and nonalcoholic steatohepatitis (NASH) [9–12]. NAFL is generally a benign, nonprogressive clinical entity, while NASH can progress to cirrhosis or even hepatocellular carcinoma. NASH is found in 10–20% of patients with NAFLD. Diagnosis of NAFLD is based on the following: (1) nonalcoholic, alcoholic liver disease that can occur when daily alcohol consumption exceeds 20 g in women or 30 g in men (thus "nonalcoholic" indicates lower levels of these alcohol consumptions), (2) hepatic steatosis diagnosed by histology or imaging modalities, and (3) appropriate exclusion of other liver diseases. NASH has emerged as a distinct clinicopathological concept, but given the lack of surrogate markers for making a diagnosis, histology is still considered the "gold standard" for a definitive diagnosis. NASH is defined as the presence of hepatic steatosis, inflammation, and hepatocyte injury (ballooning degeneration) with or without fibrosis (Figs. 7.8 and 7.9). NAFL encompasses steatosis alone or steatosis with inflammation. Most practice guidelines for diagnosis and management of NAFLD have proposed that NAFLD should only be used to define only fatty disorders of the liver based on insulin resistance, with exclusion of other causes of hepatic steatosis/steatohepatitis, such as Wilson's disease, starvation, parenteral nutrition, and drug-induced liver injury, etc. Ultrasonography is the preferred first-line diagnostic procedure for diagnosing steatosis.

The definition of NAFLD is problematic. Sensitivity to alcoholic liver injury varies; then there is no clear consensus regarding the threshold of alcohol intake to that defines "nonalcoholic."

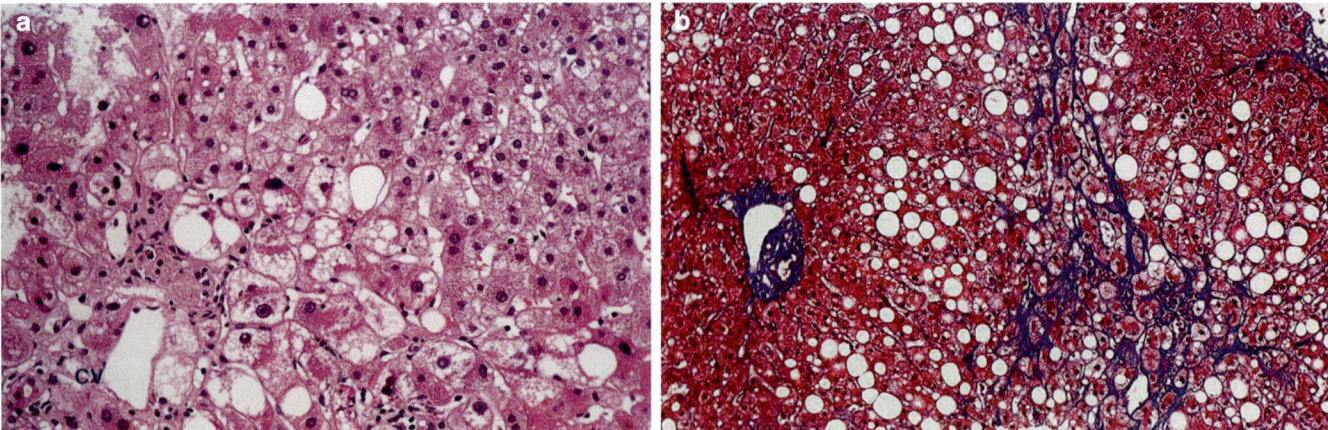

Fig. 7.8 (**a**) Liver biopsy shows macrovesicular steatosis, inflammatory infiltrates, and ballooning degeneration. There are normal-sized hepatocytes in the upper right corner, while ballooning of hepatocytes, indicating necrotic change, can be seen on the left side. (Hematoxylin-eosin stain). (**b**) Mallory staining for fibrosis shows prominent pericellular fibrosis in zone 3, while portal fibrosis is mild. In NASH, fibrosis extends from around central veins

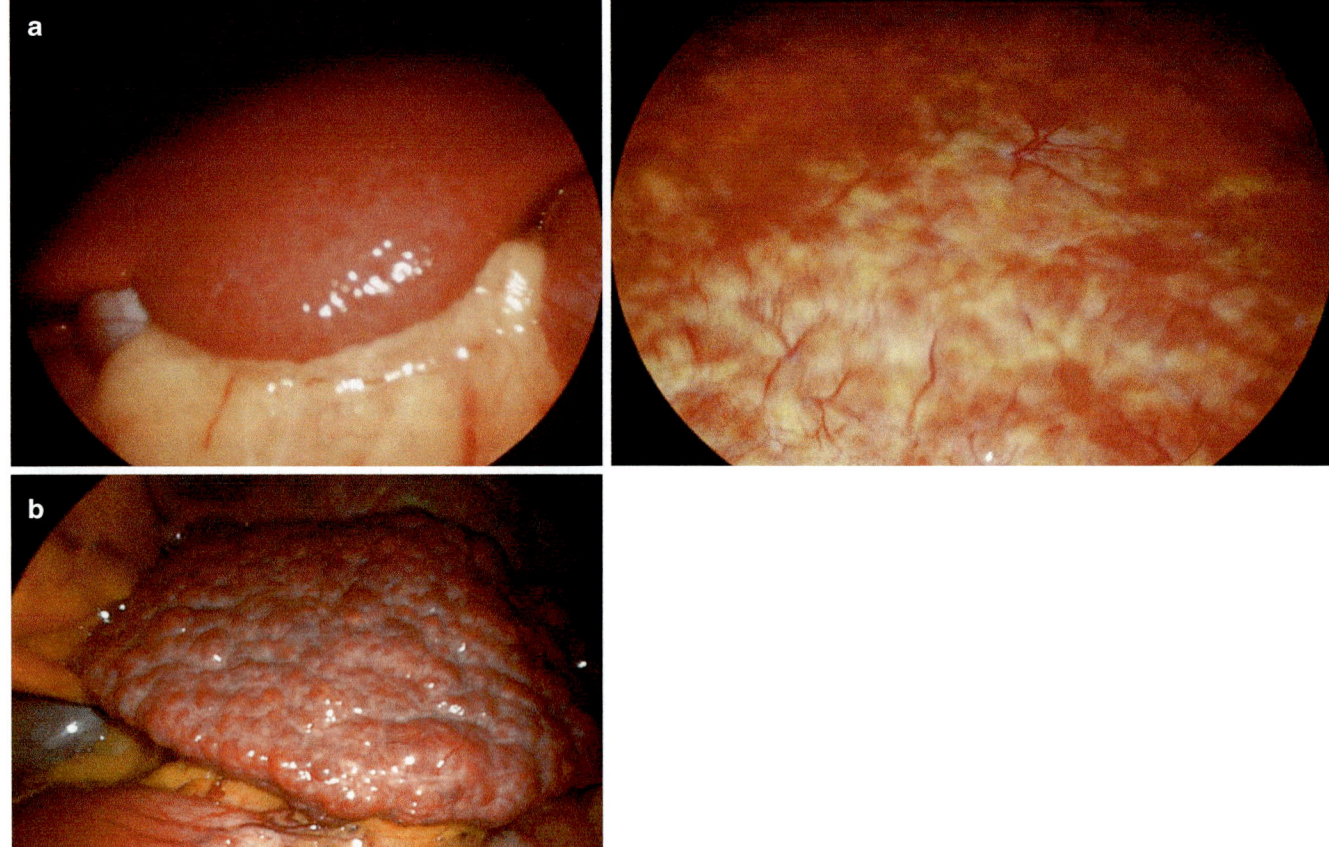

Fig. 7.9 (**a**) Peritoneoscopy shows an enlarged yellow liver with smooth surface; fatty liver. (**b**) Liver surface shows micronodular formation in a cirrhotic stage

Moreover, it is difficult to determine the exact amount of alcohol intake, and we should also consider the pattern of drinking, including binge drinking. Obesity and excess alcohol intake frequently occur in combination. The diagnostic definition and

ability of steatosis are different between liver pathology and imaging modalities; histologically, the minimum threshold for steatosis is the finding of fat droplets in 5% of hepatocytes; however, imaging modalities can identify steatosis when more than

10% of hepatocytes have fat droplets. Sampling error is inevitable in liver biopsy. There is no clear consensus regarding the histological definition of NASH. The interpretation of histology is subjective. The characteristic features of NASH disappear when cirrhosis is advanced (i.e., burned-out NASH). Lastly, contrary to current dogma, recent studies have reported that a substantial proportion of NAFL patients can progress to NASH [13]. Accordingly, Dufour commented in an editorial: "In hepatology, the worst name is NASH. Time to Abandon NASH?" [14].

There are four important pathological classifications of NAFLD/NASH: Matteoni's classification, Brunt's classification, the NAFLD activity score (NAS), the fatty liver inhibition of progression (FLIP) algorithm, and the steatosis, activity, and fibrosis (SAF) score [15–21].

In 1999, Matteoni et al. [17] described a classification that distinguished between NASH and non-NASH based on the relationship between histological characteristics and outcomes. According to their classification, type 1, steatosis alone, and type 2, steatosis with lobular inflammation, are considered non-NASH; type 3, steatosis with ballooning degeneration, and type 4, which is a type 3 plus either Mallory-Denk bodies or fibrosis, are classified as NASH. Brunt et al. [18] proposed a semiquantitative grading and staging system for NASH. Grading consists of steatosis, inflammation, and ballooning degeneration, while staging is based on fibrosis. This classification is only applicable to NASH. In 2005, the NASH Clinical Research Network Pathology Committee developed and validated a histological score for NAFLD based on Brunt's classification [19]. The NAFLD activity score (NAS) addresses the full spectrum of NAFLD and is applicable to both adult and pediatric patients. The score is determined by the unweighted sum of the scores for steatosis (0–3), lobular inflammation (0–3), and ballooning degeneration (0–2). A score ≥ 5 is diagnostic of NASH, a score of less than 3 is non-NASH, and scores of 3 or 4 are borderlines. Concerning fibrosis, stage 1 indicates perisinusoidal fibrosis in zone 3 (perivenular area), either delicate, 1A, or dense, 1B; detection of portal fibrosis without perisinusoidal fibrosis is defined as 1C (an atypical feature in pediatric and morbidly obese patients). Stage 2 is characterized by perisinusoidal and portal/periportal fibrosis. Stage 3 is defined as bridging fibrosis, and stage 4 is cirrhosis. The authors recommended the NAS system for use in research and not as a diagnostic tool for NASH. The recently reported FLIP algorithm and SAF score increase observer agreement [20, 21]. The FLIP algorithm is based on evaluation of steatosis, hepatocellular ballooning, and lobular inflammation to distinguish between normal liver, NAFLD, and NASH. The semiquantitative SAF score evaluates steatosis (S), activity (A), and fibrosis (F). The activity score consists of ballooning degeneration and lobular inflammation. It is important to note that steatosis does not include activity, but this is reported separately in the SAF score, as the degree of steatosis is not a histological marker of ongoing liver damage, i.e., necroinflammatory changes. Fibrosis staging basically relies on the Kleiner classification [19]. Based on the distinctive histological pattern, a specific histological score (Pediatric NAFLD Histological Score, PNHS) has been validated for better classification of children with/without NASH.

NAFLD/NASH patients are usually asymptomatic until the stage of decompensated cirrhosis. Blood chemistry shows mild elevation of transaminases; however substantial numbers of patients have normal levels of transaminases. There has been considerable interest in the development of biochemical markers and scoring systems for diagnosing NASH or fibrosis stages. There are no practically useful surrogate markers for diagnosing NASH. However, scoring systems for fibrosis, the NAFLD fibrosis scoring system and FIB-4 index, as well as transient elastography, are acceptable noninvasive procedures for evaluation of fibrosis stages. Fibrosis is the most important prognostic factor in NAFLD/NASH and is strongly correlated with liver-related outcomes and mortality [22].

NAFLD is associated with an increase in the standardized mortality ratio compared with the general population due to an increased liver- and cardiovascular-related mortality rate. The most common causes of death in patients with NAFLD are cardiovascular disease or malignancy. Overall, NAFLD appears to be slowly progressive, with liver-related morbidity and mortality occurring in a small number of patients. However, patients with cirrhotic NASH/NAFLD showed a survival rate similar to that of patients with cirrhosis caused by hepatitis C virus, although the rate of development of hepatocellular carcinoma was lower (5-year development rate, about 10%; 5-year survival rate, 70–80%) [23–25]. Patients with NAFLD/NASH cirrhosis should be screened for gastroesophageal varices and development of hepatocellular carcinoma.

The mainstays of prevention and treatment of NAFLD/NASH include dietary restriction and exercise. Weight reduction of 3–5% is associated with improved steatosis; reductions of 5–7% are necessary for decreased inflammation; with 7–10%, individuals may experience NAFLD/NASH remission and regression of fibrosis [26]. However, only 30–40% of NAFLD/NASH patients succeed in weight loss. Currently, vitamin E and thiazolidinedione derivatives are the most evidence-based therapeutic options, although the clinical evidence for long-term efficacy and safety is limited. Bariatric surgery may be considered in morbidly obese NASH patients who cannot reduce weight. End-stage cirrhotic NAFLD/NASH is an indication for liver transplantation. Patients with NAFLD/NASH have a high prevalence of cardiovascular complication and diabetes, and clinicians should be aware of these complications.

Case 7.4

Hematemesis was developed in a 67-year-old woman with BMI 21.6% due to rupture of esophageal varices [27]. She had no history of alcohol intake and lifestyle-related disease. Serum examination showed TBil 1.0 mg/dl, AST 34 IU/l, ALT 29 IU/l, GGT 29 IU/l, HbA1c 6.0%, Hb 12.0 g/dl, Plats 5.9 × 10^4/mm^3, and PT 71.8%. HBsAg and HCV Ab were negative. She was urgently rescued by endoscopic sclerotherapy. Peritoneoscopy showed an enlarged yellow liver with irregular surface. Her liver biopsy showed moderate steatosis, inflammation, and ballooning degeneration; she was diagnosed as having NASH (Fig. 7.10a,b). Two years later hepato-

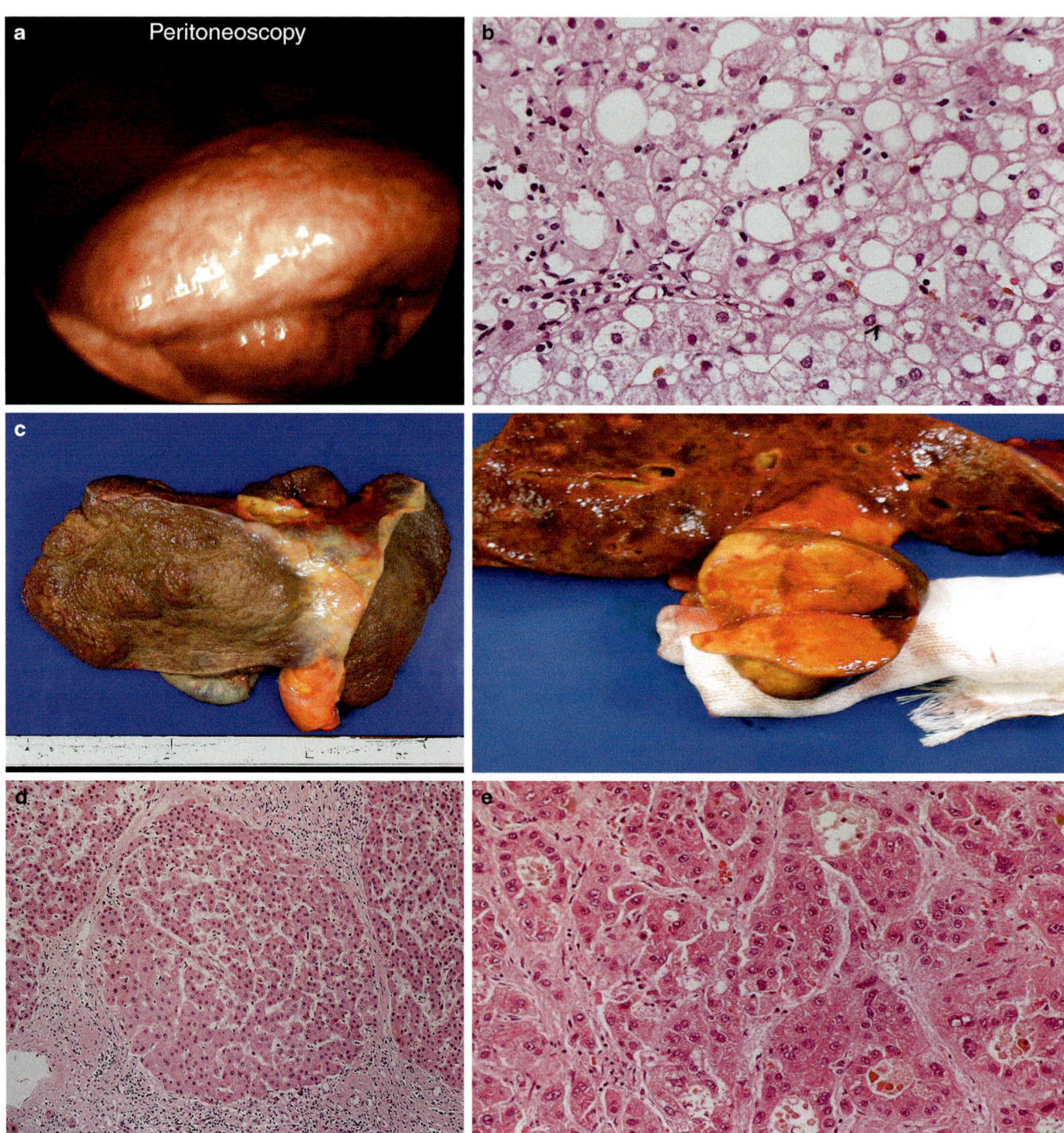

Fig. 7.10 (**a**) Peritoneoscopy showed an enlarged yellow liver with irregular surface. (**b**) Her liver biopsy showed severe steatosis with moderate inflammatory changes and ballooning degeneration. (Hematoxylin-eosin stain). (**c**) Cirrhotic liver with hepatocellular carcinoma (autopsy). (**d**) Noncancerous lesions showed cirrhosis without steatosis; burned-out NASH. (Hematoxylin-eosin stain). (**e**) The tumor showed moderately differentiated hepatocellular carcinoma with trabecular type. (Hematoxylin-eosin stain)

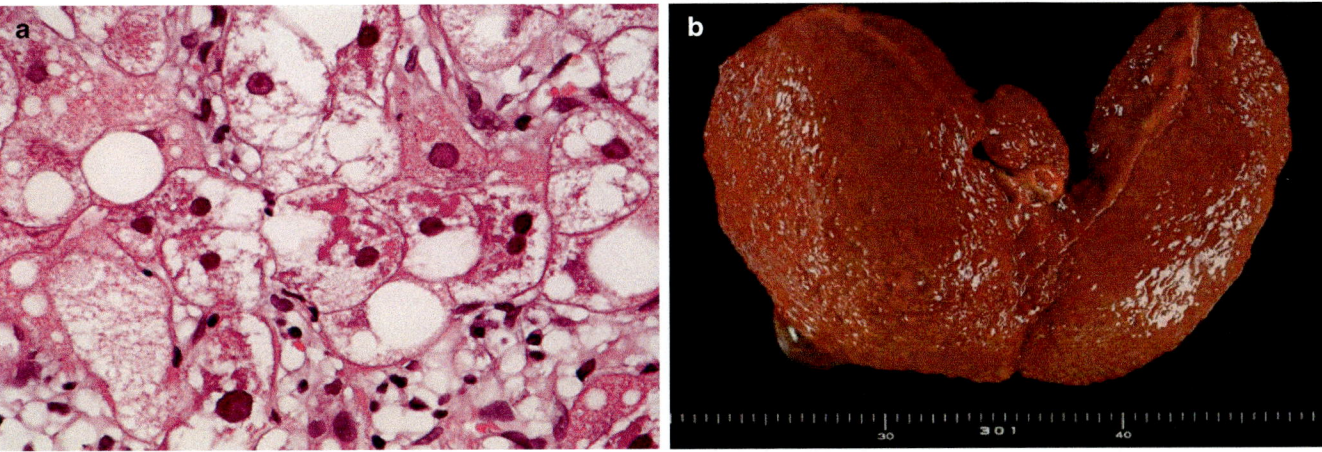

Fig. 7.11 (**a**) The liver biopsy showed macrovesicular steatosis with ballooning hepatocyte containing Mallory-Denk hyaline. (Hematoxylin-eosin stain). (**b**) His enlarged liver showed micronodular cirrhosis. (Autopsy)

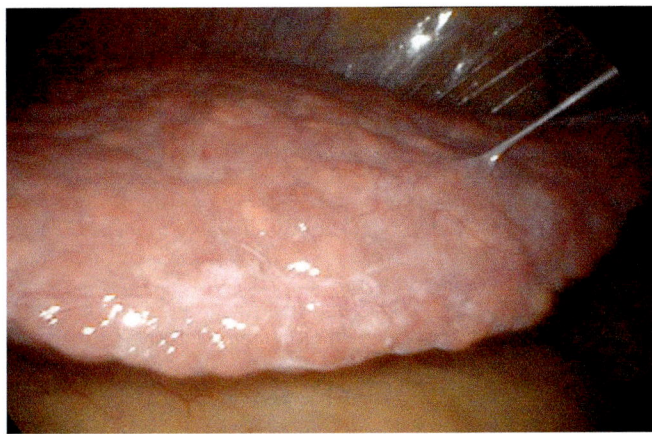

Fig. 7.12 (**a**) Her liver was yellow and micronocular formation; cirrhotic stage

cellular carcinoma was diagnosed by imaging modalities, and she died of multiple hepatocellular carcinomas in 4 years after repeated therapy for them. Autopsy showed burned-out NASH and moderately differentiated hepatocellular carcinoma (Fig. 7.10c,d,e). In cirrhotic NAFLD/NASH, screening for hepatocellular carcinoma should be performed.

Case 7.5

A 32-year-old morbid obese man was admitted in our hospital due to fatigability. He had been obese from the age of 6 [28]. He had no history of alcohol intake and complications of lifestyle-related diseases. His laboratory tests showed TBil 1.9 mg/dL, AST 64 IU/L, ALT 35 IU/L, ALP 316 IU/L, GGT 38 IU/L, Hb 13.4 g/dl, Plats 10.9×10^4/mm^3, and PT 72.4%. HBsAg and HCV Ab were negative. His liver biopsy showed moderate macrovesicular steatosis, ballooning degeneration, Mallory-Denk bodies, and pericellular fibrosis with cirrhosis (Fig. 7.11a). The features are diagnostic of NASH. Two years later, he died of liver failure. Autopsy

showed an enlarged micronodular cirrhosis (Fig. 7.11b). It is very important to note that morbid obesity is the most important risk factor of NASH and it progresses insidiously.

Case 7.6

A 59-year-old obese woman had been suffering from diabetes mellitus for 10 years and had no history of drinking. Her laboratory tests showed T.Bil 0.3 mg/dL, AST 51 IU/L, ALT 48 IU/L, ALP 250 IU/L, GGT 56 IU/L, albumin 4.2 g/dl, HbA1c 6.8%, Hb 12.4 g/dl, Plats 16.2×10^4/mm^3, and PT 100%. HBsAg and HCV Ab were negative. Her peritoneoscopy showed an enlarged yellow liver with fine nodular surface, and liver biopsy showed severe macrovesicular steatosis, inflammatory infiltrates, and ballooning hepatocytes with cirrhosis (Fig. 7.12). The features are diagnostic of NASH. Vitamin E and pioglitazone were administered, and her laboratory tests showed slight improvement. It is important to note that substantial numbers of patients with cirrhotic NASH have normal liver function with mild elevation of transaminases. It is not easy to diagnose obese cirrhotic NASH among so many NAFLD patients.

Acknowledgments Prof. Paul Y. Kwo is acknowledged for his contribution in editing this chapter.

References

1. O'Shea RS, Dasarathy S, McCullough AJ, et al. AASLD practice Guildelines; alcoholic liver disease. Hepatology. 2010;51:307–28.
2. Singal AK, Bataller R, Ahn J, et al. ACG clinical guideline: alcoholic liver disease. Am J Gastroenterol. 2018;113:175–94.
3. European Association for the Study of the Liver. EASL clinical practical guidelines: management of alcoholic liver disease. J Hepatol. 2012;57:399–420.
4. Nakano M, Worner TM, Lieber CS. Perivenular fibrosis in alcoholic liver injury: ultrastructural and histologic progression. Gastroenterology. 1982;83:777–85.

5. Goodman ZD, Ishak KG. Occlusive venous lesions in alcoholic liver disease. A study of 200 cases. Gastroenterology. 1982;83:786–96.

6. Jensen K, Gluud C. The Mallory body: morphological, clinical and experimental studies (part 1 of a literature survey). Hepatology. 1994;20:1061–77.

7. Younossi ZM, Koenig AB, Abdelatif D, et al. Global epidemiology of nonalcoholic fatty liver disease—meta-analytic assessment of prevalence, incidence, and outcomes. Hepatology. 2016;64:73–84.

8. Sookoian S, Pirola CJ. Meta-analysis of the influence of I148M variant of Patatin-like phospholipase domain containing 3 gene (PNPLA3) on the susceptibility and histological severity of nonalcoholic fatty liver disease. Hepatology. 2011;53:1883–94.

9. Watanabe S, Hashimoto E, Ikejima K, et al. Evidence-based clinical practice guidelines for nonalcoholic fatty liver disease/nonalcoholic steatohepatitis. J Gastroenterol. 2015;50:364–77.

10. easloffice@easloffice.eu EAftSotLEEa, (EASD) EAftSoD, (EASO) EAftSoO. EASL-EASD-EASO clinical practice guidelines for the management of non-alcoholic fatty liver disease. J Hepatol. 2016;64:1388–402.

11. Wong VW, Chan WK, Hashimoto E, et al. The Asia-Pacific working party on nonalcoholic fatty liver disease guidelines 2017 part 1: definition, risk factors and assessment. J Gastroenterol Hepatol. 2018;33(1):70–85.

12. Chalasani N, Younossi Z, Lavine JE, et al. The diagnosis and Management of Nonalcoholic Fatty Liver Disease: practice guidance from the American Association for the Study of Liver Diseases. Hepatology. 2017;67:328. https://doi.org/10.1002/hep.29367.

13. McPherson S, Hardy T, Henderson E, et al. Evidence of NAFLD progression from steatosis to fibrosing-steatohepatitis using paired biopsies: implications for prognosis and clinical management. J Hepatol. 2015;62:1148–55.

14. Dufour JF. Time to abandon NASH? Hepatology. 2016;63:9–10.

15. Ludwig J, Viggiano TR, McGill DB, et al. Nonalcoholic steatohepatitis. Mayo Clinic experiences with a hitherto unnamed disease. Mayo Clinic proc. 1980;55:434–8.

16. Hashimoto E, Tokushige K, Ludwig J. Diagnosis and classification of non-alcoholic fatty liver disease and non-alcoholic steatohepatitis: current concepts and remaining challenges. Hepatol Res. 2014:1–9.

17. Matteoni CA, Younossi ZM, Gramlich T, et al. Nonalcoholic fatty liver disease: a spectrum of clinical and pathological severity. Gastroenterology. 1999;116:1413–9.

18. Brunt EM, Janney CG, DiBisceglie AM, et al. Nonalcoholic steatohepatitis: a proposal for grading and staging the histological lesions. Am J Gastroenterol. 1999;94:2467–74.

19. Kleiner DE, Brunt EM, Van Natta M, et al. Design and validation of a histological scoring system for nonalcoholic fatty liver disease. Hepatology. 2005;41:1313–21.

20. Bedossa P, Poitou C, Veyrie N, et al. Histopathological algorithm and scoring system for evaluation of liver lesions in morbidly obese patients. Hepatology. 2012;56:1751–9.

21. Bedossa P. FLIP pathology consortium. Utility and appropriateness of the fatty liver inhibition of progression (FLIP) algorithm and steatosis, activity, and fibrosis (SAF) score in the evaluation of biopsies of nonalcoholic fatty liver disease. Hepatology. 2014;60:565–75.

22. Angulo P, Kleiner DE, Dam-Larsen S, et al. Liver fibrosis, but no other histologic features is associated with long-term outcomes of patients with nonalcoholic fatty liver disease. Gastroenterology. 2015;149:389–97.

23. Yatsuji S, Hashimoto E, Tobari M, Taniai M, Tokushige K, Shiratori K. Clinical features and outcomes of cirrhosis due to non-alcoholic steatohepatitis compared with cirrhosis caused by chronic hepatitis C. J Gastroenterol Hepatol. 2009;24:248–54.

24. Ascha MS, Hanouneh IA, Lopez R, Tamimi TA, Feldstein AF, Zein NN. The incidence and risk factors of hepatocellular carcinoma in patients with nonalcoholic steatohepatitis. Hepatology. 2010;51:1972–8.

25. Hashimoto E, Tokushige K. Hepatocellular carcinoma in nonalcoholic steatohepatitis: growing evidence of an epidemic? Hepatol Res. 2012;42:1–14.

26. Hannah WN, Harrison SA. Noninvasive imaging methods to determine severity of nonalcoholic fatty liver disease and nonalcoholic steatohepatitis. Hepatology. 2016;64:2234–43.

27. Yoshioka Y, Hashimoto E, Yatsuji S, et al. Nonalcoholic steatohepatitis: cirrhosis, hepatocellular carcinoma, and burnt-out NASH. J Gastroenterol. 2004;39(12):1215–8.

28. Suzuki D, Hashimoto E, Kaneda H, et al. Liver failure caused by non-alcoholic steatohepatitis in an obese young male. J Gastroenterol Hepatol. 2005;20:327–9.

Drug-Induced Liver Injury

8

Bing Ren, Arief A. Suriawinata, and Masaki Iwai

Contents

Abbreviations

AIH   Autoimmune hepatitis
ALP   Alkaline phosphatase
ALT   Alanine aminotransferase
AST   Aspartate aminotransferase
DAIH   Drug-induced autoimmune hepatitis
DILI   Drug-induced liver injury
DILIN   Drug-Induced Liver Injury Network
GGT   Gamma-glutamyltransferase
HDSs   Herbal and dietary supplements
TBIL   Total bilirubin
ULN   Upper limit of normal

B. Ren, MD, PhD · A. A. Suriawinata, MD (✉)
New Hampshire, USA
e-mail: Arief.A.Suriawinata@hitchcock.org

M. Iwai, MD, PhD
Kyoto, Japan

8.1 Introduction

The liver plays an important role in drug metabolism and disposition. Hepatic uptake, biotransformation, cellular transport, and excretion in bile are important processes that clear drugs from the body, terminate their pharmacological action, and prevent accumulation of toxic metabolites. These processes are highly regulated, and—depending on the way one looks—it may be surprising to note that adverse drug reactions are quite uncommonly encountered relative to the enormous consumption of prescription and non-prescription drugs. Drug-induced liver injury (DILI) has an estimated annual incidence between 10 and 15 per 10,000 to 100,000

© Springer Nature Singapore Pte Ltd. 2019
E. Hashimoto et al. (eds.), *Diagnosis of Liver Disease*, https://doi.org/10.1007/978-981-13-6806-6_8

persons exposed to prescription medications [1]. DILI accounts for approximately 10% of all cases of acute hepatitis, and it is the most common cause of acute liver failure in the United States. DILI is the most common reason for the withdrawal of a drug from the market, not uncommonly within months to a few years after its initial approval by agencies such as the Food and Drug Administration (FDA) of the United States.

8.2　Mechanisms of DILI

DILI can be classified in several ways (Table 8.1). Based on the mechanism of drug injury DILI is classified into two types: intrinsic type with drug-associated liver injury in a predictable, dose-dependent manner and idiosyncratic type with drug-associated liver injury in an unpredictable, non-dose-dependent manner. Rigorous testing typically

helps to identify intrinsic hepatotoxic agents. In contrast, idiosyncratic toxicity is mostly unpredictable and non-dose-dependent, and individual susceptibility varies according to genetic determinants, metabolic variations, and environmental factors. For most cases of idiosyncratic hepatotoxicity, there are as yet no specific tests to predict or confirm the association with drug-induced liver injury. Thus, practitioners have little choice but to rely on circumstantial evidence and the elimination of other obvious causes. One of the more significant breakthroughs may, in this respect, come from pharmacogenomics.

Acetaminophen, as a classic example of intrinsic hepatotoxicity, is the most common cause of severe intrinsic DILI in the United States. All subjects will develop liver damage if the dosage is high enough. Regular alcohol consumption (upregulation of toxic metabolic pathways) or underlying liver disease (diminished functional reserve) may enhance susceptibility to acetaminophen. As a consequence, some

Table 8.1 Classifications of drug-induced liver injury

Type of classification	Pattern	Comments
Mechanism of hepatotoxicity	Direct/intrinsic	Predictable, dose-dependent
	Idiosyncratic	Unpredictable, non-dose-dependent
	Immunologic	Immune-mediated hypersensitivity with fever, rash, granuloma, and eosinophilia
	Metabolic	Remaining cases lack of evidence of hypersensitivity
Clinical laboratory	Hepatocellular	$ALT \geq (2–5) \times ULN$ and/or $R \geq 5$
	Cholestatic	$ALP \geq 3 \times ULN$ and/or $R \leq 2$
	Mixed hepatocellular/cholestatic	$ALT \geq (2–5) \times ULN$ and $ALP \geq 3 \times ULN$ And/or $2 < R < 5$
Histology-common patterns	Zonal coagulative necrosis	Coagulative hepatocyte necrosis within 1 of the 3 zones without significant inflammation (zone 3 is most common)
	Submassive to massive necrosis	Confluent panacinar necrosis with variable inflammation
	Acute hepatitis	Predominantly lobular inflammation and damage without cholestasis or fibrosis
	Chronic hepatitis	Predominantly portal inflammation with variable degrees of lobular inflammation and portal fibrosis, no cholestasis
	Acute cholestasis	Hepatocellular and/or canalicular cholestasis with minimal inflammation
	Chronic cholestasis	Periportal cholate stasis, periportal fibrosis, copper accumulation, duct injury (such as ductular proliferation or ductopenia)
	Cholestatic hepatitis	A combination of acute or chronic hepatitic and cholestatic patterns
Histology-uncommon patterns	Macrovesicular steatosis	Predominantly macrovesicular steatosis without significant inflammation or cholestasis
	Microvesicular steatosis	Predominantly microvesicular steatosis without significant inflammation or cholestasis
	Steatohepatitis	Steatosis with hepatocyte ballooning, variable degrees of inflammation, and fibrosis
	Granulomatous inflammation	Non-necrotizing epithelioid granulomas
	Sinusoidal obstruction syndrome/veno-occlusive disease	Occlusions or loss of central veins, thrombosis, with or without central hemorrhage and necrosis
	Hepatoportal sclerosis	Disappearance of portal veins
	Nodular regenerative hyperplasia	Diffuse nodular formation with or without inflammation and sinusoidal fibrosis
	Sinusoidal dilation/peliosis	Sinusoidal dilation and congestion with or without mild lobular inflammation, sinusoidal fibrosis
	Glycogenosis	Diffuse hepatocyte swelling with very pale bluish-gray cytoplasm
	Ground-glass change	Diffuse hepatocellular cytoplasmic homogenization due to induction of smooth endoplasmic reticulum
	Hepatocellular inclusions (poly-glucosan-like bodies)	Discrete cytoplasmic inclusions with variable periodic acid-Schiff staining

ALT serum alanine aminotransferase, *ALP* serum alkaline phosphatase, *ULN* upper limit of normal, *R* (ALT/ULN) / (ALP/ULN)

may only tolerate 1–1.5 grams daily, whereas others tolerate a few grams or more. An acetaminophen overdose death is preventable. Acute overdose can be managed with antidote N-acetyl-cysteine if administered within 8 h of ingestion [2]. A reactive metabolite (N-acetyl-p-benzoquinone imine [NAPQI]) is produced from the metabolism of acetaminophen. Intra-hepatocellular accumulation of NAPQI will reduce the capacity of glutathione, which leads to covalent modification of numerous intracellular structures and consequently causes a zone 3, centrilobular hepatocyte necrosis. N-acetyl-cysteine acts by facilitating regeneration of glutathione, leading to detoxification for accumulated NAPQI. The dose-related manner in which acetaminophen causes liver damage has facilitated the development of specific recommendations for safe usage of this widely used medication. The FDA recommends a maximum daily dose of 3250 mg and encourages manufacturers to reduce the amount of acetaminophen to 325 mg per dose and highlight the potential for severe hepatotoxicity on labeling.

Idiosyncratic drug reactions may occur in only 1 in 10,000 to 1,000,000 individuals. It is nearly impossible to predict idiosyncratic drug reactions, which draw attention to the importance of careful post-marketing surveillance of medications as clinical trials are not done on such a major scale. In the United States, antimicrobials (amoxicillin-clavulanate, nitrofurantoin, sulfamethoxazole- trimethoprim, ciprofloxacin, isoniazid) [3], anticancer agents (such as the tyrosine kinase inhibitors and temozolomide), and immunomodulating agents (such as the tumor necrosis factor-a [TNF-a] inhibitors and anti-cytotoxic T-lymphocyte antigen-4 (CTLA-4) can cause idiosyncratic drug reactions. Most idiosyncratic DILI cases are mild, self-limited injury that reverses completely when the offending agent is identified and withdrawn. Idiosyncratic DILI accounts for 13–16% of life-threatening acute/ fulminant liver failure episodes in the United States [4]. It is a common cause of the removal of drugs from the market by the FDA. Idiosyncratic DILI can be broadly divided into hypersensitivity (also called immunologic) and metabolic mechanisms of injury. Hypersensitivity-type reactions represent 23–37% of all idiosyncratic DILIs, characterized by fever, rash, granulomas, and eosinophilia in the peripheral blood or tissue biopsy sample [5]. The remaining cases are considered to be metabolic and, by default, lack the evidence supporting hypersensitivity.

Almost all the early information about DILI was obtained from case reports or small case series collected at a single or few institutions. Therefore, their impact is limited by the rare nature of idiosyncratic drug reactions. Large national registries have been created to centralize and standardize the analysis to gain a more complete understanding of DILI. In the United States, the Drug-Induced Liver Injury Network (DILIN), funded by the National Institutes of Health, began to enroll patients in prospective study and collect cases at 12 participating sites in 2004.

Several risk factors are associated with the development of DILI [6]. Age is a risk factor for DILI development. Adults generally have a higher risk for DILI than children, except valproate and aspirin, with which children are at a higher risk for developing hepatotoxicity. Women are more likely than men to progress to acute/fulminant liver failure from idiosyncratic DILI. Individual genetic components are believed to greatly contribute to the development and injury pattern for a given chemical compound. Human leukocyte antigen (HLA) genes, involved in antigen recognition and immune function, are thought to play a role in idiosyncratic DILI. HLA genotypes, HLA-DRB1*15 and HLADRB1* 06, have been shown to be more common in patients with amoxicillin-clavulanate induced DILI, although this association is influenced by other cofounders such as ethnicity [7]. Polymorphisms within drug-metabolizing enzymes, such as cytochrome P450, N-acetyltransferase 2, UDP-glucuronosyltransferases, and glutathione S-transferases, have been found to be associated with DILI [8]. Certain genetic variations of mitochondrial DNA polymerase γ gene (*POLG*) have been shown to associate with liver toxicity caused by sodium valproate [9]. Although idiosyncratic DILI is not directly related to drug dosage, study has shown that drugs commonly taken at a dose of 50 mg or more per day represent 77% of all idiosyncratic DILIs [10]. Additionally, small reports showed that decreasing the dose of a drug below 50 mg led to the resolution of DILI symptoms [11].

8.3 Biochemical Profiles of DILI

In clinical practice, DILI is initially categorized based on the clinical presentation (i.e., biochemical testing profiles) and can be further categorized based on the histologic findings if liver biopsy is available. DILI is classified into hepatocellular, cholestatic, or mixed type based on biochemical patterns of injury, which is determined by the ratio of elevation of serum level of alanine aminotransferase (ALT) to that of serum alkaline phosphatase (ALP) (R-value, defined as [ALT/ULN of ALT]/[ALP/ULN of ALP]) (Table 8.1). Hepatocellular-type DILI is defined as ALT ≥ 2 to 5 times of the upper limit of normal (ULN) and/or an R ratio ≥ 5; cholestatic-type DILI is defined as an elevated ALP ≥ 3 times of the ULN and/or an R ratio ≤ 2; and mixed hepatocellular−/cholestatic-type DILI is defined as an increase in ALT ≥ 2 to 5 times of the ULN and an elevated ALP ≥ 3 times of the ULN and/or an R ratio between 2 and 5 [12]. The presence of jaundice (serum bilirubin >2 times of ULN) in association with an elevation in ALT (>3 times of ULN) is associated with a worse prognosis [13]. Patients with an autoimmune-like presentation may have positive serologic markers of autoimmunity (e.g., an elevated antinuclear antibody). DILI is considered acute if the liver tests have been abnormal for less than 3 months and chronic if they have been abnormal for more than 3 months.

Most patients with DILI are asymptomatic or with only mildly abnormal laboratory testing. Some patients with acute DILI may have malaise, low-grade fever, anorexia, nausea, vomiting, abdominal pain, jaundice, light-colored stool, and dark urine. Cholestatic patients may have pruritus. Acute liver injury with coagulopathy and hepatic encephalopathy may be seen in severe cases. Patients with chronic DILI may develop fibrosis or cirrhosis and have symptoms associated with cirrhosis or hepatic decompensation. Patients with DILI may also have symptoms of a hypersensitivity reaction including fever, rash, or mononucleosis-like illness, and some patients may have evidence of toxicity to other organs.

A number of scales have been developed attempting to codify causality of drug toxicity into objective criteria. They include the Council for International Organizations of Medical Sciences (CIOMS)/Roussel Uclaf Causality Assessment Method (RUCAM) scale and the Maria & Victorino (M & V) clinical scale. However, they do not address all risk factors and are not used routinely in clinical practice [14]. The US DILIN causality scoring system adjudicates the causality of drug-induced injury for patients enrolled in its prospective clinical trial, but it relies on expert opinion and is not a clinically viable option.

8.4 Challenges in Diagnosis of DILI

Diagnosis of DILI is challenging since there is no specific serum biomarkers or characteristic histologic features that can reliably identify a drug as the cause of hepatic injury. Careful history-taking is essential and should include all drugs and supplements taken over the last several months. Patients tend to forget or underreport their use of medications or supplements, such as a recent course of antibiotics. Medical records and information from the pharmacy can be most revealing.

The latent period between exposure and onset of symptoms varies from several days to a few months. Viral hepatitis, alcohol abuse, extrahepatic biliary obstruction, autoimmune hepatitis, and other causes of abnormal liver tests should be excluded, and the possibility of drug-induced injury should always be considered in any patient with liver disease without an obvious cause. If testing for alternative causes for liver injury is negative and patient has a history of exposure to a drug known associated with liver injury, the patient usually will be managed without liver biopsy. Liver biopsy is necessary in the settings of uncertain diagnosis or presenting with evidence of chronic liver disease. Several key elements could be considered before rendering a diagnosis of DILI. Patients may be taking multiple medications, making identification of a single offending agent difficult. Furthermore, patients may have underlying liver disease, which can produce an acute on chronic liver disease.

8.5 Histologic Patterns of DILI

Liver biopsy is not a requirement for clinical evaluation of DILI, and it is performed in less than 50% of suspected cases. An accurate interpretation of liver biopsy can provide valuable information on the nature and severity of liver injury, the possible pathogenesis, the expected clinical outcome, and even guidance for therapy. While histologic findings are not diagnostic for a specific cause of DILI, recognizing the histologic injury pattern will help to narrow the differential diagnosis to a small group of agents causing DILI and exclude other non-DILI cause (e.g., Wilson disease and hemochromatosis) [15]. The US DILIN recognizes 18 distinct histologic damage categories (Table 8.1), which include 7 common patterns (zonal coagulative necrosis, submassive to massive necrosis, acute hepatitis, chronic hepatitis, acute cholestasis, chronic cholestasis, and cholestatic hepatitis) and 11 uncommon patterns (macrovesicular steatosis, microvesicular steatosis, steatohepatitis, granulomatous hepatitis, sinusoidal obstruction syndrome/venoocclusive disease, hepatoportal sclerosis, nodular regenerative hyperplasia, sinusoidal dilation/peliosis, glycogenosis, ground-glass change, and hepatocellular inclusions (poly-glucosan-like bodies)) [16]. Among all of them, acute and chronic hepatitic, acute and chronic cholestatic, and mixed hepatitis-cholestatic patterns are the most common patterns.

DILI leads to acute hepatocellular injury in about 90% of cases of toxicity [17]. Hepatocellular injury caused by intrinsic toxins is commonly zonal in distribution, whereas idiosyncratic injury is usually non-zonal. Therefore, zonal necrosis—either periportal (zone 1), mid-zonal (zone 2), or perivenular (zone 3)—is usually the result of intrinsic toxins. Perivenular (zone 3) necrosis is the most common type of zonal necrosis, with carbon tetrachloride and acetaminophen as prototypical examples. Idiosyncratic injury tends to cause more of an acute hepatitis-like injury, characterized by diffuse lobular lymphocytic infiltrate with scattered apoptotic hepatocytes, ballooning degeneration of hepatocytes, regeneration with rosette formation and mitoses, and sometimes an eosinophilic infiltrate. If severe, lobular inflammation may be followed by zonal necrosis. Many of the drugs that are known to cause acute hepatitis-like injury can also cause chronic hepatitis-like injury, characterized by predominant portal and periportal necroinflammatory infiltrate and relatively mild lobular inflammation.

Drug-induced chronic hepatitis may have features similar to autoimmune hepatitis (AIH) with the presence of hypergammaglobulinemia, antinuclear antibody, or anti-smooth muscle actin. Inflammatory infiltrates with a predominance of CD8 cytotoxic T cells indicate activation of the host immune response, suggestive of intrahepatic neoantigen production by the drug or its metabolite. Examples of these drugs are clometacin, infliximab, and other tumor necrosis factor-alpha-blocking agents, methyldopa, minocycline, and nitrofurantoin. A large retrospective study showed 9%

(24/216) of AIH cases were related to medication [18]. Most of the minocycline- and nitrofurantoin-associated AIH cases presented with positive serology, while only half of the hydralazine- and methyldopa-associated AIH cases had positive serology [19]. Cholestasis in suspected drug-induced AIH cases has been suggested as a finding in favor of drug etiology [20].

Five to ten percent of acute hepatocellular DILI cases can progress to chronic injury, which can histologically resemble other chronic liver disease, such as autoimmune hepatitis, viral hepatitis, or alcohol liver disease. Some agents commonly associated with chronic DILI are amoxicillin-clavulanic acid, bentazepam, atorvastatin, methotrexate, hypervitaminosis A, vinyl chloride, heroin, herbal products, and dietary supplements [17, 21]. Drugs that can lead to cirrhosis include herbal products, dietary supplements, methotrexate, isoniazid, ticrynafen, amiodarone, enalapril, and valproic acid [17].

Some drugs may produce a predominantly cholestatic injury rather than hepatocellular injury. In pure cholestasis, there is an accumulation of bile in the hepatocytes and canaliculi (prominent in zone 3) with minimal hepatocellular injury or inflammation. This type of injury is often seen with the use of anabolic steroids or oral contraceptives, causing interference with hepatocyte secretion of bile via the bile salt excretory protein (BSEP) [22]. This pattern should be distinguished from other causes of cholestasis, such as large duct obstruction with predominant portal changes including marked portal edema and a ductular reaction. Chlorpromazine, beta-lactams, and erythromycin (macrolide antibiotics) are typical examples of zone 3 cholestatic injury. When acute cholestasis is accompanied by bile duct injury (cholangitis), it may lead to chronic duct injury and bile duct loss (ductopenia or vanishing bile duct syndrome). In rare cases, there is a progression to cirrhosis and ultimately liver failure. Drugs that have been associated with ductopenia are amoxicillin-clavulanate, flucloxacillin, ACE inhibitors, and terbinafine [23].

When both acute hepatic injury and intrahepatic cholestasis are present, it is referred to as a mixed form of hepatic injury. Cholestatic hepatitis is characterized by portal inflammation, prominent cholestasis, and hepatocellular injury. Bile duct proliferation may be seen. Hepatocyte injury is usually localized to the zones of cholestasis. Drugs associated with this type of injury include erythromycin, amoxicillin-clavulanate, herbal products, and angiotensin-converting enzyme (ACE) inhibitors.

Drugs can cause various other patterns of injury, such as steatosis, steatohepatitis, granulomatous inflammation, and vascular lesions. Drugs that disrupt mitochondrial beta-oxidation of lipids and oxidative energy production lead to steatosis. Drug-induced microvesicular steatosis is commonly associated with acute presentation and is characterized by the presence of small fat droplets composed predominantly of triglycerides in the cytoplasm of the hepatocytes.

Microvesicular steatosis has been observed in association with tetracycline, valproic acid, salicylates, and amiodarone [23]. Drug-induced chronic steatosis is predominantly macrovesicular and could be associated with inflammation (steatohepatitis). The histologic features of steatohepatitis include variable steatosis, lobular inflammation (predominantly neutrophilic), and hepatocellular injury (ballooning) [23]. Acidophil bodies, Mallory hyaline, and pericellular fibrosis may also be present. Drug-induced macrovesicular steatosis and steatohepatitis are associated with amiodarone, glucocorticoids, methotrexate, sulfasalazine, spironolactone, phosphorus, tannic acid, arsenic, metoprolol, nonsteroidal anti-inflammatory drugs (NSAIDs), tamoxifen, and total parenteral nutrition [17]. When administered over the long term, some of these agents may result in fibrosis and cirrhosis.

Granulomatous inflammation, often accompanied by increased eosinophils, can be associated with other patterns of drug-induced injury such as cholestasis and steatosis. Drug-induced granulomas are generally non-necrotizing and are not associated with the bile duct injury. It is worthy to note that systemic granulomatous disease, such as sarcoidosis, does not preclude the possibility of drug-induced granulomas.

Drug-induced endothelial injury leads to vascular manifestations, including thrombosis or occlusion of hepatic veins, venules or sinusoids, perisinusoidal fibrosis, hepatoportal sclerosis, sinusoidal dilatation, and peliosis hepatis. The abnormal blood flow caused by these lesions often results in nodular regenerative hyperplasia. Androgens, contraceptive steroids, and chemotherapeutic medications can lead to peliosis hepatis.

Certain drugs may have a variety of manifestations. Azathioprine, for example, may cause pure intrahepatic (canalicular) cholestasis [24] or a more hepatitic pictures [25] that can be confusing if given in the context of autoimmune hepatitis (uncontrolled autoimmune disease versus hepatotoxicity) or veno-occlusive disease with major edema [26] that can clinically be confused with decompensated cirrhosis or right-sided heart failure.

8.6 Herbals and Dietary Supplements

DILI develops not only following the use of prescription or over-the-counter drugs but also caused by herbals and dietary supplements (s). HDSs encompass a variety of agents including vitamin and mineral supplements, fish oils, plant extracts, traditional medicines, and proprietary commercial products. In the United States, dietary supplement is consumed by more than 50% of the general population for maintaining good health or for treatment of disease [27]. In a study drawn from the US DILIN cohort, 15% (136/839) cases were caused by HDSs [28]. In this study, HDSs were divided into bodybuilding and non-bodybuilding groups. It was found that non-bodybuilding HDSs were much more likely to develop acute liver failure or undergo liver transplantation than bodybuilding or conventional medications groups. Non-bodybuilding HDSs causing severe liver injury include a variety of agents, such as weight-loss and energy-boosting supplements, Asian herbal remedies, and multivitamins. Acute hepatitis and liver failure have been reported to be associated with proprietary mixtures of HDSs, such as Herbalife [29] and OxyELITE Pro (withdrawn from the market by FDA in 2013 due to the hepatotoxicity) [30]. Bodybuilding agents sometimes contain anabolic steroids, which have been associated with acute cholestasis or cholestatic hepatitis [31] along with sinusoidal dilation and peliosis hepatis [32, 33]. They are also associated with hepatocellular adenomas.

8.7 Immunomodulating Agents

Immunomodulating agents, including methylprednisolone, the antitumor necrosis factor (TNF) agents infliximab and adalimumab, the anti-cytotoxic T-lymphocyte antigen-4 (CTLA-4) agent ipilimumab, and the anti-alpha 4 integrin antibody natalizumab, have been described in the recent literature to cause drug-induced autoimmune hepatitis (DAIH). Methylprednisolone has been shown to cause (acute) hepatitis with zonal necrosis and to be associated with an autoimmune-like hepatitis after several weeks of therapy [34]. The anti-TNF agents infliximab, adalimumab, and etanercept are anti-inflammatory drugs, which are monoclonal antibodies and soluble form of the TNF-alpha receptor that bind and block TNF alpha. They have been associated with severe acute liver injury and can cause reactivation of hepatitis B [35, 36]. Among all the published anti-TNF-induced DILI cases, infliximab was the most frequently reported. The most common histologic pattern of infliximab DILI is acute or chronic hepatitis with features of autoimmune hepatitis (AIH). Elevated titers of antinuclear antibodies can be observed. Besides DAIH, acute cholestasis and mild reactive hepatitis have been reported. Ipilimumab and tremelimumab are monoclonal antibody agents directed against CTLA-4, which inhibits the activation of cytotoxic T lymphocytes and results in persistent activation of these immune cells. Ipilimumab has been associated with a variety of autoimmune-like reactions, with a minority of cases showing pan lobular hepatitis and central vein endothelialitis [37]. About half of the cases had a prominent plasma cell infiltrate. It is worth noting that nivolumab, another type of immune checkpoint inhibitor, has been used as combination therapy in some cases. In contrast to AIH and anti-TNF agents, patients with immune checkpoint inhibitor-associated liver injury did not have autoimmune antibodies. Natalizumab, which blocks migration of lymphocytes to areas of inflammation, is used to treat multiple sclerosis and inflammatory bowel disease. It has been associated with autoimmune-like hepatitis as well as hepatocyte dropout in zone 3. Low titers of anti-smooth muscle antibody and anti-F-actin were detected in some cases [38].

8.8 Temozolomide and Bile Duct Injury

Temozolomide, an alkylating agent to treat glioma, causes cholestatic patterns of injury including acute cholestasis, cholestatic hepatitis, and chronic cholestasis with ductopenia [39]. Most temozolomide cases are present as bile duct injury with bile duct loss. Vanishing bile duct syndrome (VBDS) is associated with poor prognosis. Patient with abnormal liver enzyme persisting over a year is more likely to have chronic cholestasis with or without ductopenia than other patterns of injury [40].

8.9 Management of DILI

The management of drug-induced hepatic injury has been addressed only to a limited extent and rarely in any controlled setting. Minor transaminase elevations, such as those caused by isoniazid, tend to resolve spontaneously, whereas minor cholestatic changes are often not associated with significant disease. Statins are widely prescribed and frequently cause an increase in enzymes, but this is rarely, if ever, associated with significant liver disease. The recognition of risky patterns (such as a rapid increase in numbers after initiating isoniazid and transaminases exceeding five times ULN) and proper monitoring ought to be done in consultation with a hepatologist.

In some patients, it can take weeks and or even 1–2 years after the withdrawal of the agent before the hepatic injury and/or liver enzymes are completely resolved. Examples include injury caused by macrolide antibiotics. Specific antidotes are barely available, except timely administration of acetylcysteine in the case of acetaminophen-induced injury and L-carnitine in the cases of valproic acid overdose [41, 42]. Drug-induced injury that strongly mimics autoimmune hepatitis, steroids, and immune modulators should be considered; the duration of such therapy is the subject of major debate. Ursodeoxycholic acid and a variety of antipruritics should be considered in severe drug-induced cholestasis.

The careful documentation of drug-induced liver injury remains a major challenge. Conclusive data on severely ill patients with multi-organ disease and complications cannot easily be obtained. There are increasing efforts to improve the study of drug-induced hepatic injury, including the activity of the Drug-Induced Liver Injury Network (DILIN) established in the United States. Major underreporting is unfortunately likely, and it may take years to assess the impact of hepatotoxic potential of an agent.

8.10 Pathologist's Role in Diagnosis of DILI

Pathologist's role is to recognize the pattern of liver injury in a case suspicious for DILI. The interpretation of histologic findings can help confirm or rule out the drug effect or raise alternative causes for liver injury. Both the histologic pattern of injury and the severity of injury should be documented in the pathology report, since the information may influence clinical decision-making. Supplement of interpretation may be added as new clinical information is generated in the follow-up. As one of the challenging areas in hepatic pathology, careful examination and accurate interpretation of a liver biopsy are invaluable in the clinical suspicious DILI cases.

8.11 Example of DILI Cases

Case 8.1 Alpha Methyldopa Induced Hepatitis

Clinical and histological features of alpha-methyldopa hepatic injury, a nearly obsolete antihypertensive agent, are often indistinguishable from viral hepatitis. A prodromal period of anorexia, malaise, and fever may be followed by jaundice. Histopathologically, various degrees of acute hepatitis with bridging necrosis, chronic hepatitis with fibrosis, and moderate to severe steatosis can be seen [24–26]. The inflammatory infiltrate is concentrated in the portal and periportal regions. Prominent plasma cell infiltrate can be present in chronic injury and mimics autoimmune hepatitis.

A 50-year-old man with hypertension had taken 250 mg/dL a day of alpha-methyldopa for 3 months when severe hepatitis developed with anorexia and general malaise. His liver function test showed TBIL 3.8 mg/dL, ALT 1850 kU/L, AST 650 IU/L, ALP 14.5 KAU, LAP 640 IU/L, and GGT 380 IU/L, and lupus erythematosus and rheumatoid arthritis tests were negative. Blastoid transformation of lymphocytes in vitro by alpha-methyldopa was positive. Liver biopsy revealed submassive hepatic necrosis with steatosis in the periportal area, and electron microscopic study showed fat droplets in the vicinity of destroyed rough endoplasmic reticulum and lysosomes (Fig. 8.1). Three months after withdrawal of alpha-methyldopa, his liver function test had reverted to normal values.

Alpha-methyldopa-related liver injury ranges from mild hepatitis and patchy hepatocellular necrosis to severe hepatitis. At times, it resembles autoimmune hepatitis associated with immune hemolytic anemia, positive antinuclear antibody test, and lupus erythematosus [26]. The clinical spectrum is usually similar to that of viral hepatitis. Interestingly, when the disease resolves, the autoimmune tests tend to become negative as well.

Case 8.2 Anticancer Drug-Induced Liver Injury

Tamoxifen used to treat breast cancer. It induces liver damage [23, 43] by affecting mitochondrial function through inhibiting the electron transport chain [44], resulting in nonalcoholic steatohepatitis and is associated with liver cirrhosis.

A 51-year-old female had mastectomy for breast cancer 11 years previously. She had been taking tamoxifen for 3 years when bone metastases were discovered. She developed abdominal fullness with ascites and leg edema.

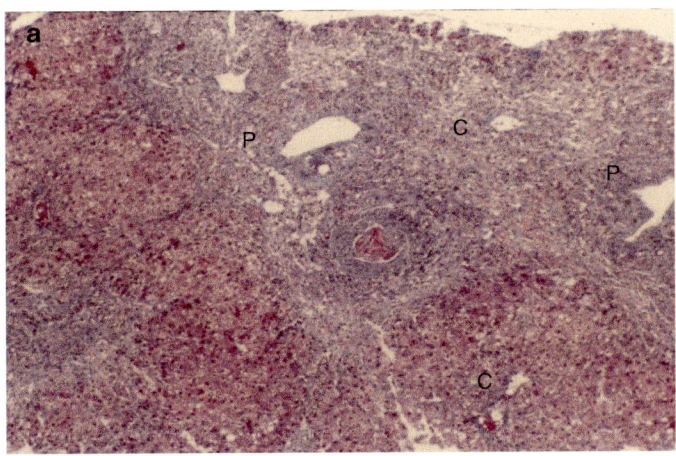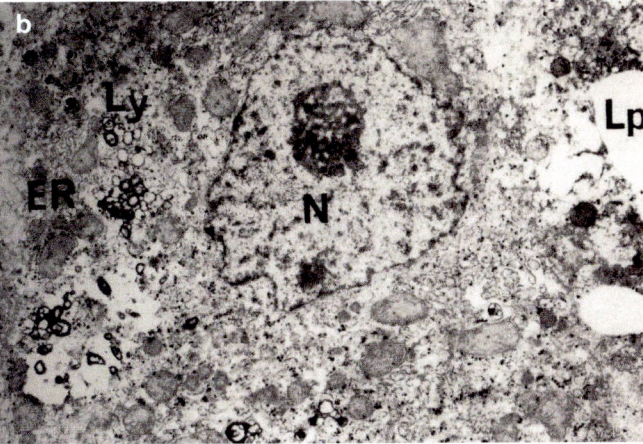

Fig. 8.1 Alpha-methyldopa-induced hepatitis. (**a**) Masson's trichrome stain shows submassive necrosis. *C* central vein, *P* portal tract. (**b**) Electron microscopy shows the presence of increased lysosomes (Ly) and fat droplets (Lp) in the vicinity of r-ER (ER). (Reuse of Iwai M, et al. Fatty metamorphosis of liver due to alpha-methyldopa. J Kyoto Pref Univ Med 1983; 92: 1427–1432., with permission of its chief editor)

CT confirmed ascites and revealed an enlarged liver with heterogeneous density. Laboratory testing showed TBIL 2.5 mg/dL, AST 108 IU/L, ALT 41 IU/L, LDH 493 IU/L, ChE 2030 IU/L, total protein 5.8 g/dL, albumin 2.9 g/dL, NH3 106 μ/dL, PLT 6.3×10^4/μL, and HPT 27%. Peritoneoscopy showed an enlarged yellow liver with dull edge and irregular surface. Liver biopsy showed nonalcoholic steatohepatitis (Fig. 8.2).

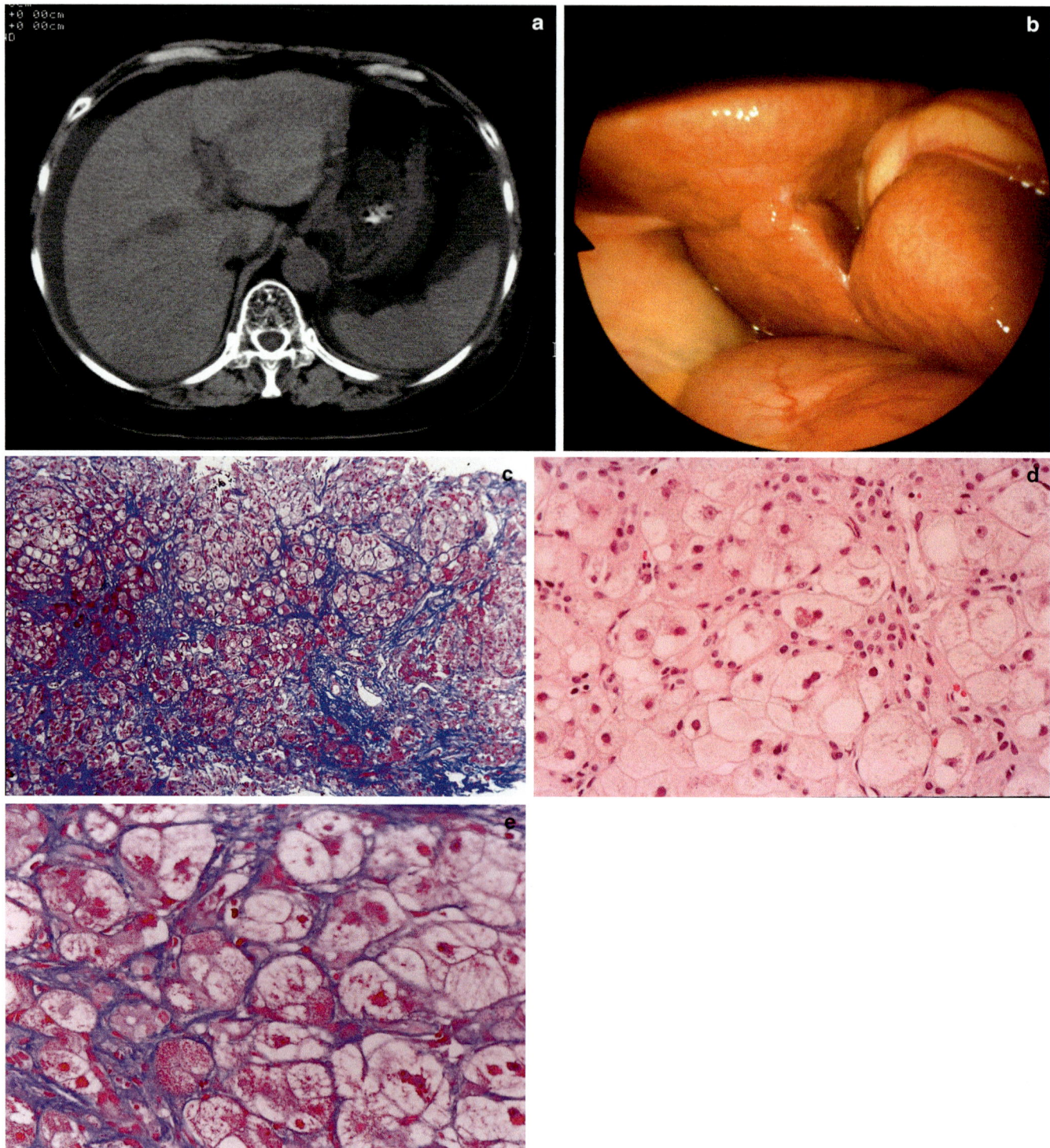

Fig. 8.2 Tamoxifen-induced liver damage. (**a**) CT shows presence of ascites, irregular surface of the liver with heterogeneous density, and mild splenomegaly. (**b**) Peritoneoscopy shows yellow liver with dull edge and enlarged left lobe. (**c**) Masson's trichrome stain shows lobular architecture disarray and bridging fibrosis. (**d**) Hepatocytes are swollen or ballooned, and mononuclear cells infiltrate the sinusoids. (**e**) Masson trichrome stain shows ballooned hepatocytes surrounded by perisinusoidal fibrosis

Case 8.3 Nutritional Supplement-Induced Liver Injury

Nutritional supplements are widely used, and their use has been linked to liver injury [45]. An interesting example is severe hepatic injury associated with intake of Herbalife products contaminated with Bacillus subtilis [46].

A 28-year-old female had been taking a weight-loss promoting agent for 3 months when she developed jaundice. Her liver function test showed TBIL 18.57 mg/dL, AST 1563 IU/L, ALT 1205 IU/L, ALP 454 IU/L, and negative IgM-HA Ab, HBsAg, HCV RNA, and ANA. Liver biopsy showed disarrayed trabecular structure and many inflammatory cells in the portal area. Periportal hepatocyte rosetting and ballooning hepatocytes in the mid-zonal to centrilobular areas were noted, and there were mixed inflammatory infiltrates including lymphocytes, neutrophils, and scattered eosinophils in the portal area, ballooning hepatocytes, and acidophilic bodies

(Fig. 8.3). After cessation of intake of supplements, liver function tests reverted to normal values 4 months later.

Case 8.4 Chlorpromazine-Induced Liver Injury

A prototypical cholestatic injury is chlorpromazine, which can cause hepatocanalicular cholestasis. Jaundice develops several weeks after its administration [47, 48].

A 77-year-old male was treated with chlorpromazine for 6 months when jaundice developed. His liver function test showed TBIL 24.03 mg/dL, ALT 60 IU/L, AST 35 IU/L, GGT 36 IU/L, LAP 294 IU/L, WBC 7100/mm³, and eosinophilia 7%. Liver biopsy showed a disarrayed trabecular structure and the presence of ballooning hepatocytes around the portal tract, and there was central parenchymal and canalicular cholestasis accompanied by scattered acidophilic bodies (Fig. 8.4).

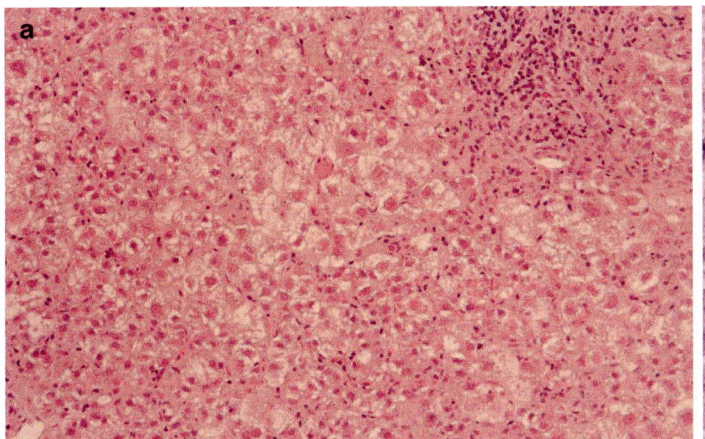 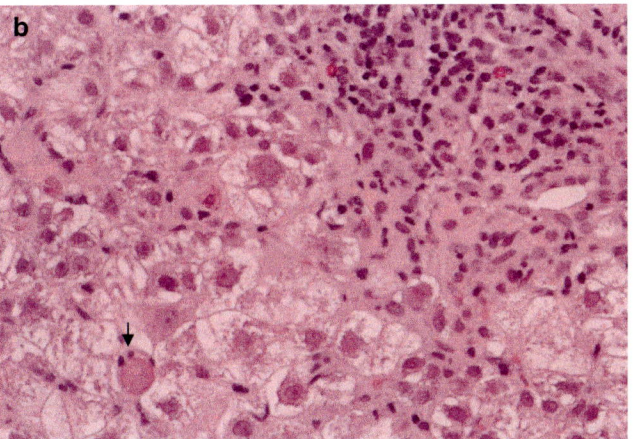

Fig. 8.3 Nutritional supplement-induced hepatitis. (**a**) Disarrayed trabecular structures with hepatocyte rosetting and portal tracts with inflammatory cell infiltrate. (**b**) Hepatocytes are ballooning and an acidophilic body (arrow) is seen, while the portal tract shows mixed infiltrate of lymphocytes, plasma cells, and eosinophils with interface hepatitis

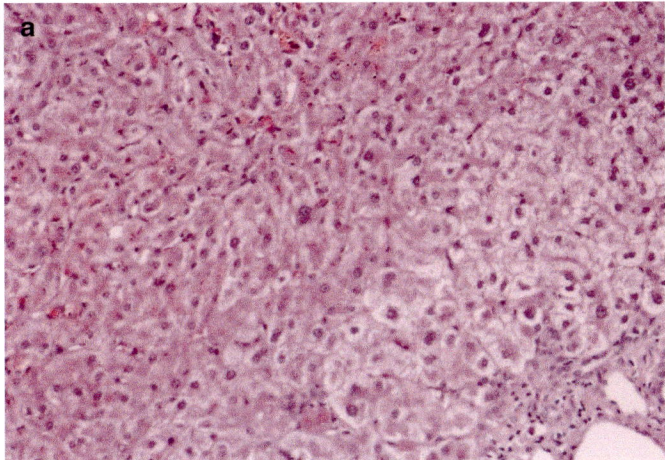 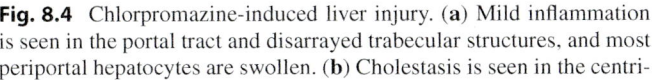 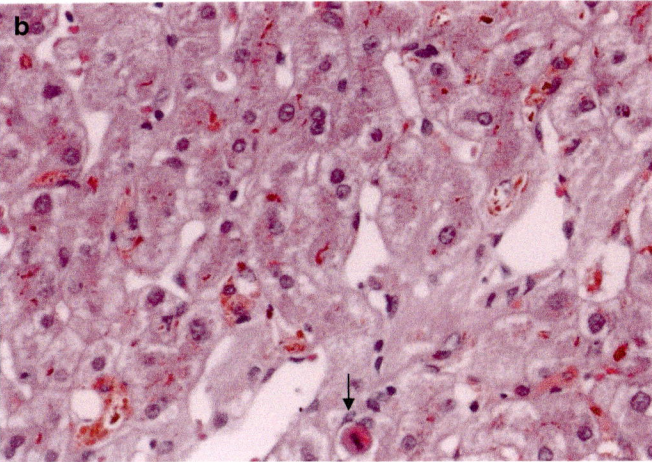

Fig. 8.4 Chlorpromazine-induced liver injury. (**a**) Mild inflammation is seen in the portal tract and disarrayed trabecular structures, and most periportal hepatocytes are swollen. (**b**) Cholestasis is seen in the centrilobular area, and bile pigments are localized in the bile canaliculi. An acidophilic body (arrow) is also noted

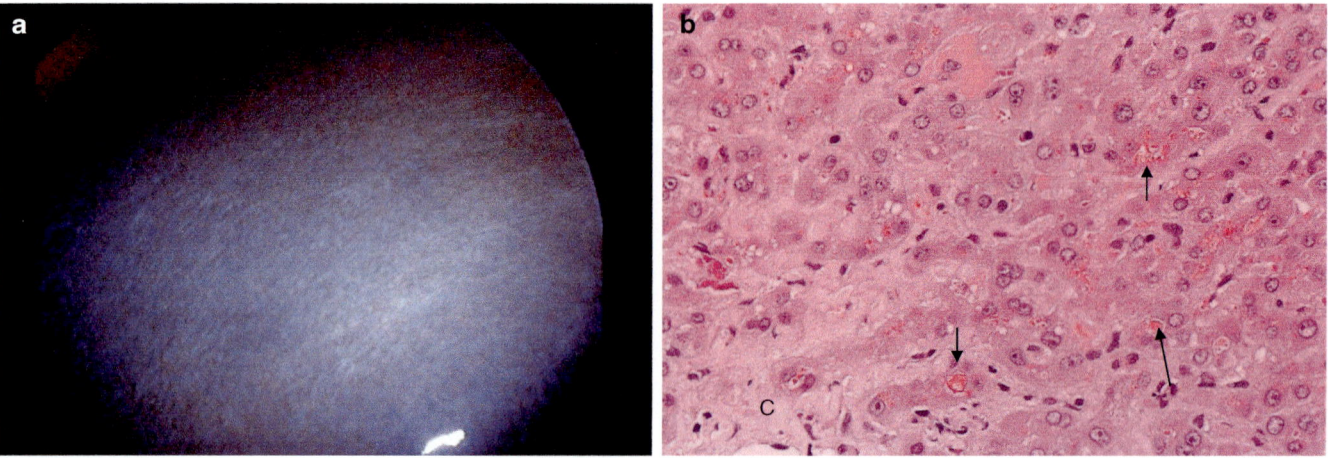

Fig. 8.5 Tiopronin-induced liver injury. (**a**) Peritoneoscopy shows green liver parenchyma with white capsule. (**b**) Cholestasis is seen in the central area (**c**), and bile plugs (arrow) are observed in the bile canaliculi

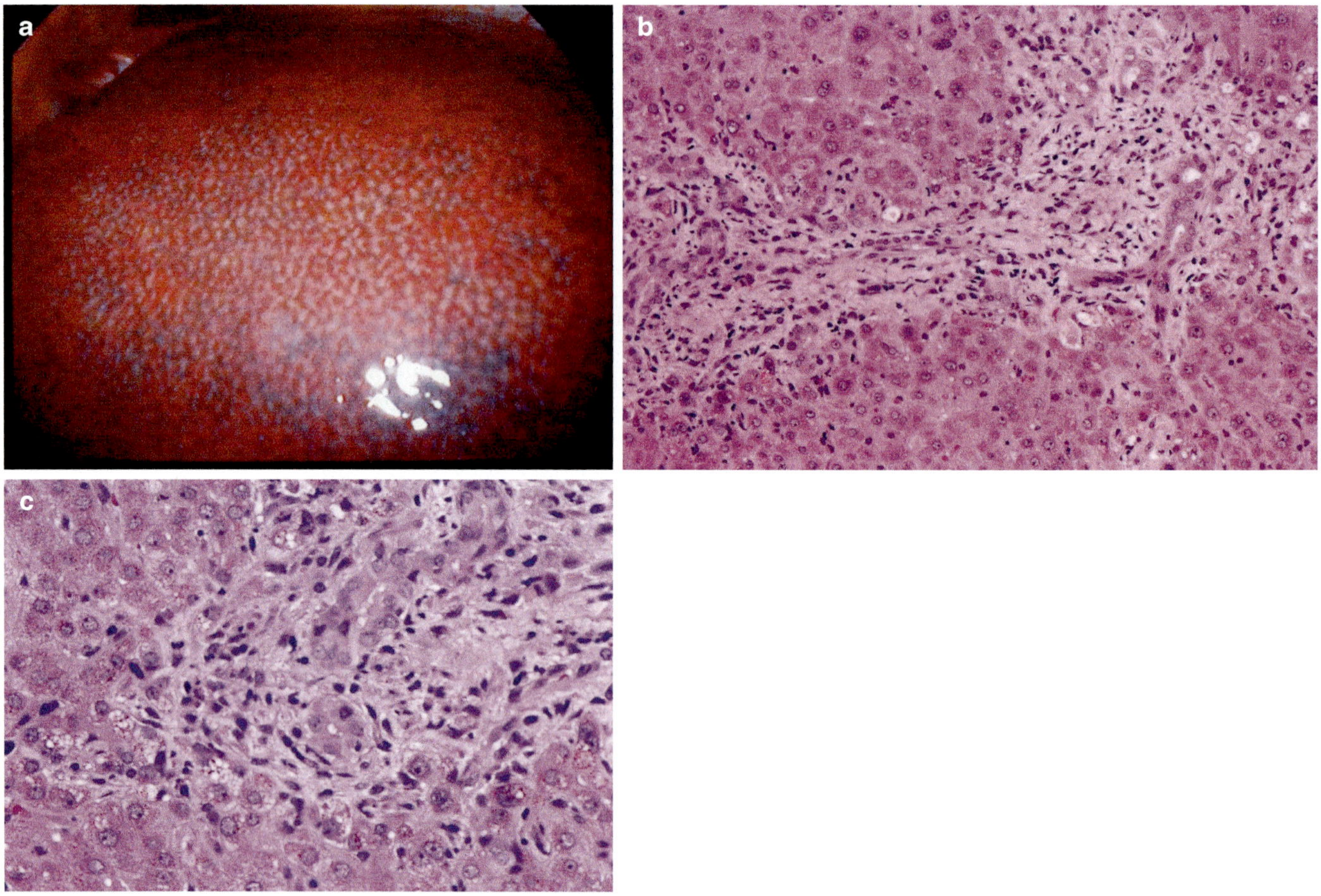

Fig. 8.6 Antibiotic-induced liver injury. (**a**) Peritoneoscopy shows clear and green prominent acinus markings. (**b**) An edematous portal tract with ductular proliferation. (**c**) Portal tract with ductular reaction and mild inflammatory cell infiltrate. Cholestasis and microvesicular steatosis are seen in the periportal hepatocytes

Case 8.5 Tiopronin-Induced Liver Injury

Tiopronin, a drug prescribed to prevent kidney stones associated with cystinuria, may induce severe cholestasis 1 month after initial administration, and the effect appears to be long-lasting [49]. Human leukocyte antigen (HLA) is reported to be associated with severe cholestasis in tiopronin-induced liver injury [50]. It is important to note that drug-induced injury can take a long time to resolve.

A 41-year-old male took tiopronin for 6 months to prevent gallstones. He developed low-grade fever and became icteric for 3 months. His liver function tests showed TBIL 17.3 mg/dL, ALT 38 IU/L, AST 42 IU/L, ALP 1022 IU/L, and GGT 526 IU/L. Peritoneoscopy showed a green liver with a white capsule; microscopic findings revealed lobular disarray with centrilobular, parenchymal damage and canalicular cholestasis; and amorphous material was seen in the perisinusoids of the centrilobular area (Fig. 8.5).

Case 8.6 Antibiotic-Induced Liver Injury

Antibiotics can induce hepatocellular injury, intrahepatic cholestasis, mixed hepatitis, chronic hepatitis, or microvesicular steatosis. Cephalosporin and its metabolites may lead to intrahepatic cholestasis with damage of the bile ducts and microvesicular steatosis [51].

A 64-year-old male had alcoholic stools, dark urine, and jaundice after administration of the antibiotic cefamezin alfa for pharyngitis. Laboratory data showed TBIL 30.89 mg/dL, AST 199 IU/L, ALT 210 IU/L, ALP 2106 IU/L, GGT 3539 IU/L, and total cholesterol 709 mg/dL. Peritoneoscopy 2 weeks after the peak of jaundice showed green liver without small excavations and scattered cholestatic acini; liver biopsy revealed expanded portal tracts with edema and proliferating bile ductules; and cholestasis was seen in hepatocytes, with microvesicular steatosis in the periportal region (Fig. 8.6).

References

1. Chalasani N, Fontana RJ, Bonkovsky HL, Watkins PB, Davern T, Serrano J, Yang H, Rochon J: Causes, clinical features, and outcomes from a prospective study of drug-induced liver injury in the United States. Gastroenterology 2008, 135:1924–34, 34.e1–4.
2. Williamson K, Wahl MS, Mycyk MB. Direct comparison of 20-hour IV, 36-hour oral, and 72-hour oral acetylcysteine for treatment of acute acetaminophen poisoning. Am J Ther. 2013;20:37–40.
3. Kleiner DE, Chalasani NP, Lee WM, Fontana RJ, Bonkovsky HL, Watkins PB, Hayashi PH, Davern TJ, Navarro V, Reddy R, Talwalkar JA, Stolz A, Gu J, Barnhart H, Hoofnagle JH. Hepatic histological findings in suspected drug-induced liver injury: systematic evaluation and clinical associations. Hepatology (Baltimore, MD). 2014;59:661–70.
4. Bower WA, Johns M, Margolis HS, Williams IT, Bell BP. Population-based surveillance for acute liver failure. Am J Gastroenterol. 2007;102:2459–63.
5. Bjornsson E, Kalaitzakis E, Olsson R. The impact of eosinophilia and hepatic necrosis on prognosis in patients with drug-induced liver injury. Aliment Pharmacol Ther. 2007;25:1411–21.
6. Yamashita YI, Imai K, Mima K, Nakagawa S, Hashimoto D, Chikamoto A, Baba H. Idiosyncratic drug-induced liver injury: a short review. Hepatol Commun. 2017;1:494–500.
7. Stephens C, Lopez-Nevot MA, Ruiz-Cabello F, Ulzurrun E, Soriano G, Romero-Gomez M, Moreno-Casares A, Lucena MI, Andrade RJ. HLA alleles influence the clinical signature of amoxicillin-clavulanate hepatotoxicity. PLoS One. 2013;8:e68111.
8. Daly AK, Day CP. Genetic association studies in drug-induced liver injury. Drug Metab Rev. 2012;44:116–26.
9. Stewart JD, Horvath R, Baruffini E, Ferrero I, Bulst S, Watkins PB, Fontana RJ, Day CP, Chinnery PF. Polymerase gamma gene POLG determines the risk of sodium valproate-induced liver toxicity. Hepatology (Baltimore, MD). 2010;52:1791–6.
10. Lammert C, Einarsson S, Saha C, Niklasson A, Bjornsson E, Chalasani N. Relationship between daily dose of oral medications and idiosyncratic drug-induced liver injury: search for signals. Hepatology (Baltimore, MD). 2008;47:2003–9.
11. Chalasani N, Bjornsson E. Risk factors for idiosyncratic drug-induced liver injury. Gastroenterology. 2010;138:2246–59.
12. Sundaram V, Bjornsson ES. Drug-induced cholestasis. Hepatol Commun. 2017;1:726–35.
13. Bjornsson E. Drug-induced liver injury: Hy's rule revisited. Clin Pharmacol Ther. 2006;79:521–8.
14. Lucena MI, Camargo R, Andrade RJ, Perez-Sanchez CJ. Sanchez De La cuesta F: comparison of two clinical scales for causality assessment in hepatotoxicity. Hepatology (Baltimore, MD). 2001;33:123–30.
15. Kleiner DE. Drug-induced liver injury: the hepatic Pathologist's approach. Gastroenterol Clin N Am. 2017;46:273–96.
16. Kleiner DE. Recent advances in the histopathology of drug-induced liver injury. Surg Pathol Clin. 2018;11:297–311.
17. Zhang X, Ouyang J, Thung SN. Histopathologic manifestations of drug-induced hepatotoxicity. Clin Liver Dis. 2013;17:547–64.. vii-viii
18. de Boer YS, Kosinski AS, Urban TJ, Zhao Z, Long N, Chalasani N, Kleiner DE, Hoofnagle JH. Features of autoimmune hepatitis in patients with drug-induced liver injury. Clin Gastroenterol Hepatol. 2017;15:103–12.. e2
19. Bjornsson E, Talwalkar J, Treeprasertsuk S, Kamath PS, Takahashi N, Sanderson S, Neuhauser M, Lindor K. Drug-induced autoimmune hepatitis: clinical characteristics and prognosis. Hepatology (Baltimore, MD). 2010;51:2040–8.
20. Suzuki A, Brunt EM, Kleiner DE, Miquel R, Smyrk TC, Andrade RJ, Lucena MI, Castiella A, Lindor K, Bjornsson E. The use of liver biopsy evaluation in discrimination of idiopathic autoimmune hepatitis versus drug-induced liver injury. Hepatology (Baltimore, MD). 2011;54:931–9.
21. Andrade RJ, Lucena MI, Kaplowitz N, Garcia-Munoz B, Borraz Y, Pachkoria K, Garcia-Cortes M, Fernandez MC, Pelaez G, Rodrigo L, Duran JA, Costa J, Planas R, Barriocanal A, Guarner C, Romero-Gomez M, Munoz-Yague T, Salmeron J, Hidalgo R. Outcome of acute idiosyncratic drug-induced liver injury: Long-term follow-up in a hepatotoxicity registry. Hepatology (Baltimore, MD). 2006;44:1581–8.
22. Stieger B, Fattinger K, Madon J, Kullak-Ublick GA, Meier PJ. Drug- and estrogen-induced cholestasis through inhibition of the hepatocellular bile salt export pump (Bsep) of rat liver. Gastroenterology. 2000;118:422–30.
23. Ramachandran R, Kakar S. Histological patterns in drug-induced liver disease. J Clin Pathol. 2009;62:481–92.
24. Arranto AJ, Sotaniemi EA. Histologic follow-up of alpha-methyldopa-induced liver injury. Scand J Gastroenterol. 1981;16:865–72.

25. Rodman JS, Deutsch DJ, Gutman SI. Methyldopa hepatitis. A report of six cases and review of the literature. Am J Med. 1976;60:941–8.

26. Toghill PJ, Smith PG, Benton P, Brown RC, Matthews HL. Methyldopa liver damage. Br Med J. 1974;3:545–8.

27. Timbo BB, Ross MP, McCarthy PV, Lin CT. Dietary supplements in a national survey: prevalence of use and reports of adverse events. J Am Diet Assoc. 2006;106:1966–74.

28. Navarro VJ, Barnhart H, Bonkovsky HL, Davern T, Fontana RJ, Grant L, Reddy KR, Seeff LB, Serrano J, Sherker AH, Stolz A, Talwalkar J, Vega M, Vuppalanchi R. Liver injury from herbals and dietary supplements in the U.S. drug-induced liver injury network. Hepatology (Baltimore, MD). 2014;60:1399–408.

29. Rios FF, Rodrigues de Freitas LA, Codes L, Santos Junior GO, Schinoni MI, Parana R. Hepatoportal sclerosis related to the use of herbals and nutritional supplements. Causality or coincidence? Ann Hepatol. 2016;15:932–8.

30. Heidemann LA, Navarro VJ, Ahmad J, Hayashi PH, Stolz A, Kleiner DE, Fontana RJ. Severe acute hepatocellular injury attributed to OxyELITE pro: a case series. Dig Dis Sci. 2016;61:2741–8.

31. Elsharkawy AM, McPherson S, Masson S, Burt AD, Dawson RT, Hudson M. Cholestasis secondary to anabolic steroid use in young men. BMJ (Clinical Res ed). 2012;344:e468.

32. Brazeau MJ, Castaneda JL, Huitron SS, Wang J. A case report of supplement-induced hepatitis in an active duty service member. Mil Med. 2015;180:e844–6.

33. Kou T, Watanabe M, Yazumi S. Hepatic failure during anabolic steroid therapy. Gastroenterology. 2012;143:e11–2.

34. Davidov Y, Har-Noy O, Pappo O, Achiron A, Dolev M, Ben-Ari Z. Methylprednisolone-induced liver injury: case report and literature review. J Dig Dis. 2016;17:55–62.

35. Ghabril M, Bonkovsky HL, Kum C, Davern T, Hayashi PH, Kleiner DE, Serrano J, Rochon J, Fontana RJ, Bonacini M. Liver injury from tumor necrosis factor-alpha antagonists: analysis of thirty-four cases. Clin Gastroenterol Hepatol. 2013;11:558–64.. e3

36. Bjornsson ES, Gunnarsson BI, Grondal G, Jonasson JG, Einarsdottir R, Ludviksson BR, Gudbjornsson B, Olafsson S. Risk of drug-induced liver injury from tumor necrosis factor antagonists. Clin Gastroenterol Hepatol. 2015;13:602–8.

37. Johncilla M, Misdraji J, Pratt DS, Agoston AT, Lauwers GY, Srivastava A, Doyle LA. Ipilimumab-associated hepatitis: Clinicopathologic characterization in a series of 11 cases. Am J Surg Pathol. 2015;39:1075–84.

38. Antezana A, Sigal S, Herbert J, Kister I. Natalizumab-induced hepatic injury: a case report and review of literature. Mult Scler Relat Disord. 2015;4:495–8.

39. Grant LM, Kleiner DE, Conjeevaram HS, Vuppalanchi R, Lee WM. Clinical and histological features of idiosyncratic acute liver injury caused by temozolomide. Dig Dis Sci. 2013;58:1415–21.

40. Fontana RJ, Hayashi PH, Barnhart H, Kleiner DE, Reddy KR, Chalasani N, Lee WM, Stolz A, Phillips T, Serrano J, Watkins PB. Persistent liver biochemistry abnormalities are more common in older patients and those with cholestatic drug induced liver injury. Am J Gastroenterol. 2015;110:1450–9.

41. Polson J, Lee WM. AASLD position paper: the management of acute liver failure. Hepatology (Baltimore, MD). 2005;41:1179–97.

42. Bohan TP, Helton E, McDonald I, Konig S, Gazitt S, Sugimoto T, Scheffner D, Cusmano L, Li S, Koch G. Effect of L-carnitine treatment for valproate-induced hepatotoxicity. Neurology. 2001;56:1405–9.

43. Saphner T, Triest-Robertson S, Li H, Holzman P. The association of nonalcoholic steatohepatitis and tamoxifen in patients with breast cancer. Cancer. 2009;115:3189–95.

44. Begriche K, Igoudjil A, Pessayre D, Fromenty B. Mitochondrial dysfunction in NASH: causes, consequences and possible means to prevent it. Mitochondrion. 2006;6:1–28.

45. Takikawa H, Murata Y, Horiike N, Fukui H, Onji M. Drug-induced liver injury in Japan: an analysis of 1676 cases between 1997 and 2006. Hepatol Res. 2009;39:427–31.

46. Stickel F, Droz S, Patsenker E, Bogli-Stuber K, Aebi B, Leib SL. Severe hepatotoxicity following ingestion of Herbalife nutritional supplements contaminated with Bacillus subtilis. J Hepatol. 2009;50:111–7.

47. Hollister LE. Allergy to chlorpromazine manifested by jaundice. Am J Med. 1957;23:870–9.

48. Ishak KG, Irey NS. Hepatic injury associated with the phenothiazines. Clinicopathologic and follow-up study of 36 patients. Arch Pathol. 1972;93:283–304.

49. Chitturi S, Farrell GC. Drug-induced cholestasis. Semin Gastrointest Dis. 2001;12:113–24.

50. Watanabe N, Takashimizu S, Kojima S, Kagawa T, Nishizaki Y, Mine T, Matsuzaki S. Clinical and pathological features of a prolonged type of acute intrahepatic cholestasis. Hepatol Res. 2007;37:598–607.

51. Westphal JF, Vetter D, Brogard JM. Hepatic side-effects of antibiotics. J Antimicrob Chemother. 1994;33:387–401.

Autoimmune Liver Disease

9

Mikio Zeniya, Masaki Iwai, and Arief A. Suriawinata

Contents

Abbreviations

AIH	Autoimmune hepatitis
ALP	Alkaline phosphatase
AMA	Anti-mitochondrial antibody
ANA	Antinuclear antibody
ASMA	Anti-smooth muscle antibody
CNSDC	Chronic nonsuppurative destructive cholangitis
ERCP	Endoscopic retrograde cholangiopancreatography
GGTP	Gamma-glutamyltranspeptidase
GOT	Glutamic oxaloacetic transaminase
GPT	Glutamic pyruvic transaminase
GVHD	Graft-versus-host disease
HLA	Human leucocyte antigen
Ig	Immunoglobulin
MRCP	Magnetic resonance cholangiopancreatography
PBC	Primary biliary cholangitis
PSC	Primary sclerosing cholangitis
UDCA	Ursodeoxycholic acid

M. Zeniya, MD, PhD, FAASLD (✉)
Tokyo, Japan
e-mail: zeniya@xk9.so-net.ne.jp

M. Iwai, MD, PhD
Kyoto, Japan

A. A. Suriawinata, MD
New Hampshire, USA

9.1 Introduction

Autoimmunity of the human body can be directed toward the hepatocytes or toward the bile ducts. Autoimmune disease affecting the hepatocytes (with elevation of hepatocellular enzymes—AST, ALT) is called autoimmune hepatitis (AIH), whereas the classical example of autoimmune disease affecting small bile ducts is called primary biliary cholangitis (PBC). The latter is associated with elevation of cholestatic liver enzyme (ALP, gamma-GT). The role of autoimmunity in primary sclerosing cholangitis (PSC) affecting the large bile ducts is rather unclear, although in recent years a variant of PSC is certainly caused by IgG4-mediated bile duct injury. Finally, sometimes features of both AIH and PBC or PSC can be present, producing so-called overlap syndrome.

9.2 Autoimmune Hepatitis

Autoimmune hepatitis (AIH) is a chronic self-perpetuating inflammatory disease with a female predominance occurring in all ages and races that may start with an episode of acute hepatitis and may lead to liver cirrhosis, liver cancer, liver transplantation, or death. The etiology of autoimmune hepatitis

© Springer Nature Singapore Pte Ltd. 2019
E. Hashimoto et al. (eds.), *Diagnosis of Liver Disease*, https://doi.org/10.1007/978-981-13-6806-6_9

is unknown, though both genetic and environmental factors are likely to be involved. An immune response targeting liver autoantigens is thought to initiate and perpetuate the liver damage. There are particularly strong associations within the HLA-DRB1 locus, with the HLA-DR3 (DRB1/0301) and HLA-DR4 (DRB1/0401) molecules conferring susceptibility to AIH-1 in Europe and North America and DR4 in Japan [1], and susceptibility to AIH type 2 is associated with HLA-DR3 and HLA-DR7 in the United Kingdom and Brazil [2].

The criteria for the diagnosis of autoimmune hepatitis (AIH) are evolving. An initial attempt to define this disease by the International Autoimmune Hepatitis Group [3] was followed by validation studies, a redefinition with still an extensive scoring system [4] and more recently a strong simplification of criteria, [5] and recently EASL published a well-summarized review [6].

AIH is in fact a syndrome, and the diagnosis is based on a combination of clinical features suggesting liver disease, the absence of other causes in conjunction with the presence of autoimmune markers (ANA, SMA, IgG), and typical features on liver biopsy. Autoantibodies are normally detected by indirect immunofluorescence on a rodent substrate that includes the kidney, liver, and stomach.

Severe liver injury and its repeated attack in AIH cause significant parenchymal loss and extinction, resulting in liver failure. Therefore, glucocorticoid with or without other immunosuppressants, such as azathioprine or cyclosporine, should be administered as soon as the diagnosis of AIH is established [7, 8] to achieve normalization of transaminases and immunoglobulin G levels in serum. Liver transplantation may be needed when treatment is delayed or ineffective [9].

Definite diagnosis requires (1) the absence of markers suggesting active viral hepatitis, abstinence from alcohol, no recent blood transfusion, and no recent exposure to hepatotoxic drugs, (2) the presence of autoimmune markers and elevated gamma-globulin, and (3) compatible histological patterns of liver injury

[1, 3–5]. The histology in AIH includes interface and panlobular hepatitis, lymphoplasmacytic infiltrate, rosette formation of the periportal hepatocytes, and absence of biliary injury. Interface hepatitis is necroinflammation at the interface between the portal tract stroma and hepatic lobule and is recognized as chronic feature; however, in some patients with acute onset, this finding is less observed, and centrilobular necrosis is the dominant findings [10, 11]. The precise mechanism of autoimmune-related liver damage has not been elucidated in the liver that is known as tolerated organ [12, 13]. Clinically, AIH is classified into acute and chronic types, with or without acute exacerbation. Central necrosis with plasma cell infiltrate is frequently seen in the "acute" phase or acute exacerbation of AIH [14, 15], and syncytial giant cells are sometimes seen in severe AIH [16–19]. Cautiously, "acute" onset AIH frequently shows negative for autoantibodies and elevation of serum immunoglobulin, resulting in a much difficult diagnosis [20]. The histology of AIH varies depending on when the biopsy is taken during the disease. It is important to understand that biopsy cannot lead the definite diagnosis; however, biopsy is essential for ruling out other diseases. There are also various overlap forms of AIH with other autoimmune diseases, including primary biliary cirrhosis (PBC), primary sclerosing cholangitis (PSC) and outliers, autoimmune cholangitis [1], and AIH with bile duct injuries [21, 22]. Especially in child the differentiation between AIH and PSC is difficult, suggesting that MRCP should be done in child case. For the diagnosis of such so-called overlap syndrome, initial diagnosis is important and should be diagnosed as AIH with bile duct injury or PBC with liver injury except for overlap syndrome.

Disease severity assessment is important especially at the initial diagnosis [23]. Peritoneoscopy reveals red swollen liver in an acute AIH with fissuring excavation, while chronic AIH demonstrates red mottling on the surface of the enlarged liver and white markings due to dilatation of the peripheral portal vein (Fig. 9.1).

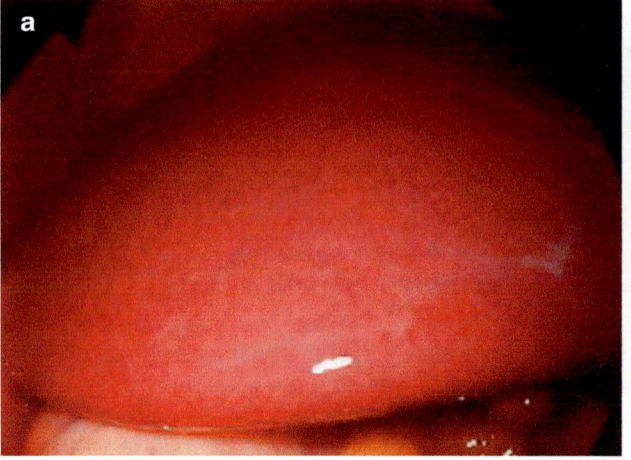
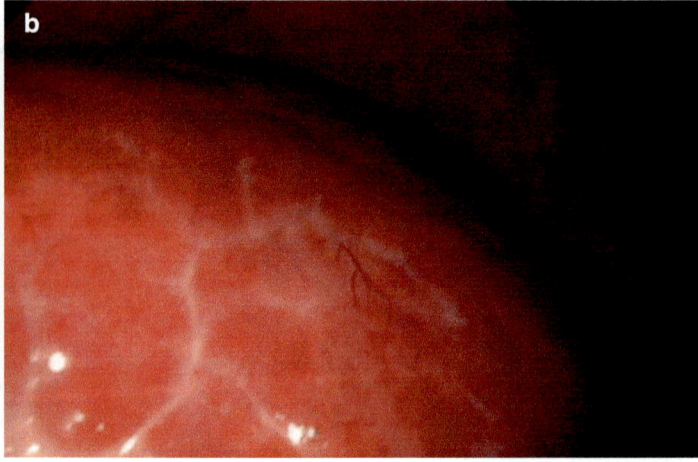

Fig. 9.1 Macroscopic findings of the liver with autoimmune hepatitis. (a) Peritoneoscopy shows swollen red liver with red markings in a patient with acute autoimmune hepatitis. (b) Peritoneoscopy in a patient with chronic autoimmune hepatitis shows fissure excavation with red markings on the surface of the enlarged liver, and white markings are visible with dilatation of the peripheral portal vein

Case 9.1

A 59-year-old male complained of general malaise, arthralgia, jaundice, and brown urine. His liver function test showed ALT 144 IU/L, AST 121 IU/L, GGT 76 IU/L, IgG 2322 mg/dL, ANA × 160, ASMA × 20, and negative AMA. Liver biopsy showed severe interface hepatitis and dense inflammatory infiltrates in the portal tract, consisting of plasma cells, lymphocytes, and rare eosinophils (Fig. 9.2). Prednisolone 30 mg/day was administered; arthralgia improved, and his liver function test reverted to normal values with maintenance dose. A variety of complications are often associated with AIH. Polyarthralgia, thyroiditis, and ulcerative colitis frequently occur in AIH, and the administration of glucocorticoid generally reduces their symptoms and signs.

Case 9.2

A 74-year-old female complained of general malaise for 6 months, and her liver function test showed ALT 673 IU/L, AST 756 IU/L, ALP 281 IU/L, GGT 420 IU/L, IgG 1361 mg/dL, ANA × 40, and negative AMA. Liver biopsy showed not only severe interface hepatitis but also central necrosis with plasma cell infiltrate (Fig. 9.3a). Prednisolone was administered, and her liver function test improved. Central necrosis with infiltration of plasma cells, such as seen in this case, is often observed in the acute phase of AIH [14, 15, 24].

Case 9.3

A 15-year-old female complained of general malaise and developed jaundice. Liver function test showed TBIL 11.5 mg/dL, AST 1185 IU/L, and ALT 1297 IU/L, and TBIL peaked

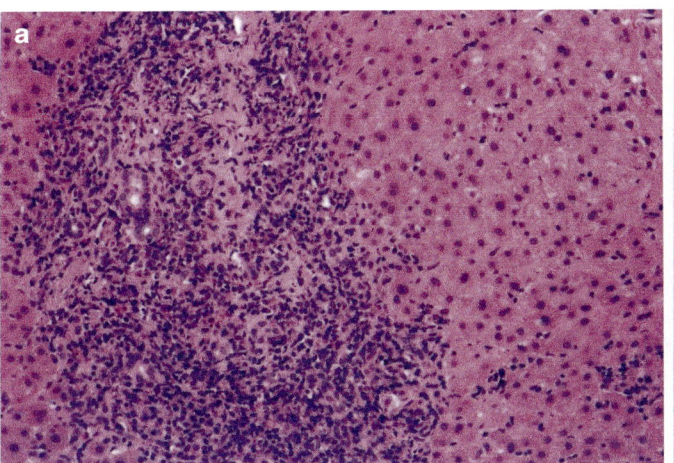
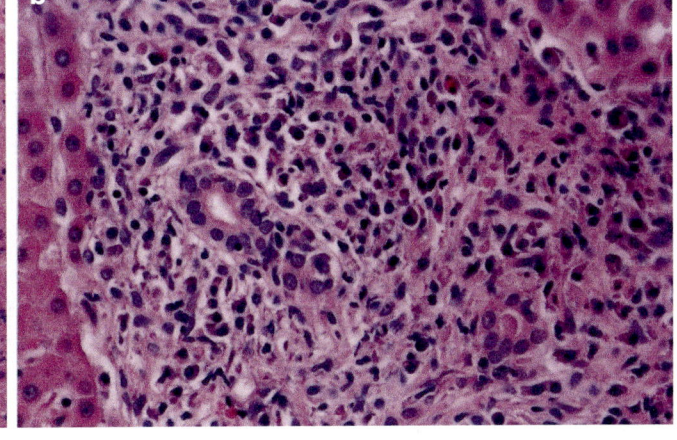

Fig. 9.2 Histological findings in autoimmune hepatitis. (**a**) Interface hepatitis is seen in the periportal area with many inflammatory cells in or around the portal tract. (**b**) The inflammatory cells in the portal tract consist of plasma cells, lymphocytes, and eosinophils. Bile ductules are damaged

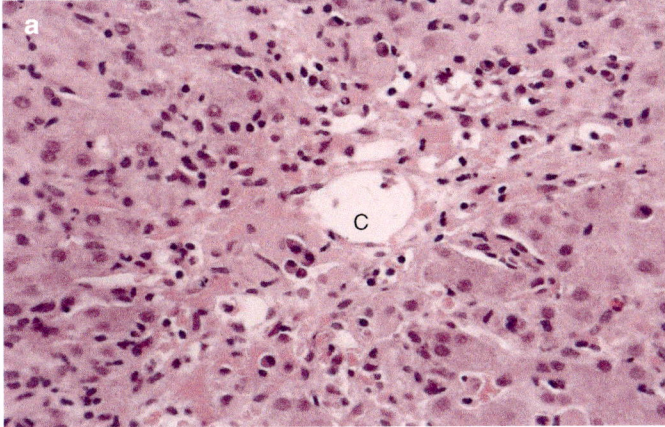
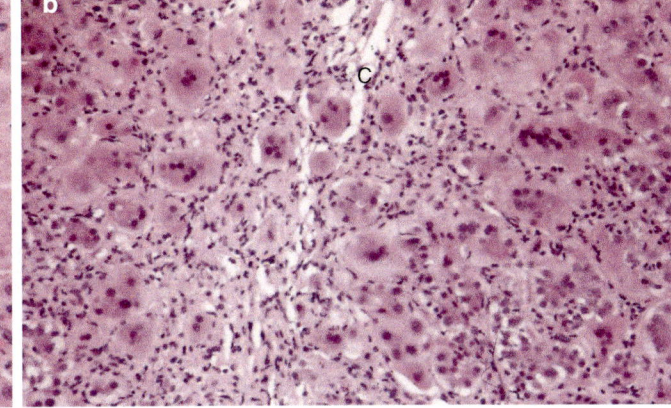

Fig. 9.3 Histological findings in autoimmune hepatitis. (**a**) Central necrosis with infiltration of plasma cells. (**b**) Multinucleated giant cells around the central vein (arrow), surrounded by plasma cells and neutrophils. Small hepatocytes are distributed in a rosette formation in the periportal area. *P* portal tract

36.4 mg/dL in a month, and PT was 55%. Liver biopsy showed syncytial giant cells in the centrilobular area, rosetting of hepatocytes in the periportal area, and neutrophilic and plasma cell infiltrate in the portal tract (Fig. 9.3b). Prednisolone 30 mg/day and azathioprine 50 mg/day were simultaneously administered, and her liver function test reverted to normal values after 3 months. Although giant cell hepatitis is a frequent pattern of liver injury in neonates, multinucleated syncytial giant cells can also be observed in AIH. Their appearance is associated with severe liver injury in AIH [18].

Case 9.4

A 51-year-old male underwent a health examination and was found to have TBIL 0.89 mg/dL, AST 95 IU/L, ALT 128 IU/L, ALP 394 IU/L, IgG 3800 mg/dL, ANA × 1280, and PLT 7.4 × 104/μL. Liver biopsy under peritoneoscopy showed nodular formations with lymphoid follicles and red markings on the surface of the liver. Liver histology showed irregularly sized pseudolobules with massive necrosis, broad septa, and a fibrotic area infiltrated with many lymphoplasmacytic cells

(Fig. 9.4). The prognosis of AIH is poor if liver cirrhosis has occurred at the time of diagnosis of AIH [25], unless prednisolone is promptly administered. The patient was treated with 30 mg prednisolone, and his liver function test improved [26].

Case 9.5

A 56-year-old male complained of abdominal discomfort with brown urine. Liver function test showed TBIL 8.5 mg/dL, AST 1173 IU/L, ALT 2236 IU/L, PT 65%, thrombocyte 10.4 × 10 [4]/μL, and ANA × 40. Repeat liver function test 1 month later did not show any improvement. Echo-guided liver biopsy showed lobular disarray with abundant inflammatory cells in the portal tracts and central necrosis, and high magnification showed interface hepatitis with mononuclear cell infiltrate comprising CD138-positive plasma cells (Fig. 9.5). Administration of prednisolone and repeat plasma exchange did not improve liver failure after 4 months. Upper abdominal CT showed a reduction in liver size compared to that seen on admission, accompanied by decreasing consciousness. He underwent liver transplantation 5 months after

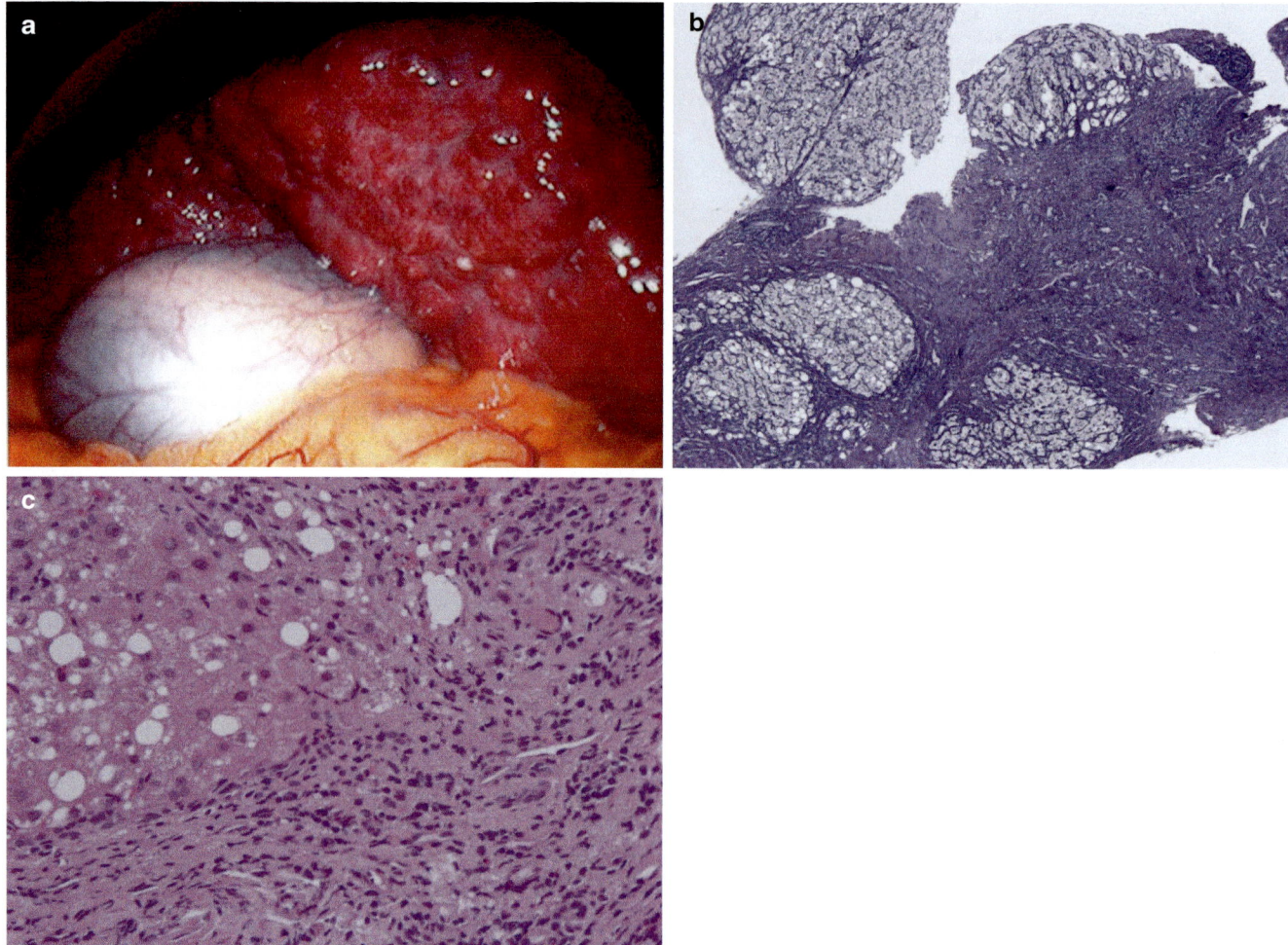

Fig. 9.4 Liver cirrhosis due to autoimmune hepatitis. (**a**) Peritoneoscopy shows irregularly sized nodules on the liver surface with intermittent large excavation. (**b**) Nodules of remaining liver parenchyma (pseudolobules) separated by wide areas of collapse fibrosis. (**c**) Lymphoplasmacellular infiltrate in broad band of fibrosis

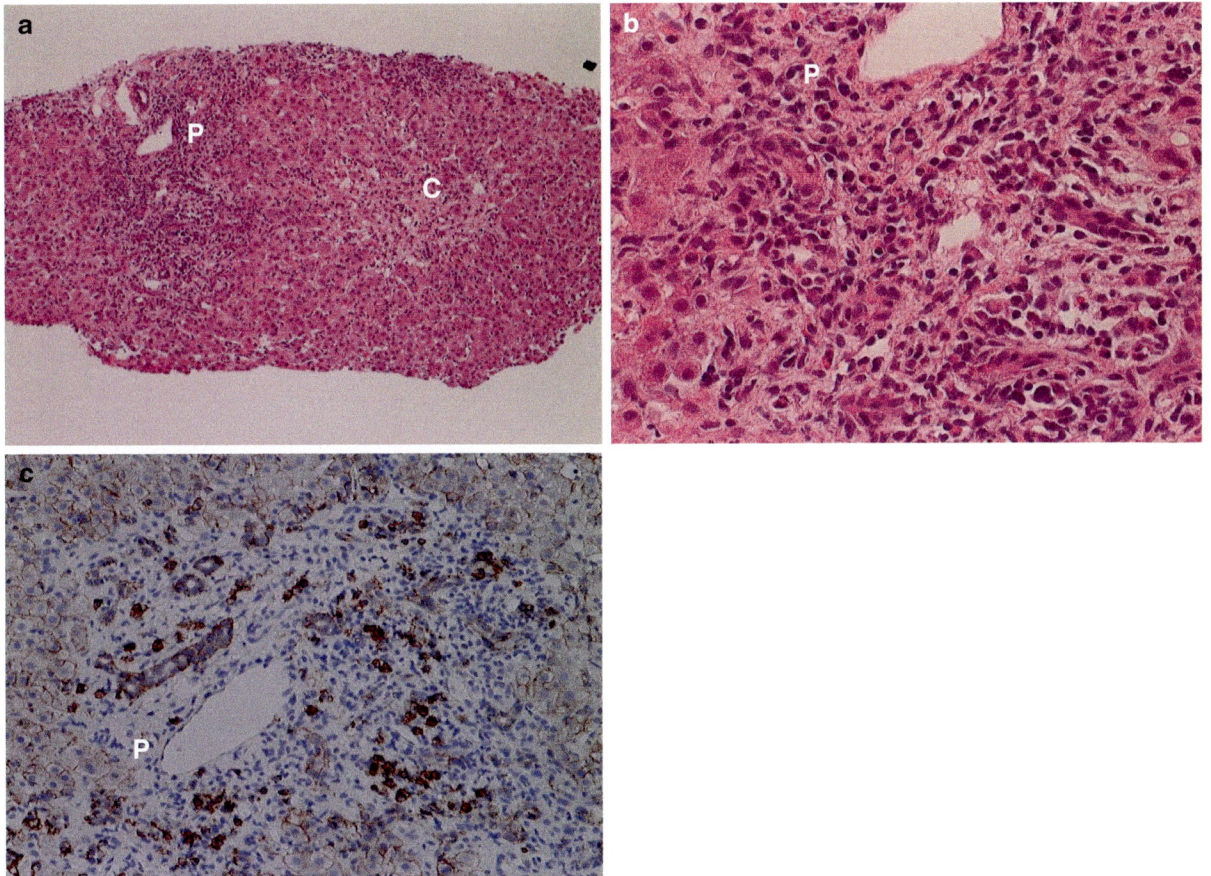

Fig. 9.5 Autoimmune hepatitis. (**a**) Liver histology at admission shows architectural disarray of the lobule, abundant inflammatory cells in the portal tract, and centrilobular necrosis. (**b**) Many inflammatory cells, including plasma cells and lymphocytes, are seen. (**c**) CD138 immunoreactivity is seen in plasma cells. *C* central vein, *P* portal tract

initial treatment. The explanted liver showed submassive hepatic necrosis with abundant ductular reaction and roset-ting of hepatocytes in the necrotic area (Fig. 9.6). Liver trans-plantation is indicated in acute liver failure due to AIH. The patient survived 4.5 years after liver transplantation.

Systemic lupus erythematosus (SLE) is an autoimmune dis-ease characterized by disorders of multiple organs, including the liver [27, 28]. The frequency of hepatic involvement in SLE is about 8–23% [28, 29]. Fatty change or congestion of the liver is frequently seen in patients with SLE [30], but concurrent AIH and SLE is quite rare [31, 32]. Furthermore, a differential diagnosis of SLE-associated hepatitis and AIH is clinically dif-ficult [33, 34]. Here, we present a case of SLE with periportal hepatitis and plasma cell infiltrate and discuss the histologic differential diagnosis of SLE-associated hepatitis and AIH.

Case 9.6

A 60-year-old woman complained of fever and fatigue and developed proteinuria and polyarthralgia. Liver function test showed slight elevation of AST and ALT. A diagnosis of SLE was established according to the criteria of the American College of Rheumatology. She was treated with low-dose prednisolone therapy for 6 months and was asymptomatic for 4 years. Subsequently, she developed new onset of polyar-thralgia, fatigue, and myalgia and had dark urine and jaundice. There was no history of drug-taking, alcohol abuse, or paren-teral exposure to blood products. On admission, her liver func-tion test revealed TBIL 3.28 mg/dL, DBIL 2.11 mg/dL, AST 192 IU/L, ALT 231 IU/L, ALP 1063 IU/L, GGT 332 IU/L, and LDH 253 IU/L. Immunological tests showed ANA × 640, IgG 2130 mg/dL, IgM 148 mg/dL, positive lupus erythematosus cell test, anti-double-stranded DNA, anti-single-stranded DNA, and HLA typing for DR4 and negative anti-ribosomal P antibody. Anti-smooth muscle antibody, anti-mitochondria antibody, and anti-LKM 1 antibody were negative. HBsAg, IgM-HA Ab, and HCV RNA were negative. Serological tests for hepatotropic viruses, including cytomegalovirus and Epstein-Barr virus, were also negative. Peritoneoscopy revealed mild excavations on the liver surface with diffuse white markings, but without any red mottling. Liver biopsy showed fatty metamorphosis in the hepatic lobules, and the portal tracts were fibrotic but without bridging fibrosis; there was mild interface hepatitis with lymphoplasmacytic infiltrate without rosetting of the hepatocytes (Fig. 9.7). After admission,

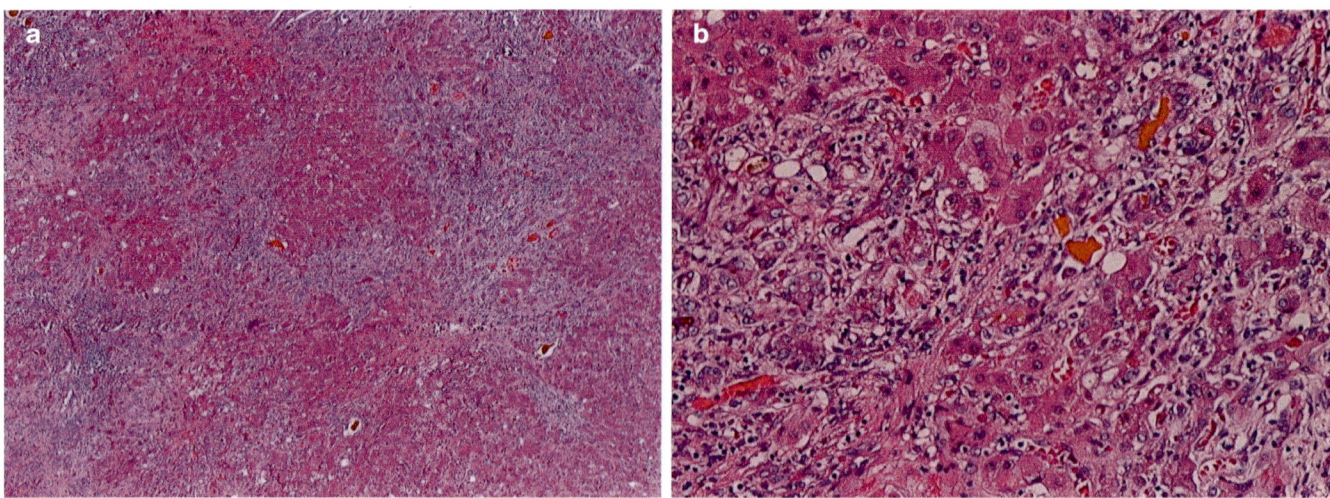

Fig. 9.6 Autoimmune hepatitis. (**a**) Submassive hepatic necrosis in the recipient liver. (**b**) Oval cells or small hepatocytes are seen around the portal tract

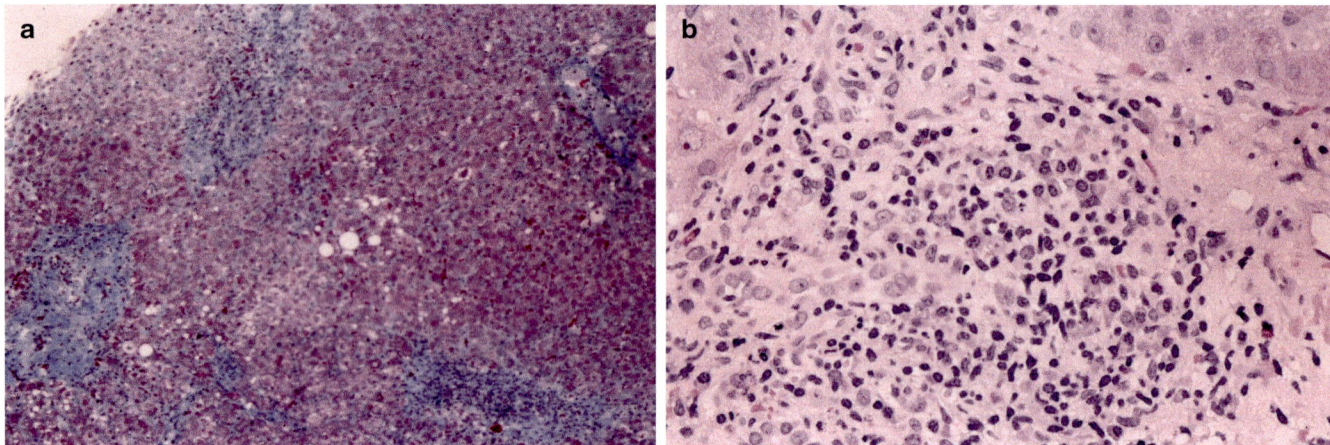

Fig. 9.7 Autoimmune hepatitis in systemic lupus erythematosus. (**a**) Mallory-Azan stain shows the portal tract is enlarged, with portal tract fibrosis. Neither bridging fibrosis nor pseudolobular formation is seen. Fatty metamorphosis is seen in hepatocytes. (**b**) Hematoxylin and eosin stain shows the portal tract is infiltrated with many plasma cells and lymphocytes, and configuration of the biliary epithelium is irregular. *C* central vein, *P* portal tract. (Reuse of Iwai M, et al. Autoimmune hepatitis in a patient with systemic lupus erythematous. Clin Rheumatol 2003; 22: 234–6., with permission from Springer)

her ALT and AST were elevated to 422 IU/L and 347 IU/L, respectively. Massive proteinuria (11 g/day), fever, massive pleural effusion, and pericardial effusion developed. Prednisolone was administered orally at an initial dose of 40 mg/day and tapered to a maintenance dose of 10 mg over a period of 3 months. Subsequently, pericarditis, pleuritis, and proteinuria disappeared, and her liver function tests reverted to normal levels. A seropositive lupus erythematosus test became negative, and serum complements returned to normal levels. Serum IgG and the ANA titers were decreased. Her AIH score was 19 before treatment and 21 after treatment. Pericarditis and pleuritis resolved after administration of prednisolone, and her liver function tests reverted to normal values for 4 years. SLE is sometimes complicated by liver injury, and it is difficult to distinguish chronic hepatitis in SLE from AIH [34, 35]. The histologic findings of interface hepatitis with lymphoplasmacytic infiltrate are those of AIH in SLE [36].

9.3   Primary Biliary Cholangitis

Primary biliary cirrhosis is recently renamed as primary biliary cholangitis (PBC) and generally regarded as an autoimmune disease. PBC is histologically characterized as chronic nonsuppurative destructive cholangitis [37]. The disease affects the small bile ducts (interlobular or septal bile ducts) in contrast to sclerosing cholangitis that affects mostly the large bile ducts.

Serum anti-mitochondrial antibody is the major marker of PBC and is positive in 90% of patients with PBC [38]. The disease usually affects middle-aged to elderly women, with a peak incidence between 40 and 60 years old. PBC is clinically classified into asymptomatic PBC (a-PBC), PBC with esophageal varices (v-PBC) [39], and symptomatic PBC (s-PBC). With the increasing number of medical checkups including laboratory testing, PBC is now frequently diagnosed at an early and completely asymptomatic stage. Most patients with a-PBC remain stable for long periods of time, but some may gradually progress to s-PBC. The presenting features in s-PBC are intense pruritis, lethargy, skin pigmentation, and cholestatic jaundice, occasionally followed by liver failure, and some patients are associated with the Sjogren disease with or without CREST (calcinosis, Raynaud's phenomenon, esophageal dysfunction, sclerodactyly, and telangiectasia) syndrome [40].

Histological staging [37] can be summarized as follows:

- Stage 1 = inflammation and nonsuppurative destructive cholangitis (florid bile duct lesion).
- Stage 2 = destruction of parenchymal limiting plates with variable degrees of ductular proliferation and early short radiating septa.
- Stage 3 = extension of the portal-septal fibrosis to include portal to portal bridging septa (biliary fibrosis).
- Stage 4 = fully developed biliary cirrhosis.

Recently more clinical scoring system for both staging and grading has been shown, and this scoring is much practical and useful for assessing the disease [41].

Ursodeoxycholic acid (UDCA) is the treatment of choice for early-stage PBC [42]. Monotherapy of UDCA improves serum biochemical markers of bilirubin, alkaline phosphatase, γ-GTP, cholesterol, and IgM levels [43, 44] and slows down histological progression to liver cirrhosis, [45] and obeticholic acid and bezafibrate, probably by activating nuclear receptor, have shown promising results for non-responders of UDCA [46, 47]. Combination therapy of UDCA with bezafibrate is reported to improve biochemical tests in patients with PBC, with partial response to UDCA [48].

Case 9.7

A 73-year-old female underwent a health examination and was found to have AST 25 IU/L, ALT 14 IU/L, ALP 358 IU/L, and GGT 73I U/L. Further examination showed IgG 1113 mg/dL, IgM 205 mg/dL, AMA ×40, and ANA ×1280. Liver biopsy under peritoneoscopy showed small scattered excavations on the liver surface with white capsular thickening, infiltration of the portal tracts by inflammatory cells, and bile duct proliferation accompanied by many inflammatory cells including lymphocytes and plasma cells (Fig. 9.8).

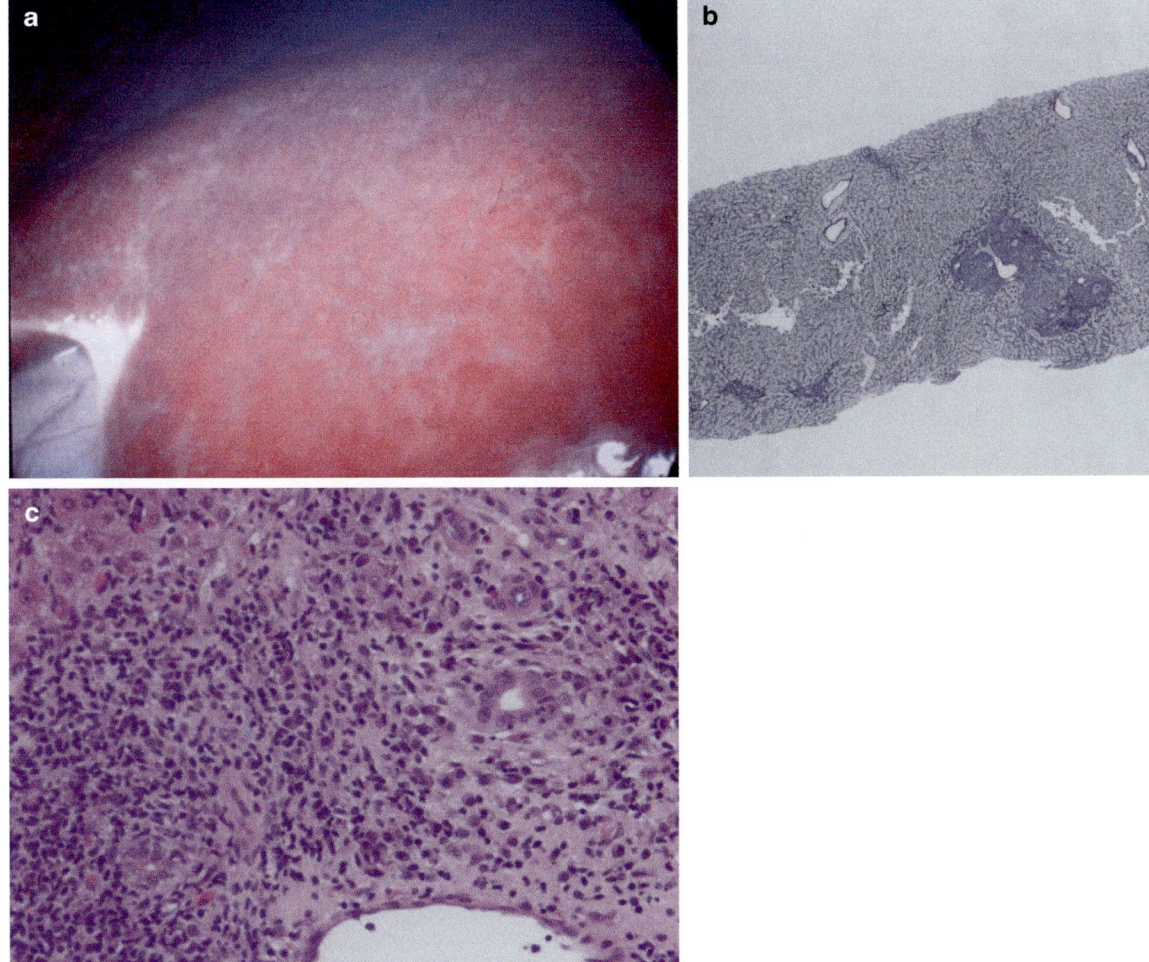

Fig. 9.8 Primary biliary cholangitis. (**a**) Peritoneoscopy shows small excavations of the liver surface, with white capsules. (**b**) Silver-stained liver tissue shows the presence of an enlarged portal tract. (**c**) Proliferating bile ductules and many lymphocytes and plasma cells in the enlarged portal tract are seen

UDCA 600 mg/day was administered, and ALP and GGT reverted to normal values after 2 months. Her liver function test remained within normal limits for a long time, which proved the efficacy of UDCA in treating a-PBC.

Patients with PBC have a complication of Sjogren syndrome, and PBC should be also considered the main cause of liver disease in primary Sjogren syndrome [49].

Case 9.8

A 45-year-old female usually complained of dry eye or mouth and Raynaud' phenomenon in cold season. Physical examination showed AST 55 IU/L, ALT 62 IU/L, ALP 525 IU/L, and GGT 198 IU/L, and detailed examinations showed AMA ×1280, ANA ×1280, thyroid test ×6400, microsomal test ×100, SS-A Ab negative, SS-B Ab negative, and HLA-DR2 positive. Peritoneoscopy with liver biopsy showed mosaic pattern of leopard with acinus markings on the surface, and there are histologically, enlarged portal tracts with infiltration of inflamma-

tory cells and neither infiltration nor necrosis was seen in central area. In portal tract bile ducts were destructed with degeneration of epithelial cells, and lymphoplasmacytic infiltration was observed (Fig. 9.9). UDCA of 300 or 600 mg/day was administered, and serum value of ALP/GGT was reverted to normal value as well as that of AST/ALT for 3 years.

Clinical manifestations and histological features in PBC with or without Sjogren syndrome were not different, and stage 1 PBC is considered to be one of the first extraglandular manifestations in patients with primary Sjogren syndrome [49], and then relation between PBC and Sjogren syndrome should be studied more in detail.

Case 9.9

A 34-year-old female complained of general malaise and itching for 2 years, which was exacerbated after the delivery of her second child [50]. After delivery, her liver function tests reverted to normal values, but were elevated later. Liver

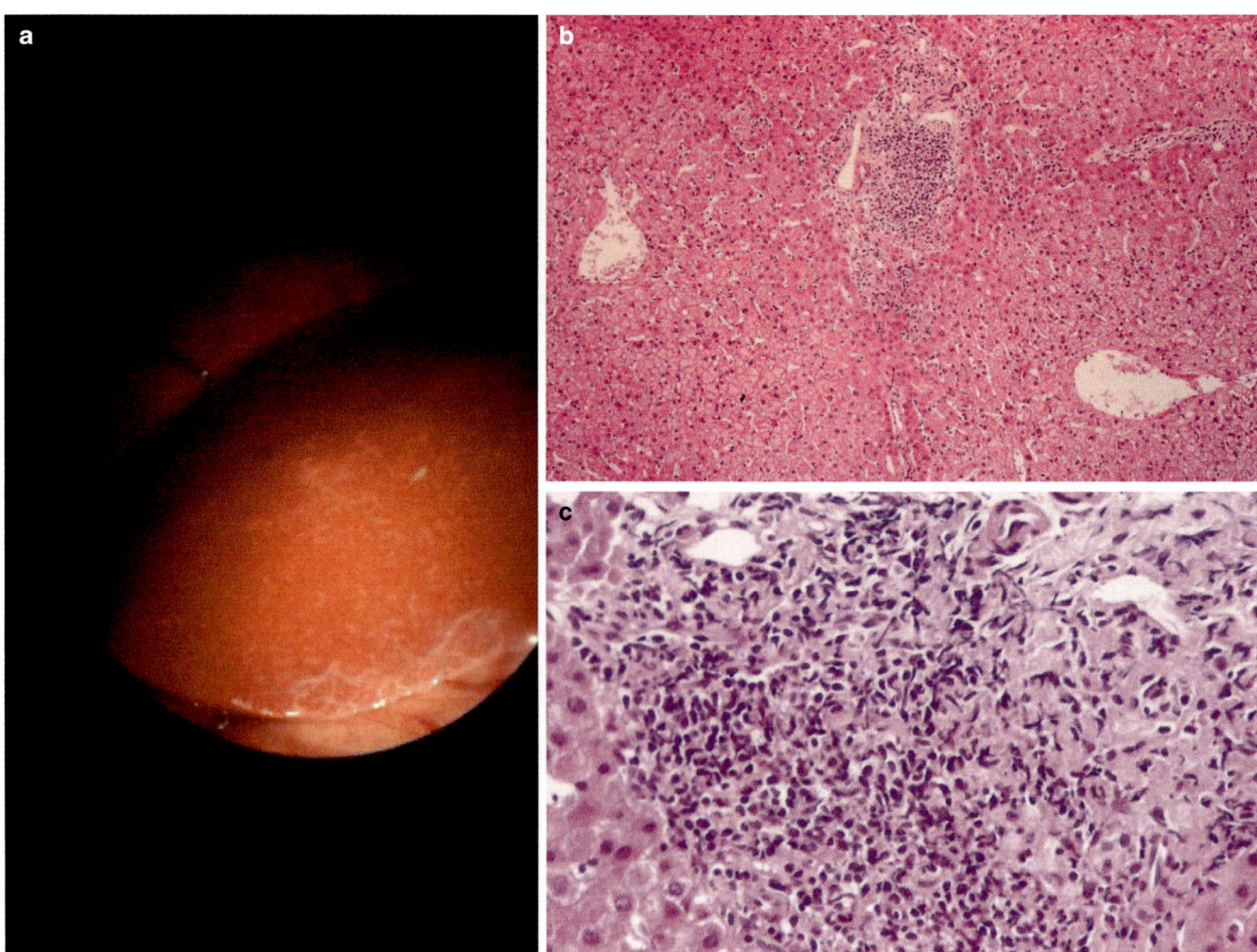

Fig. 9.9 Primary biliary cholangitis in a patient with Sjogren syndrome. (**a**) Peritoneoscopy shows appearance of leopard crest with white markings on the liver surface. (**b**) Microscopic view shows an enlarged porta tract with infiltration of inflammatory cells, and there are few necrotic areas. (**c**) There are lymphoplasmacytic cells in portal tract, and bile ducts are destructed with degenerated epithelial cells

function tests showed TBIL 0.74 mg/dL, AST 89 IU/L, ALT 131 IU/L, ALP 416 IU/L, GGT 177 IU/L, IgM 689 mg/dL, and AMA × 320. Peritoneoscopy showed a patchy liver surface, and liver biopsy showed an enlarged portal tract and fibrosis; the bile duct was damaged, with ductular proliferation accompanied by many lymphocytes and plasma cells (Fig. 9.10). UDCA 600 mg/day was effective, and the ALP, ALT, AST, and GGT levels were decreased to some extent.

Case 9.10

A 62-year-old female suffering from arthralgia with abnormal liver function tests for 10 years had TBIL 0.96 mg/dL, AST 164 IU/L, ALT 196 IU/L, ALP 483 IU/L, GGT 422 IU/L, IgM 345 mg/dL, and AMA ×320. Peritoneoscopy with liver biopsy showed early nodular formation on the liver, liver biopsy showed bridging fibrosis, and bile duct loss, interface, and intralobular hepatitis were noted (Fig. 9.11). The findings in liver biopsy were consistent with PBC stage 3. The administration of UDCA with and without bezafibrate did not improve liver chemistry. Ascites

and leg edema followed by liver failure occurred 6 years later. The levels of ALP, ALT, AST, and GGT in serum were high, and UDCA did not improve liver chemistry in this a-PBC patient.

Clinical manifestations and liver histology with peritoneoscopic findings in a patient of s-PBC is demonstrated in Chap. 6 (Case 6.2), and the patient died of hepatic failure with encephalopathy 3.5 years after initial presentation.

The PBC-AIH overlap syndrome is defined by the association of PBC and AIH in a patient, either simultaneously or consecutively [51]. The overlap syndrome has been applied to some cases with aggregate scores of definite or probable AIH using the modified scoring system of the International Autoimmune Hepatitis Group and cholestatic state of biochemical study combined with seropositivite-AMA [51]. Other study suggests requirement for two out of three diagnostic criteria of AIH and PBC among patients suspecting of overlap syndrome (Table 9.2) [52], and about 10% of AIH and PBC belongs in the overlap category [53]. The histological features include a variable combination of inflammatory

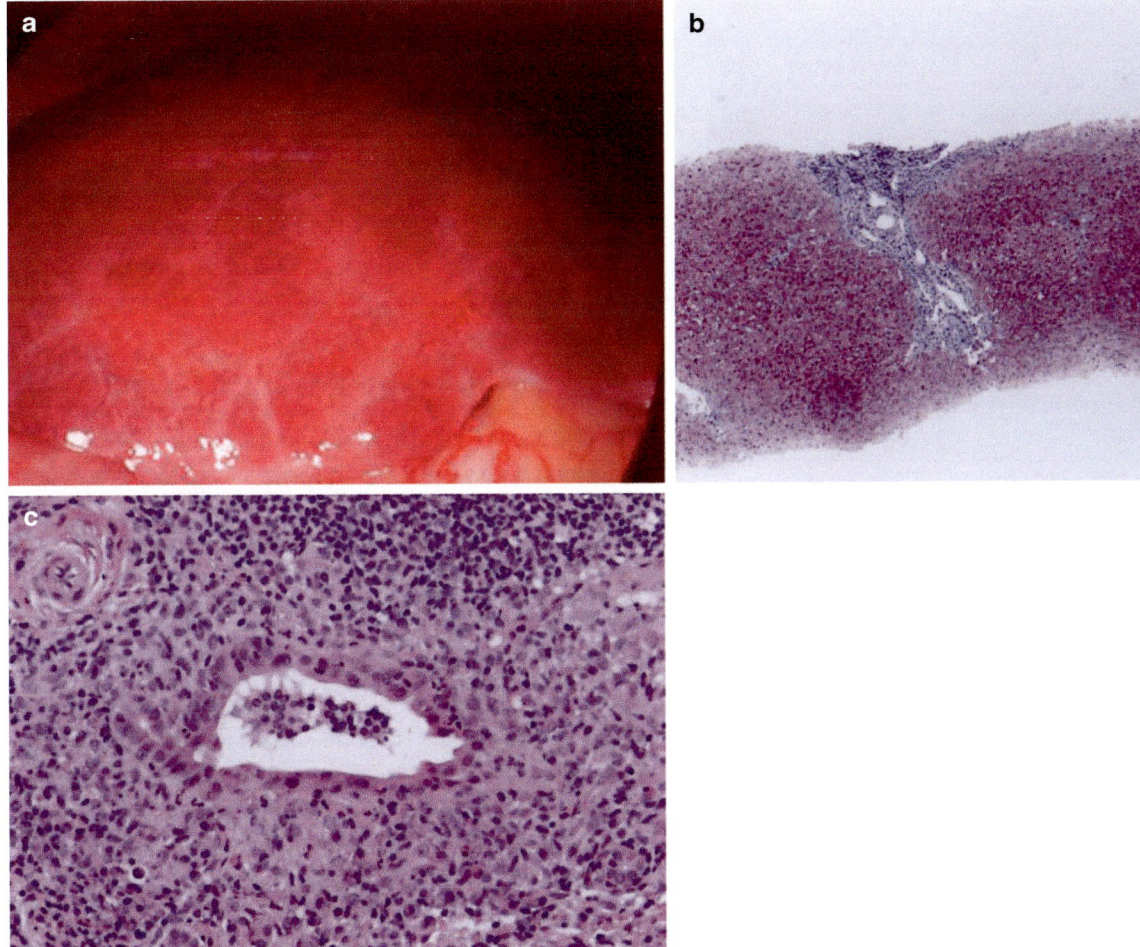

Fig. 9.10 Primary biliary cholangitis. (**a**) Peritoneoscopy shows patchy markings on the liver surface. (**b**) The portal tract is enlarged, and fibrosis extends into the lobules. (**c**) The interlobular bile duct is damaged, with an aggregate of lymphocytes, neutrophils, and eosinophils surrounding the damaged bile duct. Their inflammatory cells infiltrate beyond the basement membrane of the bile duct

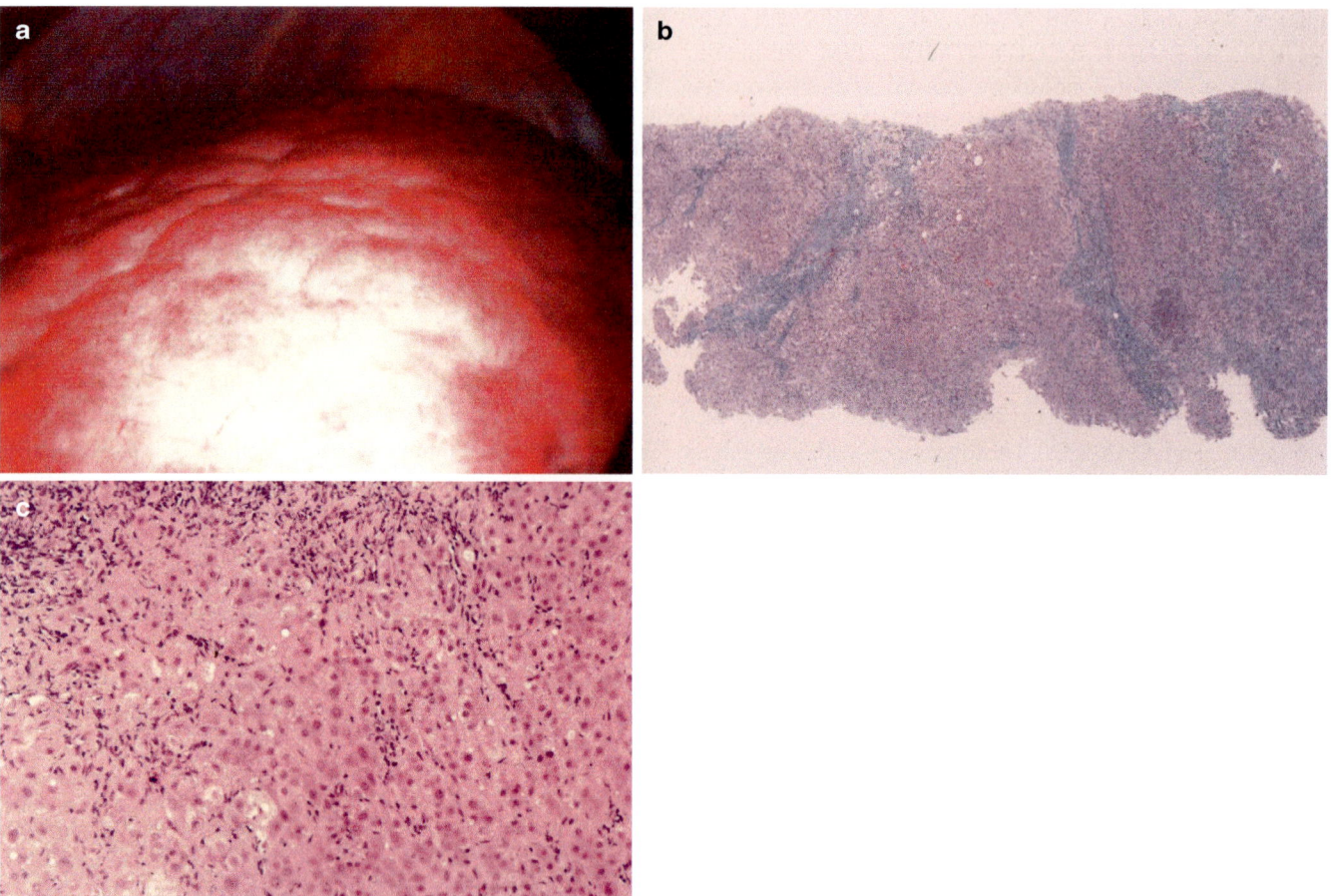

Fig. 9.11 Primary biliary cholangitis. (**a**) Peritoneoscopy shows early nodular formation and deep fissuring excavation on the liver surface. (**b**) Masson's trichrome stained liver biopsy shows bridging fibrosis, and the portal tract is expanded. (**c**) Interface or intralobular hepatitis is seen

Table 9.2 Diagnostic criteria of overlap syndrome (Paris criteria)

AIH	1.	ALT>5 times upper limit of normal
	2.	IgG > 2 times upper limit of normal, or anti-SMA positive
	3.	Chronic hepatitis pattern of injury on liver biopsy
PBC	1.	Alkaline phosphatase>2 times upper limit of normal
	2.	AMA positive
	3.	Florid duct lesion on liver biopsy

cell infiltrates directed at the bile ducts and hepatocytes, and development of superimposed AIH can result in rapid progression toward cirrhosis and liver failure [54].

Case 9.11

A 67-year-old male was found to have AST 447 IU/L, ALT 712 IU/L, ALP 266 IU/L, GGT 247 IU/L, ANA × 1280, and AMA × 40. Peritoneoscopy showed an irregular surface with red markings, formation of large nodules, and lymphangiectasia; liver biopsy showed nodule formation separated by broad septa and lymphoplasmacytic infiltration from the portal tracts, while the bile ducts decreased in number (Fig. 9.12). Administration of UDCA reduced the ALP, ALT, AST, and GGT levels for a while, but transaminase was then elevated

again. Prednisolone and UDCA administration reverted both ALT/AST and ALP/GGT to near-normal values and reduced ANA titer. UDCA and a small dosage of prednisolone maintained normal liver function in the long term.

9.4 Primary Sclerosing Cholangitis

Primary sclerosing cholangitis (PSC) is a chronic cholestatic liver disease caused by chronic inflammatory destruction of intrahepatic or extrahepatic bile ducts (large duct), and is frequently accompanied by inflammatory bowel disease, usually chronic ulcerative colitis [55]. Many patients are <50 years old at the time of diagnosis, with a male preponderance of 3 to 1. There is a variant form of small duct PSC in which findings from cholangiographic study are normal [56] and of PSC overlapped with autoimmune hepatitis [57].

Genetic and environmental factors contribute to the pathogenesis of PSC, and genome-wide association studies identified genomic region of HLA antigen-B locus most important for its development, and several other genomic regions are said to associate with disturbance of immune self-recognition and adaptive immunity in PSC [58]. Microbial component

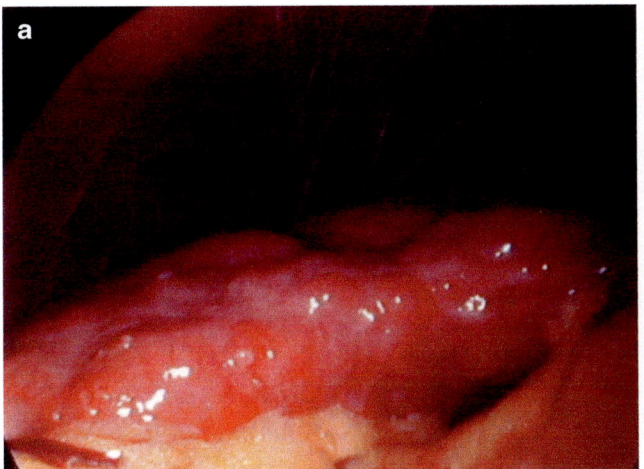
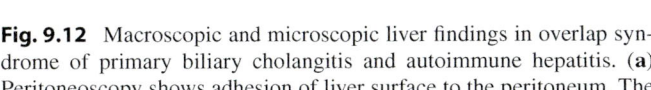
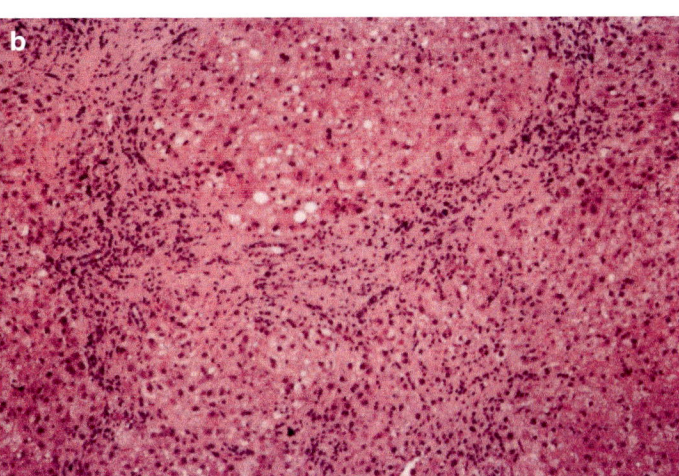

Fig. 9.12 Macroscopic and microscopic liver findings in overlap syndrome of primary biliary cholangitis and autoimmune hepatitis. (**a**) Peritoneoscopy shows adhesion of liver surface to the peritoneum. The liver surface is wavy. Large and irregularly sized nodules are visible, with red markings. (**b**) Liver histology reveals broad septum fibrosis, and inflammatory cells are seen in the portal tract

entering into the portal circulation from the gut could contribute to biliary inflammation [59]. Moreover gut-derived activated T lymphocytes may home to the liver during the development of PSC [60], and cholangiocytes undergo the phenomenon of cellular senescence influenced by various cytokines [61] and participate in pathogenesis of PSC [62].

In the early stage, PSC is asymptomatic in some patients, and 5–25% of them are discovered because of elevated serum alkaline phosphatase. In some cases, the disease progresses, and biliary cirrhosis develops; this is followed by liver failure [63].

Follow-up studies have shown considerable variations in the clinical course. The diagnosis of PSC is based on clinical, laboratory, and morphological findings as well as by endoscopic retrograde cholangiopancreatography (ERCP). Serum biliary enzyme is elevated, and protoplasmic-staining antineutrophil cytoplasmic antibodies are positive. ERCP or magnetic resonance cholangiopancreatography (MRCP) [64] shows irregular wall contour and stenosis of intrahepatic or extrahepatic bile ducts with prestenotic dilatation.

Liver biopsy is rarely done in these patients unless issues remain. Histological features are classified into four stages. In stage 1, changes are confined within the portal boundaries, with infiltration of lymphocytes, plasma cells, and neutrophils. Lymphoid follicles or aggregates are occasionally present. Small bile ducts are degenerated, and the portal stroma is edematous. In stage 2, the portal tracts are swollen, with disruption of the parenchymal limiting plates and cholangitis. Biliary interface activity is accompanied by focal ductular proliferation. In stage 3, portal fibrosis develops with formation of portal-to-portal fibrous septa and, in stage 4, biliary cirrhosis. The natural course of PSC shows different survival rates—depending on the histological stage—and its association with autoimmune diseases is far less than in PBC. It is complicated by cholecystolithiasis or choledocholithiasis and cholangiocarcinoma. However, the disease may reappear in about 25% of patients after transplantation [65].

Treatment varies from conservative therapy with UDCA [66] to invasive therapy using balloon and stent insertion to reduce isolated stenosis of intrahepatic or extrahepatic stenosis of bile ducts [67]. Liver transplantation is the therapy of choice in late-stage PSC [68] and may have a role in treatment of cholangiocarcinoma.

Case 9.12

A 20-year-old male came to our clinic complaining of epigastric pain, fever, and bloody stools. Laboratory data showed TBIL 0.32 mg/dL, ALT 32 IU/L, AST 23 IU/L, ALP 587 IU/L, GGT 130 IU/L, IgG 2270 mg/dL, ANA ×40, and negative AMA. ERCP showed irregularly narrowed and dilated intrahepatic bile ducts (Fig. 9.13). Laparoscopy showed white markings with dilated peripheral portal veins on the liver surface, and liver biopsy revealed onion-skin fibrosis surrounding small bile ducts (Fig. 9.14). UDCA was administered orally. Ulcerative colitis was diagnosed by colonoscopy.

Case 9.13

An asymptomatic 66-year-old female has TBIL 0.93 mg/dL, ALT 55 IU/L, AST 40 IU/L, ALP 674 IU/L, and GGT 390 IU/L. ERCP showed stenosis or stricture of the intrahepatic or extrahepatic bile ducts (Fig. 9.15). Peritoneoscopic findings revealed a wide excavation at the edge of the left lobe and a thick hepatic capsule with white markings (Fig. 9.16a). UDCA was administered. Excavation developed extensively on the liver surface, with increased white markings after 7 years (Fig. 9.16b). Liver biopsy from the first peritoneoscopy showed proliferating bile ducts with lymphocytic and eosinophilic infiltrate in the portal tract (Fig. 9.17).

To investigate liver fibrogenesis in PSC, we examined the expression of stem cell factor (SCF), a ligand of c-kit, in the injured bile ducts of four patients with overt PSC and histologically classified as stage 2 or 3. Mast cells were identified by immunohistochemistry using anti-human mast cell tryptase

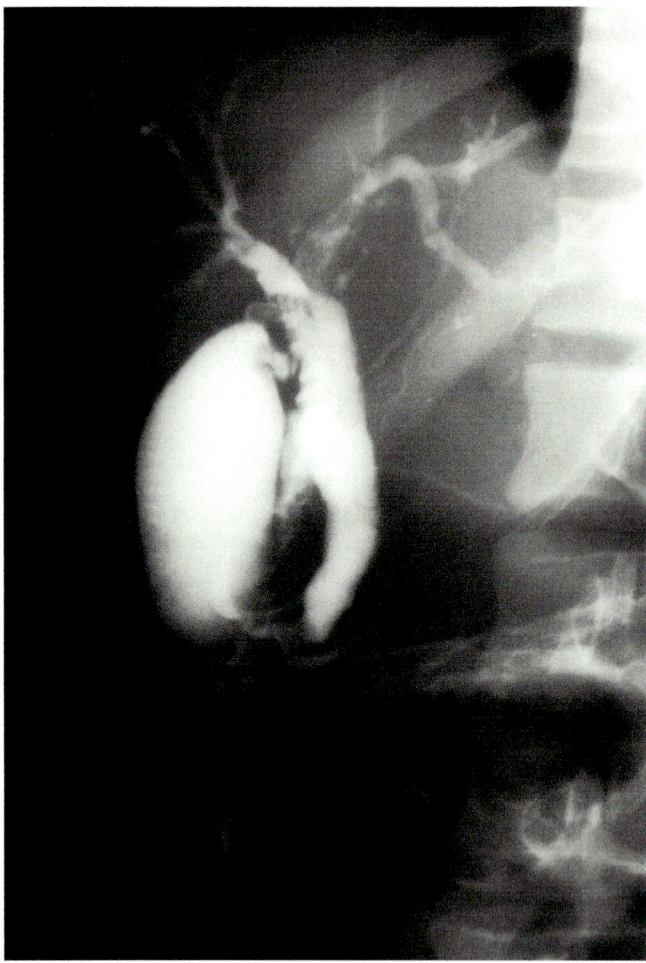

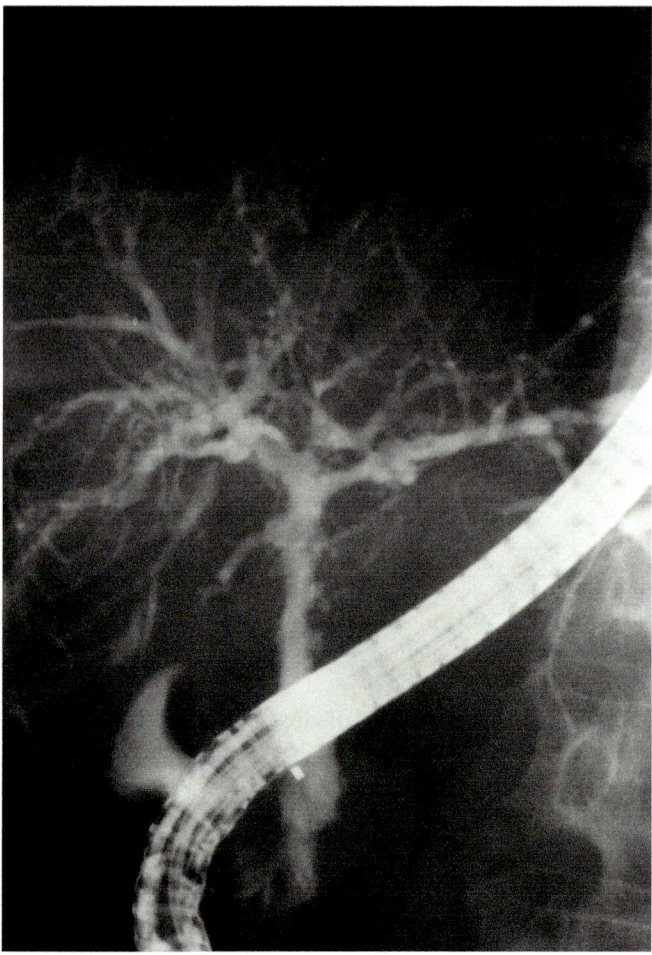

Fig. 9.13 Early-stage primary sclerosing cholangitis. Endoscopic retrograde cholangiopancreatography shows narrowing and dilatation of intrahepatic bile ducts

Fig. 9.15 Late-stage primary sclerosing cholangitis Endoscopic retrograde cholangiopancreatography shows irregular and narrowing wall of the intrahepatic or extrahepatic bile duct

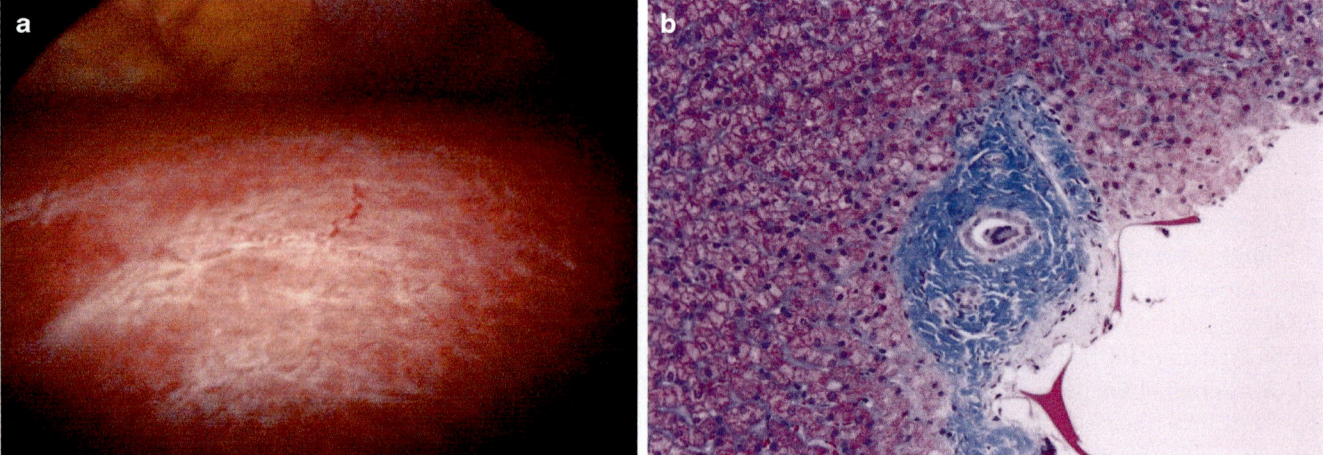

Fig. 9.14 Early-stage primary sclerosing cholangitis (**a**) Peritoneoscopy shows white markings on the smooth surface of enlarged liver. (**b**) Masson's trichrome stain shows onion-skin fibrosis in the portal tract

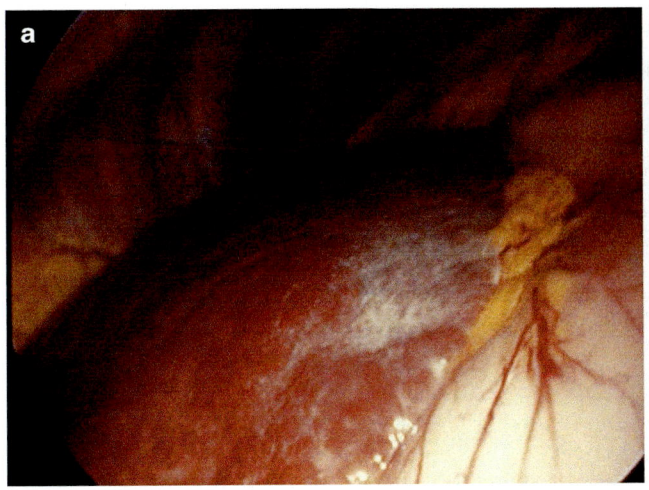
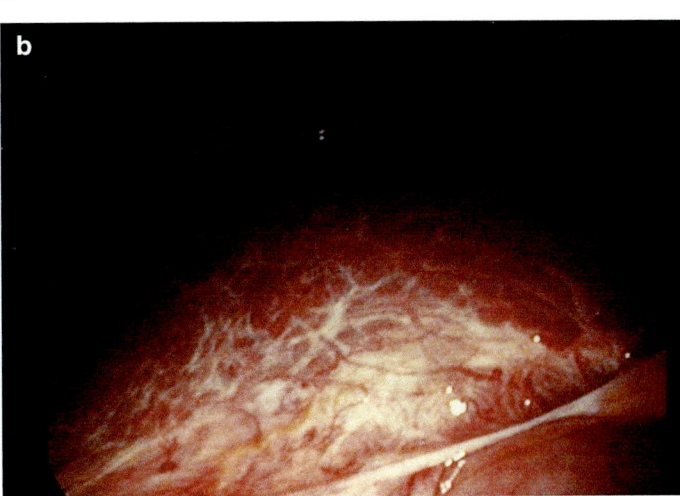

Fig. 9.16 Peritoneoscopic findings in advanced primary sclerosing cholangitis (**a**) Peritoneoscopy shows large excavation on the edge of the left lobe, and white markings are clearly demarcated on the surface.

(**b**) Repeat peritoneoscopy shows wide development of excavation on the left lobe, and the liver surface is more irregular. The liver capsule has become thick

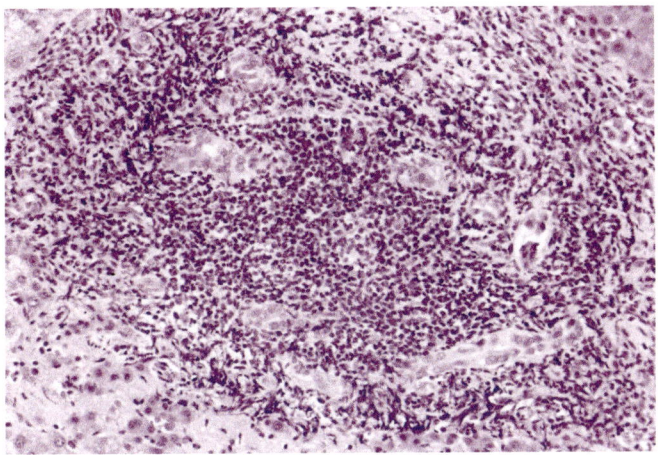

Fig. 9.17 Liver histology from the first peritoneoscopy. The portal tract is infiltrated with many lymphocytes and lymphoid follicles. Proliferating bile ductules and damaged bile duct are visible

(HMCT) and anti-c-kit antibodies to clarify their relationship with portal fibrosis and damaged bile ducts. SCF was detected in the epitheliums of most bile ducts in PSC, and many HMCT- and c-kit-positive mast cells were found in the portal tracts (Fig. 9.18). Image analysis showed more significant numbers of c-kit-positive mast cells per area of portal tract in PSC than in chronic hepatitis C, which may be increased from stage 2 to 3. The infiltration of c-kit-positive cells in SCF-positive portal tracts destroyed bile ducts, and c-kit mast cells were suggested to associate closely with hepatic fibrosis in PSC [69–73].

The overlap syndrome of primary sclerosing cholangitis and AIH is defined as meeting criteria of probable or definite AIH with cholangiographic evidence of PSC and characterized by ANA- or SMA-seropositive, interface hepatitis and hypergammaglobulinemia in mixture with cholestatic change of serum alkaline phosphatase, occurrence of inflammatory bowel disease, and fibrous obliterative cholangitis. The overlap syndrome of PSC and AIH is in general resistant to corticosteroid.

9.5 IgG4-Related Sclerosing Cholangitis

IgG4-related sclerosing cholangitis is referred to the biliary manifestation of IgG4-related systemic disease [74] and is an autoimmune inflammatory condition associated with autoimmune pancreatitis [75]. This type of sclerosing cholangitis involves the extrahepatic ducts, is characterized by IgG4-positive lymphoplasmacytic infiltrate, and is steroid-responsive [76]. It should be distinguished from PSC (Table 9.1) [77].

The clinical presentation of IgG4-related cholangitis is different from PSC. Diabetes mellitus, pseudotumor in the lung or pancreas [78, 79], and multifocal fibrosclerosis often precede or follow IgG4-related sclerosing cholangitis, and autoimmune hepatitis is rarely seen [80, 81]. The typical imaging findings of intrahepatic or extrahepatic bile ducts and pancreas in IgG4-related sclerosing cholangitis and autoimmune pancreatitis [82], and the histological findings of autoimmune pancreatitis, are fairly well recognized. However, the pathogenesis remains unclear.

Glucocorticoid therapy reduces IgG4-positive plasma cell infiltrate [80], and a consensus on the treatment of IgG4-related sclerosing cholangitis has been reached: an initial dose of prednisolone 30–40 mg/day and long-term administration are recommended [83]. Azathioprine appears useful in patients with partial response to prednisolone [84]. There are cases of IgG4-associated autoimmune hepatitis, [85] which should be distinguished from classical one. Further study is needed on this new disease entity.

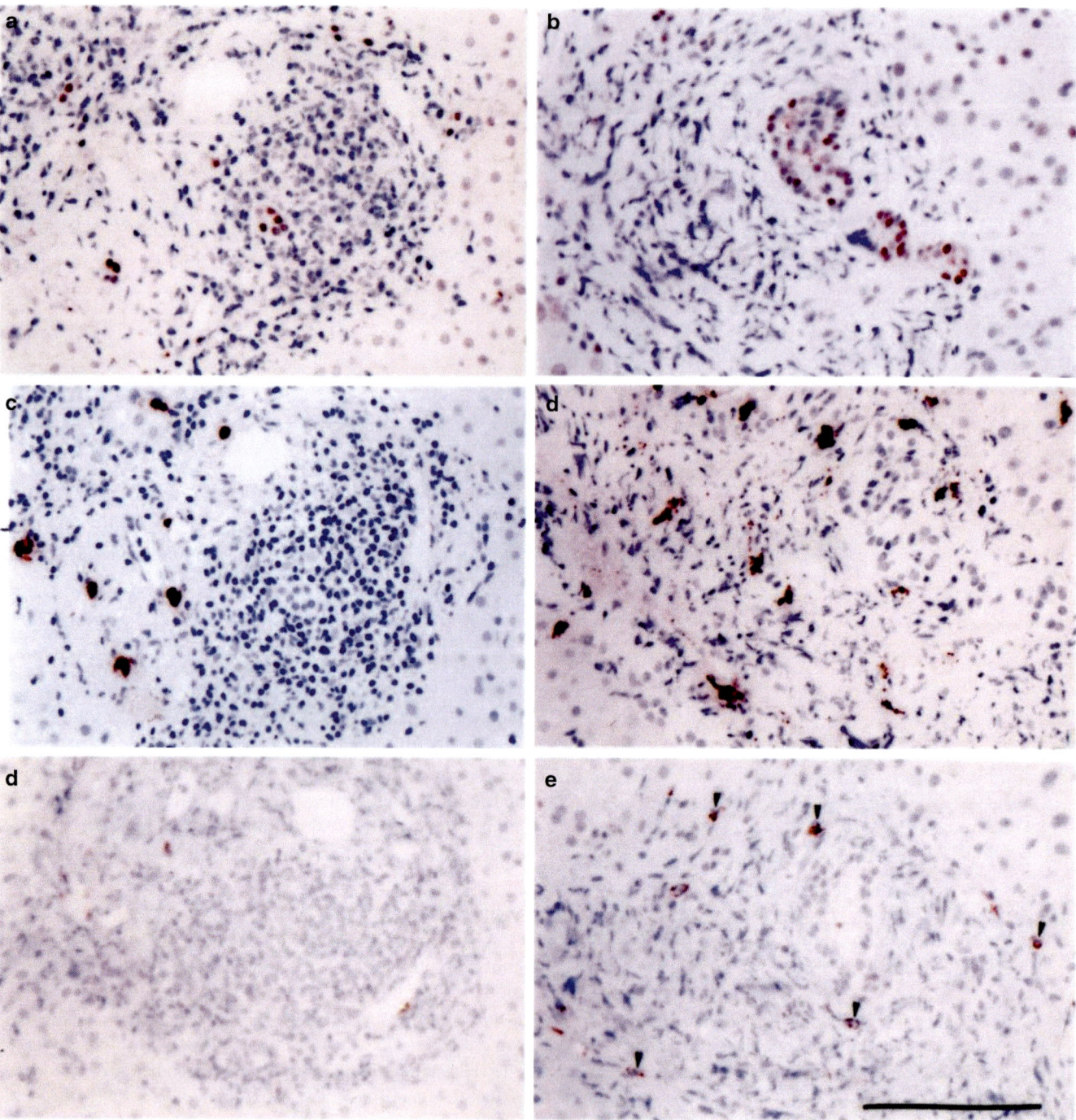

Fig. 9.18 Expression of stem cell factor, human mast cell tryptase, and c-kit in patients with chronic hepatitis C and primary sclerosing cholangitis. (**a**) Biliary epithelial cells in a portal tract show weak staining of stem cell factor in chronic hepatitis C. (**b**) Immunoreactivity of stem cell factor in most epithelial cells of bile ducts in primary sclerosing cholangitis. (**c**) Several positive human mast cells are shown in the portal tract in chronic hepatitis C. (**d**) Many positive human mast cells are visible in the portal tract in primary sclerosing cholangitis. (**e**) Few c-kit-positive cells are seen in the portal tract in chronic hepatitis C. (**f**) Several c-kit-positive cells (arrowheads) are visible in the portal tract in primary sclerosing cholangitis. Bar = 100 μm. Reuse of Ishii M, et al. A role of mast cells for hepatic fibrosis in primary sclerosing cholangitis. Hepatol Res 2005; 31: 127–31., with permission from Wiley

Case 9.14

A 77-year-old male suffered from chronic pancreatitis and complained of anorexia.

Jaundice was indicated, and serum examination showed TBil 1.92 mg/dl, DBil 1.58 mg/dl, AST 137 IU/l, ALT 186 IU/l, ALP 2227 IU/l, GGT 871 IU/l, P-amy 54 IU/l, CA19–9185 U/ml, IgG 2124.8 mg/dl, and IgG4 471 mg/dl. US and CT with contrast medium revealed enlarged pancreas, dilation of choledochus and intrahepatic bile ducts, and enlarged gall bladder (Fig. 9.19a–d). MRCP and

Table 9.1 Clinicopathological difference between IgG4-related sclerosing cholangitis and primary sclerosing cholangitis

Variable	IgG4-related sclerosing cholangitis	Primary sclerosing cholangitis
Age	Old	Young and old
Sex	Male > female	Male = female
Liver chemistry	Jaundice	Liver functional disturbance
IgG4 in serum	High	Normal
Complication	Diabetes mellitus, pancreatitis, multifocal fibrosclerosis, interstitial pneumonia	Irritable bowel syndrome
Therapy	Glucocorticoid	Transplantation
Prognosis	Good	Worse
IgG4-positive cells	Positive	
Obliterative phlebitis	Positive	Negative
Onion-skin lesion	Rare	Positive
Stage (Ludwig criteria)	I–II	I–IV

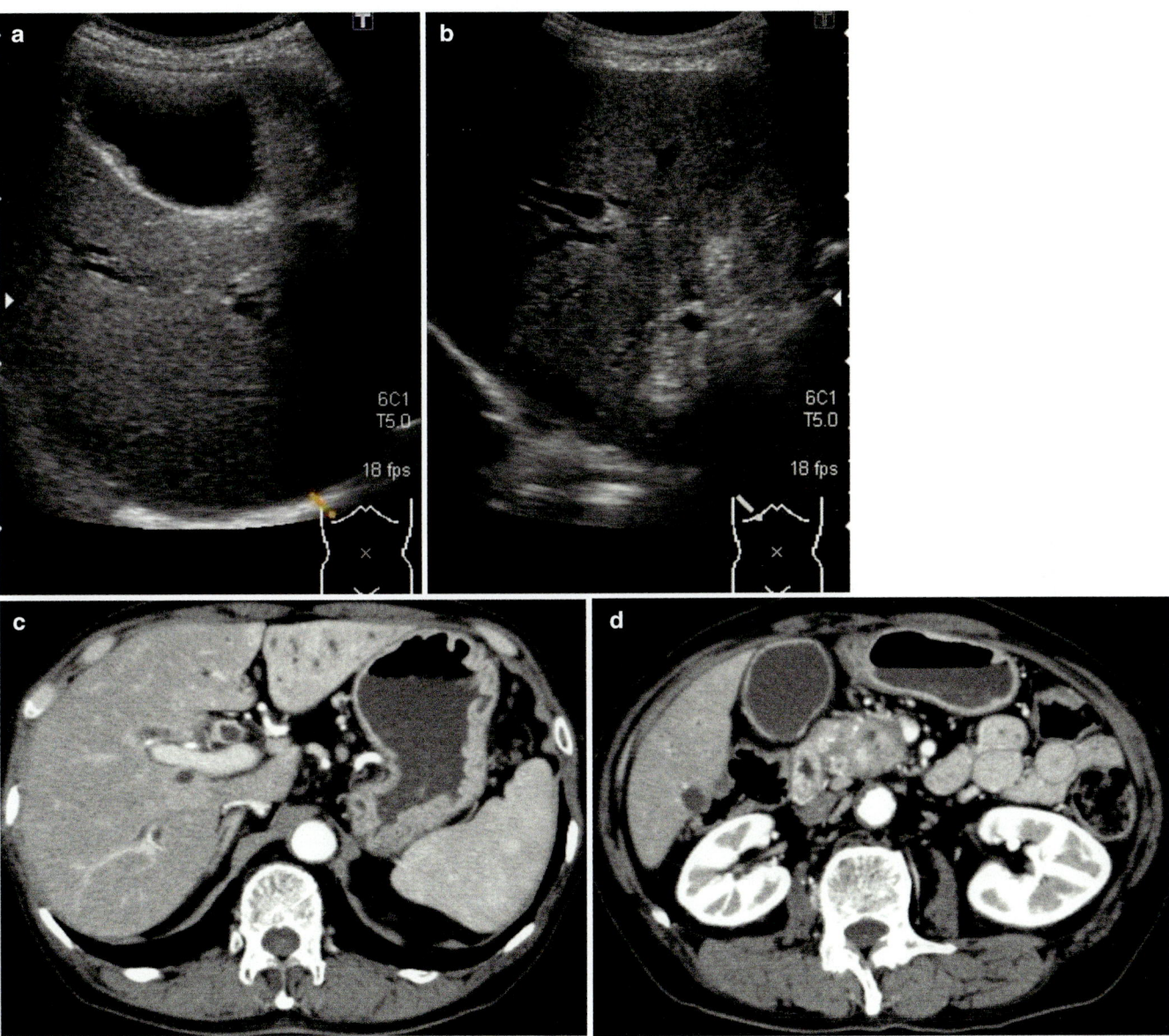

Fig. 9.19 (**a**, **b**) US shows enlarged gall bladder with stone shadow and dilated bile ducts. (**c**, **d**) CT present thickened wall of gall bladder, and dilated common and intrahepatic bile ducts are found. Head of pancreas is swollen. (b, c & d. Reuse of Douhara A, et al. Gastroenterol Endosc 2011; 53: 1617–25., with permission from Jpn Soc Gastroenterol Endosc)

ERCP presented dilated middle portion and stenotic lower portion of choledochus, and main duct of pancreas was irregularly dilated. Enlarged papilla Vater was detected by ERCP (Fig. 9.20a–d). Biopsied tissue from papilla Vater showed normal arrangement of columnar epitheliums and edematous submucosa area with infiltration of inflammatory cells. Magnified view revealed abundant plasma cells and eosinophilic leukocytes in submucosal area, and many of plasma cells contain IgG4-positive immunoreaction (Fig. 9.21a–d).

Case 9.15

A 65-year-old male had obstructive jaundice, and cholangiocarcinoma was suspected by abdominal ultrasound. Percutaneous transhepatic cholangiodrainage and endoscopic retrograde biliary drainage reduced jaundice, and his general status was stable for 1.5 years. MRCP showed reduced tail size of pancreas, and liver chemistry showed TBIL 1.39 mg/dL, AST 99 IU/L, ALT 77 IU/L, ALP 1135 IU/L, GGT 737 IU/L, IgG 2307 mg/dL, and IgG4 165 mg/dL. ERCP revealed stricture and dilatation of intrahepatic bile ducts.

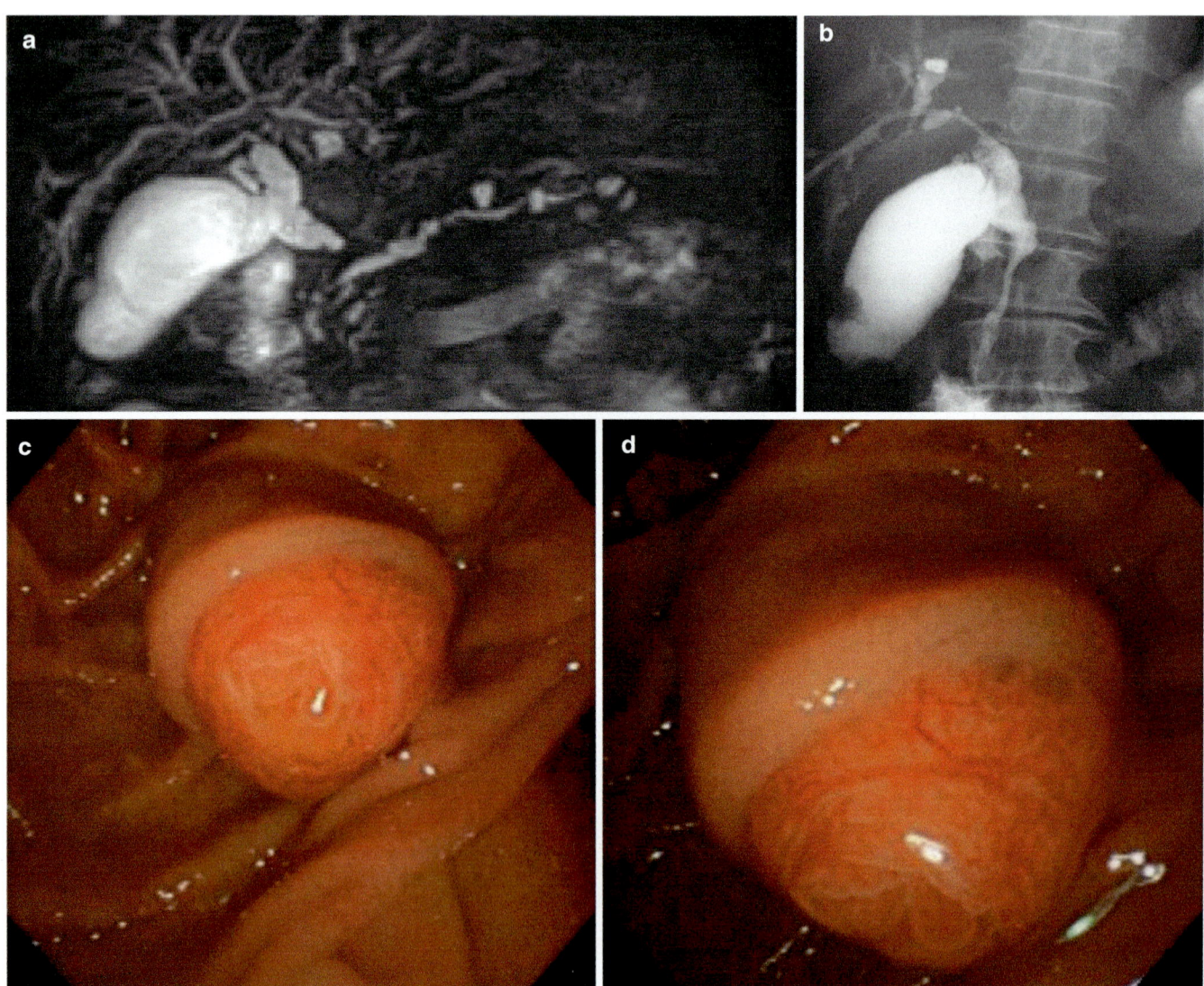

Fig. 9.20 (a, b) MRCP and ERCP shows dilated common in upper portion and intrahepatic bile ducts, and irregularly dilated pancreatic duct is seen. c.d. ERCP shows hyperemic and enlarged papilla Vater (a,

b & d. Reuse of Douhara A, et al. Gastroenterol Endosc 2011; 53: 1617–25., with permission from Jpn Soc Gastroenterol Endosc)

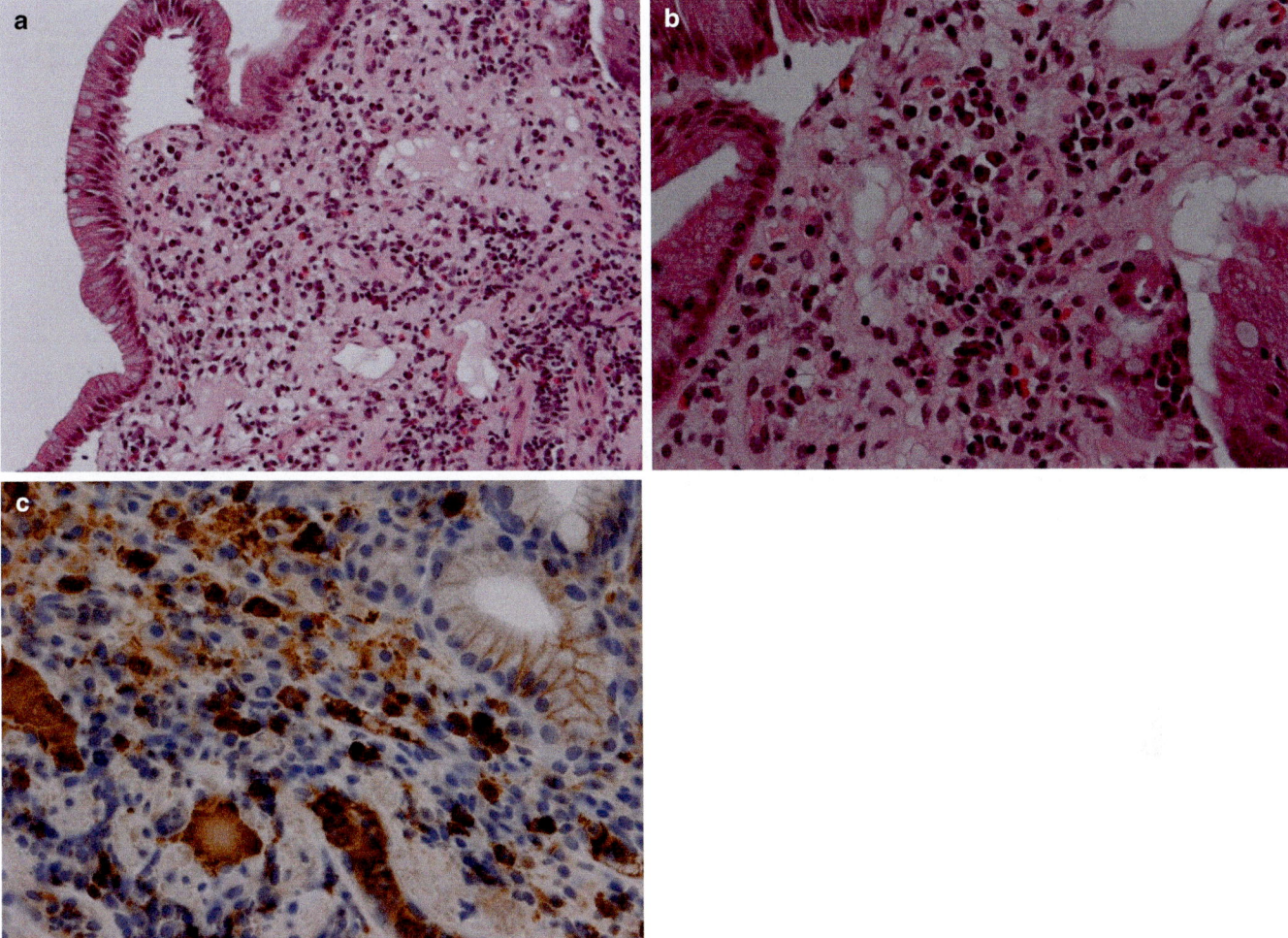

Fig. 9.21 (**a**) HE staining of papillae Vater shows edematous submucosa with many inflammatory cells. (**b**) Magnified view shows many plasma cells and eosinophilic leukocytes. (**c**) Immunohistochemistry shows IgG4 immunoreactivity in plasma cells. (a, b & c. Reuse of Douhara A, et al. Gastroenterol Endosc 2011; 53: 1617–25., with permission from Jpn Soc Gastroenterol Endosc)

The lower portion of the common bile duct was narrowed, and liver biopsy showed an enlarged portal tract with bile ductular proliferation and cluster of plasma cells and lymphocytes (Fig. 9.22). Prednisolone 20 mg/day was administered. Gradually, the dosage was tapered and ceased after 34 months, and liver function tests reverted to normal values.

Case 9.16
An 81-year-old male complained of appetite loss, weight loss, and general malaise. His liver tests showed AST 63 IU/L, ALT 54 IU/L, ALP 583 IU/L, GGT 373 IU/L, IgG 2437 mg/dL, and IgG4 487 mg/dL. ERCP showed stricture or dilatation of intrahepatic biliary ducts and strictured lower portion of the common bile duct with an irregularly sized pancreatic duct, and liver tissue showed an enlarged and inflamed portal tract with fibrous bands, neutrophils, eosinophils, and lymphoplasmacytic cells (Fig. 9.23). Prednisolone 25 mg/day was administered. The dosage was gradually tapered and ceased after 5 months, and his liver function returned to normal.

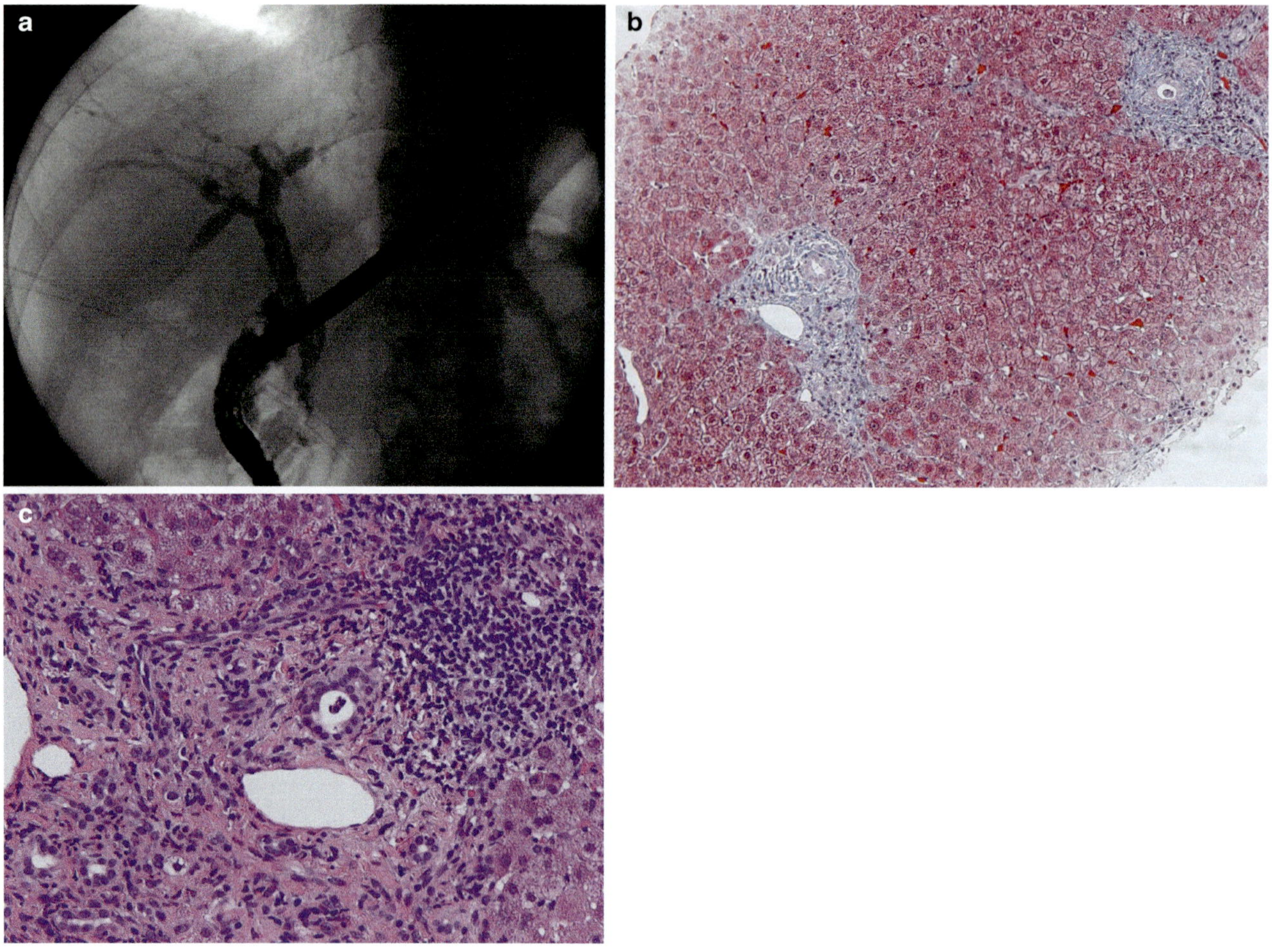

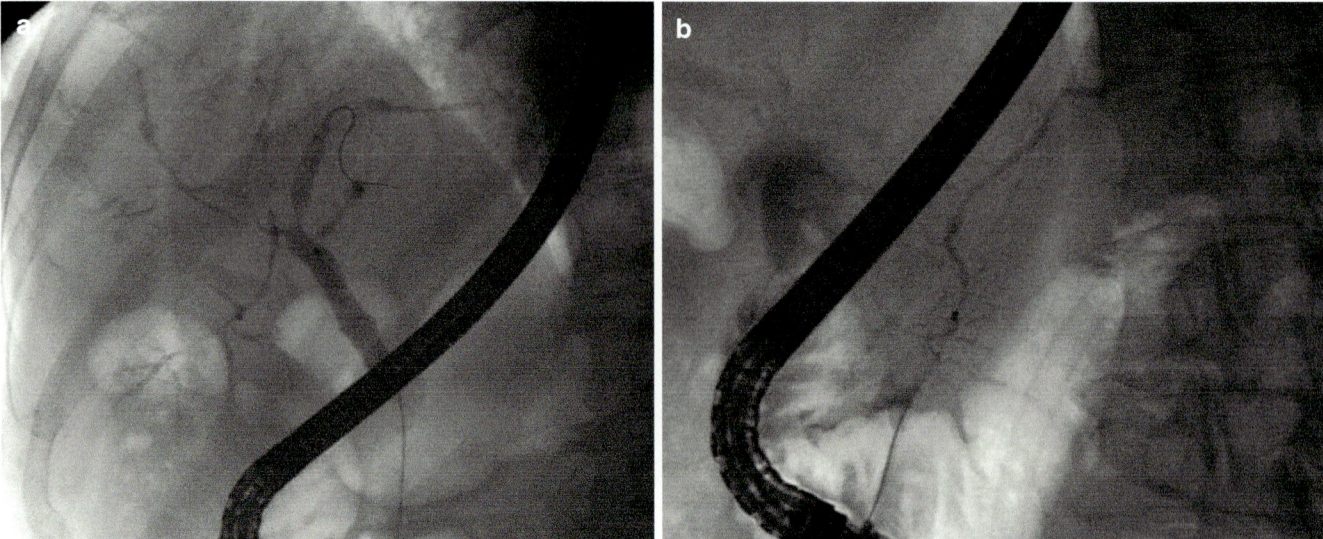

Fig. 9.22 IgG4-related sclerosing cholangitis. (**a**) Endoscopic retrograde cholangiopancreatography shows irregular stenosis of intrahepatic bile ducts, and stenotic area is seen in the lower portion of the choledochus. (**b**) Liver tissue stained by Masson's trichrome stain shows a portal tract enlarged by fibrosis. (**c**) The portal tract is enlarged by fibrosis, and proliferating bile ductules are seen. Clusters of lymphocytes are present with scattered plasma cells

Fig. 9.23 IgG4-related sclerosing cholangitis. (**a**) Endoscopic retrograde cholangiopancreatography shows irregular stenosis of the intrahepatic bile ducts. (**b**) Endoscopic retrograde cholangiopancreatography shows irregular stenosis of the pancreatic duct. (**c**) Masson's trichrome stained liver tissue shows proliferating fibrosis from an enlarged portal tract, and inflammatory cells are present along the fibrotic area. (**d**) Interface hepatitis is seen, and the epitheliums of the bile ductule are damaged, with lymphoplasmacytic and eosinophilic infiltrate

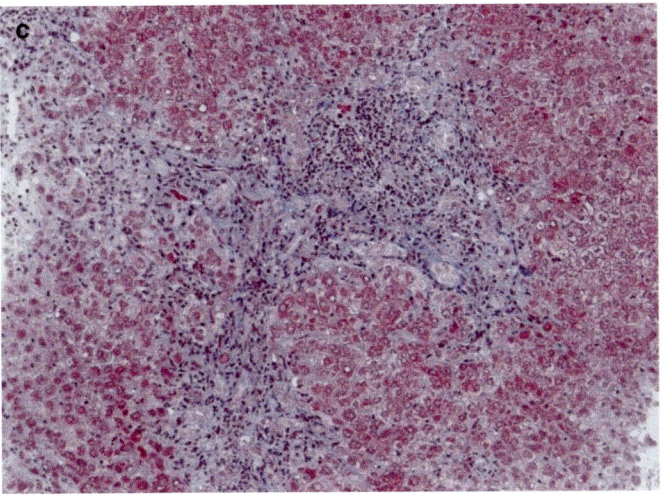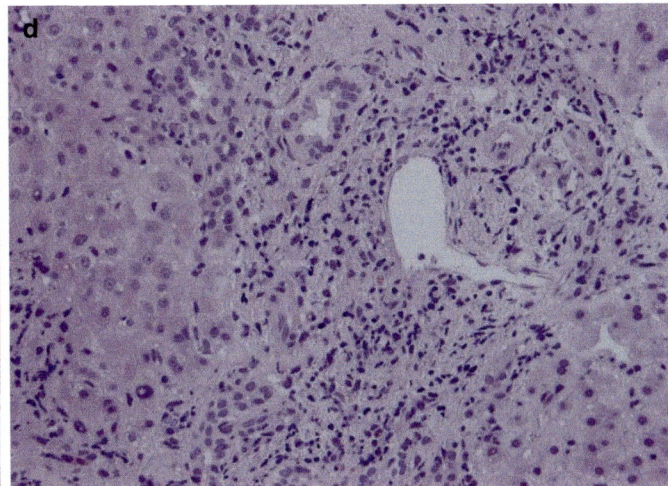

Fig. 9.23 (continued)

Acknowledgments Prof. Dirk J. van Leeuwen was a coauthor of the first edition of this chapter.

References

1. Zeniya M, Watanabe F, Aizawa Y, Toda G. Genetic background of autoimmune hepatitis in Japan. In: Nishioka M, Toda G, Zeniya M, editors. Autoimmune hepatitis. Amsterdam: Elsevier Science Publishers B.V.; 1994. p. 267–79.
2. DjilaliSaiah I, Fakhfakh A, Louafi H, CaillatZucman S, Debray D, Alvarez F. HLA class II influences humoral autoimmunity in patients with type 2 autoimmune hepatitis. J Hepatol. 2006;45:844–50.
3. Johnson PJ, McFarlane IG. Meeting report: international autoimmune hepatitis group. Hepatology. 1993;18:998–1005.
4. Alvarez F, Berg PA, Bianchi FB, Bianchi L, Burroughs AK, Cancado EL, et al. International autoimmune hepatitis group report: review of criteria for diagnosis of autoimmune hepatitis. J Hepatol. 1999;31:929–38.
5. Hennes EM, Zeniya M, Czaja AJ, Parés A, Dalekos GN, Krawitt EL, et al. Simplified criteria for the diagnosis of autoimmune hepatitis. Hepatology. 2008;48:169–76.
6. Journal of Hepatology 2015 vol. 62 j S100–S111.
7. Krawitt EL. Autoimmune hepatitis. N Engl J Med. 2006;354:54–66.
8. Sherman KE, Narkewicz M, Pinto PC. Cyclosporine in the management of corticosteroid-resistant type 1 autoimmune chronic active hepatitis. J Hepatol. 1994;21:1040–7.
9. Reich DJ, Fiel I, Guarrera JV, Emre S, Guy SR, Schwartz ME, et al. Liver transplantation for autoimmune hepatitis. Hepatology. 2000;32:693–700.
10. Stravits RT, Lelfkowitch JH, Fontana RJ, Gershwin ER, Leung PS, Steerling RK, Manns MP, Norman GL, Lee WM, Acute Liver failure Study Group. Autoimmune acute liver failure: Proposed clinical and histological criteria. Hepatology. 2011;53:517–26.
11. Canh HN, Harada K, Ouchi H, Sato Y, Tsuneyama K, Kage M, Nakano M, Yoshizawa K, Takahashi A, Abe M, Kang J-H, Koike K, Inui A, Fujisawa T, Takaki A, Arinaga-Hino T, Torimura T, Suzuki Y, Fujiwara K, Zeniya M, Ohira H, Tanaka A, Takikawa H, Intractable Liver and Biliary Diseases, Study Group of Japan. Acute presentation of autoimmune hepatitis: a multicentre study with detailed histological evaluation in a large cohort of patients. J Clin Pathol. 2017;70:961–9.
12. Crispe IN. The liver as a lymphoid organ. Annu Rev Immunol. 2009;27:147–63.
13. Kubes P, Jenne C. Immune responses in the liver. Annu Rev Immunol. 2018;36:247–77.
14. Te HS, Koukoulis G, Ganger DR. Autoimmune hepatitis: a histological variant associated with prominent centrilobular necrosis. Gut. 1997;41:269–71.
15. Canh HN, Harada K, Ouchi H, et al. Acute presentation of autoimmune hepatitis: a multicentre study with detailed histological evaluation in a large cohort of patients. J Clin Pathol. 2017;70:961–9699.
16. Devaney K, Goodman ZD, Ishak KG. Postinfantile giant-cell transformation in hepatitis. Hepatology. 1992;16:327–33.
17. Lau JYN, Koukoulis G, Mieli-Vergani G, Portman BC. Syncytial giant-cell hepatitis—a specific disease entity? J Hepatol. 1992;15:216–9.
18. Philips MJ, Blendis LM, Poucell S, Patterson J, Petric M, Roberts E, et al. Sporadic giant-cell hepatitis with distinctive pathological features, a severe clinical course, and paramyxoviral features. N Engl J Med. 1991;324:455–60.
19. Hicks J, Barrish J, Zhu SH. Neonatal syncytial giant cell hepatitis with paramyxoviral-like inclusions. Ultrastruct Pathol. 2001;25:65–71.
20. Joshita S, Yoshizawa K, Umemura T, et al. Clinical features of autoimmune hepatitis with acute presentation: a Japanese nationwide survey. J Gastroenterol. 2018;53:1079–88.
21. Lacerda MA, Ludwig J, Dickson ER, Jorgensen RA, Lindor KD. Antimitochondria antibody-negative primary biliary cirrhosis. Am J Gastroenterol. 1995;90:247–9.
22. Czaja AJ, Carpenter H. Autoimmune hepatitis with incidental histologic features of bile duct injury. Hepatology. 2001;34:659–65.
23. Onji M, Zeniya M, Yamamoto K, Tsubouchi H. Autoimmune hepatitis: diagnosis and treatment guide in Japan, 2013. Hep Res. 2014;44:368–70.
24. Misdraji J, Thiim M, Graeme-Cook FM. Autoimmune hepatitis with centrilobular necrosis. Am J Surg Pathol. 2004;28:471–8.
25. Schvarcz R, Glaumann H, Weiland O. Survival and histological resolution of fibrosis in patients with autoimmune chronic active hepatitis. J Hepatol. 1993;18:15–23.
26. Kogan J, Safadi R, Ashur Y, Shouval D, Ilan Y. Prognosis of symptomatic versus asymptomatic autoimmune hepatitis: a study of 68 patients. J Clin Gastroenterol. 2002;35:75–81.
27. Tan EM, Cohen AS, Fries JF, Masi AT, McShane DJ, Rothfield NF, et al. The revised criteria for the classification of systemic lupus erythematous. Arthritis Rheum. 1982;25:1271–7.

28. Miller AH, Urowitz MB, Gladman DD, Blendis LM. The liver in systemic lupus erythematosus. Q J Med. 1984;53:401–9.

29. van Hoek B. The spectrum of liver disease in systemic lupus erythematous. Nether J Med. 1996;46:244–53.

30. Matsumoto T, Yoshimine T, Shimouchi K, Shiotsu H, Kuwabara N, Fukuda Y, et al. The liver in systemic lupus erythematosus: pathologic analysis of 52 cases and review of Japanese autopsy registry data. Human Pathol. 1992;23:1151–8.

31. Moriwaki Y, Maebo A, Yamada W, Yamamoto T, Amuro Y, Hada T, et al. Autoimmune hepatitis or hepatic involvement in SLE? A case report. Gastroenterol Jpn. 1987;22:222–7.

32. Kooy A, de Heide LJM, Engelkens HJH, Mulder AH, van Hagen M, Schalm SW. Hepatitis in a patient with SLE: is it autoimmune hepatitis? Nether J Med. 1996;48:128–32.

33. Leggett B, Collins R, Pentice R, Powell LW. CAH or SLE? Hepatology. 1986;6:341–2.

34. Kooy A, de Heide Loek JM, Engelkens HJK, Mulder AH, van Hagen M, Schalm SW. How to diagnose autoimmune hepatitis in systemic lupus erythematosus? Hepatology. 1995;23:936–8.

35. Kojima H, Uemura M, Sakurai S, Ann T, Ishii Y, Imazu H, et al. Clinical features of liver disturbance in rheumatoid diseases: clinicopathological study with special reference to the cause of liver disturbance. J Gastroenterol. 2002;37:617–25.

36. Runyon BA, LaBreque DR, Anuras S. The spectrum of liver disease in systemic lupus erythematosus. Report of 33 histologically-proved cases and review of the literature. Am J Med. 1980;69:187–94.

37. Rubin E, Schaffner F, Popper H. Primary biliary cirrhosis. Chronic non-suppurative destructive cholangitis. Am J Pathol. 1965;46:387–407.

38. Leung PSC, Coppel RL, Anari A, Munoz S, Gershwin ME. Antimitochondria antibodies in primary biliary cirrhosis. Semin Liver Dis. 1997;17:61–9.

39. Nurata Y, Abe M, Furukawa S, Kuamagai T, Matsui H, Matsuura K, et al. Clinical features of symptomatic primary biliary cirrhosis initially complicated with esophageal varices. Hepatol Res. 2006;12:1220–6.

40. Heathcote J. Primary biliary cirrhosis. Clin Perspect Gastroenterol. 2001;1:39–46.

41. Nakanuma Y, Zen Y, Harada K, et al. Application of a new histological staging and grading system for primary biliary cirrhosis to liver biopsy specimens: Interobserver agreement. Pathol Int. 2010;60:167–74.

42. Corpechot C, Carrat F, Bahr A, Chretien Y, Poupon RE, Poupon R. The effect of ursodeoxycholic acid therapy on the natural course of primary biliary cirrhosis. Gastroenterology. 2005;128:297–303.

43. Lindor KD, Dickson ER, Baldus WP, Jorgensen RA, Ludwig J, Murtaugh PA, et al. Ursodeoxycholic acid in the treatment of primary biliary cirrhosis. Gastroenterology. 1994;106:1284–90.

44. Heathcote EJ, Cauch-Dudek K, Walker V, Bailey RJ, Blendis LM, Ghent CN, et al. The Canadian multicenter double-blind randomized controlled trial of ursodeoxycholic acid in primary biliary cirrhosis. Hepatology. 1994;19:1149–56.

45. Corprechot C, Carrat F, Bonnand AM, Poupon RE, Poupon R. The effect of ursodeoxycholic acid therapy on liver fibrosis progression in primary biliary cirrhosis. Hepatology. 2000;32:1196–9.

46. Corprechot C. Promary biliary cirrhosis and bile acids. Clin Res Hepatol Gastroenterol. 2012;36(suppl 1):S12–20.

47. Lens S, Leoz M, Nazal L, Bruguera M, Pares A. Bezafibrate normalizes alkaline phosphatase in primary biliar cirrhosis patients with incomplete response to ursodeoxychoclic acid. Liver Int. 2014;34:197–203.

48. Iwasaki S, Ohira H, Nishiguchi S, Zeniya M, Kaneko S, Onji M, et al. The efficacy of ursodeoxycholic acid and bezafibrate combination therapy for primary biliary cirrhosis: a prospective, multicenter study. Hepatol Res. 2008;38:557–64.

49. Zeron PB, Retamozo S, Bove A, Kostov BA, Siso A, Ramos-Casais M. Diagnosis of liver involvement in primary Sjogren syndrome. J Clin Trans Hepatol. 2013;1:94–102.

50. Rabinovitz M, Appasamy R, Finkelstein S. Primary biliary cirrhosis diagnosed during pregnancy. Does it have a different outcome? Dig Dis Sci. 1995;40:571–4.

51. Czaja AJ. Frequency and nature of the variant syndrome of autoimmune liver disease. Hapatology. 1998;28:360–5.

52. Chazouilleres O, Wendum D, Serfatty L, et al. Primary biliary cirrhosis-autoimmune hepatitis overlap syndrome: clinical features and response to therapy. Hepatology. 1998;28:296–301.

53. Heurgue A, Vitry F, Diebold MD, et al. Overlap syndrome of primary biliary cirrhosis and autoimmune hepatitis: a retrospective study of 115 cases of autoimmune liver disease. Gastroenterol Clin Biol. 2007;31:17–25.

54. Poupon R, Chauzouilleres O, Corpechot C, Chretien Y. Development of autoimmune hepatitis in patients with typical primary biliary cirrhosis. Hepatology. 2006;44:85–90.

55. Chapman R, Fevery J, Kalloo A, et al. Diagnosis and management of primary sclerosing cholangitis. Hepatology. 2010;51:660–78.

56. Bjornsson E. Small-duct primary sclerosing cholangitis. Curr Gastroenterol Rep. 2009;11:l37–41.

57. Floreani A, Rizzotto ER, Ferrara F, et al. Clinical course and outcome of autoimmune hepatitis/primary sclerosing cholangitis overlap syndrome. Am J Gastroenterol. 2005;100:1516–22.

58. Melum E, Franke A, Schramm C, et al. Genome-wide association analysis in primary sclerosing cholangitis identifies two non-HLA susceptibility loci. Nat Genet. 2011;43:17–9.

59. O'Mahony CA, Vierling JM. Etiopathogenesis of primary sclerosing cholangitis. Semin Liver Dis. 2006;26:3–21.

60. Grant AJ, Lalor PF, Salmi M, Jalkanen S, Adams DH. Homing of mucosal lymphocytes to the liver in the pathogenesis of hepatic complications of inflammatory bowel disease. Lancet. 2002;359:150–7.

61. Roder F, Coppe JP, Patil CK, et al. Persistent DNA damage signaling triggers senescence-associated inflammatory cytokine secretion. Nat Cell Biol. 2009;11:973–9.

62. Tabibian JH, O'Hara SP, Splinter PL, Trussoni CE, LaRusso NF. Cholangiocyte senescence by way of N-ras activation is a characteristic of primary sclerosing cholangitis. Hepatology. 2014;59:2263–75.

63. Eaton JE, Talwalker JA, Lazaridis KN, Gores GJ, Lindor KD. Pathogenesis of primary sclerosing cholangitis and advances in diagnosis and management. Gastroenterology. 2013;145:521–36.

64. Colle I, Van Vlierberghe H. Diagnosis and therapeutic problems of primary sclerosing cholangitis. Acta Gastroenterol Belg. 2003;66:155–9.

65. Fosby B, Karlsen TH, Melum E. Recurrence and rejection in liver transplantation for primary sclerosing cholangitis. World J Gastroenterol. 2012;18:1–15.

66. Mitchell SA, Bansi DS, Hunt N, Von Bergmann K, Fleming KA, Chapman RW. A preliminary trial of high-dose ursodeoxycholic acid in primary sclerosing cholangitis. Gastroenterology. 2001;121:900–7.

67. Wagner S, Gebel M, Meier P, Trautwein C, Bleck J, Nashan B, et al. Endoscopic management of biliary tract strictures in primary sclerosing cholangitis. Endoscopy. 1996;28:546–51.

68. Chapman WC. Primary sclerosing cholangitis: role of liver transplantation. J Gastrointest Surg. 2008;12:426–8.

69. Yamashiro M, Kouda W, Kono N, Tsuneyama K, Matsui O, Nakanuma Y. Distribution of intrahepatic mast cells in various hepatobiliary disorders. An immunohistochemical study. Virchows Arch. 1998;433:471–9.

70. Farell DJ, Hines JE, Walls AF, Kelly PJ, Bennett MK, Burt AD. Intrahepatic mast cells in chronic liver diseases. Hepatology. 1995;22:1175–81.

71. Armbrust T, Batusic D, Ringe B, Ramadori G. Mast cells distribution in human liver disease and experimental rat liver fibrosis. Indications for mast cell participation in development of liver fibrosis. J Hepatol. 1997;26:1042–54.

72. Nakamura A, Yamazaki K, Suzuki K, Sato S. Increased portal tract infiltration of mast cells and eosinophils in primary biliary cirrhosis. Am J Gastroenterol. 1997;92:2245–9.

73. Matsunaga Y, Kawasaki H, Terada T. Stromal mast cells and nerve fibers in various chronic liver diseases: relevance to hepatic fibrosis. Am J Gastroenterol. 1999;94:1923–32.

74. Bjomsson E, Chari ST, Smyrk TC, et al. IgG4 associated cholangitis: description of an emerging clinical entity based on review of the literature. Hepatology. 2007;45:1547–54.

75. Kamisawa T, Okamoto A, Funata N. Clinicopathological features of autoimmune pancreatitis in relation to elevation of serum IgG4. Pancreas. 2005;31:23–31.

76. Bjornsson E, Chari ST, Smyrk TC, Lindor K. Immunoglobulin G4-associated cholangitis: description of an emerging clinical entity based on review of the literature. Hepatology. 2007;45:1547–54.

77. Kumagi T, Alswat K, Hirschfield GM, Heathcote J. New insights into autoimmune liver diseases. Hepatol Res. 2008;38:745–61.

78. Kamisawa T, Funata N, Hayashi Y, Eishi Y, Koike M, Tsuruta K, et al. A new clinicopathological entity of IgG4-related autoimmune disease. J Gastroenterol. 2003;38:982–4.

79. Deheragoda MG, Church NI, Rodriguez-Justo M, Munson P, Sandanayake N, Seward EW, et al. The use of immunoglobulin g4 immunostaining in diagnosing pancreatic and extrapancreatic involvement in autoimmune pancreatitis. Clin Gastroenterol Hepatol. 2007;5:1229–34.

80. Umemura T, Zen Y, Hamano H, Kawa S, Nakanuma Y, Kiyosawa K. Immunoglobulin G4 hepatopathy: association of immunoglobulin G4-bearing plasma cells in liver with autoimmune pancreatitis. Hepatology. 2007;46:463–71.

81. Chung H, Watanabe T, Kudo M, Maenishi O, Chiba T. Identification and characterization of IgG4-associated autoimmune hepatitis. Liver Int. 2010;30:222–31.

82. Nakazawa T, Ohara H, Sano H, et al. Cholangiography can discriminate sclerosing cholangitis with autoimmune pancreatitis from primary sclerosing cholangitis. Gastrointest Endosc. 2004;60:937–44.

83. Ito T, Nishimori I, Inoue N, Kawabe K, Gibo J, Arita Y, et al. Treatment for autoimmune pancreatitis: consensus on the treatment for patients with autoimmune pancreatitis in Japan. J Gastroenterol. 2007;42(Suppl 18):50–8.

84. Hirano K, Tada M, Isayama H, Yagioka H, Sasaki T, Kogure H, et al. Long-term prognosis of autoimmune pancreatitis with and without corticosteroid treatment. Gut. 2007;56:1719–24.

85. Umemura T, Zen Y, Hamano H, Ichijyo T, Kawa S, Nakanuma Y, Kiyosawa K. IgG4 associated autoimmune hepatitis: a differential diagnosis for classical autoimmune hepatitis. Gut. 2007;56:1471–2.

Developmental Abnormalities of the Bile Duct and Foregut

10

Masaki Iwai, Takahiro Mori, and Wilson M. S. Tsui

Contents

Abbreviations

ADPKD	Autosomal dominant polycystic kidney disease
ADPLD	Autosomal dominant polycystic liver disease
ARPKD	Autosomal recessive polycystic kidney disease
CHF	Congenital hepatic fibrosis
Erb-B2	Erythroblastic oncogene B2
Gd-EOB-DTPA-MRI	Gadolinium ethoxybenzyl diethylenetriaminepentaacetic acid magnetic resonance imaging
MEK	MAP (Mitogen-Activated Protein) / ERK (Extracellular Signal-Regulated Kinase) kinase
mTOR	Mechanistic target of rapamycin
SOL	Space-occupying lesion
Srk kinase	S-receptor kinase

M. Iwai, MD, PhD
Kyoto, Japan

T. Mori, MD, PhD
Hyogo, Japan

W. M. S. Tsui, MD, FRCPath (✉)
Hong Kong, China
e-mail: mstsui@ha.org.hk

Extrahepatic biliary atresia, paucity of intrahepatic bile ducts, viral hepatitis, and malformations of bile ducts are the main causes of neonatal cholestasis. Biliary atresia occurs due to inflammation and destruction of extrahepatic bile duct systems in utero and during the perinatal period. Malformations of bile ducts are associated with abnormal remodeling of embryonic bile duct plate and fibrocystic lesions are developed, and they include congenital hepatic fibrosis [1], Caroli's disease [2], microhamartoma [3], and choledochal cyst, and they carry an increased risk of bile duct carcinoma. Differing from other cystic lesions, ciliated hepatic cyst arising from embryonic foregut is detected incidentally in adults and should be differentiated from bile duct lesions [4]. Infantile and adult types of hereditary polycystic disease cause renal failure, and hepatic failure is rare [5, 6].

10.1 Biliary Atresia

Biliary atresia may involve the entire extrahepatic biliary tree or only proximal or distal segments of bile ducts [7, 8]. Intrahepatic bile ducts are rarely affected early in the disease, but they may be gradually destroyed by fibrosis due to prolonged biliary obstruction. If biliary atresia is not diagnosed and treated, biliary cirrhosis develops early in life, and median age of death is 12 months [9]. Biliary atresia is classified into two patterns: early one (embryonal/fetal) accounting for 15–35% and late one (perinatal) for 65–85% of cases. About 20% of cases are associated with congenital anomalies of cardiovascular or digestive system and spleen [10]. Patients are anicteric at birth and develop jaundice in the first weeks of life, accompanied by dark urine and pale stools. Liver is enlarged and hard at presentation, and laboratory examinations show elevation of serum bilirubin, alkaline phosphatase, and gamma-glutamyltransferase.

It is hypothesized that prenatal or postnatal viral infection may initiate cholangiocyte apoptosis and trigger immune response of T-helper cell lymphocytes which amplify bile duct injury, inflammation, and obstructive fibrosis [11]. Regulatory T cells and genetic factors play a role in destructive autoimmune mechanisms in biliary atresia [12, 13].

Histological change of extrahepatic bile ducts is classified into three types: [1] atretic with no inflammatory cells in surrounding connective tissue, [2] cleft-like lumen lined by cuboidal epithelium, and [3] altered bile duct incompletely lined by columnar epithelium. The pathological features of liver include cholestasis, periportal ductular proliferation, and presence of bile plugs in cholangioles and interlobular bile ducts.

Hepatoportoenterostomy (Kasai procedure) [14] is the first-line surgical approach for biliary atresia, but it should be performed before 30–45 days of life to prevent worsening of the disease [15]. Even after successful hepatoportoenterostomy, more than 70% of the patients develop liver cirrhosis and require liver transplant by adulthood [11].

Case 10.1

A 1-month-old girl was icteric and her stool was acholic. Liver chemistry showed TBIL 11.9 mg/dL, DBIL 8.78 mg/dL, ALT 42 IU/L, AST 80 IU/L, ALP 1441 IU/L, and GGT 395 IU/L. Computed tomogram (CT) with contrast medium did not show dilatation of intrahepatic or extrahepatic bile

ducts, and portal veins were seen. Percutaneous transhepatic cholangiography showed fine intrahepatic bile ducts, but no extrahepatic bile ducts (Fig. 10.1). Wedge biopsy of liver during Kasai enterostomy showed portal and bridging fibrosis. Magnified view of portal tract revealed proliferating bile ductules. Their epithelia were degenerated, with congestion mixed with fibrosis and infiltration of neutrophilic leukocytes and lymphocytes (Fig. 10.2).

10.2 Fibropolycystic Diseases

Fibropolycystic diseases include congenital hepatic fibrosis, Caroli's disease, microhamartoma (von Meyenburg complex), choledochal cyst, and both infantile and adult forms of polycystic disease, which represent a number of congenital abnormalities involving the bile ducts related to abnormal remodeling of the embryonic bile duct plate [16].

10.2.1 von Meyenburg Complex

Usually, Caroli's disease and von Meyenburg complex cannot be easily distinguished. However, cystic malformation affects different parts of the intrahepatic biliary trees with or without surrounding fibrosis in Caroli's disease, and portal tract bile ducts are affected in von Meyenburg complex.

Von Meyenburg complex is often multiple and distinct from congenital hepatic fibrosis. CT shows presence of multiple low-density areas, MRI demonstrates multiple high-intensified small lesions, and peritoneoscopy reveals diffuse distribution of white maculae with small cystic lesions on liver surface (Fig. 10.3a,b,c). Morphologically, there are small nodules with inspissated bile in the lumen, which are portal-based lesions comprising angulated, ectatic, branching

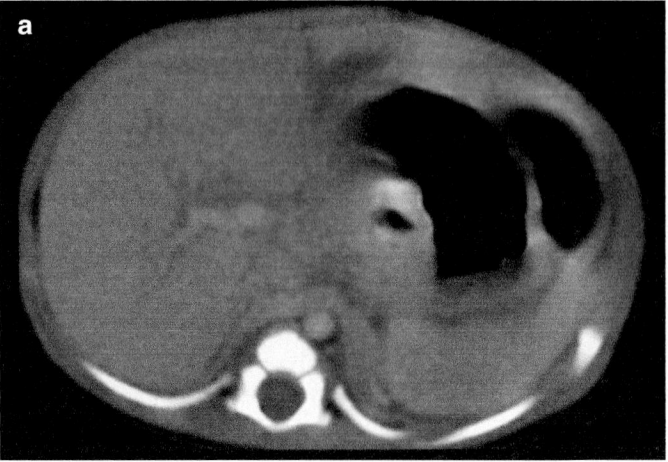
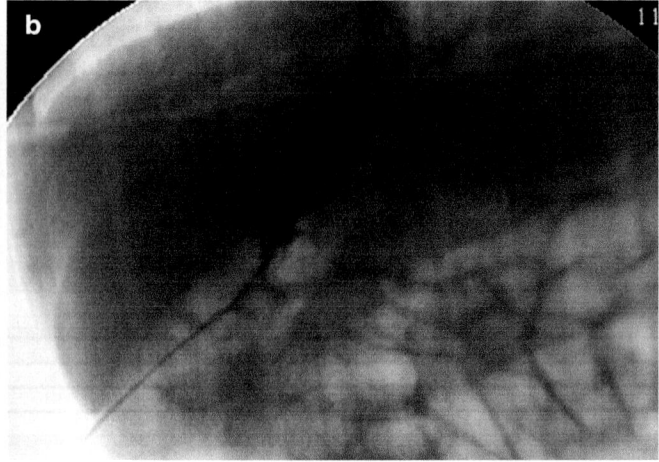

Fig. 10.1 Biliary atresia. (**a**) CT with contrast medium does not show dilatation of intrahepatic or extrahepatic bile duct, and portal trunk and veins are seen. (**b**) Percutaneous hepatic cholangiography shows immature intrahepatic bile ducts, but extrahepatic bile duct is not detected

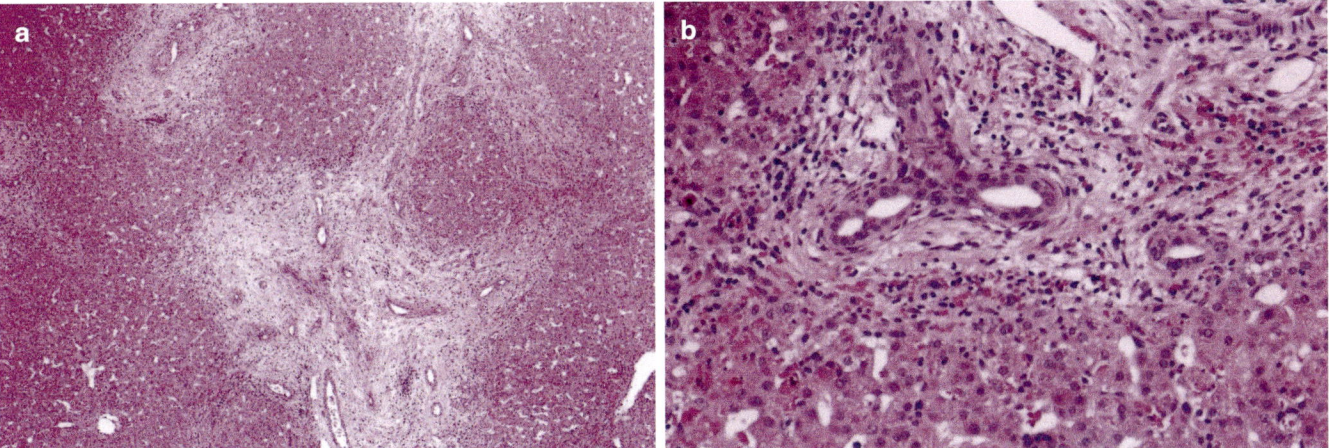

Fig. 10.2 Biliary atresia. (**a**) Fibrosis develops from periportal area and is bridged among portal tracts. (**b**) Bile ductular proliferation is accompanied by fibrosis. Congestion is seen in portal tract, and lymphocytes or neutrophilic leukocytes infiltrate in the portal tract

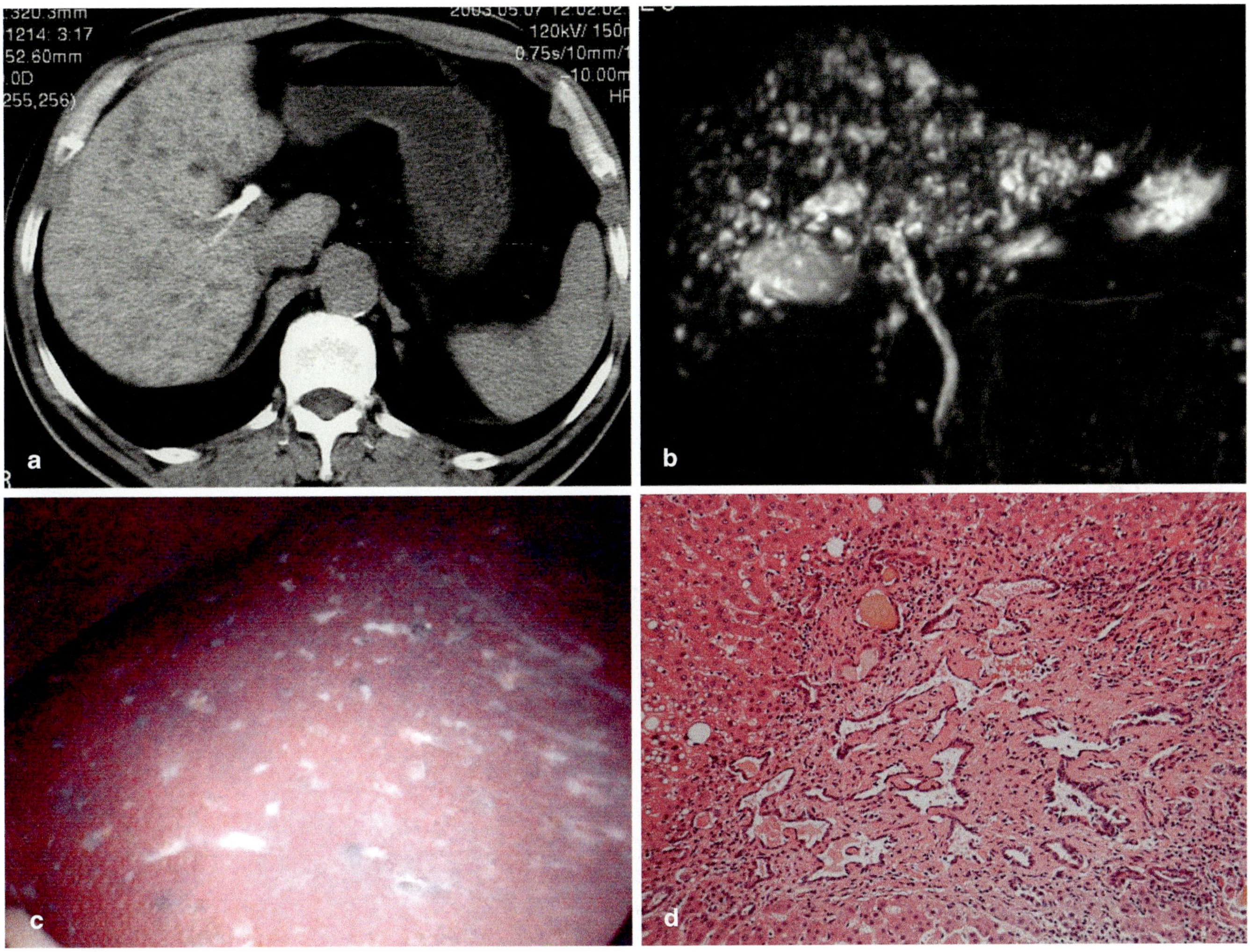

Fig. 10.3 von Meyenburg complex. (**a**) Multiple low-density areas are seen in right lobe of liver in CT image. (**b**) MRI for cholangio-pancreatic ducts shows multiple high-intensified small lesions in liver. (**c**) Peritoneoscopy shows white maculae with small cyst on liver surface. (**d**) Portal-based lesion consists of angulated, ectatic, and branching bile ducts in fibrous stroma. The ducts are lined by columnar or cuboidal epithelium and contain amorphous pink material or inspissated bile

bile ducts in fibrous stroma, and ducts lined by columnar or cuboidal epithelium containing amorphous pink material or inspissated bile (Fig. 10.3d).

10.2.2 Caroli's Disease

Caroli's disease is characterized by segmental or lobar cystic dilatation of bile ducts [17], and cysts are round or lanceolate. The inheritance is autosomal recessive, and the patients suffer from fever and pain when cholelithiasis develops. Liver test is always normal, and biliary duct enzymes are only elevated when obstruction of biliary ducts occurs. Transluminal fibrovascular bridges are visualized in cysts as central dot sign by CT [18, 19] or abdominal ultrasound (US), and cystic lesions are shown by endoscopic retrograde cholangiography to communicate with biliary ducts (Fig. 10.4). Macroscopic findings of liver in Caroli's disease show cystically dilated bile ducts traversed by fibrovascular

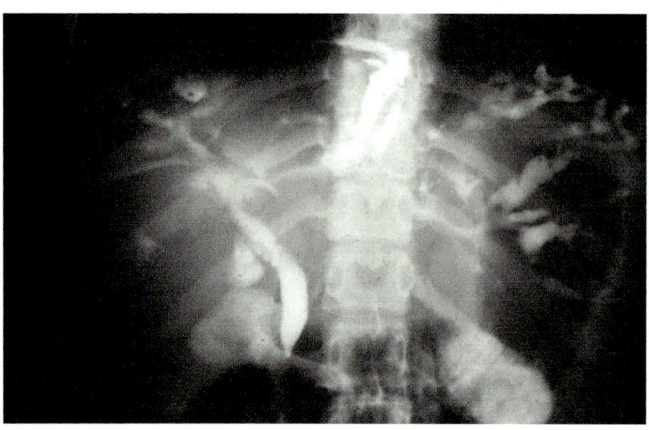

Fig. 10.4 Endoscopic retrograde cholangiography in Caroli's disease. There is cystic and irregular dilatation of intrahepatic bile ducts

bridges. Microscopic findings reveal dark bilirubinate calculi in the lumen and dilated bile ducts arranged around the central vessels (ductal plate malformation) and lined by mucin-secreting columnar epithelium (Fig. 10.5).

Due to communication of the abnormal dilated bile ducts with bowel, Caroli's disease is complicated by cholangitis and cholelithiasis [2], and treatment consists of biliary drainage, administration of antibiotics, surgical procedures, and liver transplantation.

Case 10.2

A 26-year-old female complained of right hypochondralgia and vomiting. She had a history of infection in the biliary tree 12 years ago. Her liver chemistry showed ALT 6 IU/L, AST 13 IU/L, ALP 187 IU/L, and GGT 48 IU/L. US showed multiple low-echoic lesions communicating with biliary trees in liver, MRI showed high signal intensity in cystic lesions, and abdominal CT showed cystic dilatation of intrahepatic bile ducts (Fig. 10.6). There were no abnormal liver values, except for elevated ALP. Peritoneoscopy showed dark blue lesions mixed with white maculae of various sizes on liver surface (Fig. 10.7). Histology showed irregularly configured bile ducts surrounded by broad band of fibrosis, and columnar epithelium of bile ducts was flattened and desquamated into bile duct lumen, consistent with ductal plate malformation (Fig. 10.8).

10.3 Ciliated Hepatic Foregut Cyst

The cyst is generally found incidentally by imaging studies or during surgery, seen more frequently in men, and commonly detected in the medial segment of left lobe. It is proposed that the cyst is originated from the detachment and migration of buds from esophagus or bronchial regions of foregut and subsequent entrapment by the liver [20]. In most

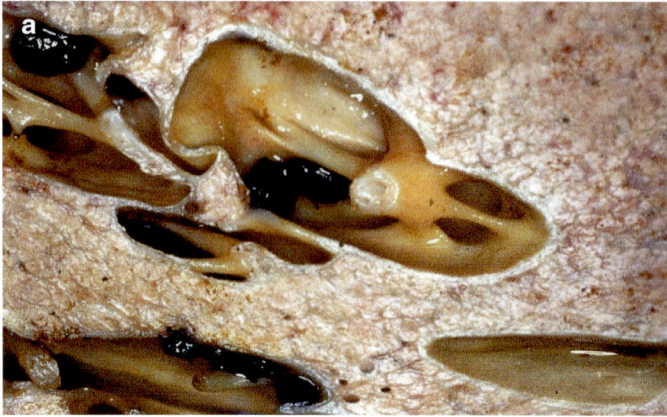
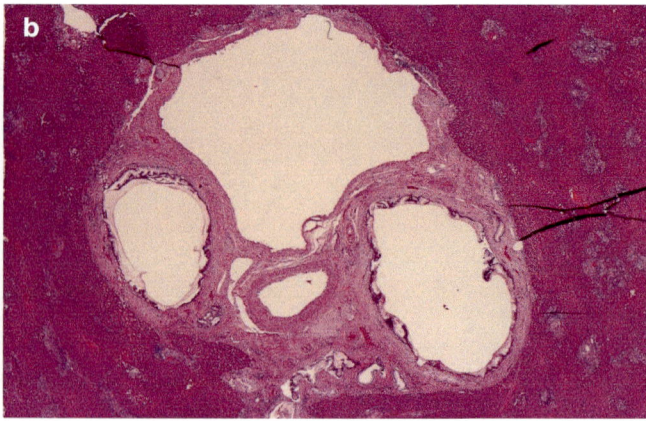

Fig. 10.5 Macroscopic and microscopic findings of liver in Caroli's disease. (**a**) Cystically dilated bile ducts are traversed by fibrovascular bridges. Dark bilirubinate calculi are present in lumen of bile ducts. (**b**) Dilated bile ducts are arranged around central vessels (ductal plate malformation) and lined by mucin-secreting columnar epithelium

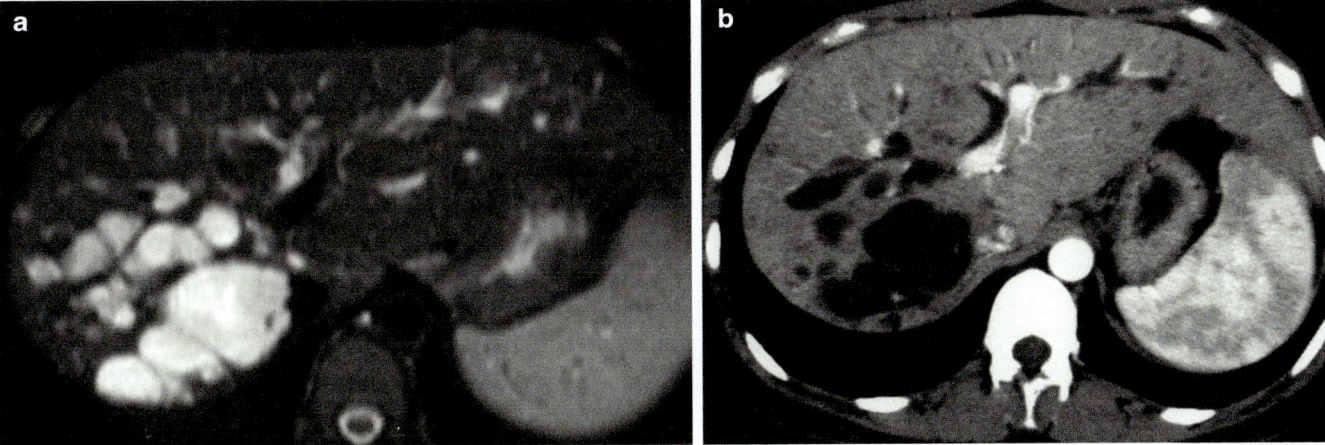

Fig. 10.6 Caroli's disease. (**a**) T2-weighted magnetic resonance image shows multiple lesions with high intensity in liver. (**b**) CT with contrast medium shows multiple cystic dilatations of intrahepatic bile ducts

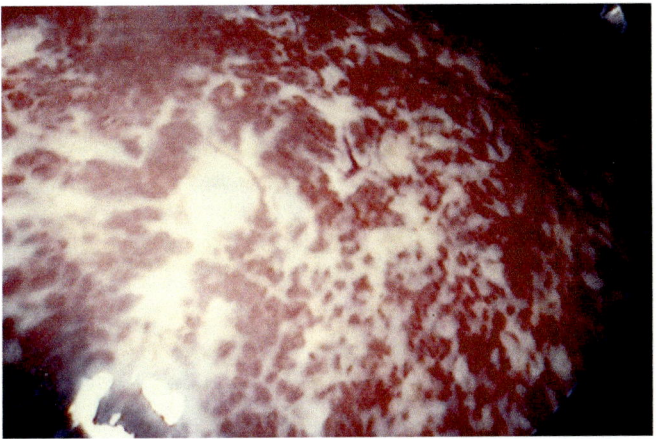

Fig. 10.7 Caroli's disease. Peritoneoscopy shows dark blue lesions mixed with white maculae of varying sizes and dilated peripheral portal veins

cases, it is unilocular and its diameter is about 3 cm. It should be differentiated from solitary bile duct cysts, hepatobiliary cystadenomas, or echinococcal cysts. There are a few reports of squamous cell carcinoma arising from a ciliated foregut cyst [21].

Case 10.3
An 80-year-old male suffering from advanced gastric cancer was hospitalized for preoperative examination. Abdominal US showed a protrusive space-occupying lesion (SOL) in S4 area of left lobe, and its circumference was low-echoic and inner area of SOL isoechoic (Fig. 10.9a). Doppler-echo showed no signal of vasculature (Fig. 10.9b). His laboratory test showed neither HBsAg nor anti-HCV in serum, and CEA, CA19–9, and AFP were within normal limits. CT without contrast medium showed high-density area detected by US (Fig. 10.9c), and CT with contrast

medium revealed low-density area in the early phase (Fig. 10.9d). MRI intensified by T1 showed high-intensified tumor (Fig. 10.10a), MRI intensified by T2 showed low-intensified tumor and high intensity in its surrounding area (Fig. 10.10b), and Gd-EOB-DTPA-MRI in phase of hepatocytes showed slightly high intensity in comparison with non-tumor area and high intensity in its surrounding area (Fig. 10.10c). Tumor resected by partial hepatectomy showed a cystic lesion containing mass of yellow jerry-material in transparent and viscus liquid (Fig. 10.11a). Histologically the cystic lesion was surrounded by a thick capsule composed of connective tissues, muscular structure, and arterioles (Fig. 10.11b). The inner surface is lined by ciliated stratified epithelium and separates from the hepatic parenchyma by connective tissue containing some inflammatory cells and muscle bundles (Fig. 10.11c). Columnar epithelium is stratified and ciliated with some mucus cells, and lymphoplasmacytic infiltrate is present beneath the epithelium (Fig. 10.11d). There was no tumor recurrence after resection.

10.4 Polycystic Kidney Disease

Autosomal recessive and dominant polycystic kidney disease (ARPKD and ADPKD) can occur in both children [5] and adults [6]. The gene for ARPKD, *PKHD1* (polycystic kidney and hepatic disease 1), is mapped to chromosome 6p 21.2-p12, and the gene encodes a 4074-amino acid protein, fibrocystin [22]. There are perinatal, neonatal, infantile, and juvenile types. The liver does not show gross cystic lesions. There is striking increase in number of portal bile ducts with intraacinar extension and little supporting connective tissue stroma. Circumferential arrangement reminiscent of the embryonic ductal plate (ductal plate malformation) and often

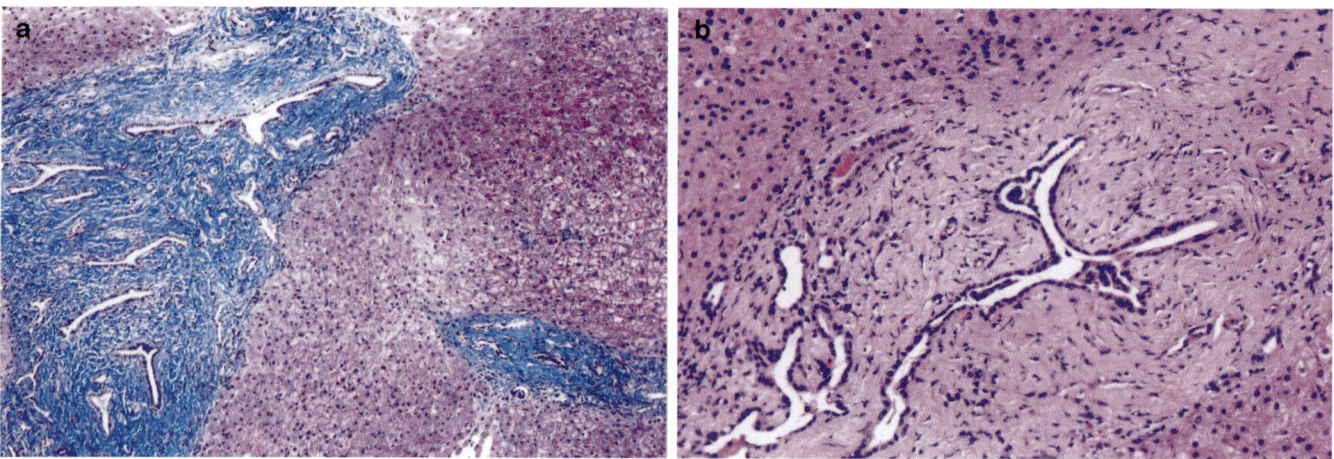

Fig. 10.8 Portal tract in Caroli's disease. (**a**) Masson's trichrome stain shows wide band of fibrosis with irregularly configured bile ducts in the portal area. (**b**) Fibrosis develops in portal tract with irregularly configured bile ducts, and lining epithelium is flattened and desquamated into lumen

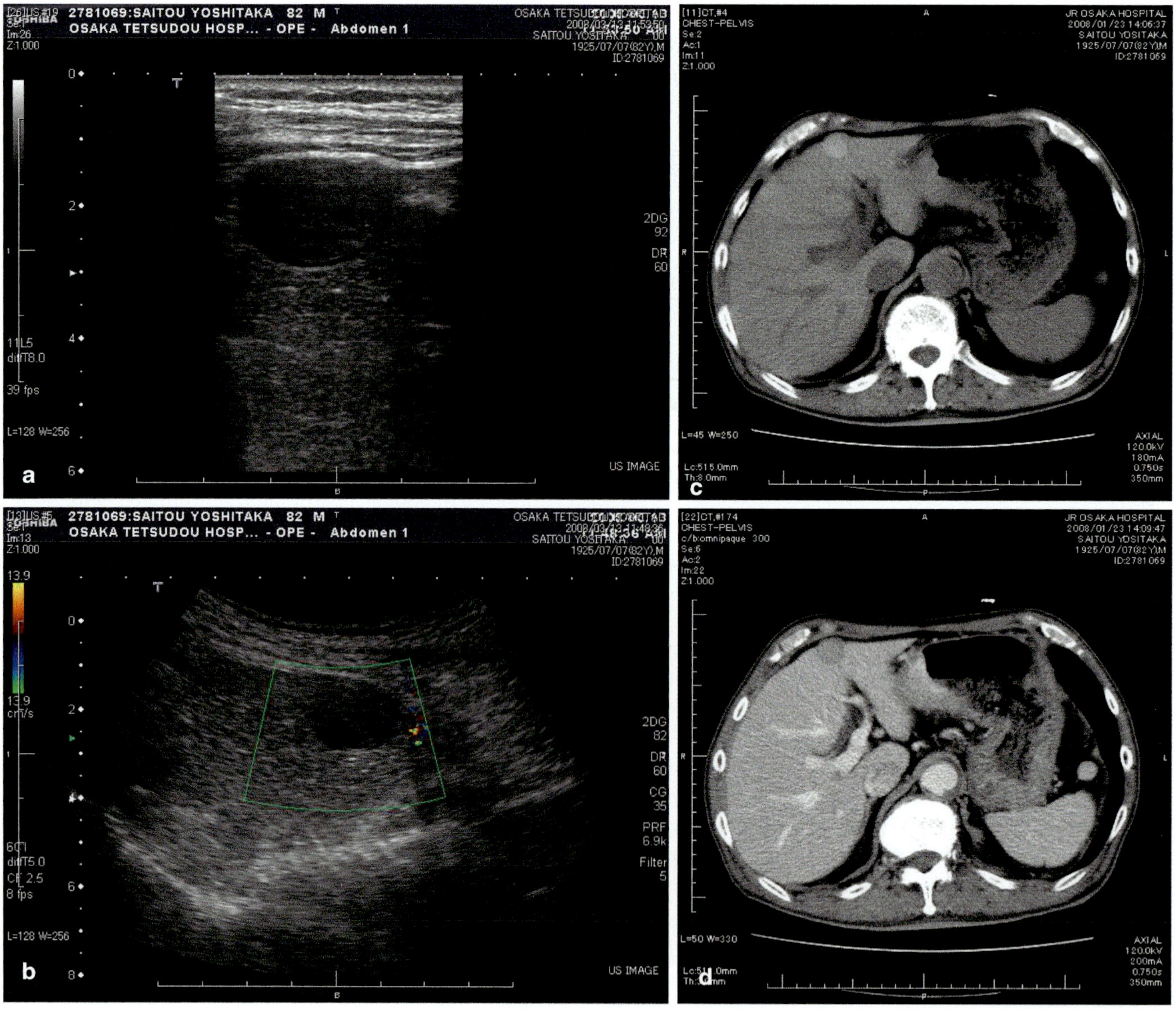

Fig. 10.9 Ciliated hepatic foregut cyst. (**a**) US shows a protrusive space-occupying lesion (SOL) in S4 area of left lobe, and its circumference is low-echoic and inner area of SOL isoechoic. (**b**) Doppler-echo shows no signal of vasculature. (**c**) CT without contrast medium shows high-density area in tumor. (**d**) CT with contrast medium reveals low-density area in the early phase

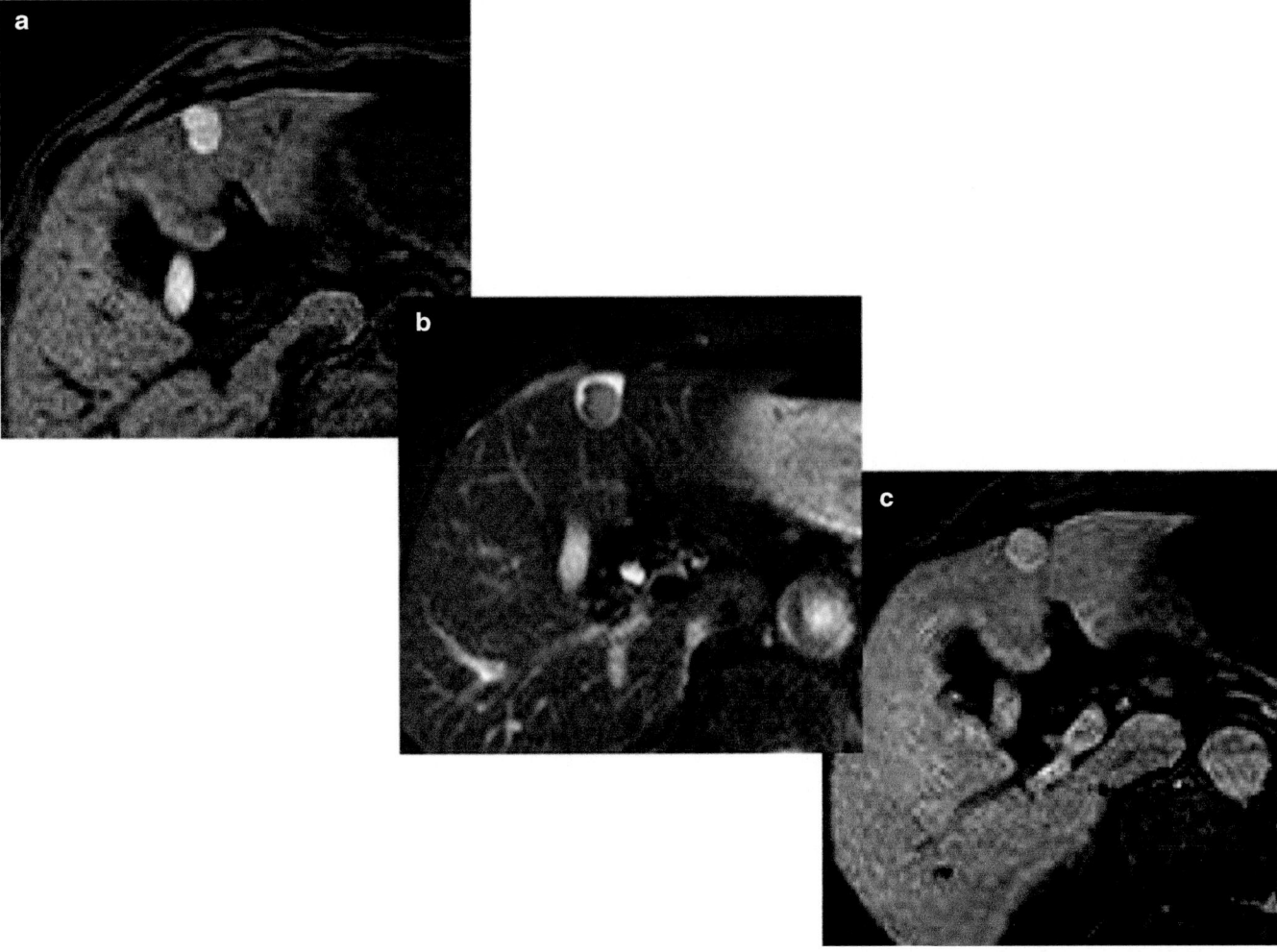

Fig. 10.10 Ciliated hepatic foregut cyst. (**a**) MRI intensified by T1 shows high-intensified tumor. (**b**) MRI intensified by T2 shows low-intensified tumor and high-intensified area in its surrounding. (**c**) Gd-EOB-DTPA-MRI in phase of hepatocytes shows slightly high intensity in tumor in comparison with non-tumor area and higher intensity in its surrounding

polypoid fibrovascular projections into microcystically dilated ducts are present (Fig. 10.12). Increasing portal fibrosis develops, evolving into a pattern of congenital hepatic fibrosis (CHF) .

ADPKD is associated with mutations of *PKD1* or *PKD2*, located on chromosome 16 (16p13) or chromosome 4 (4q21), and encoding for polycystin 1 and polycystin 2, respectively [23]. Autosomal dominant polycystic liver disease (ADPLD) with isolated liver involvement and no kidney disease has also been identified and is genetically distinct from ADPKD [24]. Multiple cystic lesions of various sizes are seen in liver, and cystic bile ducts are dilated and lined with bile duct epithelium (Fig. 10.13). Rupture of a large cyst may lead to acute abdomen. The large cyst causes portal hypertension, cholestasis [25], and leg edema. Renal insufficiency due to the development of multiple cysts is a dangerous complication [26]. Treatment includes laparoscopic or surgical fenestration [27], injection of minocycline hydrochloride [28] or alcohol [29], and surgical management [30]. There is no clear role for medical therapy for polycystic diseases, but somatostatin analogs, vasopressin, vitamin K3, mTOR inhibitors, inhibitors of Erb-B2 tyrosine kinase, Srk kinase, and MEK have been investigated to decrease size of cysts and to reduce symptoms.

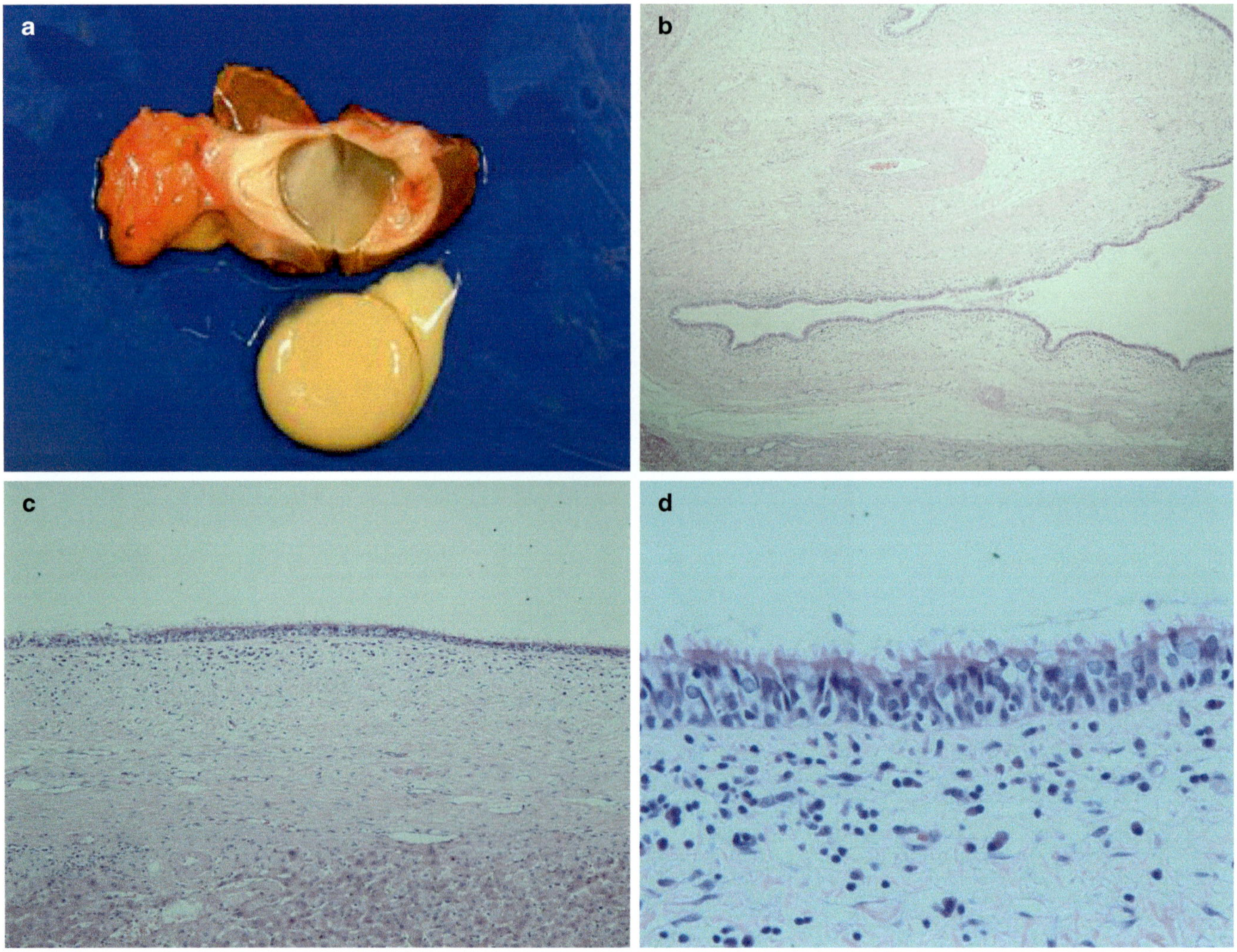

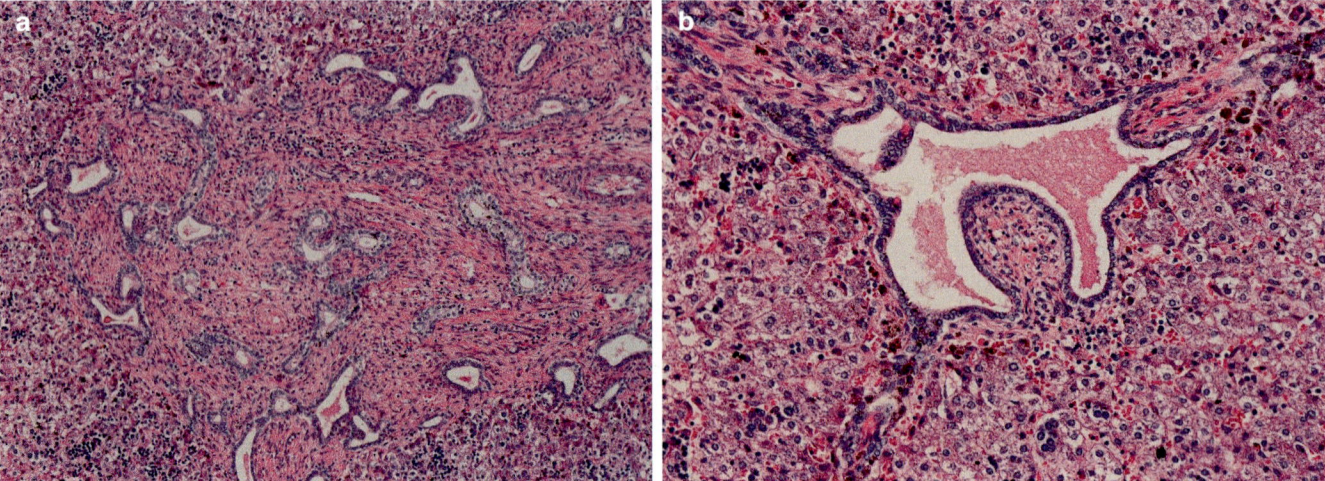

Fig. 10.11 Ciliated hepatic foregut cyst. (**a**) Tumor resected by partial hepatectomy shows a cystic lesion containing yellow jerry-material in transparent and viscus liquid. (**b**) Tumor is cystic and surrounded by thick capsule composed of connective tissue, muscular structure, and arterioles.

(**c**) Lining epithelium is ciliated and stratified, and inflammatory cells and muscle bundles are present in the connective tissue wall. (**d**) Stratified columnar epithelium is mucinous and ciliated, and lymphocyte and plasma cells are infiltrating between the epithelium and connective tissue

Fig. 10.12 Autosomal recessive type of polycystic disease. (**a**) Enlarged portal tract contains increased numbers of bile ducts arranged circumferentially (ductal plate malformation). (**b**) There is polypoid fibrovascular projection into microcystically dilated duct

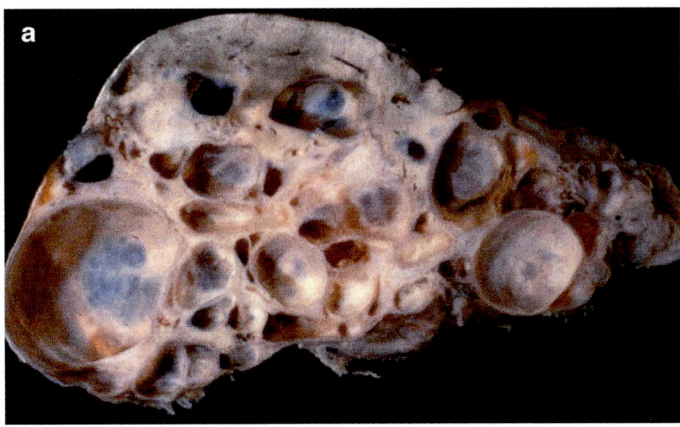
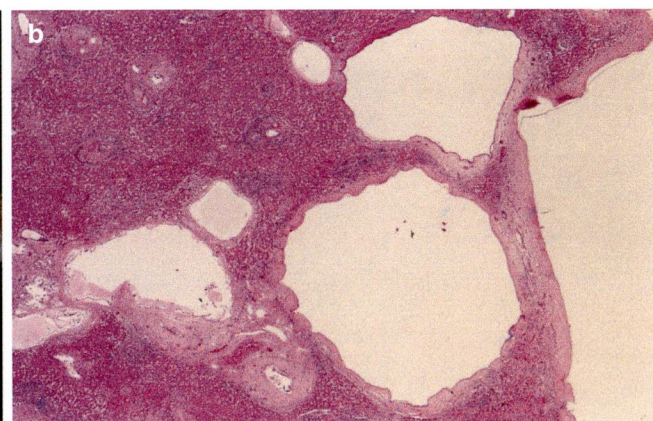

Fig. 10.13 Autosomal dominant type of polycystic disease. (**a**) Numerous cysts of various sizes are present throughout liver. (**b**) Multiple cysts of various sizes are lined by flattened epithelium

References

1. De Vos BF, CuveLier C. Congenital hepatic fibrosis. J Hepatol. 1988;6:222–8.
2. Dagli U, Atalay F, Sasmaz N, Bostanoglu S, Temucin G, Sahin B. Caroli's disease: 1977–1995 experiences. Eur J Gastroenterol Hepatol. 1998;10:109–12.
3. Thommesen N. Biliary hamartomas (von Meyenburg complexes) in liver needle biopsies. Acta Pathol Microbiol Sacd Sect A. 1978;86:93–9.
4. Vick DJ, Goodman ZD, Deavers MT, et al. Ciliated foregut cyst. A study of six cases and review of the literature. Am J Surg Pathol. 1999;23:671–7.
5. Everson GT, Taylor MR, Doctor RB. Polycystic disease of the liver. Hepatology. 2004;40:774–82.
6. Krohn PS, Hillingso JG, Kirkegaard P. Liver transplantation in polycystic liver disease: a relevant treatment modality for adults? Scad J Gastroenterol. 2008;43:89–94.
7. Lefkowitch JH. Biliary atresia. Mayo Clin Proc. 1998;73:90–5.
8. Balistreri WF, Grand R, Hoofnagle JH, Suchy FJ, Ryckman FC, Perlmutter DH, et al. Biliary atresia: current concepts and research directions. Summary of a symposium. Hepatology. 1996;23:1682–92.
9. Adelman S. Prognosis of uncorrected biliary atresia: an update. J Pediatr Surg. 1978;13:389–91.
10. Carmi R, Magee CA, NEILL CA, Karrer FM. Extrahepatic biliary atresia and associated anomalies: etiologic heterogeneity suggested by distinctive patterns of associations. Am J Med Genet. 1993;45:683–93.
11. Petersen C, Davenport M. Aetiology of biliary atresia: what is actually known? Orphanet J Rare Dis. 2013;8(1):128.
12. Brindley SM, Lanham AM, Karrer FM, Tucker RM, Fontenor AP, Mack CI. Cytomegalovirus-specific T-cell reactivity in biliary atresia at the time of diagnosis is associated with deficits in regulatory T cells. Hepatology. 2012;55:1130–8.
13. Miethke AG, Sexena V, Shivakumar P, Sabla GE, Simmons J, Chougnet CA. Post-natal paucity of regulatory T cells and control of NK cell activation in experimental biliary atresia. J Hepatol. 2010;52:718–26.
14. Kasai M, Suzuki H, Ohashi E, et al. Technique and results of operative management of biliary atresia. World J Surg. 1978;2:571–9.
15. Mack CL, Feldman AG, Sokol RJ. Clues to the etiology of bile duct injury in biliary atresia. Semin Liver Dis. 2012;32:307–16.
16. Summerfield J, Nagafuchi Y, Sherlock S, et al. Hepatobiliary fibro-polycystic diseases. A clinical and histological review of 51 patients. J Hepatol. 1986;2:141–56.
17. Caroli J. Diseases of the intrahepatic biliary tree. Clin Gastroenterol. 1973;2:147–61.
18. Choi BI, Mo-Yeon K, Kim SH, Han MC. Caroli disease: central dot sign in CT. Radiology. 1990;174:161–3.
19. Brancatelli G, Federle MP, Vilgrain V, Vullierme MP, Marin D, Lagalla R. Polycystic liver disease: CT and MRI imaging findings. Radiographics. 2005;25:659–70.
20. Wheeler DA, Edmondson HA. Ciliated hepatic foregut cyst. Am J Surg Pathol. 1984;8:467–70.
21. Farlanetto A, Dei Tos AP. Squamous cell carcinoma arising in a ciliated hepatic foregut cyst. Virchows Arch. 2002;441:296–8.
22. Ward CJ, Hogan MC, Rossetti S, et al. The gene mutated in autosomal recessive polycystic kidney disease encodes a large, receptor-like protein. Nat Genet. 2002;30:259–69.
23. Torres VE, Harris PC, Pirson Y. Autosomal dominant polycystic kidney disease. Lancet. 2007;369:1287–301.
24. Pirson Y, Lannoy N, Peters D, et al. Isolated polycystic liver disease as a distinct genetic disease, unlinked to polycystic kidney disease 1 and polycystic kidney disease 2. Hepatology. 1996;23:249–52.
25. Dmitrewski J, Olliff S, Buckels JA. Obstructive jaundice associated with polycystic liver disease. HPB Surg. 1996;10:117–20.
26. Cowles RA, Mulholland MW. Solitary hepatic cysts. J Am Coll Surg. 2000;191:311–21.
27. Garcea G, Pattenden CJ, Stephenson J, Dannison AR, Berry DP. Nine-year single-center experience with non-parasitic liver cysts: diagnosis and management. Dig Dis Sci. 2007;52:185–91.
28. Yoshida H, Onda M, Tajiri T, Arima Y, Mamada Y, Taniai N, et al. Long-term results of multiple minocycline hydrochloride injections for the treatment of symptomatic solitary hepatic cyst. J Gastroenterol Hepatol. 2003;18:595–8.
29. Okano A, Hajiro K, Takakuwa H, Nishio A. Alcohol sclerotherapy of hepatic cysts: its effect in relation to ethanol concentration. Hepatol Res. 2000;17:179–84.
30. Russell RT, Pinson CW. Surgical management of polycystic liver disease. World J Gastroenterol. 2007;13:5052–9.

Vascular Disorders in the Liver

11

Masahiko Koda, Tomomitsu Matono,
Makiko Taniai, and Masaki Iwai

Contents

Abbreviations

APF	Arterioportal fistula
AVM	Arteriovenous malformations
BCS	Budd-Chiari syndrome

M. Koda, MD, PhD (✉)
Tottori, Japan

T. Matono, MD, PhD
Tottori, Japan

M. Taniai, MD, PhD
Tokyo, Japan

M. Iwai, MD, PhD
Kyoto, Japan

CDUS	Color Doppler ultrasonography
CV	Central vein
EHPVO	Extrahepatic portal venous obstruction
FALD	Fontan-associated liver disease
FNH	Focal nodular hyperplasia
HA	Hepatic artery
HCC	Hepatocellular carcinoma
HHT	Hereditary hemorrhagic telangiectasia
HSCT	Hematopoietic stem cell transplantation
HV	Hepatic vein
INCPH	Idiopathic non-cirrhotic portal hypertension
IVC	Inferior vena cava
MOVC	Idiopathic membranous obstruction of IVC
PV	Portal vein
PVT	Portal vein thrombosis

© Springer Nature Singapore Pte Ltd. 2019
E. Hashimoto et al. (eds.), *Diagnosis of Liver Disease*, https://doi.org/10.1007/978-981-13-6806-6_11

RA	Right atrium
SMAV fistula	Superior mesenteric arteriovenous fistula
SMV	Superior mesenteric vein
SV	Splenic vein
TIPS	Transjugular intrahepatic portosystemic shunt

11.1 Introduction

The liver has a dual blood supply: 60–70% from portal vein and 30–40% from hepatic artery. Arterioportal mixed blood in sinusoids streams to terminal hepatic veins from the periportal zone, and the venous blood collected in three hepatic veins is carried to inferior vena cava and right-sided atrium. Vascular disorders of the liver can be classified into three groups, the impairments of blood flow into (prehepatic), through (intrahepatic), or from (posthepatic) the liver (Table 11.1, Fig. 11.1). Then disturbance of blood flow in cardiovascular system (acute or chronic heart failure), hepatic veins or arteries, portal veins, and sinusoids must affect liver function, and these vascular lesions are closely associated

Table 11.1 Classification of vascular disorders of the liver

Posthepatic
1. Right hepatic failure
• Congestion heart failure
• Constructive pericarditis
• Intracardiac neoplasia
• Fontan procedure
2. Budd-Chiari syndrome
• Hepatic vein obstruction
• Inferior vena cava obstruction at its hepatic portion (obliterative hepatocavopathy)
Intrahepatic
1. Presinusoidal
• Non-cirrhotic portal fibrosis (idiopathic portal hypertension)
• Hepatic arteriovenous fistula
• Hepatic arterioportal fistula
• Schistosomiasis
• Nodular hyperplasia
• Caroli's disease (ductal plate abnormalities)
2. Sinusoidal
• Cirrhosis
• Peliosis hepatis
• Hereditary hemorrhagic telangiectasia (Osler-weber-Rendu disease)
3. Postsinusoidal
• Sinusoidal obstruction syndrome (veno-occlusive disease)
Prehepatic
1. Portal vein
• Portal thrombosis
• Portal tumor thrombus
• Phlebitis
• Congenital portal atresia
• Portal vein aneurysm
2. Hepatic artery
• Polyarteritis nodosa
• Hepatic artery aneurysm
3. Portal vein and hepatic artery
• Hepatic infarction

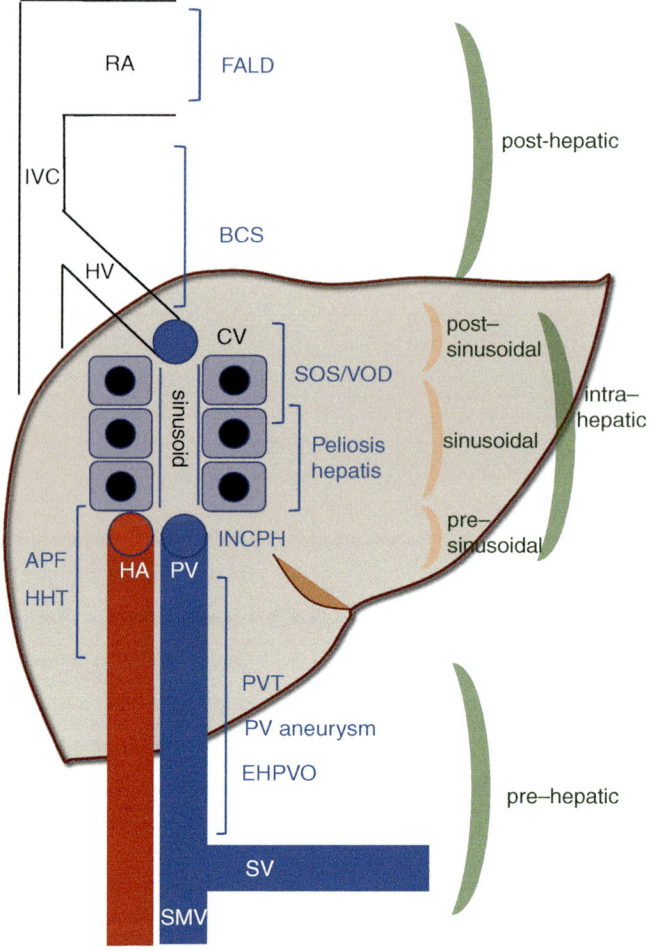

Fig. 11.1 Schematic representative of the anatomic classification of hepatic vascular disorders. Hepatic vascular disorders can be classified into prehepatic, intrahepatic (presinusoidal, sinusoidal, postsinusoidal), and posthepatic lesions. *APF* arterioportal fistula, *BCS* Budd-Chiari syndrome, *CV* central vein, *EHPVO* extrahepatic portal venous obstruction, *FALD* Fontan-associated liver disease, *HA* hepatic artery, *HHT* hereditary hemorrhagic telangiectasia, *HV* hepatic vein, *INCPH* idiopathic non-cirrhotic portal hypertension, *IVC* inferior vena cava, *PV* portal vein, *PVT* portal vein thrombosis, *RA* right atrium, *SMV* superior mesenteric vein, *SV* splenic vein

with development of acute and chronic liver diseases. This chapter describes liver disorders caused by abnormal stream or obstruction of hepatic artery, portal or hepatic veins, and sinusoids.

11.2 Hepatic Veins

The hepatic venous flow begins in terminal hepatic veins; drains into the intercalated veins, from there into the collecting veins and truncal veins; and reaches the inferior vena cava. Congestive cardiac failure (acute or chronic type), stenosis or obstruction of inferior vena cava, hepatic vein thrombosis, veno-occlusion, and endophlebitis obliterans cause acute or chronic liver disease and cirrhosis.

11.3 Budd-Chiari Syndrome (BCS)

Budd-Chiari Syndrome [1–4] is a rare disease with an estimated prevalence of 1/100,000 [5] and is a disorder caused by obstruction of hepatic veins and inferior vena cava (IVC). Primary BCS is due to endoluminal venous lesions such as thrombus or web. Secondary BCS is due to a lesion outside the venous system such as tumor, abscess, or cysts. Obstruction of a single hepatic vein out of three hepatic veins is clinically silent. The obstruction of 2–3 hepatic veins induces hepatic dysfunction and becomes symptomatic. According to the location of obstruction, BCS is classified into three types: pure obstruction of hepatic veins, pure obstruction of IVC, and combined obstruction of hepatic veins and IVC. Clinical manifestations are characterized by abdominal pain, edema, ascites, jaundice, hepatomegaly, hepatic encephalopathy, variceal bleeding, and/or formation of collateral circulation pathways in abdominal and chest walls. However, they vary according to whether the disorder is acute, subacute, or chronic [6].

On etiology, the primary BCS is associated with hypercoagulable states leading to vascular thrombosis and develops from hereditary conditions such as Factor V Leiden, protein C, S, or antithrombin deficiency [7]. Pregnancy and estrogen intake can promote or trigger BCS especially in the presence of an underlying risk factor of thrombosis. The secondary BCS is associated with invasion or extrinsic compression of the hepatic veins and/or IVC. Causes of vascular compression are a pyogenic infectious process, amoebas, hydatid disease or echinococcosis, and benign and/or malignant tumors. Idiopathic membranous obstruction of IVC (MOVC) is frequently seen in South Africa [8], India [9], Nepal [10], and Japan [11].

The clinical diagnosis of BCS can be accurately assessed with imaging modalities. Color Doppler ultrasonography (CDUS) [12] is a noninvasive technique and has high sensitivity and specificity. Typical findings are absence of flow or flat wave form without fluttering as against a triphasic pattern observed in patent hepatic vein. Small and tortuous intrahepatic or subcapsular collaterals are seen in about 80% patients. Abdominal computed tomography (CT) and magnetic resonance imaging (MRI) are also used as diagnostic tools. Triple-phase CT [13] shows the absence of hepatic vein opacity and a mottled appearance along with late enhancement of the hepatic periphery. MRI [13] is helpful for visualizing the entire length of IVC or intrahepatic collaterals and for differentiating acute from subacute or chronic BCS. In acute form, post-contrast MR show decreased T1 signal intensity and heterogeneously increased T2 signal intensity in the hepatic periphery. In the chronic form, T1 and T2 signal intensity are decreased on unenhanced MR imaging due to hepatic fibrosis. Noninvasive imaging modalities are sufficient for the diagnosis of BCS at most cases. However, if inadequate, venography and liver biopsy should be performed. Venograohy [13] is a useful modality for assessing extension and location of obstruction and measuring hepatic venous pressure.

Liver biopsy is not required to confirm BCS and insufficient to assess the severity of BCS due to sampling errors but is useful for the differential diagnosis of veno-occlusive disease. As histologic findings in BCS have previously been described [14–16], zone 3 sinusoidal congestion and dilatation may be the only findings in the early stage. Centrilobular fibrosis and nodular regenerative hyperplasia may develop over time in chronic stage and may lead to cirrhosis.

Laparoscopy is a useful tool in the diagnosis of BCS, but only a few reports have described macroscopic findings in the liver [17]. We describe the laparoscopic appearance of the liver in BCS with MOVC to clarify the macroscopic features associated with liver histology.

Treatment depends on the causes, anatomic location, extent of thrombotic process, and functional capacity of the liver. The primary goal of the treatment is relieving hepatic venous outflow obstruction and improving liver perfusion, leading to preserve functioning hepatocytes. It is divided into medical treatment, including anticoagulation and thrombolysis, interventional procedures such as angioplasty and transjugular intrahepatic portosystemic shunt (TIPS), and surgical interventions including orthotopic or living donor liver transplantation. BCS should manage stepwise [18, 19]. The first-line treatment is medical therapy which uses heparin or vitamin K antagonist. The second step is percutaneous transluminal angioplasty for patients with short-length stenosis of either the hepatic veins or IVC. TIPS is the third step in patients not responding to medical therapy and without response to or stenosis unsuitable for angioplasty/stenting. A transcaval approach has been found to be successful in most patients using covered stents [20]. The last step is liver transplantation. The remaining 10–20% of patients with BCS treated with a stepwise management strategy need rescue transplantation. A large series of transplanted patients have shown 5-year survival rates of up to 80% [21].

We present four cases of acute (case 11.1), subacute (case 11.2), and chronic BCS (cases 11.3 and 11.4) including the clinical manifestations, image analyses, and liver histology results with or without macroscopic findings to derive an accurate diagnosis. The clinical signs and symptoms may be caused either by a large, sudden blockage of hepatic veins or by portal hypertension due to differentiate chronic BCS from liver cirrhosis. Therefore, cirrhotic patients with negative hepatitis B and C tests should be examined by US, CT, and MRI to detect obstruction of IVC or thrombus in hepatic veins. In subacute phase, sinusoids become collagenized, and hepatocytes become atrophic and are lost. In chronic BCS, small hepatic veins disappear as they are incorporated into septa that eventually link hepatic veins to form cirrhosis with relative sparing of portal triads, also known as reversed lobulation cirrhosis or venocentric cirrhosis.

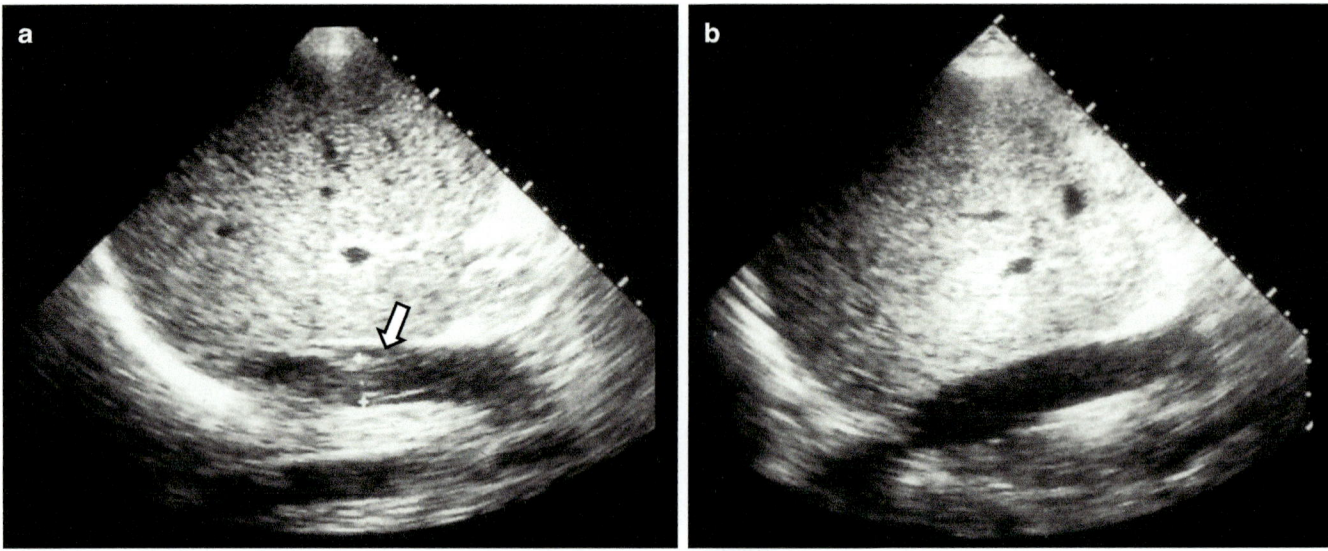

Fig. 11.2 Ultrasonographic findings in acute BCS without MOVC. (**a**) Thrombus (arrow) is seen in IVC. (**b**) No thrombus is detected in subdiaphragmatic area of IVC

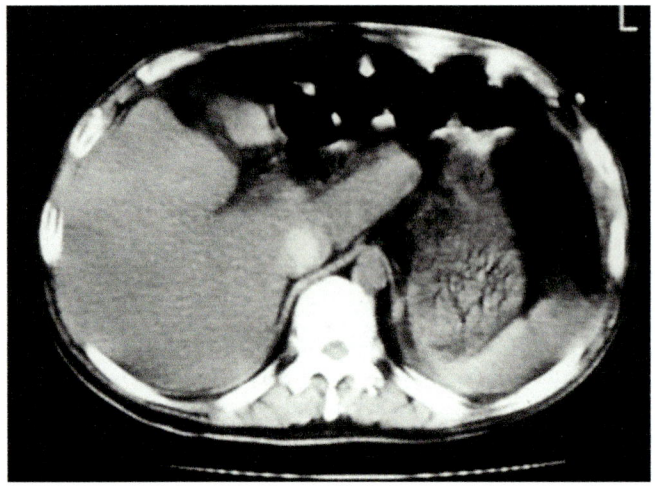

Fig. 11.3 CT in acute BCS without MOVC. High-density thrombus material is seen in IVC

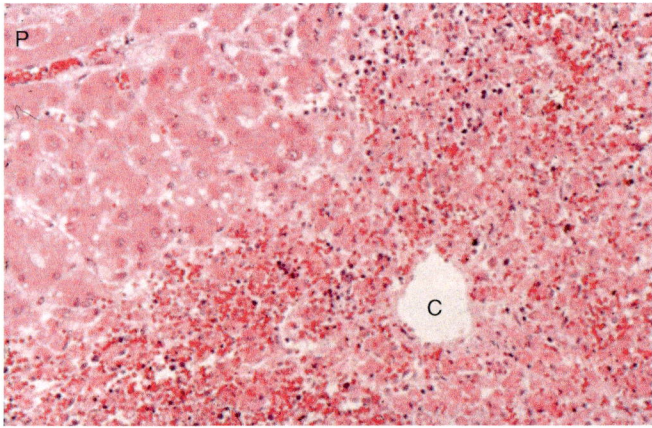

Fig. 11.4 Histological appearance of autopsied liver in acute BCS. Massive hemorrhagic necrosis is seen in zones 2 and 3, but hepatocytes in zone 1 remain intact. No fibrotic change is seen in portal tract (P). *C* central vein

Acute BCS is associated with various conditions, including malignancy, myeloproliferative disorders, infection, pregnancy, oral contraceptives, Bechet's disease, and hypercoagulable state. The patient described in case 11.1 had leukocytosis, high transaminase levels, and prolonged prothrombin time; he rapidly developed hepatic failure. High serum aminotransferase levels are considered ominous in acute BCS. Hypercoagulable state after operation might cause the thrombosis of IVC or hepatic veins and pulmonary artery, leading to respiratory and hepatic failure. Autopsy of the liver in case 11.1 showed massive hemorrhagic necrosis in zones 2 and 3.

Case 11.1

A 44-year-old male had surgery for a herniated cervical disc and was on complete bed rest for 1 week. He experienced vertigo upon standing and was in shock. He had no history of autoimmune, myeloproliferative, or infectious disease and had not taken any hormonal drugs. His serum and blood examination showed TBIL 2.1 mg/dL, SGOT 1250 KU, SGPT 1130 KU, PT 13%, PLT 5.7×10^4/μL, total cholesterol 169 mg/dL, WBC 30,600/mm³, and serum creatinine 3.8 mg/dL. He developed hepatic failure, and abdominal US revealed thrombus in IVC (Fig. 11.2). He was transferred to the intensive care unit. CT revealed high-density material in IVC at the hepatic vein ostia (Fig. 11.3), and acute BCS was diagnosed. Anticoagulants were administered, and plasmapheresis and hemodialysis were initiated. However, he died from multiorgan failure due to a hypercoagulable state. Autopsy showed massive hemorrhagic necrosis in zones 2 and 3, while hepatocytes in zone 1 remained intact (Fig. 11.4).

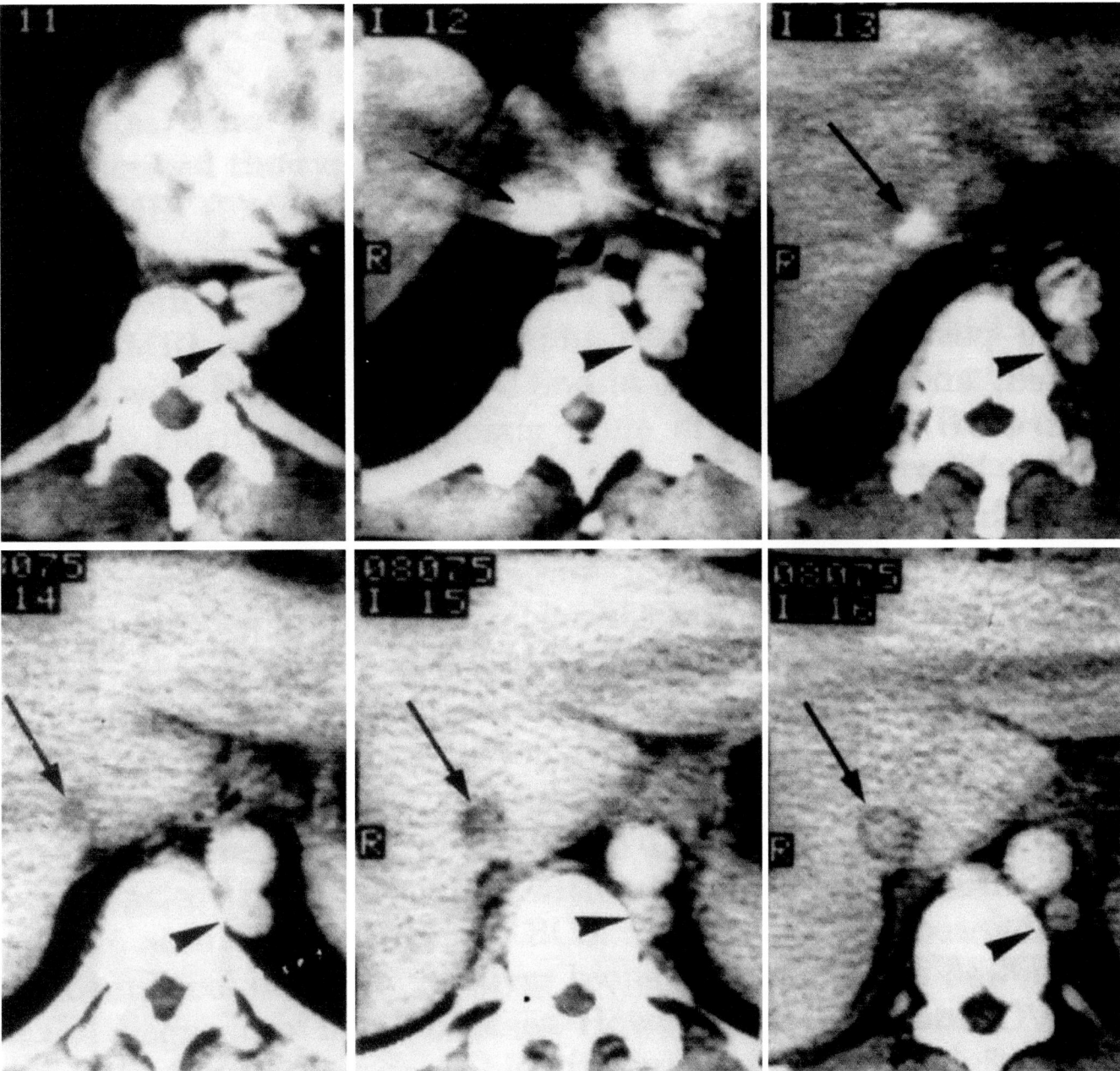

Fig. 11.5 CT in subacute BCS with MOVC. Serial CT shows IVC (arrow) as a low-density or high-density area, and thrombus is seen in IVC. Collateral vein (arrow head) is next to thoracic or abdominal aor-tic artery. (Redrawn from Iwai M, et al. Clinical features, image analysis, and laparoscopic and histological liver findings in Budd-Chiari syndrome, Hepato-Gastroenterol 1998; 45: 2359–68)

Thrombus was seen in the pulmonary artery, along with microthrombi in the adjacent small arteries and hemorrhage in surrounding tissues.

Case 11.2

A 37-year-old male had complained of leg edema for 6 months and developed epigastralgia and brown urine. On admission, his laboratory data were TBIL 2.1 mg/dL, SGOT 32 IU/L, SGPT 37 IU/L, ALP 13.9 KAU, total cholesterol 138 mg/dL, PLT 11.1×10^4/μL, and $ICGR_{15}$ 38.5%. Enhanced serial CT showed disappearance of IVC, presence of a throm-bus in the IVC, dilated collateral veins, and enlarged caudate lobe (Fig. 11.5). Simultaneous inferior and superior venocavography showed a complete obstruction of the IVC and at the entry of the right and middle hepatic veins into the IVC (Fig. 11.6). Laparoscopy revealed enlarged liver with a dusky green color, and blue maculae and white markings were detected on the surface; numerous lymphatic cysts were seen, and small amount of ascites were present in the abdominal cavity; and laparoscopy-guided liver biopsy revealed a dilated portal vein and increasing fibrosis in the portal tract, and congestion was seen around the central vein (Fig. 11.7).

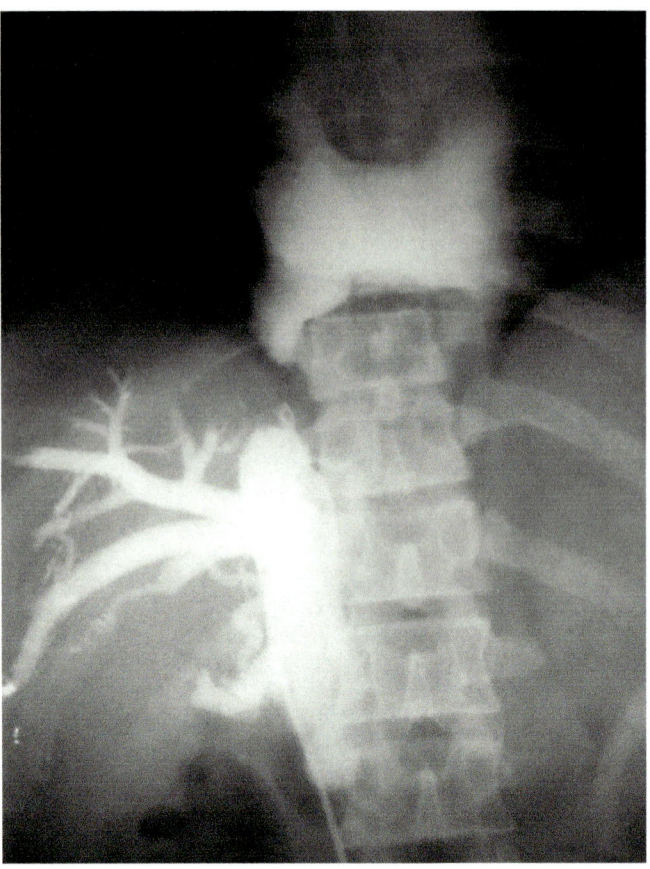

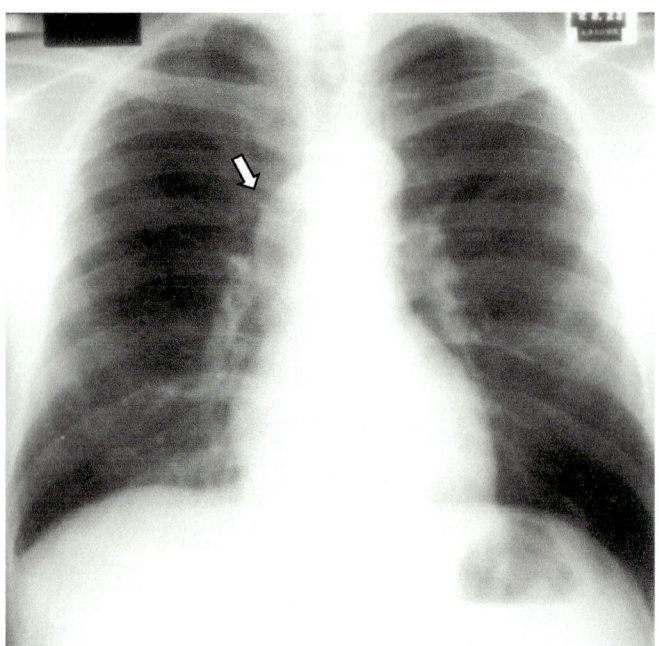

Fig. 11.8 Chest radiograph in an asymptomatic BCS patient. Shadow of enlarged azygos vein (arrow) is seen in paratracheal area. (Redrawn from Iwai M, et al. Clinical features, image analysis, and laparoscopic and histological liver findings in Budd-Chiari syndrome, Hepato-Gastroenterol 1998; 45: 2359–68)

Fig. 11.6 Simultaneous superior and inferior venocavography. IVC is obstructed in right subatrium, and right and middle hepatic veins drain into IVC. (Redrawn from Iwai M, et al. Clinical features, image analysis, and laparoscopic and histological liver findings in Budd-Chiari syndrome, Hepato-Gastroenterol 1998; 45: 2359–68)

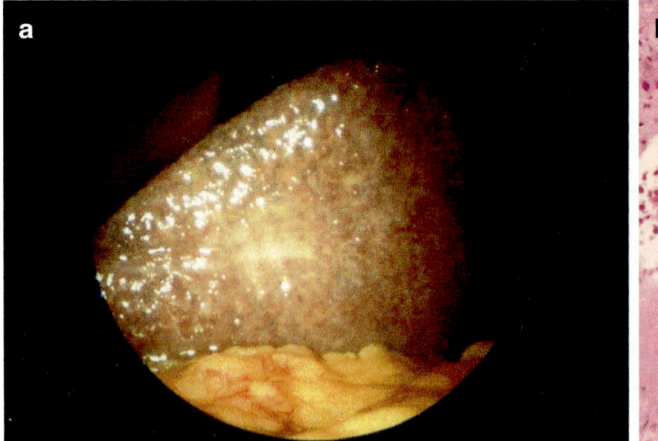

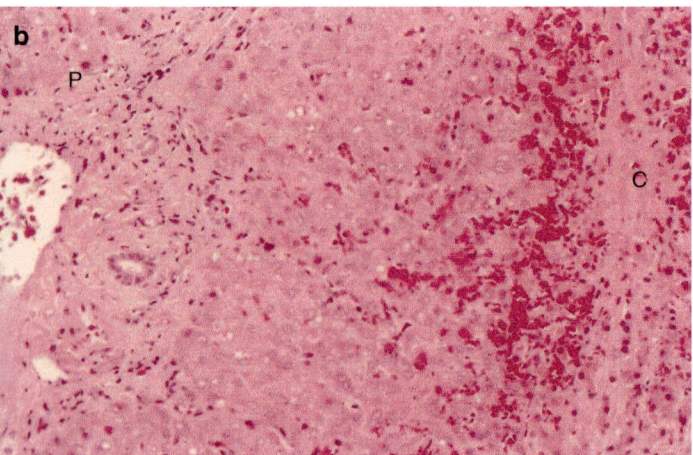

Fig. 11.7 Macroscopic and histological findings of liver in subacute BCS with MOVC. (**a**) Greenish liver is enlarged, white markings are visible with blue maculae, and numerous lymphatic vesicles are visible on liver surface. (**b**) Hematoxylin eosin stain shows congestion around central vein, and portal tract is enlarged. *C* central vein, *P* portal tract

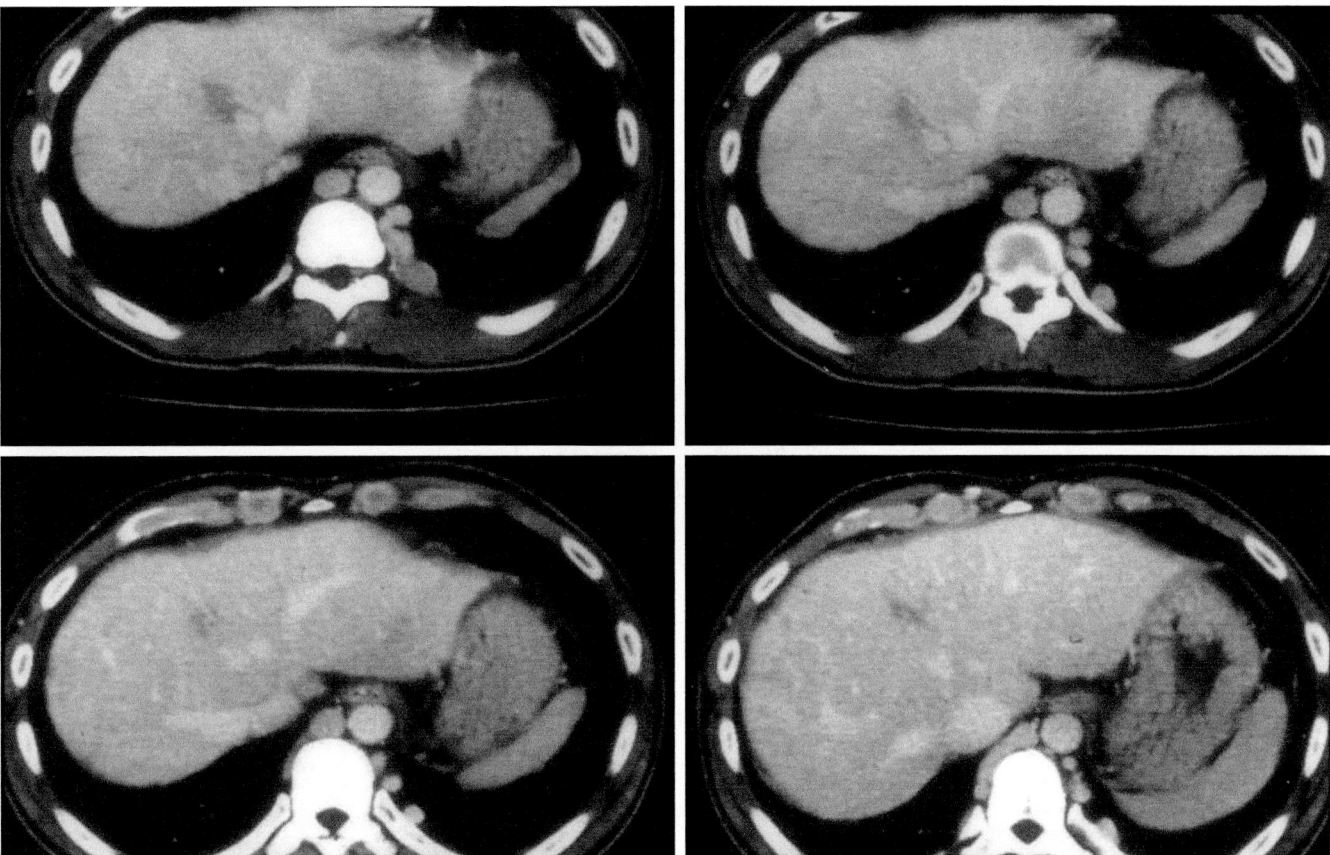

Fig. 11.9 Serial enhanced CT in BCS. Narrowing of IVC is seen at hepatic vein ostia. Middle and left hepatic veins are visible, but there is no clear communication between both veins and IVC. Entry of right hepatic vein into IVC is visible, and IVC is dilated distant to occlusion. Azygos vein is dilated, and other collateral veins are seen. (Redrawn from Iwai M, et al. Clinical features, image analysis, and laparoscopic and histological liver findings in Budd-Chiari syndrome, Hepato-Gastroenterol 1998; 45: 2359–68)

Case 11.3

The chest radiograph of an asymptomatic 42-year-old male showed the shadow of an enlarged azygos vein in the right paratracheal area (Fig. 11.8). His liver chemistries were TBIL 1.0 mg/dL, SGOT 19 IU/L, SGPT 19 IU/L, ALP 9.4 KAU, total cholesterol 123 mg/dL, PLT $11.0 \times 10^4/\mu$L, and ICGR$_{15}$ 23.5%. BCS was suspected. Superior and inferior venocavography showed complete obstruction of IVC and drainage of the right hepatic vein into IVC. Serial enhanced CT showed the presence of left, middle, and right hepatic veins. The right hepatic vein communicated with the IVC, but the connection of the middle and left hepatic veins with the IVC was not clear; the lumen of the IVC in the hepatic vein ostia was narrow, the post-occlusion portion of IVC was dilated, and dilated collateral veins were also seen (Fig. 11.9). Laparoscopy revealed enlarged, purplish liver with white markings and dilated peripheral portal veins, while liver biopsy revealed capsular thickening and subcapsular hemorrhage; the sinusoids were dilated and congested in the subcapsular area (Fig. 11.10). Routine chest radiograph showed the shadow of a dilated azygos vein, and this finding could be a valuable tool in the diagnosis of BCS [16].

Case 11.4

A 66-year-old male with a 3-year history of liver cirrhosis underwent enhanced CT, which showed a thrombus in the hepatic portion of IVC. BCS was the suspected diagnosis. The sagittal view of his abdominal MRI showed obstruction of IVC, entry of right hepatic vein into IVC, and high-intensity thrombus in the hepatic vein ostia; MRI angiography revealed stenosis of IVC and dilated collateral veins communicating with the femoral vein (Fig. 11.11). Simultaneous inferior and superior venocavography showed obstruction at the hepatic vein ostia, nozzle-like tapering of IVC from the right atrium, and entry of right hepatic vein into IVC. Laparoscopy showed liver atrophy with formation of multiple nodules, capsular thickening, and numerous lymphatic cysts; the nodules were low in height, internodular space was wide, and scattered subcapsular hemorrhages were visible (see Fig. 4.9 in Chap. 4). Liver biopsy showed pseudolobular formation with wide septum of fibrosis, capsular thickening, and subcapsular hemorrhage; hemorrhaging was evident in the interspace between parenchymal cells and septal fibrosis in the portal area, and dilated portal veins were surrounded by increased fibrosis (Fig. 11.12).

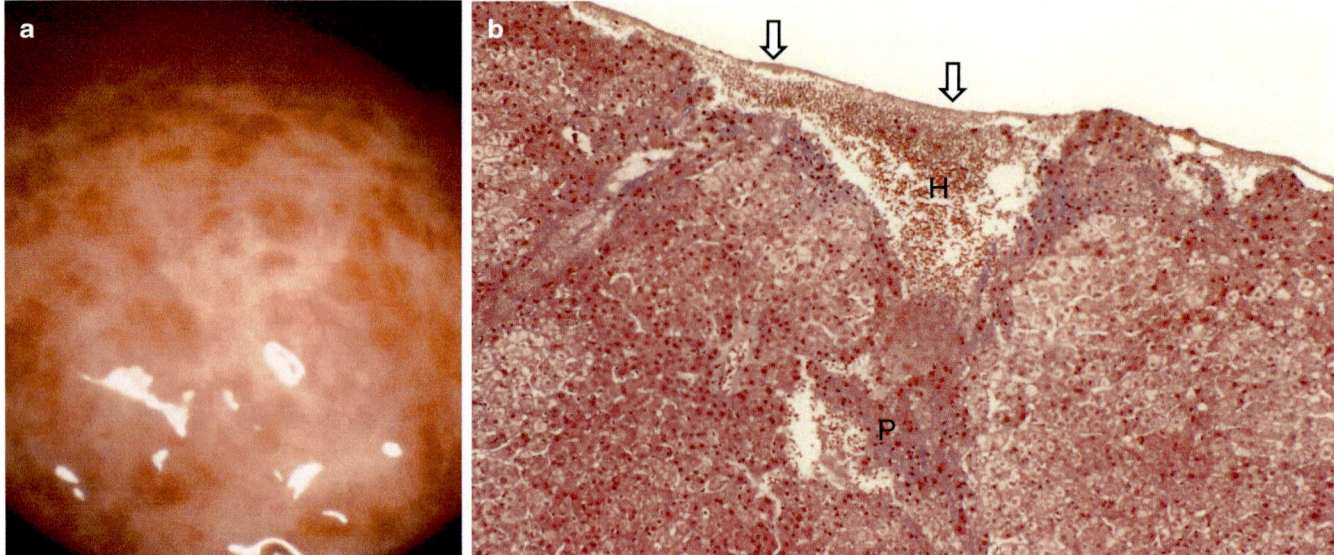

Fig. 11.10 Macroscopic and microscopic appearance of liver in an asymptomatic BCS patient. (**a**) Surface of enlarged liver is purplish red in color with white markings, and dilated peripheral portal veins are visible. (Redrawn from Iwai M, et al. Clinical features, image analysis, and laparoscopic and histological liver findings in Budd-Chiari syndrome, Hepato-Gastroenterol 1998; 45: 2359–68). (**b**) Histological appearance of the liver shows capsule of liver surface (arrow) to be thick, and subcapsular hemorrhage (H) is visible. Mallory-Azan stain shows peliosis (P) communicates with subcapsular hemorrhage

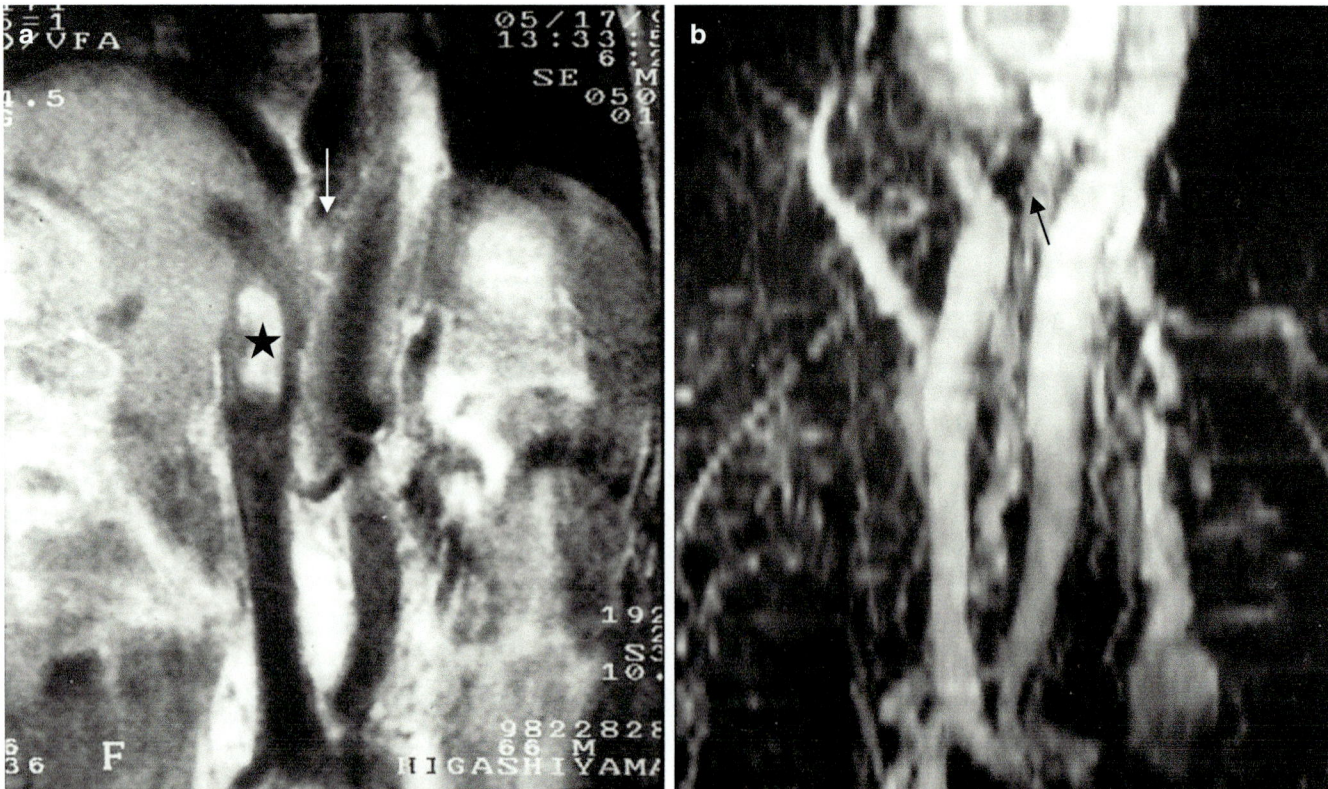

Fig. 11.11 MRI in chronic BCS with MOVC. (**a**) Sagittal MRI shows obstruction of IVC (arrow), entry of right hepatic vein into IVC, and highly intense thrombus (star) in hepatic vein ostia. (**b**) MRI angiography shows obstruction of IVC (arrow) in hepatic vein ostia, entry of right hepatic vein in IVC, and formation of collateral circulation. (Redrawn from Iwai M, et al. Clinical features, image analysis, and laparoscopic and histological liver findings in Budd-Chiari syndrome, Hepato-Gastroenterol 1998; 45: 2359–68)

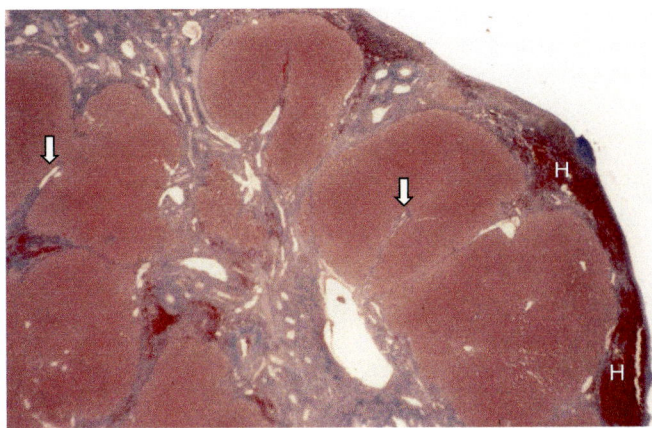

Fig. 11.12 Mallory-Azan stain of liver in chronic BCS. Thick capsule and subcapsular hemorrhage are visible. Hemorrhage is also visible around portal fibrosis. There is pseudolobular formation, and wide septum formation is seen between regenerating nodules. Portal veins are dilated, and lumen of central veins (arrow) is narrow. (Redrawn from Iwai M, et al. Clinical features, image analysis, and laparoscopic and histological liver findings in Budd-Chiari syndrome, Hepato-Gastroenterol 1998; 45: 2359–68)

11.4 Fontan-Associated Liver Disease (FALD)

In 1971, Fontan and Baudet reported an effective palliative operation for tricuspid atresia, and it is currently the most common surgical procedure performed in patients with single-ventricle physiology or when biventricular repair is not feasible. Advances in perioperative management have contributed to an improved outcome of the Fontan operation and an increase of long-term survivors. Venous congestion and decreased cardiac output are the hallmarks of Fontan circulation, and then it is rational that long-term survivors of Fontan surgery commonly progress to congestive hepatopathy [22]. FALD can be defined as abnormalities in liver structure and function that result from the Fontan circulation. FALD arises due to chronic congestion of the liver created by the elevated venous pressure and low cardiac output. Main pathologic features are massive or universal sinusoidal dilatation, centrilobular and /or sinusoidal fibrosis, and cardiac cirrhosis [23].

Elevated hepatic venous pressure due to Fontan circulation may diminish portal flow, and portal vein saturation can be decreased by the hepatic arterial buffering response. These changes may promote the development of focal nodular hyperplasia (FNH), since it arises secondary to arterial hyperperfusion. Recently, hepatocellular carcinoma (HCC) after Fontan operation has been reported [24]. There is a well-documented multistep process of progression to hepatocellular carcinoma. A subgroup of hyperplastic nodules may have malignant potential. The development of HCC gives a great impact for the prognosis of patients with FALD.

Noninvasive imaging modalities are useful for detecting FALD [25]. US can identify in liver parenchymal changes (parenchymal heterogeneity, liver surface irregularity), cirrhotic findings (hepatomegaly, splenomegaly, ascites), and liver tumors. CT and MRI can demonstrate IVC engorgement, hepatic vein dilatation, and hypervascular tumors. Hepatic elastography is a noninvasive tool for assessing hepatic fibrosis and hepatic congestion. Because it is not able to determine the true hepatic fibrosis excludes the effect of hepatic congestion, we should keep in mind that the elastography may overestimate hepatic fibrosis. Increased central venous pressure has been shown to be associated with increased morbidity and mortality in patients undergoing Fontan procedure. All Fontan patients should undergo the surveillance for FALD and HCC.

Case 11.5

This case was a 31-year-old man who was referred to our division for evaluation of liver nodules detected on US. He had undergone the Fontan procedure for a single ventricle at the age of 10 years, which was his second operation for congenital heart disease. He had also received insertion of a permanent pacemaker for sick sinus syndrome. When liver cirrhosis and esophageal varices were diagnosed at the age of 29 years, he was on treatment with diuretics, antiarrhythmic agents, and antithrombotic drugs, with his cardiac status being NYHA class III. On admission, he was cyanotic and showed poor growth with a reduced exercise capacity. He had moderate ascites and a pleural effusion. Laboratory tests revealed a hemoglobin 11.7 g/dL, platelet count 13.2 × 10,000/μL, AST 38 IU/L, ALT 21 IU/L, T-bil 1.8 mg/dL, and albumin 3.3 mg/dL. Serum AFP level was 4.0 ng/mL. US showed characteristic features of cirrhosis and several nodules ranging in size from 10 to 35 mm that were suspected to be regenerative nodules or FNH. CT demonstrated diffuse patchy enhancement of the hepatic parenchyma, as well as hypervascular nodules ranging from 10 to 35 mm in size (Fig. 11.13a). Most of the nodules displayed enhancement in the arterial phase and contrast retention in the portal venous phase, which are characteristics consistent with FNH. However, the 23 mm mosaic pattern nodule with a halo in S2 showing early arterial uptake followed by washout in the portal venous phase was suspected of hepatocellular carcinoma (Fig. 11.13b). Liver biopsy was contraindicated due to ascites and anticoagulant therapy. One year and a half later, follow-up imaging showed enlargement of the suspected hepatocellular carcinoma from 23 to 35 mm in diameter, while the other nodules were unchanged in size. The serum AFP level remained in the normal range. This patient died of combined hepatic and cardiac failure.

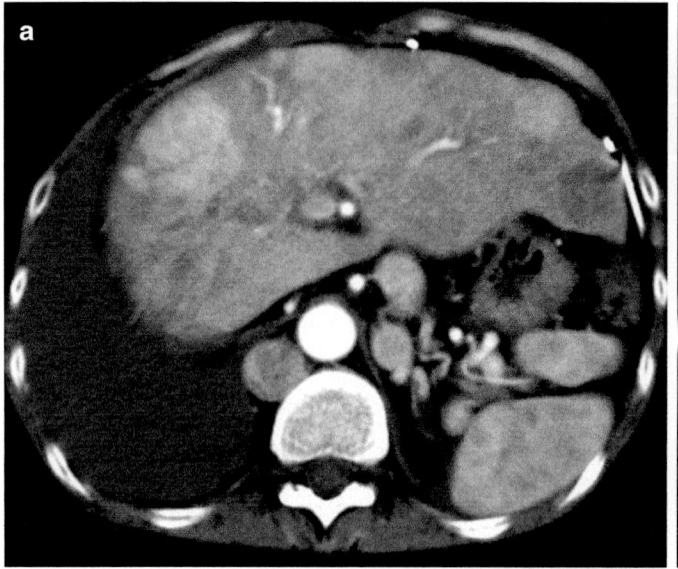 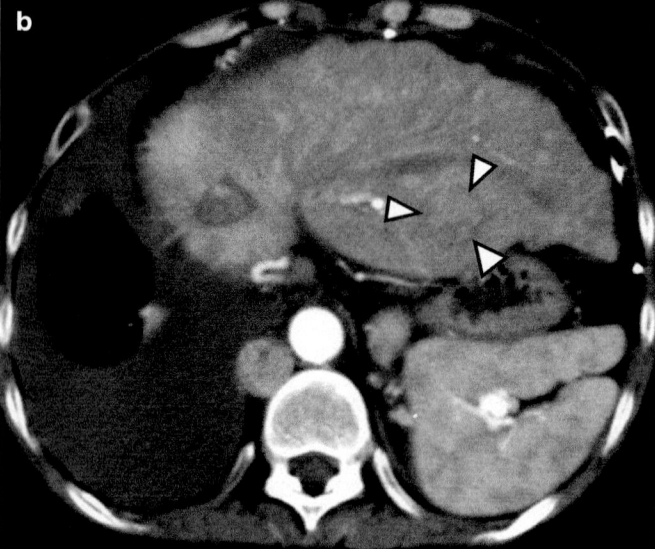

Fig. 11.13 CT in a patient with FALD and HCC. (**a**) CT demonstrated diffuse patchy enhancement of the hepatic parenchyma, as well as hypervascular nodules ranging from 10 to 35 mm in size. (**b**) The 23 mm mosaic pattern nodule with a halo in S2 showing early arterial uptake followed by washout in the portal venous phase was suspected of hepatocellular carcinoma (arrowheads)

11.5 Sinusoidal Obstruction Syndrome (SOS)/Veno-Occlusive Disease (VOD)

Sinusoidal obstructive syndrome (SOS) known as veno-occlusive disease (VOD) is a condition characterized by toxic destruction of hepatic sinusoidal endothelial cells with sloughing and downstream occlusion of terminal hepatic venules. Initially, VOD was well-established as a hepatic complication by either chemical or radiation. In the 1970s, hepatic VOD in patients undergoing bone marrow transplantation was reported. A large number of drugs and toxins have been associated with SOS/VOD. Causal factors include hematopoietic stem cell transplantation, adjuvant or neoadjuvant chemotherapy with hepatectomy for metastatic liver diseases, radiation (total body or hepatic) chemotherapy for acute leukemia, liver transplantation, use of herbal remedies, and VOD with immunodeficiency. The presentation mimics BCS. In its acute form, presentation may include hepatomegaly, ascites, and liver failure. The chronic form leads to cirrhosis and portal hypertension with esophageal varices. Liver biopsy typically shows striking centrilobular congestion around the hepatic venule with centrilobular hepatocellular necrosis in acute phase (Fig. 11.14). The terminal hepatic venules exhibit subintimal edema without obvious fibrin deposition or thrombosis. This is accompanied by dissection of erythrocytes into the space of Disse and downstream accumulation of cellular debris in the terminal vein. In the subacute phase, collagen deposition occurs in and around the terminal venules, resulting in progressive obliteration of the venule. In the chronic phase, dense perivenular fibrosis radiating out into the parenchyma develops [26]. Currently, no effective therapy is available other than to remove the etiologic agent, typically a drug. As a medical treatment, defibrotide has shown the most promising results in clinical trials, which showed 32% of patients who underwent hematopoietic stem cell transplantation (HSCT) achieved complete response [27]. High-dose methylprednisolone has also been used. Liver transplantation should be considered only in patients who are expected to have a good outcome [28]. The prevention is needed for patients at high risk for developing SOS. Ursodeoxycholic acid or low-dose heparin prophylaxis and aggressive fluid management during HSCT are available.

11.6 Hepatic Artery

Forty to 50% of the oxygen requirement and 35% of the blood volume of the liver are supplied by hepatic artery. The common hepatic artery continues as the proper hepatic artery and branches into the right and left hepatic artery. Clinical disorders of the hepatic artery are aneurysm [25], occlusion or infarction [26], and arteriovenous fistula [27, 28]. Some of these diseases should be diagnosed immediately to prevent circulatory insufficiency and liver failure by using image analysis of US, CT with contrast medium, and angiography.

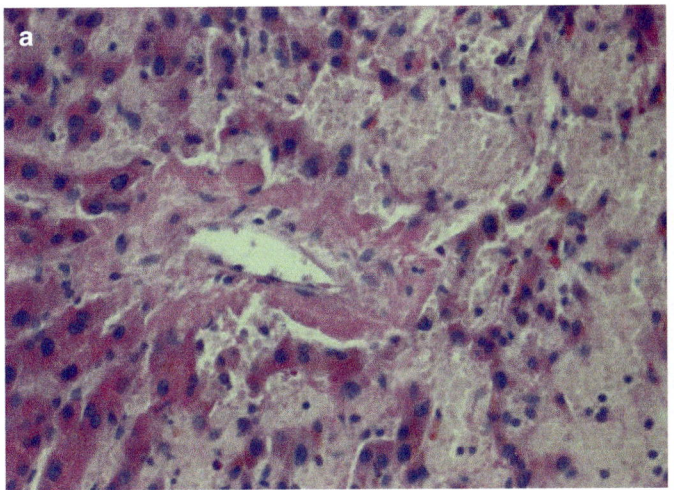
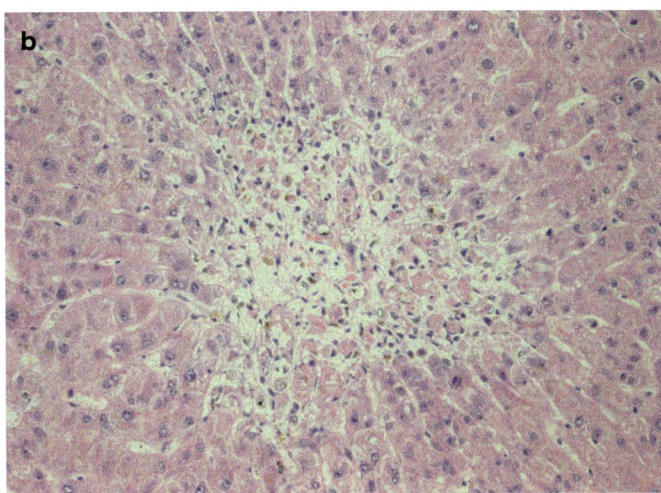

Fig. 11.14 Sinusoidal obstruction syndrome. (**a**) Periodic acid Schiff's stain in SOS shows zone 3 hepatocytes have been replaced by blood cells. A small vein contains macrophages and fibrous tissue. (**b**) Hematoxylin eosin stain shows loss of hepatocytes around the hepatic vein in SOS. (Courtesy of Professor Michael A Kern)

11.7 Arterioportal Fistulas (APFs)

APFs are fistulas between any of the splanchnic arteries and the portal veins and represent an infrequent cause of presinusoidal portal hypertension. They can be acquired or congenital. Acquired APFs can be by liver trauma, interventional procedures (liver biopsy, percutaneous transhepatic catheterization of bile duct, radiofrequency ablation, etc.), artery aneurysm, and hepatic tumors (hepatocellular carcinoma). Many patients with APF are asymptomatic. Symptoms depend on the location of APF and the amount of shunted blood. They are usually secondary to portal hypertension. Common manifestations include gastrointestinal bleeding, ascites, congestive heart failure, and diarrhea. The pathologic features of APFs are the dilation of the sinusoids and portal branches in the early stage and venous intimal hyperplasia and arterialization of the portal branches, called hepatoportal sclerosis after persistent portal hypertension. Doppler US is the first-choice tool for the diagnosis or a screening of APFs. Doppler US demonstrates pulsatile flow in the portal system with or without hepatofugal flow. On triple-phase enhanced CT, the early filling of the portal vein and the presence of wedge-shaped, transient peripheral enhanced area are observed in the arterial phase. Hepatic arteriography reveals early visualization of the portal system after celiac or hepatic artery injection. Superior mesenteric arteriovenous fistulas (SMAVF) are usually caused by iatrogenic or traumatic damage, though a few congenital cases have also been reported [29, 30]. Fistula formation originates from a transfixion suture through the artery and vein simultaneously or via mass ligation in the mesentery [31, 32]. Some

patients with SMAVF have suffered cardiac failure or liver failure [33, 34]. Treatment indication is to prevent the development of portal hypertension. Extrahepatic APFs should be treated because of no spontaneous closure of APFs. Arterial embolization is effective in treating single or a few APFs. Next options are hepatic artery ligation or fistula resection. Liver transplantation may be the last possible therapy in patients with extensive involvement, especially congenital multiple APFs.

We present a case of SMAVF occurring after small bowel resection to treat an ileus.

Case 11.6

A 38-year-old woman was admitted for watery and bloody diarrhea and abdominal distension for several weeks. She had undergone a wide resection of the small bowel to relieve intestinal obstruction 6 years earlier. Physical examination revealed massive ascites, and a bruit was audible in the periumbilical area. On admission, her heart rate was 98/min, and blood pressure was 110/70 mmHg. Her hemoglobin level was 10.6 g/dL and hematocrit 33.2%. Liver chemistries revealed TBIL 0.6 mg/dL, GOT 34 IU/L, GPT 34 IU/L, TP 6.7 g/dL, and gamma globulin 11.5%. US examination revealed massive ascites, dilated intrahepatic and extrahepatic portal veins, and "rabbit tail" appearance of the superior mesenteric vein communicating with some vessels (Fig. 11.15). Conventional enhanced CT showed a dilated portal vein in parallel with the superior mesenteric artery, and the bowel wall was enhanced by contrast medium (Fig. 11.16); a connection between the portal vein and superior mesenteric artery was suspected. Superior mesenteric arteriography revealed

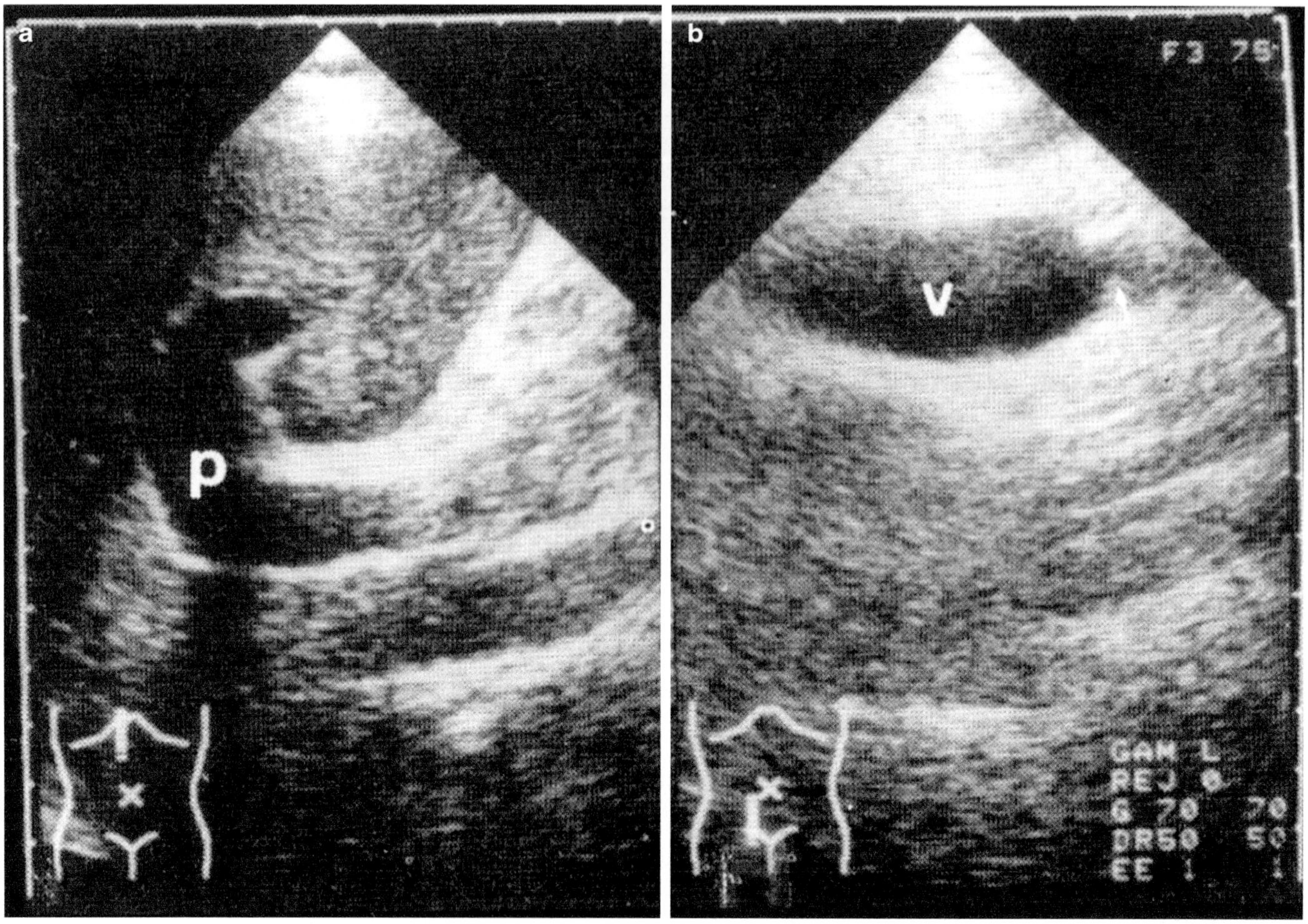

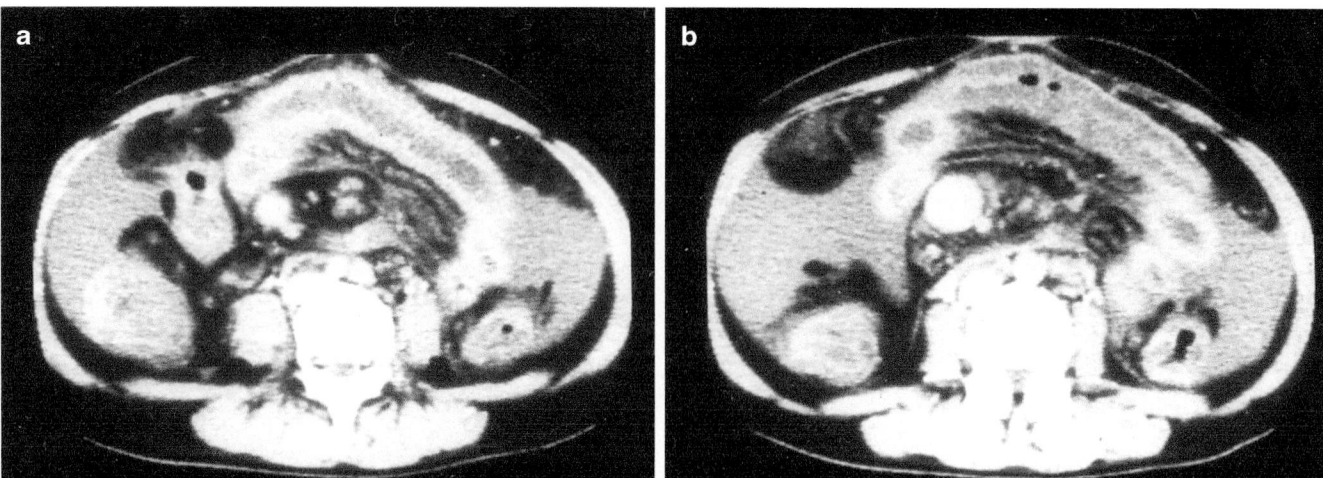

Fig. 11.15 US in SMAV fistula. (**a**) The extrahepatic and intrahepatic portal vein (P) is dilated. (**b**) The superior mesenteric vein (V) is dilated and is connected to a stenotic vessel. (Reuse of Iwai M, et al. Iatrogenic superior mesenteric arteriovenous fistula: Ultrasonographic, CT and angiographic features and histological findings of the liver biopsy. J Gastroenterol Hepatol 1990; 5: 586–9, with permission of Wiley)

Fig. 11.16 Enhanced CT in SMAV fistula. The dilated superior mesenteric vein is contiguous to the superior mesenteric artery (**a**), and the vein makes a fistula with the artery (**b**). The small intestine is enhanced by contrast medium. (Reuse of Iwai M, et al. Iatrogenic superior mesenteric arteriovenous fistula: Ultrasonographic, CT and angiographic features and histological findings of the liver biopsy. J Gastroenterol Hepatol 1990; 5: 586–9, with permission of Wiley)

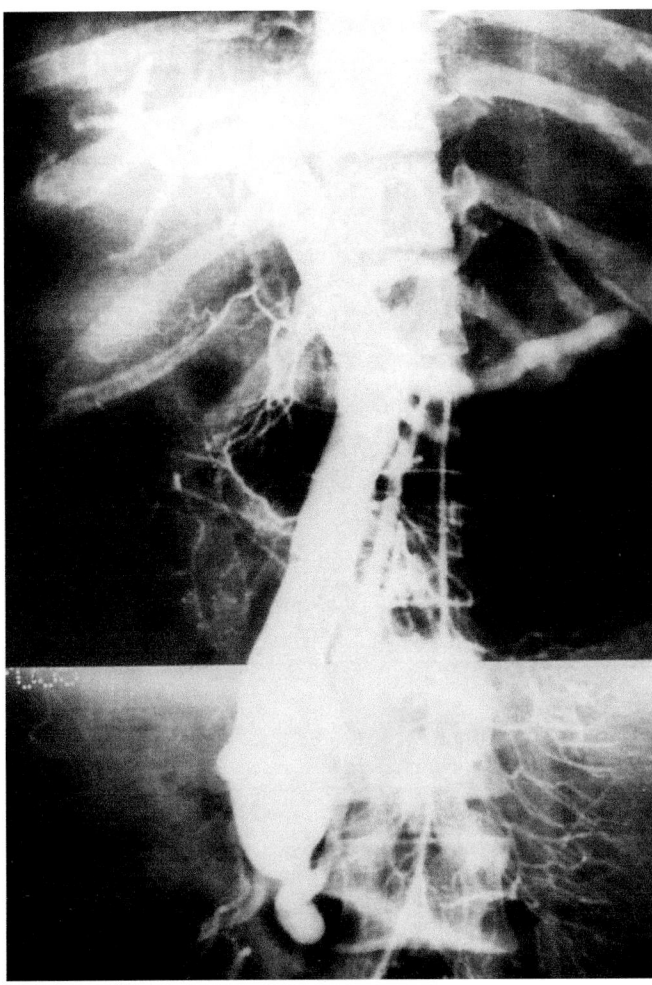

Fig. 11.17 SMAV fistula. Superior mesenteric arteriography shows a fistula of the dilated mesenteric vein. (Reuse of Iwai M, et al. Iatrogenic superior mesenteric arteriovenous fistula: Ultrasonographic, CT and angiographic features and histological findings of the liver biopsy. J Gastroenterol Hepatol 1990; 5: 586–9, with permission of Wiley)

a fistula of the dilated mesenteric vein, with its artery at the level of the fourth lumbar vertebra (Fig. 11.17). Hematochezia was frequent, and hematemesis occurred due to rupture of esophageal varices. Cardiac output was measured via isotope dilution, and the cardiac index was 7.78 L/mm/m². Cardiac failure occurred, and blood urea nitrogen and creatinine were elevated to 85 and 4.7 mg/ dL, respectively. The fistula between the superior mesenteric artery and vein was ligated as an emergency procedure. The pressure in the superior mesenteric vein before and after ligation was 56 and 47 mmHg, respectively. No regenerating nodules were seen on the liver surface, and a wedge biopsy of the liver showed arteriolized portal veins surrounded by increasing fibrosis (Fig. 11.18). Neither septum nor pseudolobular formation was seen.

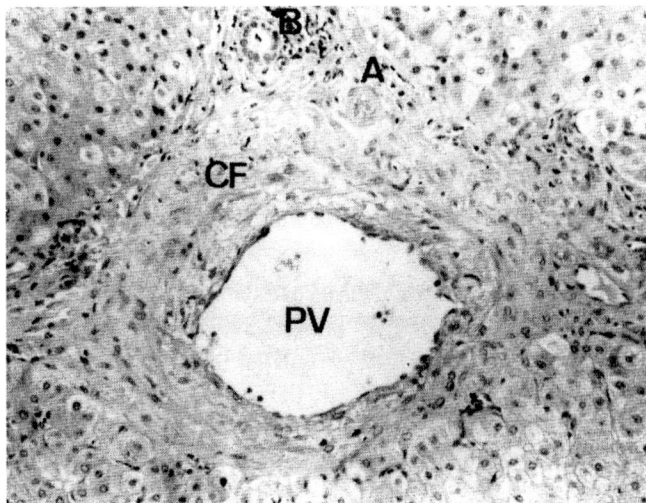

Fig. 11.18 SMV fistula. Liver histology shows deposition of collagen fibers (CF) surrounding the portal vein (PV). *A* artery, *B* bile duct. (Reuse of Iwai M, et al. Iatrogenic superior mesenteric arteriovenous fistula: Ultrasonographic, CT and angiographic features and histological findings of the liver biopsy. J Gastroenterol Hepatol 1990; 5: 586–9, with permission of Wiley)

11.8 Portal Vein

Portal vein is formed by gastric or pyloric and superior or inferior mesenteric and splenic veins. The portal vein divides into left and right branch, and the branch reaches interlobular veins and interlobular venules and continues into afferent venules and into sinusoids.

There are congenital or acquired diseases of portal veins, and their diseases cause portal hypertension. Portal hypertension arises due to obstruction of hepatic blood flow, and patients with portal hypertension are classified as having either presinusoidal or postsinusoidal obstruction. Congenital anomalies of the portal vein, portosystemic shunts, or arterioportal fistula cause portal hypertension, and acquired diseases of large or small portal veins (idiopathic portal hypertension) lead to liver disturbance with or without cirrhotic change.

11.9 Idiopathic Non-cirrhotic Portal Hypertension (INCPH)

Idiopathic non-cirrhotic portal hypertension has been recently proposed to replace terms, for example, hepatoportal sclerosis, idiopathic portal hypertension, and so on [35]. INCPH is defined as a presinusoidal non-cirrhotic portal hypertension of unknown etiology with a patent extrahepatic portal vein and hepatic veins. Anemia, thrombocytopenia, and esophageal or gastric varices are clinically manifested, and splenomegaly is always detected. Liver biopsy should be performed for the diagnosis of INCPH. Pathological features are (1) obliterative portal venopathy, (2) portal fibrosis without inflammation, (3) paraportal shunting vessels, (4) enlarged portal branches, and (5) increased number of portal vascular channels [36, 37].

The diagnosis of INCPH is based on the portal hypertension with patent portal and hepatic veins in the absence of known causes of liver damage. In patients with INCPH, hepatic synthetic capacity is usually preserved. Imaging modalities have poor sensitivity and specificity. These modalities demonstrated portal hypertension findings such as splenomegaly, collateral shunts, and enlarged caudate lobe. US shows thickened PV with echogenic walls, normal liver size, and normal echotexture.

Variceal bleeding is a life-threatening complication [38], and combined pharmacological and endoscopic therapy is effective to control acute bleeding [39]. Endoscopic variceal ligation [40] and transjugular intrahepatic portosystemic shunt [41] are applied for prophylaxis of bleeding, and balloon-occluded retrograde transvenous obliteration is indicated to prevent gastric variceal bleeding [42]. The natural course of INCPH is good except for uncontrolled gastrointestinal bleeding. Long-term survival after eradication of esophagogastric varices is nearly 100% [43]. Hepatic reserve usually remains well preserved, but 20% of patients develop parenchymal atrophy with subsequent decompensation.

Case 11.7

A 58-year-old female complained of melena and was found to have anemia. Her liver test showed AST 23 IU/L, ALT 18 IU/L, ALP 495 IU/L, GGT 73 IU/L, and PLT 11.7×10^4/μL. Upper abdominal CT with contrast medium showed esophageal varices in the venous phase, and another slice of

CT revealed splenomegaly and development of a collateral portal vein around the stomach (Fig. 11.19). Upper gastrointestinal fiberscope showed esophageal varices with RC sign. Three-dimensional CT showed presence of esophageal varices, collateral portal branch around the stomach, and splenomegaly (Fig. 11.20). Liver biopsy showed non-cirrhotic liver, bile ducts and artery in a portal tract, and herniated portal vein (Fig. 11.21). Thrombocytopenia and anemia are found in idiopathic portal hypertension, and hematemesis or melena develops. Histological findings show non-cirrhotic

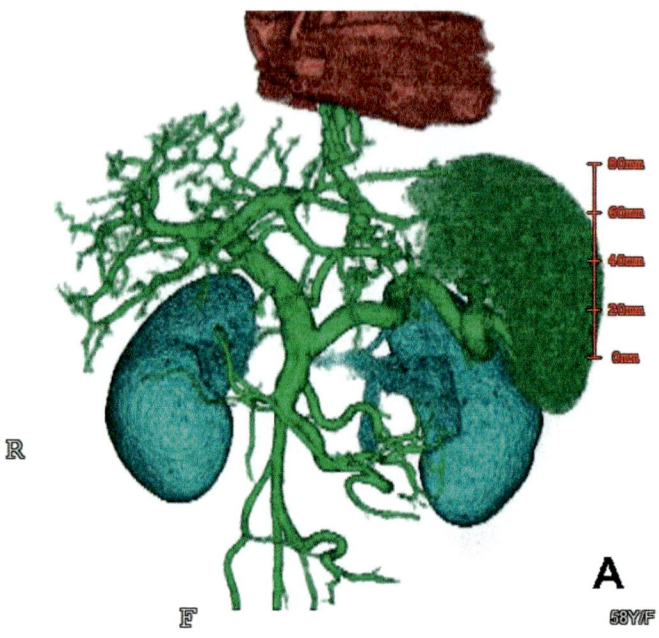

Fig. 11.20 Three-dimensional analysis by CT. CT shows esophageal varices, dilatation of perigastric veins, and splenomegaly

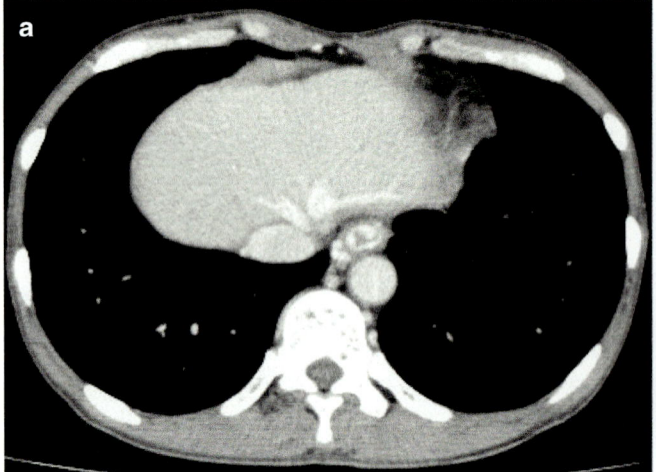
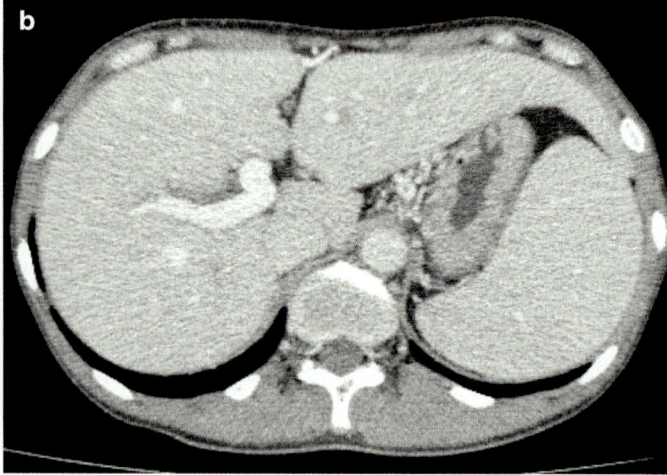

Fig. 11.19 Idiopathic portal hypertension. (**a**) CT with contrast medium shows presence of *esophageal varices and paraesophageal veins* in the venous phase. (**b**) CT with contrast medium shows splenomegaly and dilatation of perigastric veins

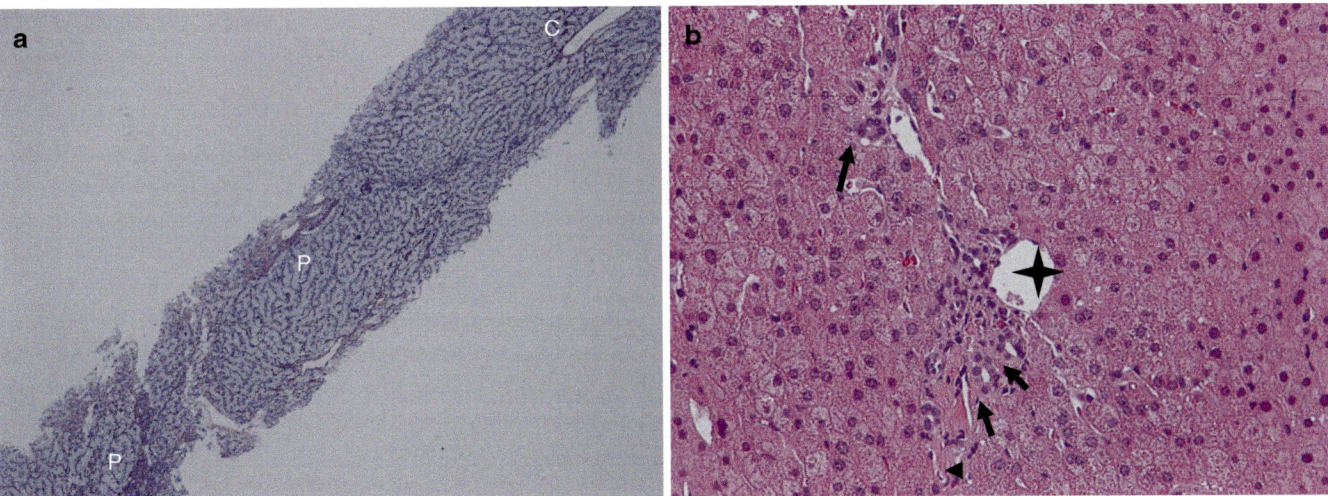

Fig. 11.21 Idiopathic portal hypertension. (**a**) Silver stain shows non-cirrhotic liver with mild fibrosis in the portal tract. *P* portal tract, *C* central vein. (**b**) Bile duct (arrow) and arterial structure (arrow head) are observed, and portal vein (star) is herniated from the portal tract

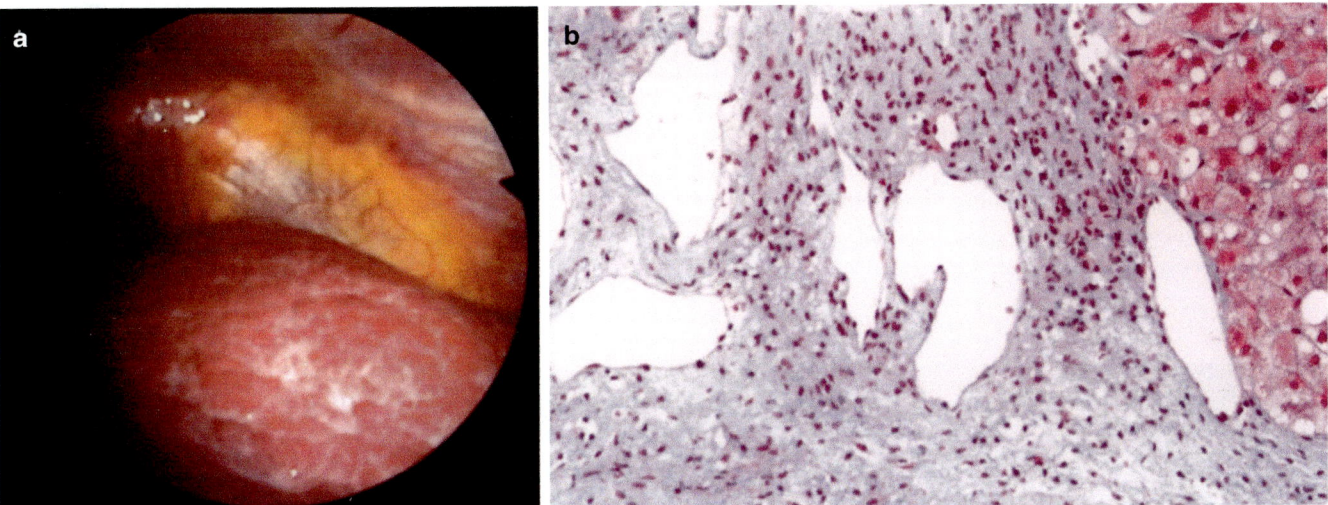

Fig. 11.22 Laparoscopic and histological findings of liver in idiopathic portal hypertension. (**a**) The liver surface is wavy and excavated with a thick white capsule and white markings. (**b**) The peripheral portal vein is branched and dilated in the portal tract and herniated. Fibrosis has developed

liver, narrow lumen or destruction of the portal vein, and herniation of the portal vein.

Case 11.8

A 53-year-old female was diagnosed with esophageal varices. Her liver function tests showed ALT 14 IU/L, AST 21 IU/L, LDH 303 IU/L, gamma globulin 23.3%, and $ICGR_{15}$ 9.8%. Neither HBsAg nor HCV Ab were present. Her thrombocyte level was $6.1 \times 10^4/\mu L$. US revealed splenomegaly with collateral vein formation, and splenectomy was performed to reduce portal hypertension. MRI revealed dilatation of the portal trunk and tapering of the intrahepatic portal veins.

Regenerating hyperplastic nodules were laparoscopically seen on the liver surface, but no cirrhotic nodules were detected, and liver biopsy showed portal fibrosis and dilated peripheral portal veins with herniated abnormal vessels (Fig. 11.22).

11.10 Portal Vein Thrombosis (PVT)

Portal vein thrombosis refers to thrombosis that develops in the portal trunk including its right and left branches and extends to the splenic or superior mesenteric veins [44]. The pathogenesis of PVT is reduced portal flow, a hypercoagulable state and vascular endothelial injury. Etiology of PVT is cirrhosis, primary hepatobiliary malignancy, secondary hepatobiliary malignancy, abdominal infection including pancreatitis and cholangitis, and a myeloproliferative disorder. Cirrhosis is associated with increased intrahepatic vascular resistance and reduced portal flow, leading to venous stasis. Levels of both pro- and anticoagulant factors are reduced in cirrhosis. Its balance may often tilt toward hypercoagulability in cirrhotic patients. Bacterial translocation and endotoxemia lead to portal endothelial injury and the activation of coagulation cascade. Cirrhotic patients are higher risky due to these three pathogeneses.

On the diagnosis of PVT [45], US is the first-choice diagnostic modality. It shows hypo (recent thrombus)-, iso-, or hyperechoic (elderly) material within portal vein either filling the lumen partially or completely. Color Doppler US and contrast-enhanced US allow the diagnosis of an occlusion of the veins by an elimination of the flow signal. They can reveal collateral flows such as in a portal cavernoma, which is multiple tortuous small vessels with hepatopetal flow or varices. Enhanced CT shows a bland thrombus as a low density, non-enhancing defect within portal veins. CT and MRI can provide additional information such as extension of thrombus, collaterals, differentiation from tumor thrombus, and status of adjacent organs. The variations of T1- and T2-weighted signals allow defining the age of thrombus formations. The increase of both signal intensity is due to fresh thrombus. The aim of the treatment is to reverse or prevent advancement of PVT. Anticoagulation therapy should be initiated with heparin or low molecular weight heparin and maintained 2–3 weeks [46]. Later, oral vitamin K antagonists should be given to maintain an INR of 2–3. Thrombolytic therapy with recombinant tissue plasminogen activator, urokinase, for very fresh PVT can be done via indirect intra-arterial infusion into the superior mesenteric artery or directly into portal vein and might improve regional clot lysis. However, there is a high rate of bleeding.

Extrahepatic portal venous obstruction (EHPVO) refers to chronic portal obstruction in the absence of associated liver disease [47]. EHPVO should be considered as a separate entity. Etiology of EHPVO in children is infection, congenital anomaly, or a primary thrombotic disorder. Infections include omphalitis, neonatal umbilical sepsis, repeated abdominal infection, or umbilical vein catheterization. However, 50% of patients still remain idiopathic. EHPVO in adult is due to prothrombotic disorders, intra-abdominal infection, pregnancy, or oral contraceptives.

Case 11.9

A 21-year-old female using low-dose pill for premenstrual syndrome complained acute severe stomachache. Her liver function test showed ALT 16 IU/L, AST 17 IU/L, ALP 161 IU/L, GGT 15 IU/L, and PLT $18.0 \times 10^4/\mu L$. Abdominal enhanced CT showed persistent well-defined filling defect within superior mesenteric vein to extrahepatic portal vein (Fig. 11.23a). She was diagnosed

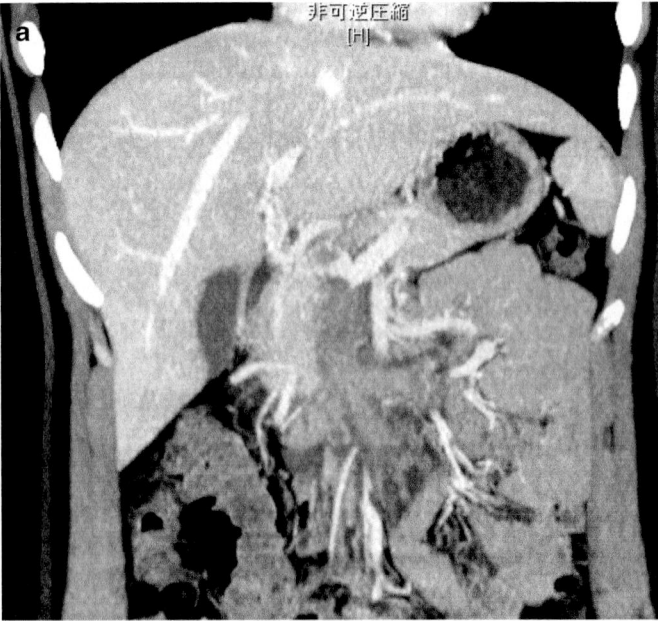
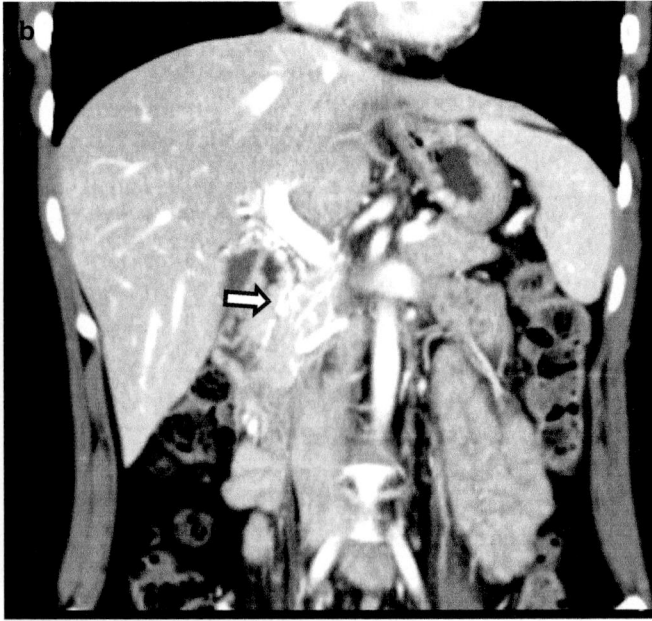

Fig. 11.23 Portal vein thrombosis. (**a**) Portal vein thrombosis on coronal section. Contrast-enhanced CT showed filling defect from superior mesenteric vein to intrahepatic portal vein in the portal phase. (**b**) Portal cavernoma (arrow) around the pancreas on coronal section. Contrast-enhanced CT showed collaterals with hepatopetal flow around pancreas in the portal phase

portal vein thrombosis and underwent anticoagulant therapy. Enhanced CT after anticoagulant therapy revealed hepatopetal collaterals (portal cavernoma) around pancreas (Fig. 11.23b). Portal vein thrombi disappeared after anticoagulant therapy, but superior mesenteric vein remained narrowed.

11.11 Pylephlebitis

Pylephlebitis is characterized by suppurative thrombosis of the portal vein and is a deadly complication of intra-abdominal infections such as appendicitis, diverticulitis, pancreatitis, peritonitis, or cholangitis [48]. An uncontrolled infection in the regions neighboring or drained by the portal system induces thrombophlebitis of small mesenteric veins and can spread to the portal system and to the liver. It is not easy in clinical settings to get the culture-positive fluid from the portal system for its diagnosis. As an alternative method, it is defined as the presence of portal mesenteric venous thrombosis with or without bacteremia within 30 days of intra-abdominal infection. It is advocated to use broad-spectrum antibiotics for pylephlebitis, even without bacteremia.

11.12 Portal Vein Aneurysm (PVA)

PVA is an unusual vascular dilatation of the portal vein with an incidence of 0.06% and defined as a diameter exceeding 15 mm in normal liver and 19 mm in cirrhosis [49]. Etiology of PVA is still unclear but considered to be congenital or acquired. The congenital cause is the incomplete regression of the right primitive distal vitelline vein. Moreover, the presence of vein wall defects can facilitate the development of the aneurysm. The acquired cause is mainly portal hypertension in cirrhosis. The high splanchnic flow and hyperdynamic circulation cause the portal dilatation with weakening venous wall. Other causes are pancreatitis, trauma, and invasion of portal wall by malignancies.

One third of patients are asymptomatic. Main symptom is abdominal pain. Symptoms by the compression of adjacent organs, gastrointestinal hemorrhage, and spontaneous rupture are rare. Most of the cases are diagnosed with US or CT. US, especially color Doppler US, can show hemodynamics of the portal vein and PVA. CT is useful to evaluate the positional relationship with adjacent organs. Surgical indications are patients with complicated PVA such as rupture, high risk of the rupture, and thrombosis.

11.13 Hereditary Hemorrhagic Telangiectasia (HHT)

Hereditary hemorrhagic telangiectasia (HHT) was initially reported as Osler-Weber-Rendu disease named Rendu in 1896, Osler in 1901, and Weber in 1907. HHT is a genetic vascular disorder characterized by the primarily dominant autosomal hereditary transmission of dermal, mucosal, and visceral telangiectasia and arteriovenous malformations (AVMs). The genetic mutations lead to the impairment of blood vessel development, resulting in telangiectasia and AVMs. Liver involvement is more common with an incidence of about 75% [50–52]. Hepatic histological features are a honeycombed meshwork of dilated sinusoids or tortuous veins, adjacent arteries, and increased portal vascular channels. Portal fibrosis may be seen. Triple-phase enhanced CT demonstrates arteriovenous, arterioportal, or portovenous shunts in the liver. Arteriovenous shunt is the most common and may induce congestive heart failure, hepatomegaly, and pulmonary hypertension. Arterioportal shunt may induce portal hypertension including splenomegaly or esophagogastric varices.

The diagnosis of HHT is widely used Curaçao criteria [53] which is based on the most characteristic features of disease: (a) recurrent spontaneous epistaxis, (b) a family medical history, (c) mucocutaneous telangiectasia, and (d) the presence of visceral lesions. A definitive diagnosis of HHT is made if a patient exhibits at least three of the four criteria. If the diagnosis of HHT is proven or assumed, all patients should be screened for cerebral vascular malformations, pulmonary AVMs, and hepatic vascular malformations and annual hemoglobin examined.

The therapeutic options for hepatic involvement were limited. Complications of portal hypertension such as bleeding of varices or ascites should be treated with medical and endoscopic treatments. High-output cardiac failure can be treated with medical treatment. Liver transplantation may be the only curative option for hepatic vascular malformations and apply to uncontrolled high-output cardiac failure, cholangitis, and portal hypertension.

Case 11.10

A 60-year-old man was admitted because of iron deficient anemia. Telangiectasia in the tongue was observed. Upper gastrointestinal endoscopy showed many gastrointestinal angioectasia and esophageal varices. His blood test was hemoglobin 7.1 g/dL, platelet count 197,000/μL, albumin 4.0 g/dL, total bilirubin 0.5 mg/dL, AST 15 U/L, ALT 15 U/L, γ-GTP 73 mg/dL, Fe 28 μg/dL, TIBC 373 μg/dL,

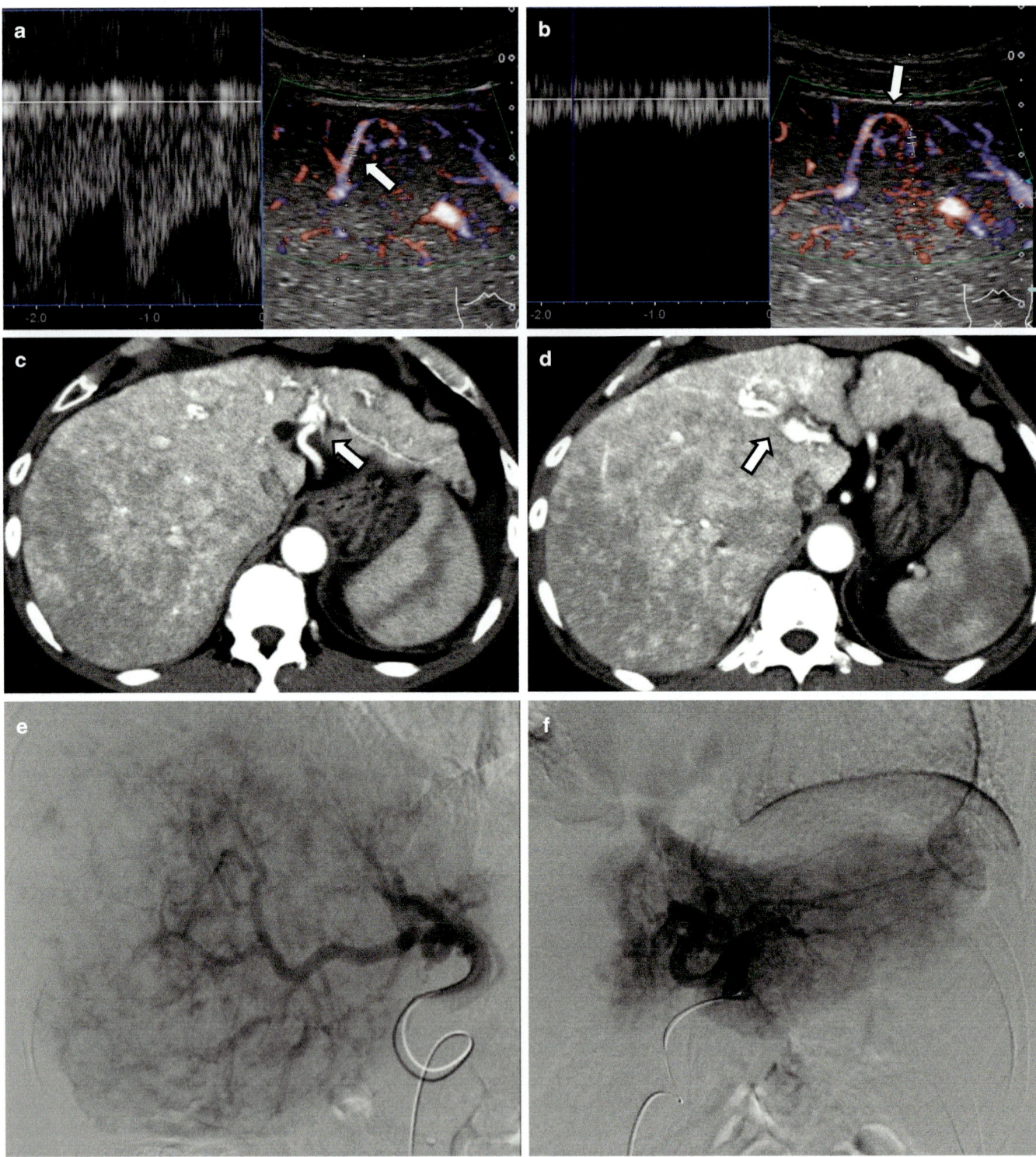

Fig. 11.24 Hereditary hemorrhagic telangiectasia. (**a**) An arteriove- nous shunt (arrow) is presented in the liver with color Doppler ultraso- nography. (**b**) A portovenous shunt (arrow) is presented in the liver with color Doppler ultrasonography. (**c**) An arterioportal shunt (arrow) is shown between a left gastric artery and portal vein with contrast- enhanced computed tomography. (**d**) A portovenous shunt (arrow) is presented between a portal vein and a middle hepatic vein with contrast- enhanced computed tomography. (**e**, **f**) Multiple arterioportal shunts are presented with angiography

ferritin 10.3 ng/mL, HBs antigen-negative, and HCV antibody-negative, antinuclear antibody-negative, and anti-mitochondrial antibody-negative. From these data, he was diagnosed iron deficient anemia. Color Doppler US showed an arterioportal shunt and a portovenous shunt in the liver (Fig. 11.24a, b). MDCT also showed an arterioportal shunt and a portovenous shunt between a left portal vein and a middle hepatic vein (Fig. 11.24c, d). Angiography revealed the multiple arterioportal shunts in both lobes (Fig. 11.24e, f).

11.14 Sinusoids

Sinusoids are lined by endothelial cells containing fenestrations, and Kupffer cells reside in the lumen, and hepatic stellate cells, natural killer cells, and mast cells are found within the space of Disse. Pericellular fibrosis, sinusoidal dilatation, peliosis hepatis, and microvascular injury may be related to drugs, toxins, and ischemia.

11.15 Peliosis Hepatis

Peliosis hepatis is defined as blood-filled cystic spaces, either nonlined or lined with sinusoidal endothelial cells in the liver [54, 55]. At gross inspection, it looks like "Swiss cheese appearance." Microscopically, it is classified into two types; the first type is designated "parenchymal peliosis" and consists of irregular cavities that are neither lined by sinusoidal cells nor by fibrous tissue. The second type is "phlebectatic peliosis" and characterized by regular spherical cavities

lined by endothelium and /or fibrosis [56]. Macroscopic peliosis hepatis is induced by anabolic, estrogenic, or adrenocortical steroids. It can also be caused by malnutrition, leukemia, tuberculosis, leprosy, vasculitis, and AIDS. Microscopic lesions are caused by the intake of drugs for organ transplantation and various malignancies.

Imaging modalities do not allow a clear diagnosis of peliosis hepatis. It should be differentially diagnosed from hemangioma, hepatocellular adenoma, hepatocellular carcinoma, focal nodular hyperplasia, abscess, and metastatic adenocarcinoma. US shows heterogenous with both hypo- and hyperechoic areas. On enhanced CT, they appear hypervascular in the arterial phase and then become isodense. On unenhanced T2-weighted MR images, they demonstrate high intensity with high-intensity multiple spots, which are attribute to hemorrhagic necrosis.

We present a case of macroscopic peliosis hepatis of unknown etiology.

Case 11.11

A 29-year-old female complained of mild fever accompanied by right-sided hypochondralgia and a backache. Contrast-enhanced abdominal CT showed a low-density area 6 cm by 4 cm in diameter in the early phase, and the area was still low in density in the late phase (Fig. 11.25). No abnormal values on liver function tests were seen, and no coagulopathy was detected. Echo-guided tumor biopsy showed dilatation of sinusoids with preservation of the portal tracts; the sinusoids were congested with red blood cells and destroyed (Fig. 11.26). Peliosis hepatis is usually of no significance, but macroscopic peliosis may rupture spontaneously [57].

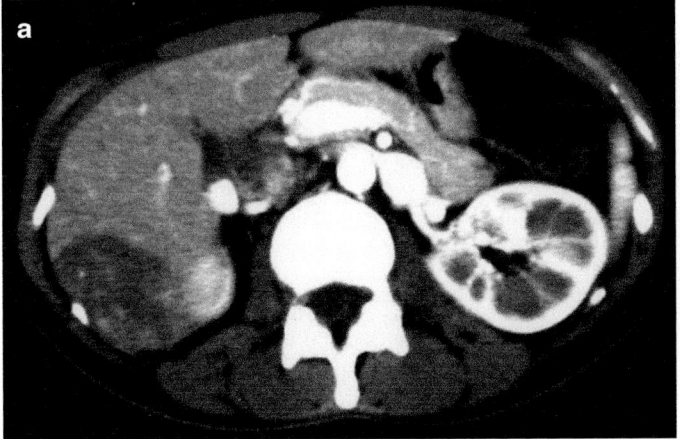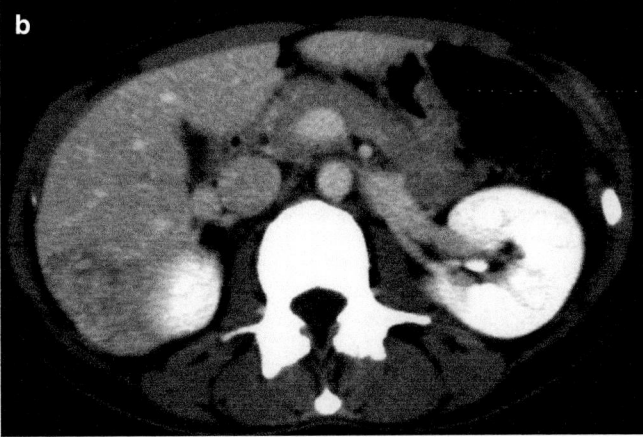

Fig. 11.25 Peliosis hepatis. (**a**) CT with contrast medium shows a low-density area in S6 in the arterial phase. (**b**) CT in the late phase shows a low-density area, and its density is heterogeneous

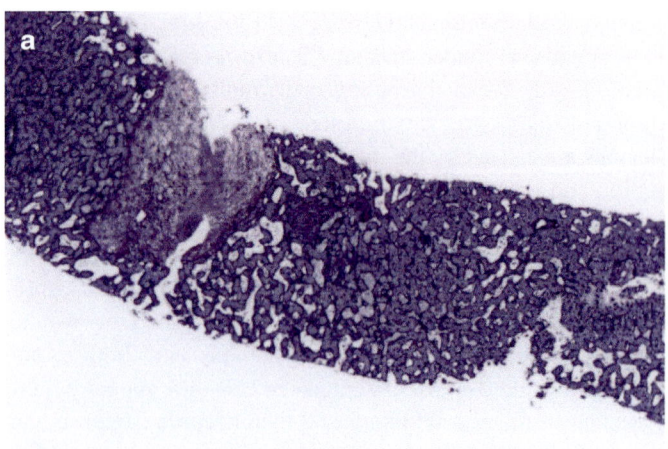 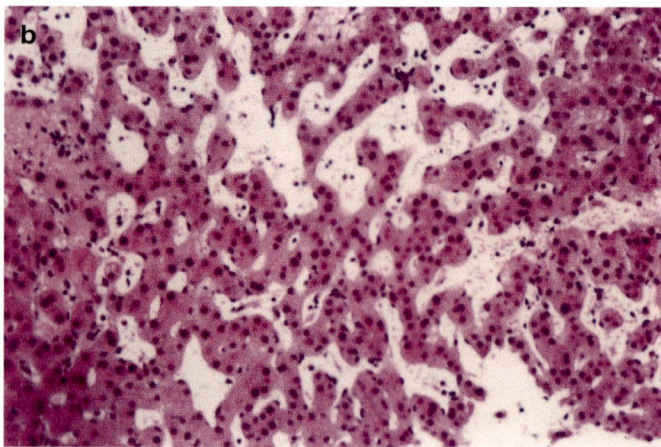

Fig. 11.26 Peliosis hepatis. (**a**) Sinusoids are dilated, and fibrosis is seen in the portal tract. (**b**) Non-parenchymal cells of the endothelium are destroyed and congested with red blood cells

Acknowledgment We are grateful to Professor Michael A. Kern for constructive advice and helpful suggestions in first edition of this chapter.

References

1. Budd G. On diseases of the liver. London: John Churchill; 1845. p. 135.
2. Chiari H. Experiences about infarction in human liver. Zeitschrift fur Hailkunde. 1898;19:475–512.
3. Rajani R, Melin T, Bjornsson E, Broome U, Sangfelt P, Danielsson A, et al. Budd-Chiari syndrome in Sweeden; epidemiology, clinical characteristics and survival – an 18-year experience. Liver Int. 2008;29:253–9.
4. Orloff MJ, Daily PO, Orloff SL, Girard B, Orloff MS. A 27-year experience with surgical treatment of Budd-Chiari syndrome. Am Surg. 2000;232:340–52.
5. Aydinli M, Bayraktar Y. Budd-Chiari syndrome: etiology, pathogenesis and diagnosis. World J Gastroenterol. 2007;13:2693–6.
6. Dilawari JB, Bambery P, Chawla Y, Kaur U, Bhusnurmath SR, Malhotra HS, et al. Hepatic outflow obstruction (Budd-Chiari syndrome). Experience with 177 patients and a review of the literature. Medicine. 1994;73:21–36.
7. Denninger MH, Chait Y, Casadevall N, Hillaire S, Guillin MC, Bezeaud A, et al. Cause of portal or hepatic venous thrombosis in adults: the role of multiple concurrent factors. Hepatology. 2003;31:587–91.
8. Simon IW. Membranous obstruction of the inferior vena cava and hepatocellular carcinoma in South Africa. Gastroenterology. 1982;68:171–8.
9. Datta DV, Saha S, Singh SA, Gupta BB, Aikat BK, Chuttani PN. Clinical spectrum of Budd-Chiari syndrome in Chandigarh with particular reference to obstruction of intrahepatic portion of inferior vena cava. Indian J Med Res. 1972;60:385–402.
10. Shrestha SM, Shrestha S. Hepatic vena cava disease: etiologic relation to bacterial infection. Hepatol Res. 2007;37:196–204.
11. Okuda H, Yamagata H, Obata H, Iwata H, Sasaki R, Imai F, et al. Epidemiological and clinical features of Budd-Chiari syndrome in Japan. J Hepatol. 1995;22:1–9.
12. Das CJ, Soneja M, Tayal S, Chahal A, Srivastava S, Kumar A, et al. Role of radiological imaging and interventions in management of Budd-Chiari syndrome. Clin Radiol. 2018. pii: S0009–9260(18)30084–9. https://doi.org/10.1016/j.crad.2018.02.003. [Epub ahead of print].
13. Copelan A, Remer EM, Sands M, Nghiem H, Kapoor B. Diagnosis and management of Budd Chiari syndrome: an update. Cardiovasc Intervent Radiol. 2015;38:1–12.
14. Henderson JM, Warren WD, Millikan WJ, Galloway JR, Kawasaki S, Stahl RL, et al. Surgical options, hematologic evaluation, and pathologic changes in Budd-Chiari syndrome. Am J Surg. 1990;159:41–50.
15. Mitchell MC, Boitnott JK, Kaufman S, Cameron JL, Maddrey WC. Budd-Chiari syndrome: etiology, diagnosis and management. Medicine. 1982;61:199–218.
16. Bourlière M, Le Treut YP, Arnoux D, Castellani P, Bordigoni L, Maillot A, et al. Acute Budd-Chiari syndrome with hepatic failure and obstruction of the inferior vena cava as presenting manifestations of hereditary protein C deficiency. Gut. 1990;31:949–52.
17. Bhargawa DK, Arova A, Dasarathy AS. Laparoscopic features of the Budd-Chiari syndrome. Endoscopy. 1991;23:259–61.
18. Mancuso A. An update on management of Budd-Chiari syndrome. Ann Hepatol. 2014;13:323–6.
19. European Association for the Study of the Liver. EASL clinical practice guidelines: vascular diseases of the liver. J Hepatol. 2016;64:179–202.
20. Tripathi D, Macnicholas R, Kothari C, Sunderraj L, Al-Hilou H, Rangarajan B, Chen F, Mangat K, Elias E, Olliff S. Good clinical outcomes following transjugular intrahepatic portosystemic stent-shunts in Budd-Chiari syndrome. Aliment Pharmacol Ther. 2014;39:864–72.
21. Mentha G, Giostra E, Majno PE, Bechstein WO, Neuhaus P, O'Grady J, Praseedom RK, Burroughs AK, Le Treut YP, Kirkegaard P, Rogiers X, Ericzon BG, Hockerstedt K, Adam R, Klempnauer J. Liver transplantation for Budd-Chiari syndrome: a European study on 248 patients from 51 centres. J Hepatol. 2006;44:520–8.
22. Deal BJ, Jacobs ML. Management of the failing Fontan circulation. Heart. 2012;98:1098–104.
23. Rychik J, Veldtman G, Rand E, Russo P, Rome JJ, Krok K, et al. The precarious state of the liver after a Fontan operation: summary of a multidisciplinary symposium. Pediatr Cardiol. 2012;33:1001–12.
24. Ghaferi AA, Hutchins GM. Progression of liver pathology in patients undergoing the Fontan procedure: chronic passive congestion, cardiac cirrhosis, hepatic adenoma, and hepatocellular carcinoma. J Thorac Cardiovasc Surg. 2005;129:1348–52.
25. Greenway SC, Crossland DS, Hudson M, Martin SR, Myers RP, Prieur T, et al. Fontan-associated liver disease: implications for heart transplantation. J Heart Lung Transplant. 2016;35:26–33.

26. Fan CQ, Crawford JM. Sinusoidal obstruction syndrome (hepatic veno-occlusive disease). J Clin Exp Hepatol. 2014;4:332–46.

27. Richardson PG, Smith AR, Triplett BM, Kernan NA, Grupp SA, Antin JH, et al. Defibrotide study group. Defibrotide for patients with hepatic Veno-occlusive disease/sinusoidal obstruction syndrome: interim results from a treatment IND study. Biol Blood Marrow Transplant. 2017;23:997–1004.

28. Norris S, Crosbie O, McEntee G, Traynor O, Molan N, McCann S, et al. Orthotopic liver transplantation for veno-occlusive disease complicating autologous bone marrow transplantation. Transplantation. 1997;63:1521–4.

29. Takehara H, Komi N, Hino M. Congenital arteriovenous fistula of the superior mesenteric vessels. J Pediatr Surg. 1988;23:1029–31.

30. Wood M, Nykamp PW. Traumatic arteriovenous fistula of the superior mesenteric vessels. J Trauma. 1980;20:378–82.

31. Benedetto JC, Liszewski RF. Superior mesenteric arteriovenous fistula: case report and literature review. J Am Osteopath Assoc. 1988;88:517–20.

32. Lee KR, Kishore P, Hardin CA. Postsurgical arteriovenous fistula. Acquired AV fistula of the mesentery. J Kans Med Soc. 1974;75:87–90.

33. Rabhan NB, Guillebeau JG, Brachney EG. Arteriovenous fistula of the superior mesenteric vessels after a gunshot wound. N Engl J Med. 1962;266:603–5.

34. Brunner JH, Stanley RJ. Superior mesenteric arteriovenous fistula. JAMA. 1973;223:316–8.

35. Riggio O, Gioia S, Pentassuglio I, Nicoletti V, Valente M, d'Amati G. Idiopathic noncirrhotic portal hypertension: current perspectives. Hepat Med. 2016;8:81–8.

36. Tsuneyama K, Ohta K, Zen Y, Sato Y, Niwa H, Minato H, et al. A comparative histological and morphometric study of vascular changes in idiopathic portal hypertension and alcoholic fibrosis/cirrhosis. Histopathology. 2003;43:55–61.

37. Ohbu M, Okudaira M, Watanabe K, Kaneko S, Takai T. Histopathological study of intrahepatic aberrant vessels in cases of noncirrhotic portal hypertension. Hepatology. 1994;20:302–8.

38. Dhiman RK, Chawla Y, Vasishta RK, Kakkar N, Dilawari JB, Trehan MS, et al. Non-cirrhotic portal fibrosis (idiopathic portal hypertension): experience with 151 patients and a review of the literature. J Gastroenterol Hepatol. 2002;17:6–16.

39. de Franchis R, Dell'Era A, Iannuzzi F. Diagnosis and treatment of portal hypertension. Dig Liver Dis. 2004;36:787–98.

40. Lay CS, Tsai YT, Lee FY, Lai YL, Yu CJ, Chen CB, et al. Endoscopic variceal ligation versus propranolol in prophylaxis of first variceal bleeding in patients with cirrhosis. J Gastroenterol Hepatol. 2006;21:413–9.

41. Patidar KR, Sydnor M, Sanyal AJ. Transjugular intrahepatic portosystemic shunt. Clin Liver Dis. 2014;18:853–76.

42. Shimoda R, Horiuchi K, Hagiwara S, Suzuki H, Yamazaki Y, Kosone T, et al. Short-term complications of retrograde transve-nous obliteration of gastric varices in patients with portal hypertension: effects of obliteration of major portosystemic shunts. Abdom Imaging. 2005;30:306–13.

43. Sarin SK, Kumar A, Chawla YK, Baijal SS, Dhiman RK, Jafri W, et al. Members of the APASL working party on portal hypertension. Noncirrhotic portal fibrosis/idiopathic portal hypertension:APASL recommendations for diagnosis and treatment. Hepatol Int. 2007;1:398–413.

44. Chawla YK, Bodh V. Portal vein thrombosis. J Clin Exp Hepatol. 2015;5:22–40.

45. Hauenstein K, Li Y. Radiological diagnosis of portal/mesenteric vein occlusion. Viszeralmedizin. 2014;30:382–7.

46. Manzano-Robleda Mdel C, Barranco-Fragoso B, Uribe M, Méndez-Sánchez N. Portal vein thrombosis: what is new? Ann Hepatol. 2015;14:20–7.

47. Khanna R, Sarin SK. Idiopathic portal hypertension and extrahepatic portal venous obstruction. Hepatol Int. 2018;12(Suppl 1):148–67.

48. Choudhry AJ, Baghdadi YM, Amr MA, Alzghari MJ, Jenkins DH, Zielinski MD. Pylephlebitis: a review of 95 cases. J Gastrointest Surg. 2016;20:656–61.

49. Laurenzi A, Ettorre GM, Lionetti R, Meniconi RL, Colasanti M, Vennarecci G. Portal vein aneurysm: what to know. Dig Liver Dis. 2015;47:918–23.

50. Ianora AA, Mememo M, Sabba C, Cirulli A, Rotondo A, Angelelli G. Hereditary hemorrhagic telangiectasia: multi-detector row helical CT assessment of hepatic involvement. Radiology. 2004;230:250–9.

51. Bernard G, Mion F, Henry L, Plauchu H, Paliard P. Hepatic involvement in hereditary hemorrhagic telangiectasia: clinical, radiological, and hemodynamic studies of 11 cases. Gastroenterology. 1993;105:482–7.

52. Piskorz MM, Waldbaum C, Volpacchio M, Sorda J. Liver involvement in hereditary hemorrhagic telangiectasia. Acta Gastroenterol Latinoam. 2011;41:225–9.

53. Shovlin CL, Guttmacher AE, Buscarini E, Faughnan ME, Hyland RH, Westermann CJ, Kjeldsen AD, Plauchu H. Diagnostic criteria for hereditary hemorrhagic telangiectasia (Rendu-Osler-weber syndrome). Am J Med Genet. 2000;91:66–7.

54. Wold LE, Ludwig J. Peliosis hepatis: two morphologic variants? Hum Pathol. 1981;12:388–9.

55. Tsokos M, Erbersdobler A. Pathology of peliosis. Forensic Sci Int. 2005;149:25–33.

56. Crocetti D, Palmieri A, Pedullà G, Pasta V, D'Orazi V, Grazi GL. Peliosis hepatis: personal experience and literature review. World J Gastroenterol. 2015;21:13188–94.

57. Choi SK, Jin JS, Cho SG, Choi SJ, Kim CS, Choe YM, et al. Spontaneous liver rupture in a patient with peliosis hepatis: a case report. World J Gastroenterol. 2009;15:5493–7.

Metabolic Disorders in the Liver

12

Masaki Iwai, Atsushi Kitamura, Hajime Isomoto,
Yutaka Horie, and Wilson M. S. Tsui

Contents

Abbreviations

AIP	Acute intermittent porphyria
ALA	δ-aminolevulinic acid
ALP	Alkaline phosphatase
ATP7B	Adenosine triphospholic acid 7B
CTLN2	Adult-onset type II citrullinemia
EPP	Erythropoietic protoporphyria
FTTDCD	Failure to thrive and dyslipidemia caused by citrin deficiency
HH	Hereditary hemochromatosis
HLA	Human leukocyte antigen
LSCs	Liver stellate cells
NADH	Reduced nicotinamide adenine dinucleotide
NICCD	Neonatal intrahepatic cholestasis caused by citrin deficiency
PBG	Porphobilinogen
PCT	Porphyria cutanea tarda
TfR2	Transferrin receptor 2

M. Iwai, MD, PhD (✉)
Kyoto, Japan
e-mail: masaiwai@koto.kpu-m.ac.jp

A. Kitamura, MD, PhD · Y. Horie, MD, PhD
Shimane, Japan

H. Isomoto, MD, PhD
Tottori, Japan

W. M. S. Tsui, MD, FRCPath
Hong Kong, China

© Springer Nature Singapore Pte Ltd. 2019
E. Hashimoto et al. (eds.), *Diagnosis of Liver Disease*, https://doi.org/10.1007/978-981-13-6806-6_12

12.1 Iron Overload

Iron overload, or siderosis, is a commonly encountered problem in clinical practice and may be classified as primary (genetic) or secondary to other diseases, such as hereditary anemias (Table 12.1). Dietary iron is absorbed primarily by enterocytes in the duodenum, transported from the intestine to the portal blood stream (where it is bound to apotransferrin), and transported to the liver. It is, therefore, not surprising that excessive deposition of iron in liver is commonly encountered in liver biopsies.

12.1.1 Hereditary Hemochromatosis

Hereditary hemochromatosis (HH) due to human hemochromatosis (HFE) mutations is one of the most common genetic disorders in Caucasians, with a prevalence of nearly 1 in 200 [1, 2]. These patients suffer from lifelong and excessive gastrointestinal absorption of iron. The two most common mutations are designated C282Y (85–90% of affected individuals)

Table 12.1 Causes of hepatic iron overload

Primary hereditary hemochromatosis
• HFE-associated hereditary hemochromatosis (type 1); autosomal recessive
• Non-HFE-associated hereditary hemochromatosis
– Juvenile hemochromatosis (type 2A, hemojuvelin; type 2B, hepcidin mutations)
– Transferrin receptor 2 mutations (type 3)
– Ferroportin mutations (type 4); autosomal dominant
Secondary hemosiderosis
• Dyserythropoietic and hemolytic anemias
– Beta-thalassemia major
– Sideroblastic anemia
– Pyruvate kinase deficiency
– Chronic hemolytic anemias
• Chronic liver disease
– End-stage cirrhosis
– Chronic viral hepatitis B and C
– Alcoholic liver disease
– Nonalcoholic steatohepatitis
– Post-portocaval shunt
• Dietary iron overload
– African "bantu" hemochromatosis
– Prolonged excessive medicinal iron ingestion
• Parenteral iron overload
– Transfusion iron overload
– Excessive parenteral iron
• Miscellaneous
– Porphyria cutanea tarda
– Neonatal hemochromatosis
– Aceruloplasminemia
– Atransferrinemia

HFE human hemochromatosis

and H63D and account for approximately 85% of autosomal recessive HH [3]. The C282Y mutation prevents formation of a disulfide bond essential for binding of the protein to beta-2-microglobulin, thus preventing transportation of the HFE protein to the cell surface. The H63D mutation affects binding of the HFE to the transferrin receptor and results in a less severe phenotype; homozygosity for H63D mutation accounts for <2% of HH. About 8–18% of Northern, Central, and Western Europeans are heterozygotes for the C282Y mutation. The high frequency of this mutation and data from population studies suggest origin from a common ancestor in Northwest Europe before 4000 BC.

Juvenile hemochromatosis and transferrin receptor 2 (TfR2)-associated hemochromatosis are inherited as autosomal recessive disorders [4]. The juvenile form has the same pattern of iron overload seen in the homozygous C282Y form. However, iron overload occurs much sooner: in the second and third decades. Ferroportin disease is inherited in an autosomal dominant fashion, and there are two phenotypes: a mild and severe form [5]. Defective hepcidin synthesis, which is a central regulator of systemic iron homeostasis, is a common mechanism underlying iron overload in HFE and non-HFE-associated HH.

Individuals with HFE HH are asymptomatic until significant accumulation of iron occurs in the liver and other organs, a process which takes decades. Men typically present in their 40s or 50s, with women presenting a decade later because of the protective effects of menstruation. Skin pigmentation is less frequently found with earlier diagnosis than in the past. Weakness, lethargy, abdominal pain, and arthropathy are common, nonspecific presenting symptoms. In late stages, iron deposition in pancreatic islets results in diabetes mellitus. Hypogonadism is very common. In young subjects, cardiac manifestations may be the presenting feature—generally as congestive cardiomyopathy—and death may result within 1 year of presentation if iron reduction is not instituted. Many patients with HFE mutations are now identified at an asymptomatic stage, when hyperferritinemia is discovered upon routine testing. Treatment is generally phlebotomy to reduce iron stores [6].

In HH due to HFE mutations, iron is preferentially deposited in hepatocytes as granular, refractile, golden-brown hemosiderin. In early stages, iron deposition is more prominent in zone 1. As the disease progresses, zone 2 and 3 hepatocytes are involved. Inflammation is not a feature of hemochromatosis, and fatty change is not specifically associated with the disorder. Iron also accumulates in biliary epithelial cells. The accumulation of iron causes necrosis of individual hepatocytes, releasing iron which is taken up by Kupffer cells. Unlike HFE HH, iron deposition in ferroportin disease and hematologic disorders occurs preferentially in Kupffer cells, involving hepatocytes only when they are present in large quantities. Fibrosis in HH occurs when a threshold of approximately 15,000 μg iron/gram dry weight liver is reached. This corresponds to grade 3 siderosis. It begins in the periportal areas, where iron deposition is greatest, thereby causing portal-to-portal septa. Early cirrhosis is typically micronodular with no significant ductular proliferation, and the liver is rust-colored. The risk for hepatocellular carcinoma is up to 200 times that of the general population, and the carcinoma almost always occurs in cirrhotic livers. It is postulated that the presence of increased iron produces oxidation stress that leads to p53 mutations [7].

Case 12.1

A 37-year-old Chinese woman was investigated for secondary amenorrhea, which was found to be related to hypogonadotropic hypogonadism. Her liver function was also slightly deranged: ALP 283 IU/L, AST 175 IU/L, ALT 85 IU/L, and normal bilirubin. Hepatitis viruses and autoimmune markers were negative. Ferritin was markedly elevated at 2220 μg/L, and the Fe/TIBC ratio increased to 86.2%. Hyperglycemia was present, and US revealed a normal-sized liver with normal echo pattern. Liver biopsy showed normal architecture tissue with abundant coarse brown pigment granules in all the hepatocytes, which were shown to be hemosiderin (Fig. 12.1). Iron was also present in some Kupffer cells and bile duct epithelium. There was periportal fibrosis with occasional fibrous bridges. Subsequently, her older brother was found to be suffering from iron overload. When genotyping was available several years later and performed, it was found that the patient did not have the typical mutations in the HFE gene (C282Y or H63D). This finding does not exclude a diagnosis of genetic hemochromatosis, since the C282Y HFE gene mutation is not found in Chinese hemochromatotics [8]. Other types of non-HFE-associated HH may be responsible.

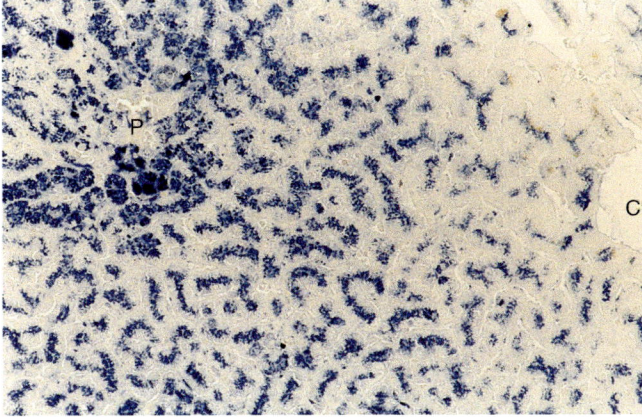

Fig. 12.1 Hereditary hemochromatosis. Perls' stain shows all hepatocytes contain hemosiderin granules in the pericanalicular area. Hepatic iron gradient (heaviest in zone 1, least in zone 3) is still identified (grade 3 iron overload). *C* central vein, *P* portal tract

12.1.2 Secondary Hemochromatosis

Iron deposits are occasionally seen in chronic hepatitis B and C [9, 10]. However, its significance has not been determined. We observed secondary hemochromatosis in a patient with chronic hepatitis B and chronic renal failure with blood transfusion.

Case 12.2

A 69-year-old female received interferon for chronic hepatitis B, and seroconversion of HBeAg to HBeAb was seen. Her liver function test showed AST 68 IU/L, ALT 47 IU/L, ferritin 7080 ng/mL, s-Fe 206 μg/dL, TIBC 238, type IV collagen 6.5 ng/mL, hyaluronic acid 149 ng/mL, and PLT 7.2×10^4. CT showed high density diffusely in the liver; MRI revealed low intensity on T1- and T2-weighted images; laparoscopic findings showed a brown-colored liver surface, and low nodules with thick capsules; fibrosis had spread from the portal tract, and a brown pigment was observed in hepatocytes and Kupffer cells (Fig. 12.2).

12.1.2.1 Transfusion Iron Overload

The clinical and pathological features of iron overload are well known in patients with HH [1, 2]. They suffer from lifelong and excessive gastrointestinal absorption of iron. Iron overload in patients with chronic renal failure is often complicated by intravenous blood transfusion or iron dextran during hemodialysis [11], and there are common liver pathology findings in advanced-stage HH and parenteral iron overload [12, 13]. It has been stated that blood transfusion results in accumulation of iron not only in the reticuloendothelial system but also in parenchymal cells [12]. Patients with chronic renal failure often have iron overload through continuous blood transfusion, and iron overload in experimental animals has a big influence on liver fibrosis [14]. Below, we report cirrhotic changes of the liver in a renal transplant recipient with a long history of blood transfusion. We observed alpha-smooth muscle actin-positive stellate cells and their ultrastructural features to investigate their role in liver fibrosis in iron overload, after reviewing the literature [15–17].

Case 12.3

A 39-year-old man with chronic renal failure complained of malaise and was referred for evaluation of abnormal liver function tests. Proteinuria was indicated, and he had chronic hemodialysis. He had received a first renal allograft, but the cadaveric transplant failed due to immunological rejection, and he was retransplanted. He received 300 units of packed red blood cells during chronic hemodialysis, but no iron dextran had been administered. He was taking prednisolone and azathioprine and did not drink alcohol. On admission, his skin was pigmented but not icteric. Elastic liver was palpable 5 cm

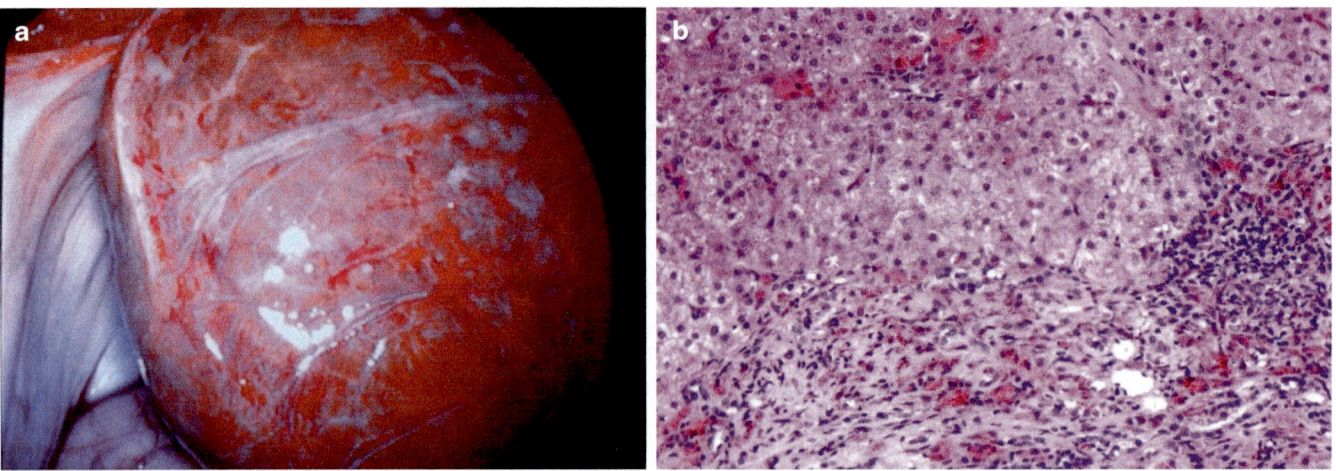

Fig. 12.2 Secondary hemochromatosis. (**a**) Dull edge of the liver and a brown-colored surface are seen, and acinus markings are clear. (**b**) Brown pigment is seen not only in hepatocytes but also in mesenchymal cells in the fibrotic area of the portal tract

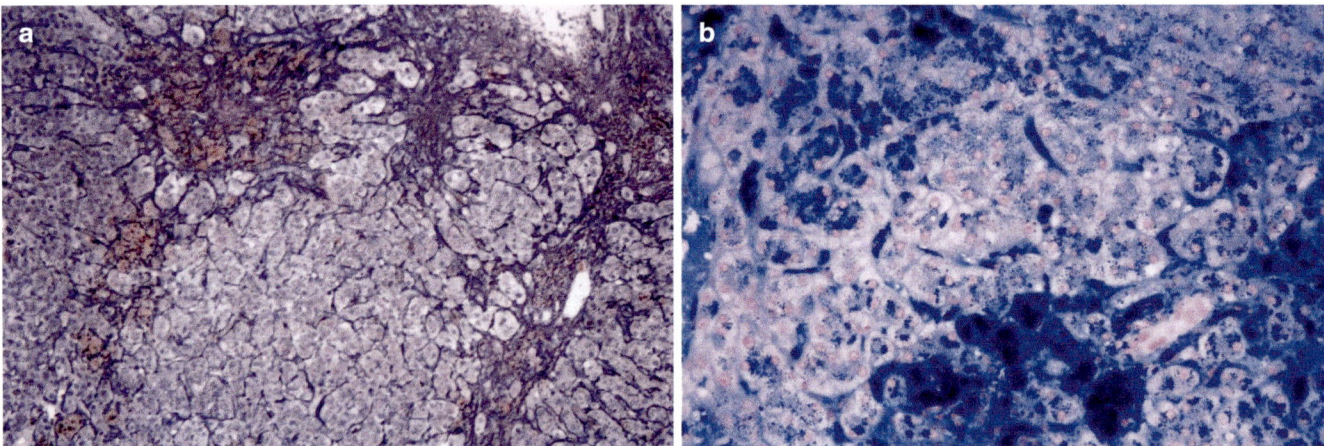

Fig. 12.3 Morphological aspects of liver with secondary hemochromatosis. (**a**) Reticulin fiber stain shows bridging fibrosis between portal tracts and little fibrosis around the central area. (**b**) Berlin blue stain shows iron is deposited not only in Kupffer cells but also in hepatocytes around the portal tracts and along the fibrotic area. Other hepatocytes contain fine iron granules

beneath the right costal margin, and extremities were edematous. The laboratory examination showed RBC 3.28×10^6/mm^3, Hb 9.7 g/dL, HT 29.6%, s-Fe 148 μg/dL, TIBC 162 μg/dL, s-ferritin 8180 ng/mL, TBIL 0.89 mg/dL, AST 92 IU/L, ALT 148 IU/L, ALP 1853 IU/L, gamma-GTP 1322 IU/L, hyaluronic acid 424 ng/mL, desferal test 5.7 mg/dL, blood urea nitrogen 52 mg/dL, creatinine 2.9 mg/dL, and HLA typing A2 AW24BW39 BW55 CW1 CW7. Neither HBsAg nor HCV Ab was present. Ultrasonography of the abdomen demonstrated an irregular liver surface, and computed tomography (CT) showed a high-density liver, spleen, and pancreas. CT density of the liver was 106 Hounsfield units (HU). Magnetic resonance imaging (MRI) showed low intensity in the liver on T1- and T2-weighted images. Laparoscopy revealed an enlarged, lobulated, and brown-colored liver. Histological features showed bridging fibrosis from the portal tract to the neighboring one, and pseudo-lobular formation was seen

(Fig. 12.3a); iron deposits were found in both Kupffer and parenchymal cells, and heavy iron-loaded hepatocytes were distributed mainly in the periportal area (Fig. 12.3b). Electron microscopy showed hepatocytes laden with iron deposits surrounded by collagen fibers, Kupffer cells, and neutrophils. Immunocytochemical study showed alpha-smooth muscle actin-positive stellate cells near fibrosis and heavy iron-deposited hepatocytes, forming a continuous network.

12.1.2.2 Liver Fibrosis

Iron is essential to life, but its excessive intake is toxic to many organs. The liver is a major organ for its storage and is susceptible to its toxic effect. Our patient had received 300 units of packed red blood cells during chronic hemodialysis. Ferritin in serum was very high, and CT density of the liver was 106 HU. It has been reported that the upper limit of 70 HU for coefficient attenuation provides 64% sensitivity and 87% specificity for hepatic iron overload [18], and high-density hepatic CT in a patient with elevated serum ferritin is suspicious of iron deposition in the liver [19]. Hepatic MRI showed low intensity on both T1- and T2-weighted images, and image analysis indicated iron deposition in the liver [20]. Laparoscopy showed a brown, lobulated liver. Biopsy showed bridging fibrosis that distorted lobular formation. Iron deposition is often seen in inherited and acquired disorders [21], and pathological features in iron overload by blood transfusion are indistinguishable from those of HH. Iron deposition in hemochromatosis is saturated not only in Kupffer cells but also in parenchymal cells [12]. The specific mechanism of hepatocellular injury in iron overload is still unknown, but in experimental studies, iron overload has caused the formation of free radicals and peroxidation of membrane lipids that are closely associated with hepatocellular injury [22, 23], eventually leading to liver fibrosis and cirrhotic change.

Recently, liver stellate cells (LSCs) have been noted to play an important role for liver fibrosis in experimental rats after administration of iron [15, 24]. Activated LSCs are reported to participate not only in a necroinflammatory reaction [25] but also in fibrosis, expressing collagen and extracellular matrix [16]. Recent studies also indicate that human-activated LSCs express alpha-isotype actin that is specific for the differentiation of smooth muscle cells [16, 25]. We identified alpha-smooth muscle actin-positive LSCs in the liver tissue, and many of them were found to coexist with fibrosis in the periportal area. There might be a significant association between them and fibrosis [26]. Activated LSCs, hypertrophic Kupffer cells, and increased collagen were ultrastructurally seen around iron-laden degenerative hepatocytes, and LSCs are reported to be activated by Kupffer cells through cytokines [27]. Subsequently, activated LSCs participate in liver fibrosis with transfusion iron overload.

12.1.3 Differential Diagnosis

Quantitative analysis of iron in the liver has long been the gold standard for the diagnosis of HH but is supplanted in some settings by genetic testing. HLA typing has been used as a surrogate test for HH within kindreds because of the tight linkage between the HFE gene and the HLA complex but has largely been replaced by testing for C282Y mutations. The role of liver biopsy in the evaluation of iron overload has also changed—it has become less of a diagnostic tool and more of a grading and staging tool, and it also serves to detect incidental diseases and complications such as hepatocellular carcinoma.

The differential diagnosis of HH primarily includes chronic liver diseases associated with hepatic iron deposition and hematologic disorders (Table 12.1). Although iron overload from transfusions and/or chronic hemolytic anemias is easily distinguished from HH by the preferential deposition

of iron in Kupffer cells rather than hepatocytes, a note of caution must be sounded here because of the recent descriptions of the hepatopathology of ferroportin disease. Clinical history should aid in making these distinctions, but in ambiguous cases, genetic testing may be indicated.

Hepatic iron overload is commonly seen in alcoholic liver disease and cirrhosis of any type [28] and may overlap morphologically with HH. The pathogenesis of iron deposition in alcoholics is largely unknown, but increased alcohol consumption may increase intestinal iron absorption in some patients. Heterozygosity for C282Y does not appear to influence hepatic iron levels or the risk of fibrosis in these patients [29]. Quantitative iron determination is usually helpful in distinguishing these entities. The hepatic iron index is determined by dividing the weight of iron (micromoles per gram) in the biopsy by the patient's age in years. A level of >1.9 reliably distinguishes homozygosity for HH from the heterozygous state and alcoholic liver disease. However, the hepatic iron index may exceed 1.9 in chronic hemolytic anemia, and levels <1.9 are seen in up to 15% of HH patients. The test may be performed on formalin-fixed, paraffin-embedded tissue or fresh tissue.

Hepatic iron deposition in chronic viral hepatitis is typically modest and is found primarily in Kupffer cells; inconspicuous deposits in endothelial cells may also be noted. The contribution of HFE heterozygosity and increased hepatic iron to nonalcoholic fatty liver disease is controversial, with some—but not all—investigators reporting increased prevalence of HFE mutations in nonalcoholic steatohepatitis [30, 31]. It should be noted that HH, by itself, does not produce an inflammatory pattern of injury in the liver; if present, it should be a prompt consideration of superimposed disease processes or alternative diagnoses.

12.2 Wilson's Disease

Wilson's disease is an autosomal recessive disorder in which there is a mutation in the ATP7B gene for copper-transporting ATPase in the liver [32], and the functional loss of ATP7B gene impairs excretion of copper into the bile, leading to accumulation of copper in the liver and other organs. Increased level of copper in tissues induces harmful reactions and oxidative stress and can damage the structure and integrity of mitochondria, leading to cell injury [33]. Patients with symptomatic Wilson's disease present with liver disease or neurologic/psychiatric symptoms and osteoarthritis, functional disturbance of kidneys, or cardiomyopathy [34]. Keizer-Fleisher rings are caused by deposition of copper in Descemet's corneal membrane [35], and their presence is confirmed by slit-lamp examination, and they are present in about 50% of patients with hepatic disease [36]. A diagnostic score was proposed by International Meeting on Wilson's disease, Leipzig, 2001 [37], and the scoring system includes the following elements, (1) serum ceruloplasmin, (2) 24-h urinary copper excretion, (3) the presence of nonimmune hemolytic anemia, (4) hepatic copper, (5) the presence of Kayser-Fleisher rings on slit-lamp examination, (6) neurologic or neuroimaging features, and (7) mutation analysis, and a score of 4 or more provides good accuracy for diagnosis of Wilson's disease, and the probable case with 2 or 3 points needs more diagnostic tests [38], and nonimmune hemolytic anemia with elevation of serum bilirubin and low serum alkaline phosphatase in young patients may predict acute liver failure [39]. There are four pathological features in the liver: acute hepatitis, fulminant hepatitis, chronic active hepatitis, and cirrhosis. In the early phase, there is fatty metamorphosis with fat granulomas [40, 41] and glycogenated nuclei in hepatocytes and focal hepatocellular necrosis, and these abnormalities are often misdiagnosed as nonalcoholic fatty liver or nonalcoholic steatohepatitis [42]. Ultrastructural findings show enlarged mitochondria with a dense matrix and vacuolated granules [43]. In the presence of acute liver failure, marked hepatocellular degeneration and parenchymal collapse are developed on a background of cirrhosis although some might show the presence of massive necrosis with only bridging fibrosis [35, 44, 45].

To treat Wilson's disease, nutrition should be low in copper, and the first choice of medication is D-penicillamine [46]. Zinc [47] or triethylenetetramine [48] is considered as an alternative therapy to penicillamine. About 3–5% of patients present with acute liver failure, and prognostic score incorporating serum bilirubin, AST, prothrombin time, and leukocytes-count is reliable to determine liver transplantation [49], and liver transplantation is the remaining therapy in a fulminant course or an advanced stage of liver cirrhosis [50, 51].

Case 12.4

A 12-year-old boy had abnormal values in his liver function test when he had a common cold. His serum examination for liver function showed GOT 47 IU/L, GPT 42 IU/L, s-Cu 26 µg/dL, ceruloplasmin 8 mg/dL, hyaluronic acid 295.4 ng/mL, type IV collagen 7S 8.0 ng/mL, and $ICGR_{15}$ 12.6%. Peritoneoscopy showed yellow liver surface with nodular formation; the nodules were homogenously equal in size, and the internodular space was narrow; and bridging fibrosis was observed with necrosis in the portal tracts. Interface hepatitis was seen in the portal tract with infiltration of lymphocytes, and microvesicular fatty metamorphosis remained (Fig. 12.4). His 11-year-old sister also had abnormal values in the liver function test: AST130 IU/L, ALT 232 IU/L, s-Cu 16 µg/dL, ceruloplasmin 2.1 mg/dL, type IV collagen 7S 8.5 ng/mL, hyaluronic acid 315 ng/mL, and $ICGR_{15}$ 4.0%. Peritoneoscopy showed smooth yellow liver surface with shallow excavations (Fig. 12.5a); liver histology showed fibrosis in the portal tract, and macrovesicular or microvesicular formation was seen in hepatocytes (Fig. 12.5b); and lobular formation was distorted by fibrosis, but no pseudo-lobular formation was present

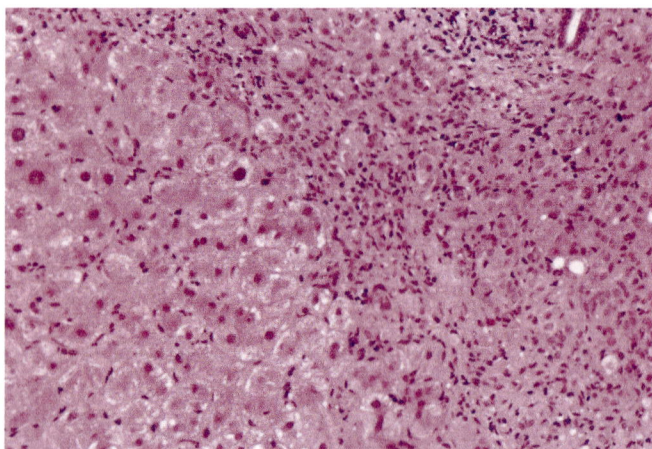

Fig. 12.4 Wilson's disease. Active inflammation is seen in the portal tract of cirrhotic liver and microvesicular fatty change is detected in hepatocytes. HE staining

(Fig. 12.5c). In the fulminant type, massive necrosis was seen, while pseudo-lobular formation was constructed in other areas. Steatosis was also seen in pseudo-lobules; electron microscopy showed electron-dense materials, and mitochondria cristae were distorted (Fig. 12.6).

12.3 Non-Wilson's Disease Form of Copper Toxicosis

12.3.1 Indian Childhood Cirrhosis

Daily ingestion of dietary in copper household utensils or drinking of milk stored in brass is the cause of copper overload, and urinary, serum, and hepatic copper concentration becomes noted; however serum ceruloplasmin is normal or elevated. The disease has been reported to present in genetically susceptible individuals at 4 months to 5 years of age, with a peak around 2 years not only in Indian subcontinent [52] but also in the USA [53]. There are clinically three stages, an early, an intermediate, and a late stage, with jaundice, hepatosplenomegaly, and progression to hepatic failure [54], but it has been rarely seen because education is widely spread. The earliest morphological change is ballooning degeneration and focal necrosis, followed by formation of Mallory-Denk bodies [54, 55]. There is inflammatory cell infiltration, periportal ductular reaction, and progressive fibrosis to the development of micronodular cirrhosis. Copper toxicosis is treated with copper chelation therapy of D-penicillamine [56].

12.3.2 Idiopathic Copper Toxicosis

Progressive cirrhosis develops by 2 years of age in the absence of neurological symptoms sporadically worldwide; however serum ceruloplasmin is normal or

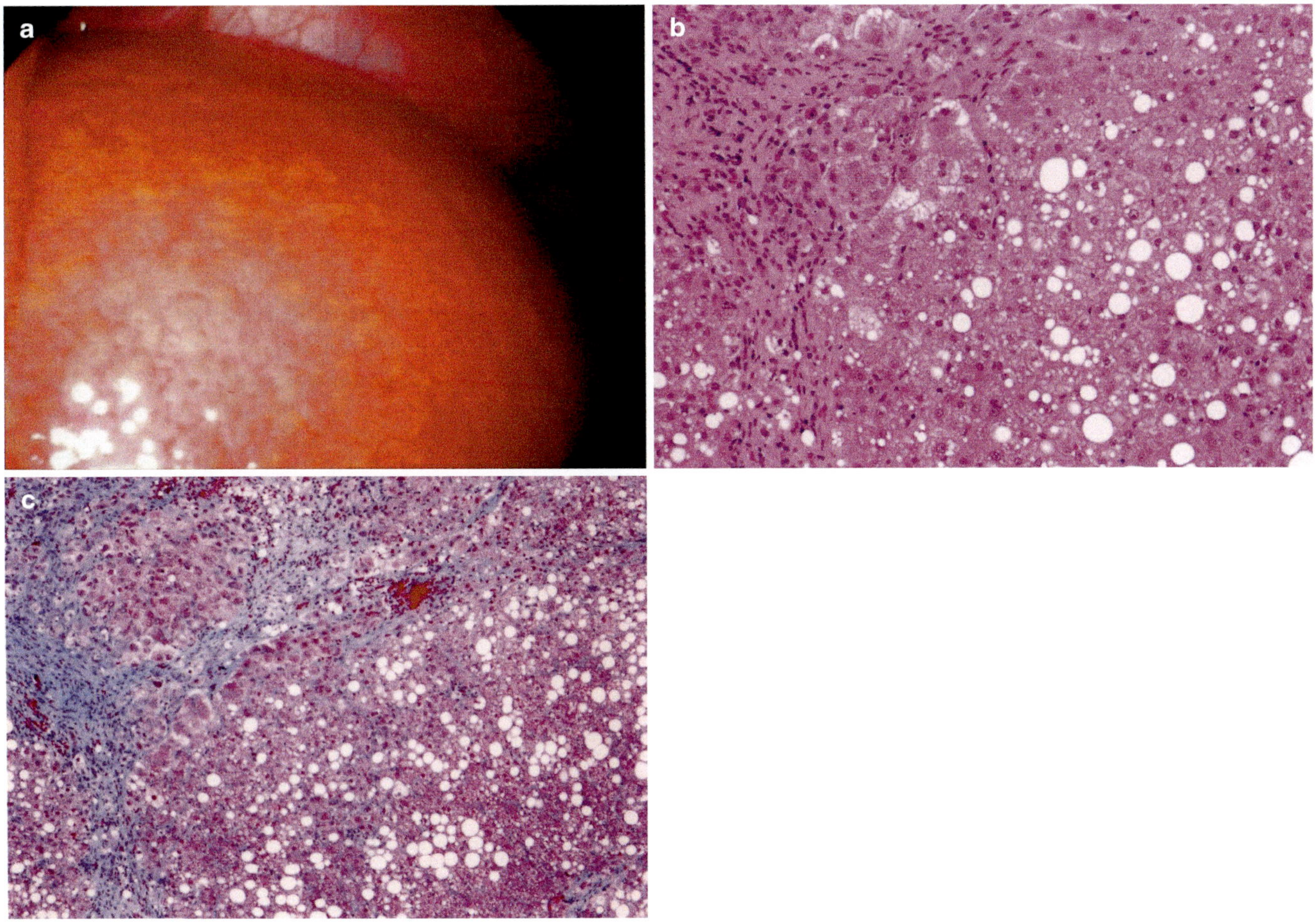

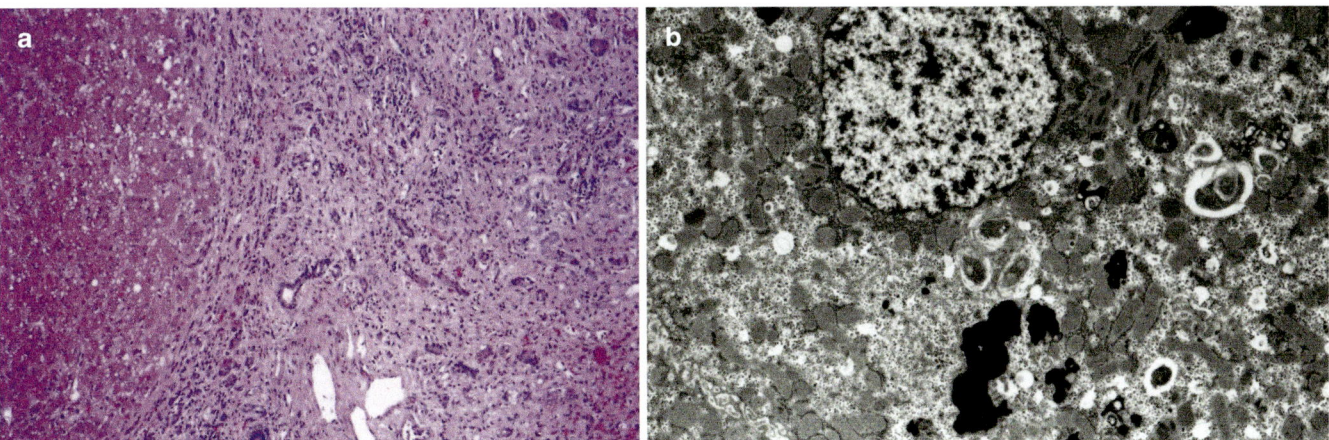

Fig. 12.5 Wilson's disease. (**a**) Peritoneoscopy shows diffuse excavations on the yellow liver. (**b**) Fibrosis is proliferated in the portal tract, and hepatocytes have macrovesicular and microvesicular formation. (**c**) Mallory-Azan stain shows bridging fibrosis from the portal tract and lobular formation is distorted, but no pseudo-lobular formation is established

Fig. 12.6 Wilson's disease. (**a**) Massive necrosis is accompanied with ductular reaction and fibrosis, and macrovesicular or microvesicular formations are seen in residual hepatocytes. (**b**) Electron microscopy shows electron-dense materials and secondary lysosomes, and mitochondria cristae are disturbed

elevated. This disease is caused by excessive amount of environmental copper exposure, for example, by drinking cow's milk from untinned copper or brass vessels or spring water contaminated with copper, and an autosomal recessive inheritance has been described in endemic Tyrolean cirrhosis (non-Indian childhood cirrhosis) [57]. Histopathology shows micronodular cirrhosis with copper overload in severely affected children [58], and combined administration of trientine and zinc can improve the decompensated function of the liver [59].

12.3.3 Menkes Disease

Menkes disease is an X-linked recessive neurodegenerative disorder, and it presents by 3 months of age and is fatal by 3–6 years of age. It is caused by mutations in ATP7A gene, homologous to ATP7B, that causes impaired copper transport across the placenta, small intestine, and blood-brain barrier and then leads to a severe copper deficiency state [60]. Affected infants develop hypotonia, seizure, and failure to thrive, and "kinky hair," hypopigmentation, osteoporosis, and arterial vascular tortuosity are characteristically detected. Serum copper or ceruloplasmin is low. Treatment of copper histidine should be instituted in the early phase of the disease and improve outcomes partially.

12.4   Porphyria

Porphyrias are disorders of the biosynthesis of porphyrins and heme synthesis, which has eight steps. They are grouped into two types: acute hepatic porphyria and cutaneous porphyria, and X-linked dominant protoporphyria is added to a category of porphyria (Fig. 12.7) [61]. The acute porphyrias are due to overproduction of the porphyrin precursors, δ-aminolevulinic acid(ALA) and porphobilinogen (PBG). The symptoms are caused by injury primarily to the nervous system. Cutaneous porphyria is due to overproduction of photosensitizing porphyrins in the liver or bone marrow, characteristically leading to skin damage following sunlight exposure.

12.4.1 Acute Intermittent Porphyria (AIP)

It is the acute type most often encountered in clinical practice [62, 63] and is due to partial deficiency of the third enzyme of heme synthesis, porphobilinogen deaminase. Attack in AIP largely occurs in women of reproductive age, presenting with unexplained abdominal pain, nausea with vomiting, constipation, and muscle weakness. Psychiatric symptoms of confusion, hallucination, and seizure are sometimes recognized as well as peripheral neuropathy. The attack is triggered by infections, smoking, excessive alcohol consumption, intake of oral contraceptives or medications, and caloric deprivation. Hepatic abnormalities range from mild elevations in AST/ALT to liver failure. The amber-colored urine is a clue to the diagnosis of AIP and can be confirmed by remarkable elevation of urinary PBG and ALA [64]. Measurement of PBG, ALA, uroporphyrin, and coproporphyrin in urine is useful to make a differential

Fig. 12.7 Pathway of heme biosynthesis

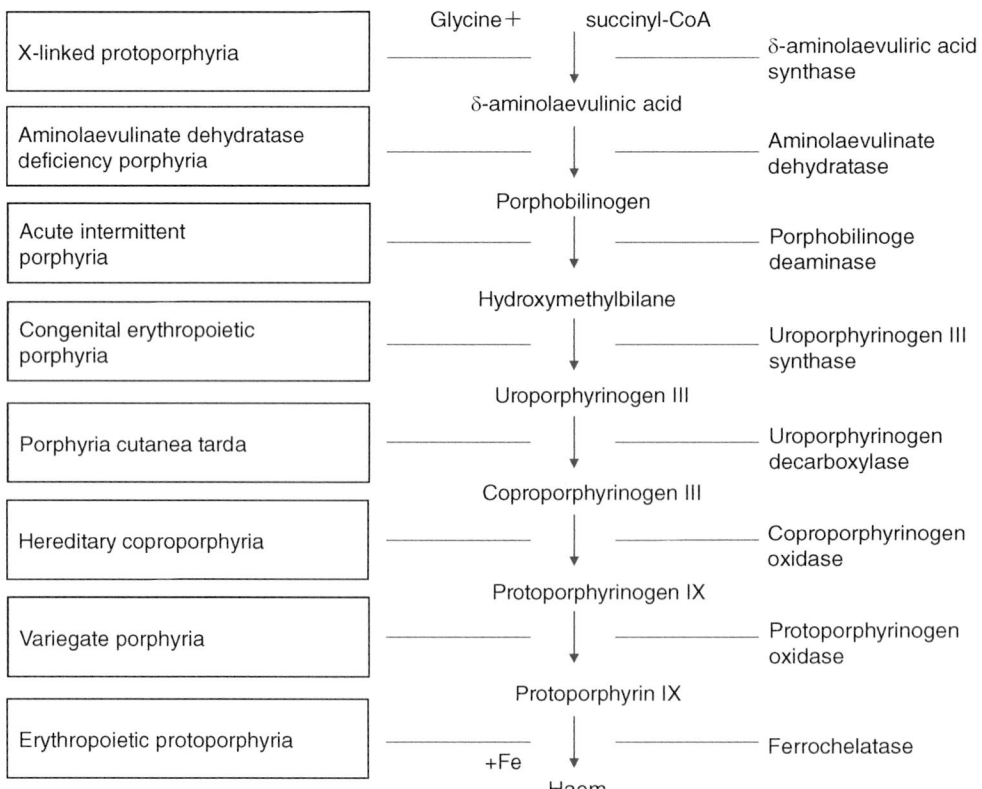

diagnosis among different types of porphyria. Estimation of erythrocyte PBG deaminase activity is available to establish the diagnosis of AIP and its carriers, and gene analysis of PBG deaminase helps to find out not only patients with AIP but also an asymptomatic carrier in family. Long-term follow-up of AIP patients reveals complications of chronic hypertension, chronic kidney insufficiency, chronic pain syndrome, and hepatocellular carcinoma [65]. Management of AIP is to provide adequate caloric intake by intravenous infusion, correct electrolyte disturbance including hyponatremia, treat pain with opiate analgesia, administer hematin, suppress ovulation with gonadorelin analogues, treat any intercurrent infections, or treat hepatic failure by liver transplantation [63].

12.4.2 Cutaneous Porphyrias

Porphyria cutanea tarda (PCT) and erythropoietic protoporphyria (EPP) are the most prevalent in cutaneous porphyrias, and the presentation typically occurs during or after puberty. They are also two of the porphyrias which importantly affect the liver. PCT is the most common form of porphyria and is due to acquired deficiency of uroporphyrinogen decarboxylase [66] and is almost always sporadic. Spontaneous PCT is reported to be associated with alcoholic liver disease, HCV infection, iron overload, and Alagille syndrome. In the liver, there is accumulation of uroporphyrin forming needle-shaped inclusions in the cytoplasm of hepatocytes detectable by light, fluorescent, and electron microscopy. Patients are at risk of developing hepatocellular carcinoma. Phlebotomy is useful for patients with PCT to reduce the iron burden. In

Japan, 85% of PCT patients suffer from HCV infection, and interferon- or direct-acting antiviral therapy is a standard method for treating PCT [67, 68].

EPP is an inherited porphyria caused by decrease of ferrochelatase activity which is a terminal enzyme of heme biosynthesis [66] and is a disorder in which accumulation of protoporphyrin in the erythrocytes, skin, liver, and other tissues leads to lifelong and acute painful photosensitivity. Presentation usually begins in childhood, with swelling, burning, itching, and redness of the skin after exposure to sunlight. The most effective treatment is the prevention of the photosensitive reaction by avoiding sunlight, and administration of carotenoids is also effective for skin lesions. Liver disease develops later, mostly after 30 years of age, and death occurs within 3–5 months following the development of jaundice due to hepatic failure as a result of excessive deposits of protoporphyrin in the hepatobiliary tract. Liver biopsy specimens show accumulation of dark brown pigment in canaliculi, interlobular bile ducts, and Kupffer cells, displaying a characteristic bright red birefringence with central dark Maltese cross (Fig. 12.8). Many patients have mild degree of anemia suggesting iron deficiency. It is important not to give excessive amount of blood transfusion to patients of EPP with anemia. Hematin is successful for treatment, and liver transplantation is required for patients with liver failure or end-stage cirrhosis [69].

Case 12.5

A 34-year-old female with a history of acute intermittent porphyria (AIP) for 15 years was admitted to a hospital with complaints of abdominal pain and sensory loss of lower extremities, and her mother also suffered from AIP. The

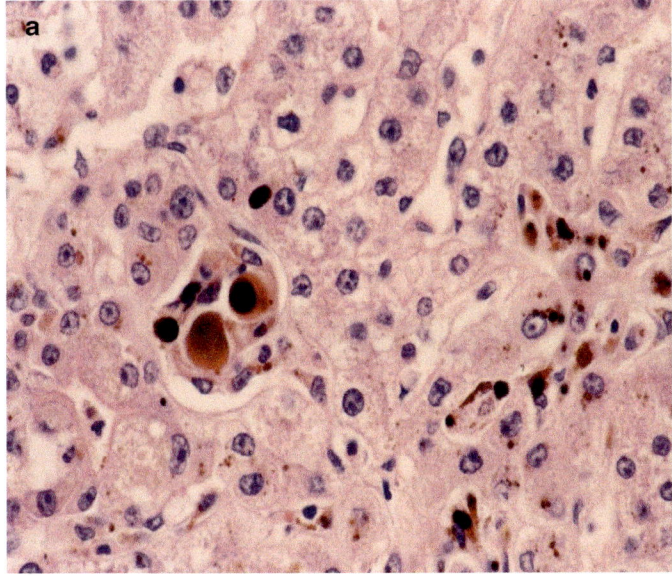
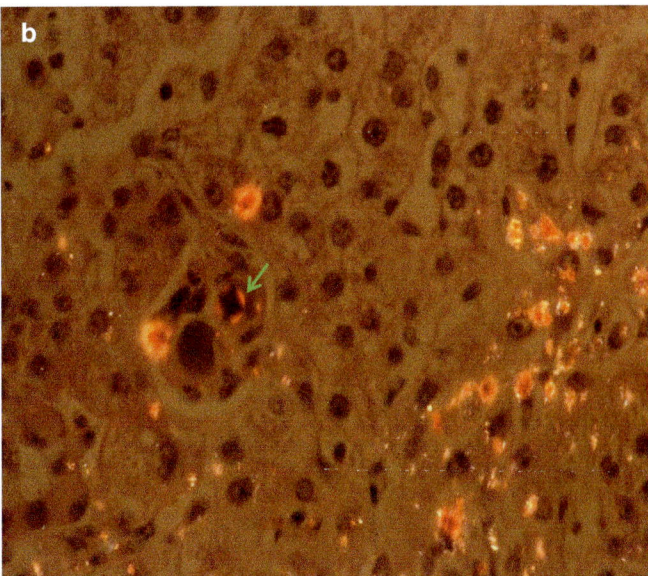

Fig. 12.8 Liver in erythropoietic protoporphyria. (**a**) Brown deposits are present in bile canaliculi, hepatocytes, and Kupffer cells. (**b**) The deposits have a yellow to red birefringence with a dark Maltese cross (arrow)

urine during her acute attack was wine-red colored (Fig. 12.9). Biochemical analysis of porphyrin and precursors in urine was porphobilinogen (PBG) 20.6 mg/day (N < 5), δ-aminolevulinate 3.5 mg/day (N<3), uroporphyrin (UP) 449 μg/gCRN (N<36), and coproporphyrin (CP) 765 μg/gCRN (N < 170). Gene analysis of porphobilinogen deaminase showed a point mutation of C to T in exon 8. After admission, intermittent attack of abdominal and limb pain occurred. To relieve the pain, morphine chloride of 30–160 mg/day was administered intramuscularly, and body weight was reduced by diet therapy. The porphyrin and its precursors were serially measured in urine, and the dosage of morphine chloride was determined by the value of PBG and ALA (Fig. 12.10). She was finally relieved from the pain and discharged.

Case 12.6

A 54-year-old male with history of heavy drinking for 30 years complained of skin lesions on the face or hands (Fig. 12.11) and was admitted to a hospital for survey of liver functional disturbance. Urine color was reddish-brown (Fig. 12.12), and his biochemical tests were AST 67 IU/mL,

ALT 54 IU/mL, GGT 191 IU/mL, HCV RNA 4.7 × 10 [6], and genotype Ib. Urinary data were ALA 2.4 mg/day (N < 3), PBG 0.8 mg/day (N < 5), UP 1029 μg/g CRN (N < 20), and CP 524 μg/g CRN (N < 170). IFNβ therapy (900 γ/day) was intravenously administered. HCV RNA became negative,

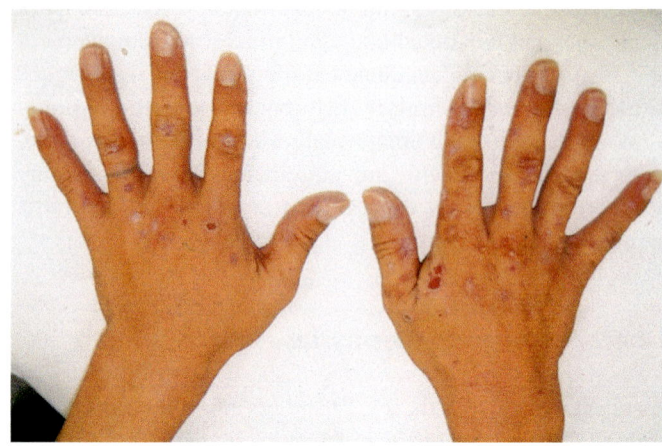

Fig. 12.11 Skin lesions on back hands in a 54-year-old male with PCT patient. There were scars, hyperpigmentation, and bullae and skin was fragile

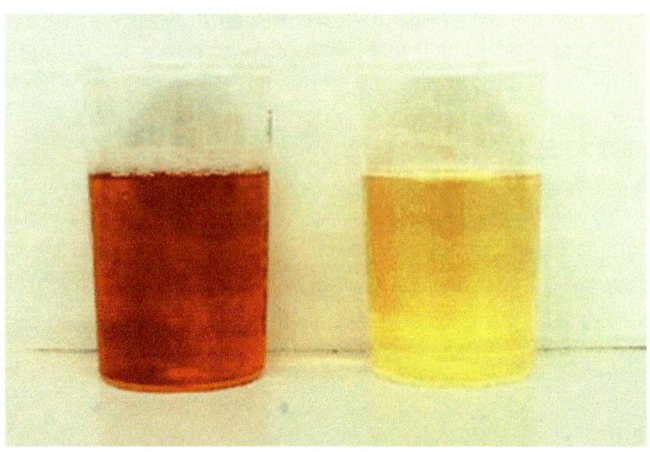

Fig. 12.9 Urine color of AIP patients. Urine color is amber in AIP patient (left) in comparison with one without porphyria (right)

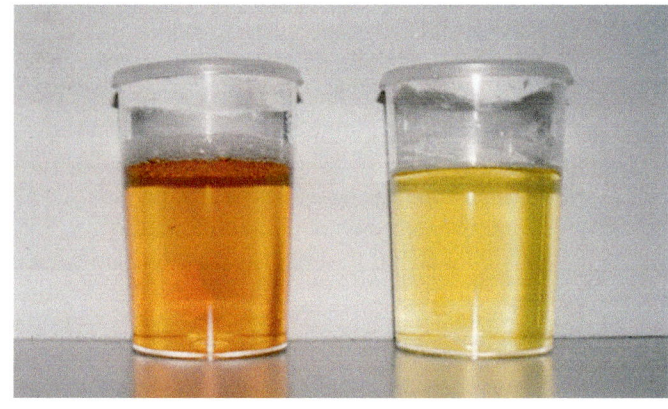

Fig. 12.12 Urine color in a patient with PCT. Urine color is reddish-brown in a patient with PCT (left) in comparison with one in a patient without porphyria (right)

Fig. 12.10 Dosage of morphine chloride related with urinary value of δ-aminolevulinic acid (ALA) and porphobilinogen (PBG) in a 34-year-old female with AIP. She had severe abdominal pain and intramuscular management of morphine chloride. Dosage of morphine chloride is closely related with urinary excretion of PBG and ALA, and PBG is closely related with dosage of morphine chloride in comparison with ALA

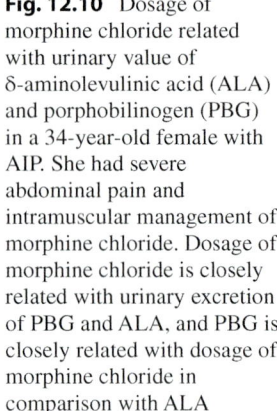
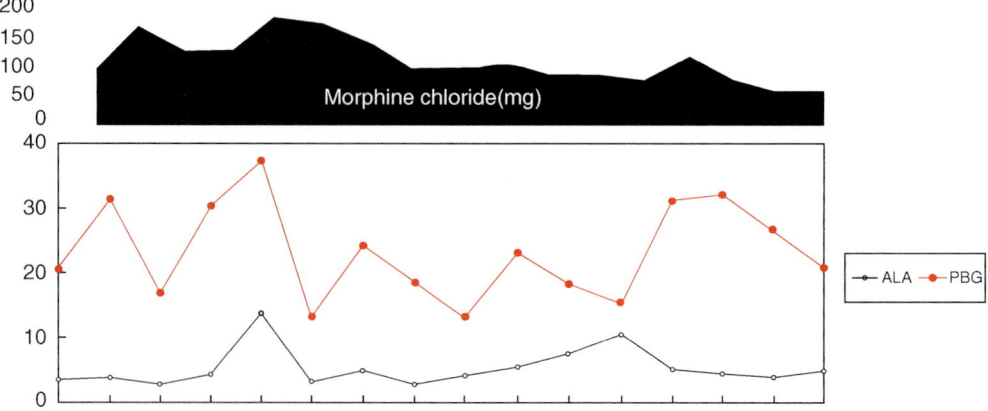

porphyrins decreased in urine, and the skin lesion disappeared. On decreasing intake of alcohol, there was no more liver functional disturbance.

12.5 Amyloidosis

Amyloid deposition occurs in the liver in primary amyloidosis, secondary amyloidosis (in response to chronic infection or inflammatory process of tuberculosis, lepromatous leprosy, osteomyelitis, rheumatoid arthritis, or Crohn's disease), and heredofamilial amyloidosis. Primary amyloidosis (amyloid light chain case) is characterized by the deposition of abnormal extracellular protein in the form of fibrils in many organs, especially the heart, kidneys, gastrointestinal tract, and peripheral nervous system [70]. Hepatic involvement is not uncommon in both secondary and primary amyloidosis [71]. Hepatomegaly occurs in >50% of patients suffering from amyloidosis, but disturbance of liver function is mild [72]. Jaundice is rare, but a primary amyloidosis patient with severe jaundice was reported in 1971 [73], and 25 cases of cholestatic jaundice were discussed by Peters and colleagues [74].

Approximately 5% of patients with primary amyloidosis have clinical evidence of cholestatic jaundice [73]. In systemic amyloidosis, death often occurs from congestive heart failure or arrhythmia and is usually due to renal failure, but a few patients die of hepatic failure with cholestatic jaundice [74–77]. Therefore, it is significant to recognize the clinical features of primary amyloidosis with cholestatic jaundice and to investigate why cholestatic jaundice develops in patients with amyloidosis. Here we describe two patients with primary amyloidosis who developed severe cholestatic jaundice. Besides the clinical and histopathological features of the syndrome, we also describe the ultrastructural findings of the liver to discuss the pathogenesis of cholestatic jaundice in primary amyloidosis.

Case 12.7

A 73-year-old male complained of hoarseness, and squamous cell cancer of the vocal cords was diagnosed. Preoperative physical examination showed elastic liver palpable 6 cm beneath the right costal margin. His laboratory data were TBIL 0.4 mg/dL, DBIL 0.3 mg/dL, GOT 25 KU, GPT 20 KU, ALP 12.9 KAU, GGT 104 IU/L, and leucine aminopeptidase 358 GRU. Neither dilated biliary ducts nor space-occupying lesions were seen on ultrasonography. A month after laryngectomy, his liver function test results were TBIL 0.6 mg/dL, DBIL 0.4 mg/dL, GOT 81 KU, GPT 55 KU, LDH 382 WU, ALP 63.2KAU, GGT 357 IU/L, and LAP 1191 IU/L. Liver scintigraphy showed irregular uptake of technetium, and CT revealed an enlarged liver, mild ascites, and splenomegaly. Peritoneoscopy showed enlarged liver with a lardaceous, smooth surface, and acinus or white markings were ambiguous (Fig. 12.13). Biopsied tissue showed amorphous eosinophilic material in the perisinusoidal space compressing hepatocytes, while fine granules were seen in hepatocytes of the pericentral veins (Fig. 12.14). Congo red staining was positive in the amorphous material, and polarized light microscopy showed green fluorescence in the perisinusoidal space. Electron microscopy showed the presence of amyloid fibrils in Disse's space, and aggregates of electron-dense fine granules were seen near bile canaliculi (Fig. 12.15). Two months after peritoneoscopy, the patient became jaundiced. The laboratory data were TBIL 17.6 mg/dL, DBIL 17.0 mg/dL, GOT 270 KU, GPT 126 KU, LDH 543 WU, ALP 181.8 KAU, GGT 674 IU/L, LAP 1662 IU/L, albumin 4.4 g/dL, gamma-globulin 0 .6g/dL, IgG 580 mg/

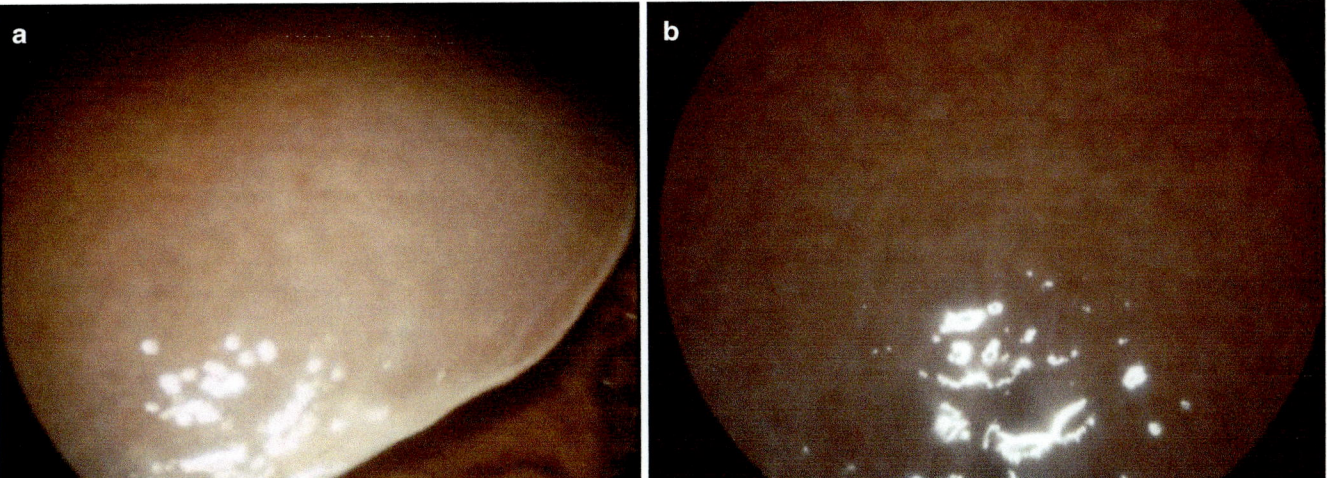

Fig. 12.13 Peritoneoscopic findings of liver with hepatic amyloidosis. (**a**) Liver surface is smooth and lardaceous. (**b**) Acinus markings are ambiguous, and peripheral portal veins are dilated

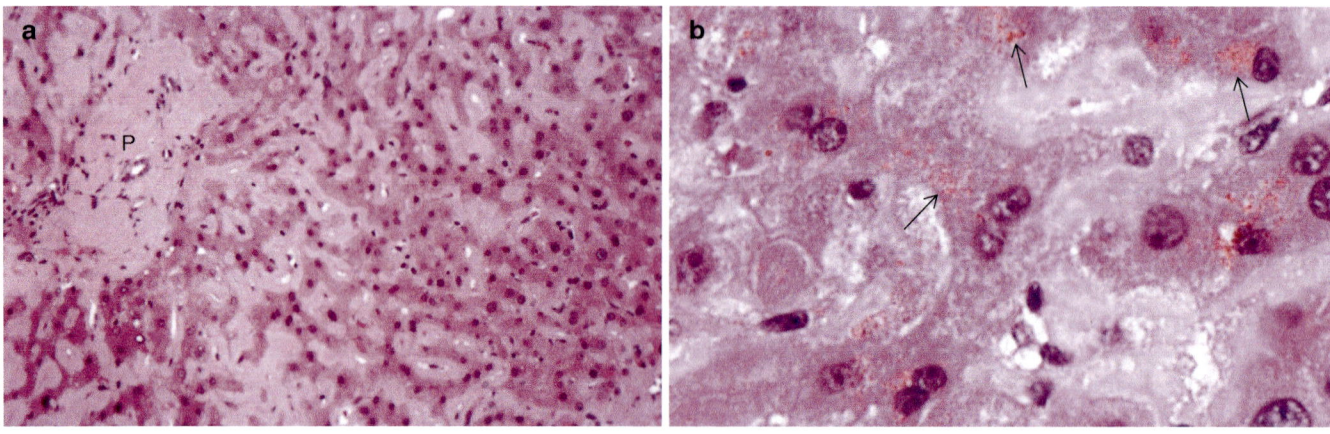

Fig. 12.14 Hepatic amyloidosis. (**a**) Amorphous eosinophilic materials are seen in the perisinusoidal space in a lobule, and the sinusoidal space is narrow. (**b**) Fine granules (arrow head) are present in hepatocytes around the central vein. *P* portal tract

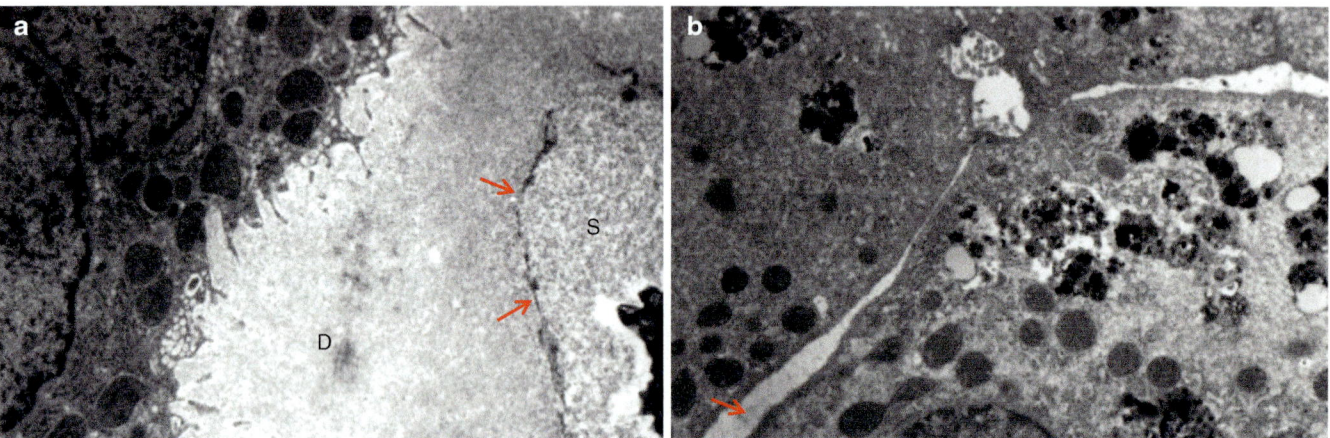

Fig. 12.15 Electron microscopic findings in liver with amyloidosis. (**a**) Amyloid fibrils are present not only in Disse's space(D), but also in sinusoid (S). Endothelial cells (arrow) along sinusoid are flattened, and materials are leaked into sinusoid. (**b**) Amyloid fibrils (arrow) infiltrate into lateral space of hepatocytes, and intercellular space becomes wide. Lysosomal granules can be seen in vicinity of bile canaliculi

dL, IgA 100.3 mg/dL, and IgM 164 mg/dL. Protein electrophoresis was normal, and Bence-Jones proteins were not detected. Bone marrow examination revealed no abnormal plasma cells. One month later, TBIL was 30.4 mg/dL (DBIL 28.6 mg/dL), pleural effusion and ascites appeared, and he died of cardiac and hepatic failure.

Case 12.8

A 58-year-old female presented with epigastralgia and hepatomegaly. Liver function tests revealed no abnormality. Three years later, TBIL was 1.1 mg/dL, DBIL 0.6 mg/dL, GOT 111 KU, GPT 84 KU, LDH 500 WU, ALP 41.6 KAU, GGT 239 IU/L, LAP 957 IU/L, ChE 0.69 ΔpH, ALB 3.6 g/dL, gamma-globulin 1.4 g/dL, IgG 1420 mg/dL, IgA 205 mg/dL, IgM 58 mg/dL, and indocyanine green test (R15) 32.4%. Protein electrophoresis was normal, and urine Bence-Jones proteins were not detected. Bone marrow examination

revealed 3% plasma cells. On physical examination, elastic liver was palpable 8 cm beneath the xiphoid process, but neither splenomegaly nor ascites were present. Scintigraphy revealed heterogeneous uptake of technetium in the liver, and CT showed enlarged liver without any defect or low attenuation. Peritoneoscopy revealed a lardaceous and irregular liver surface and dilated intracapsular vessels; liver biopsy showed deposits of amorphous eosinophilic material in the perisinusoidal space, and hepatocytes were atrophic due to compression of amyloid deposit (Fig. 12.16). Electron microscopy showed amyloid fibrils not only in the dilated Disse's space but also in the sinusoids; endothelial cells were flattened, hepatocyte microvilli facing Disse's space were spicular, and the nucleus of the hepatocyte was irregularly shaped; the intercellular space of epithelia in the bile duct was widened, and the basement membrane was destroyed due to compression of the amyloid deposit and secretory

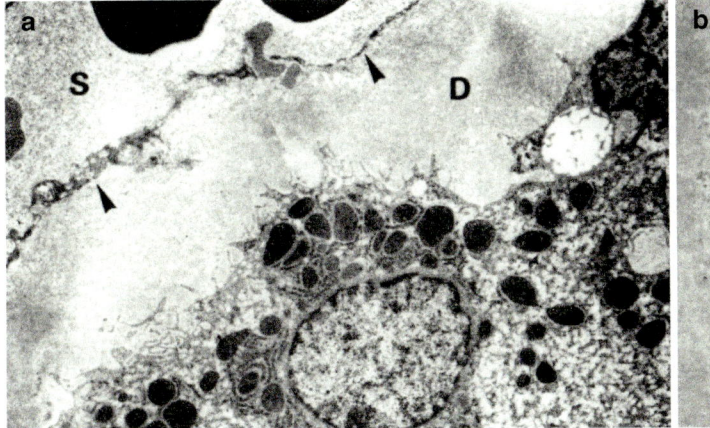

Fig. 12.16 Peritoneoscopic findings of liver with hepatic amyloidosis. (**a**) Liver is white in color, and there are small excavations and lymph vesicles on the liver surface. (**b**) Acinus markings are ambiguous, and peripheral portal veins are dilated. (**c**) Amorphous eosinophilic material is distributed diffusely in a lobule, and all hepatocytes are atrophic by compression of amyloid fibrils. *C* central vein, *P* portal tract (Reuse of Iwai M, et al. Cholestatic jaundice in two patients with primary amyloidosis. J Clin Gastroenterol 1999; 28: 162–6., with permission of Wolters Kluwer Health, Inc.)

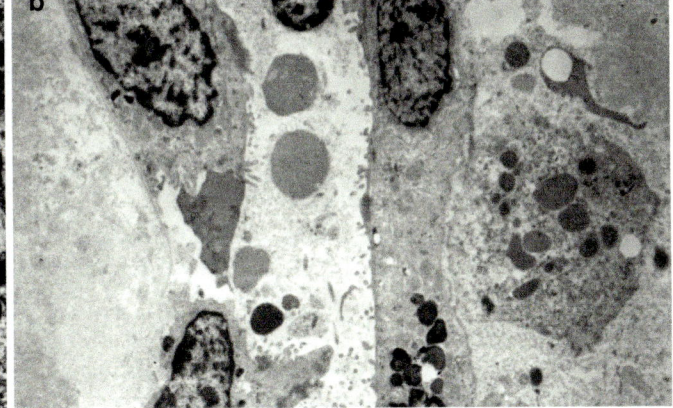

Fig. 12.17 Electron microscopic findings of liver with amyloidosis. (**a**) Amyloid fibrils are seen not only in dilated Disse's space (D) but also in the sinusoids (S). Endothelial cells (arrow head) are flattened and microvilli of cytoplasmic membranes are spicular. The nucleus is irregular in shape. (Reuse of Iwai M, et al. Cholestatic jaundice in two patients with primary amyloidosis. J Clin Gastroenterol 1999; 28: 162–6., with permission of Wolters KluwerHealth, Inc.) (**b**) Intercellular spaces of cholangiocytes are widened by compression of amyloid fibrils, and secretory materials are leaked outside. Bar = 1 μm

component leaking from the lumen (Fig. 12.17). After diagnosis of primary amyloidosis, dimethyl sulfoxide was administered. However, TBIL and DBIL reached 32.1 mg/dL and 28.3 mg/dL, respectively, 3 months after the onset of jaundice. The kidney function deteriorated, and the patient died of renal and hepatic failure.

12.6 Discussion of Amyloidosis

We treated two patients with systemic amyloidosis who developed severe cholestatic jaundice. The clinical manifestations, biochemical test results, macroscopic and microscopic appearance of the liver biopsied under peritoneoscopy, and the ultrastructural features of the hepatocytes have been described. Hepatomegaly was present without symptoms in our patients, and the median size of the liver was reported to be about 7 cm below the right costal margin [71]. Ascites were present in only one patient; it is relatively uncommon and may be associated with a good prognosis [78]. Globulin level in serum, especially IgM, was notedly low, and hypogammaglobulinemia has been detected in 34% of amyloidosis patients [71]. They indicate urinary loss or suppression of normal immunoglobulin synthesis by an abnormal plasma cell clone. Gamma-glutamyl transpeptidase, leucine aminopeptidase, and alkaline phosphatase (ALP) were elevated in both patients. However, glutamic-oxaloacetic transaminase and glutamic-pyruvic transaminase were only slightly elevated. Isolated elevation of ALP is generally found [79], and the ALP level does not correlate with survival. However, extreme elevation of ALP in one of our patients was associated with hyperbilirubinemia. Bilirubin is almost always normal, and hyperbilirubinemia has been reported in only 5% of primary amyloidosis patients [73]. Our patients died of renal, cardiac, or hepatic failure within 3 months after the onset of jaundice. Thus, hyperbilirubinemia is a sign of the approach of the preterminal stage, and a marked increase of ALP leading to jaundice is associated with a poor prognosis [74]. Image analysis showed no dilatation of intrahepatic bile ducts. Cholestasis was due to parenchymal damage or to mechanical impedance to bile flow at the level of the bile canaliculi or at the small bile ducts. Hepatomegaly and mild ascites were seen in abdominal CT, but no low attenuation in the liver was detected [80]. Scintigraphy showed low uptake of technetium in the liver, as deposits of amyloid in Disse's space disturbed the transfer of technetium into hepatocytes and the reticular endothelium system, and portal hypertension had developed [77, 81].

Peritoneoscopy showed a lardaceous liver surface and dilated peripheral portal veins or numerous lymph vesicles. These peritoneoscopic findings are typical of hepatic amyloidosis [82]. Liver biopsy is said to carry an added risk in patients with amyloidosis [83], but peritoneoscopy with liver biopsy prevents patients from bleeding because anticoagulants are injected through needle biopsy or the biopsied area can be compressed by the needle. Thus, peritoneoscopy with liver biopsy is safer than echo-guided biopsy and is a useful tool in the diagnosis of hepatic amyloidosis.

Amorphous eosinophilic materials were present in the perisinusoidal space and portal tract, and they were identified as amyloid fibrils by Congo red stain and light hemifluorescence. Hepatic amyloidosis is classified into three types—vascular pattern, parenchymal pattern, and stromal pattern—according to the topographic distribution [84]. Amyloid fibrils in our patients could be identified not only in the parenchymal sinusoid involvement of Disse's space but also in the portal tracts. Our case was a mixture of parenchymal and stromal types. The amyloid fibrils infiltrated into the sinusoidal space, and it was narrow. Hence, portal hypertension may be caused by the blockage of sinusoids by amyloid fibrils.

A few reports have described ultrastructural findings in hepatic amyloidosis [85, 86], but there are no reports on the preterminal stage of hepatic amyloidosis and no confirmatory electron microscopic data on the pathogenesis of severe cholestatic jaundice in primary amyloidosis [87, 88]. In our cases, electron microscopy showed many lysosomal granules near bile canaliculi before the onset of jaundice, and some bile canaliculi were dilated with stunting or loss of microvilli. Edematous microvilli protruded into the lumen in the preterminal stage. As a result, the secretory vesicles or bile juice may have been retained because the structure of the cytoskeletal system around the bile canaliculi may have been damaged by compression of amyloid fibrils [89]. Amyloid fibrils infiltrated into the portal tracts and compressed bile ductules and the basement membrane of bile ductules were separated from the epithelium by infiltration of amyloid fibrils. As the contact was loose, bile juice may have been retained in small bile ductules and leaked from them. Amyloid fibrils were seen not only in Disse's space but also in the sinusoids. Hepatocytes were rendered atrophic by being compressed by amyloid fibrils; hepatocyte microvilli facing Disse's space were spicular, and irregularly shaped mitochondria with disturbed arrays of cristae were present in hepatocytes.

These findings suggest the difficulty in transporting and supplying essential materials from sinusoids to hepatocytes, and the disturbance in the uptake of essential substances from sinusoids may be closely related to hepatic failure. Cholestatic jaundice must be distinguished from obstructive jaundice in primary amyloidosis [90], and the pathogenesis of cholestatic jaundice should be examined in more detail by ultrathin sections from the same patient at different stages.

Treatment for amyloidosis depends upon the type of amyloidosis. Melphalan and prednine are superior to colchicine [91], and melphalan in combination with dexamethasone is highly effective in treating AL amyloidosis [92]. Autologous stem cell transplantation is considered to be a primary option, but few patients are required [93]. Thalidomide, lenalidomide, pomalidomide, and bortezomib are examined, and non-cell transplant candidates can be offered melphalan-dexamethasone or cyclophosphamide-bortezomib-dexamethasone. Other combination chemotherapies of cyclophosphamide-thalidomide (or lenalidomide)-dexamethasone, bortezomib-dexamethasone, and melphalan-prednisone-lenalidomide have been investigated, and antibodies designed to dissolve existing amyloid deposits are under study [94].

12.7 Anorexia Nervosa

Anorexia nervosa is an eating disorder predominantly affecting young women, and hepatic dysfunction is present among the patients, and it has the highest mortality rate of all psychiatric disorders due to multiple organ failure with hepatic insufficiency by severe malnutrition [95]. Patients have elevated value of liver biochemical test, predominantly the aminotransferases [95]. Previous pathological findings show centrilobular changes (trabecular atrophy and/or sinusoidal fibrosis), nonspecific periportal inflammatory infiltrates, and fatty changes, and glycogen is depleted or accumulated depending upon the duration of starvation [96, 97]. Hepatic cytoplasm and organelles are quite low in density [97] and there are numerous autophagosomes [96]. Pathogenesis of acute liver insufficiency is not clarified yet, but two principle hypotheses, acute hypoperfusion and starvation-induced autophagy, are discussed. The treatment is hydration, correction of electrolyte and fluid imbalance, and gradual nutritional support in consideration of refeeding syndrome, and supervised increase in caloric intake and a return to healthy body weight can lead to normalization of elevated aminotransferases [95, 98].

Case 12.9

A 30-year-old female had a history of anorexia nervosa for 10 years, and general malaise and nausea with vomiting were developed a month ago, and 4 kg of body weight was additionally lost. Biochemical and blood tests after hospitalization revealed abnormal value, TBil 0.8 mg/dl, AST 5124 IU/L, ALT 4413 IU/L, PLT 13.1×10^4 ul/ml, and PT 49%. Her liver biopsy under guidance of ultrasonography showed disarrayed trabecular structure in periportal tract and hepatocytes revealed pale staining by hematoxylin and eosin (Figs. 12.18a), and sinusoidal spaces in pericentral area were dilated, and endothelial cells were decreased in number (Figs. 12.18b). Fibrosis was seen in portal tract and slightly present in perisinusoidal space (Figs. 12.18c). Electron microscopy showed presence of giant mitochondria and poor structure of endoplasmic reticulum, Golgi apparatus, and mitochondria and their low density, and a fat storing cell was seen in contact with hepatocytes (Figs. 12.18d). Hydration and intravenous infusion of electrolytes with intake of moderate calorie improved her general condition, and liver function tests were reverted to normal value, and gradual intake of food recovered her condition without refeeding syndrome.

12.8 Glycogen Storage Disease

The hepatic glycogen storage diseases are a group of inherited disorders affecting the metabolism of glycogen to glucose leading to excessive or abnormal glycogen in the tissues (Table 12.2), and there are more than ten types. Liver disease is seen in most types, and there are morphological changes of steatosis or glycogenic distension in hepatocytes and fibrosis or cirrhotic change in liver. In type 1A glycogen storage disease, deficiency of glucose-6-phosphatase leads to hypoglycemia during fasting, and patients present with lactate acidemia, hyperuricemia, hypertriglyceridemia, hypercholesterolemia with hepatomegaly, short stature, and immaturity [99]. Glycogen and fat are stored in the cytoplasm of hepatocytes, and their storage places nuclei in the periphery of the cytoplasm. There are two main complications of this disease, the development of hepatocellular adenoma and focal glomerulosclerosis [100, 101], and adenoma is reported to develop into hepatocellular carcinoma [102].

Frequent feedings of a high-starch, low-simple sugar or glucose polymer are recommended to keep glucose level at 70 mg/dl during infancy and childhood, and uncooked cornstarch is fed at night. Liver transplantation is effective for curing type 1A glycogen storage disease, and transplantation of both liver and kidney is recommended for patients with glomerulosclerosis [103].

Case 12.10

A 42-year-old male with a short stature and "doll's face" had a history of type 1A glycogen storage disease since the age of 14, and liver functional disturbance was monitored regularly. His laboratory data revealed high values of ALT and AST, and hepatomegaly was progressed, and he was admitted assessing his liver disease. His liver function test showed TBIL 0.47 mg/dL, ALT 32 IU/L, AST 79 IU/L, ALP 289 IU/L, GGT 80 IU/L, and negative HBsAg and HCV Ab. Liver biopsy showed distorted lobular formation with bridging fibrosis, but pseudo-lobules were not established; a magnified view showed enlarged pale-staining hepatocytes containing macrovesicular or microvesicular steatosis and

Table 12.2 Glycogen storage disease: enzyme defect, clinical findings, and histological features

Type	Name	Enzyme defect	Signs and symptoms	Liver histology
O	von Gierke's disease	Glycogen synthase	Ketotic hypoglycemia, alanine↓, lactate↓	Steatosis
Ia		Glucose-6-phosphatase	Hepatomegaly, lactate↑, glucose↓, uric acid↑	Steatosis, glycogenic hepatocytes
				Adenoma, hepatocellular carcinoma
Ib		Glucose-6-phosphate	Hepatomegaly, acidosis, glucose↓, neutrophils↓	Steatosis, glycogenic hepatocytes
		Translocase		Adenoma, hepatocellular carcinoma
II	Pompe's disease	Lysosomal-γ1–4 &	Cardiomyopathy, creatine	Cytoplasmic vacuoles, lysosomal mono-
		-γ1–6-glucosidase	Kinase↑	Particulate glycogen
IIIa/b	Cori's disease	Amylo-alpha-1, 6-glucosidase	Hepatomegaly, muscle weakness, glucose↓	Steatosis, glycogenic hepatocytes, fibrosis, cirrhosis (rare)
IV	Andersen's disease	Amylo-1-4 glycan6-glycosyltransferase	Hepatomegaly, cardiomyopathy, myopathy	Fibrosis, cirrhosis, ground-glass, diastase-resistant inclusions
VI	Her's disease	Liver phosphorylase E	Hepatomegaly, slow growth,	Glycogenic hepatocytes, steatosis, fibrosis, cirrhosis (rare)
			Ketotic hypoglycemia	
IX		Liver phosphorylase kinase	Hepatomegaly, hyperlipidemia	Non-uniform glycogenic hepatocytes, steatosis
XI	Fanconi-Bickel	GLUT2 transporter		Glycogenic hepatocytes

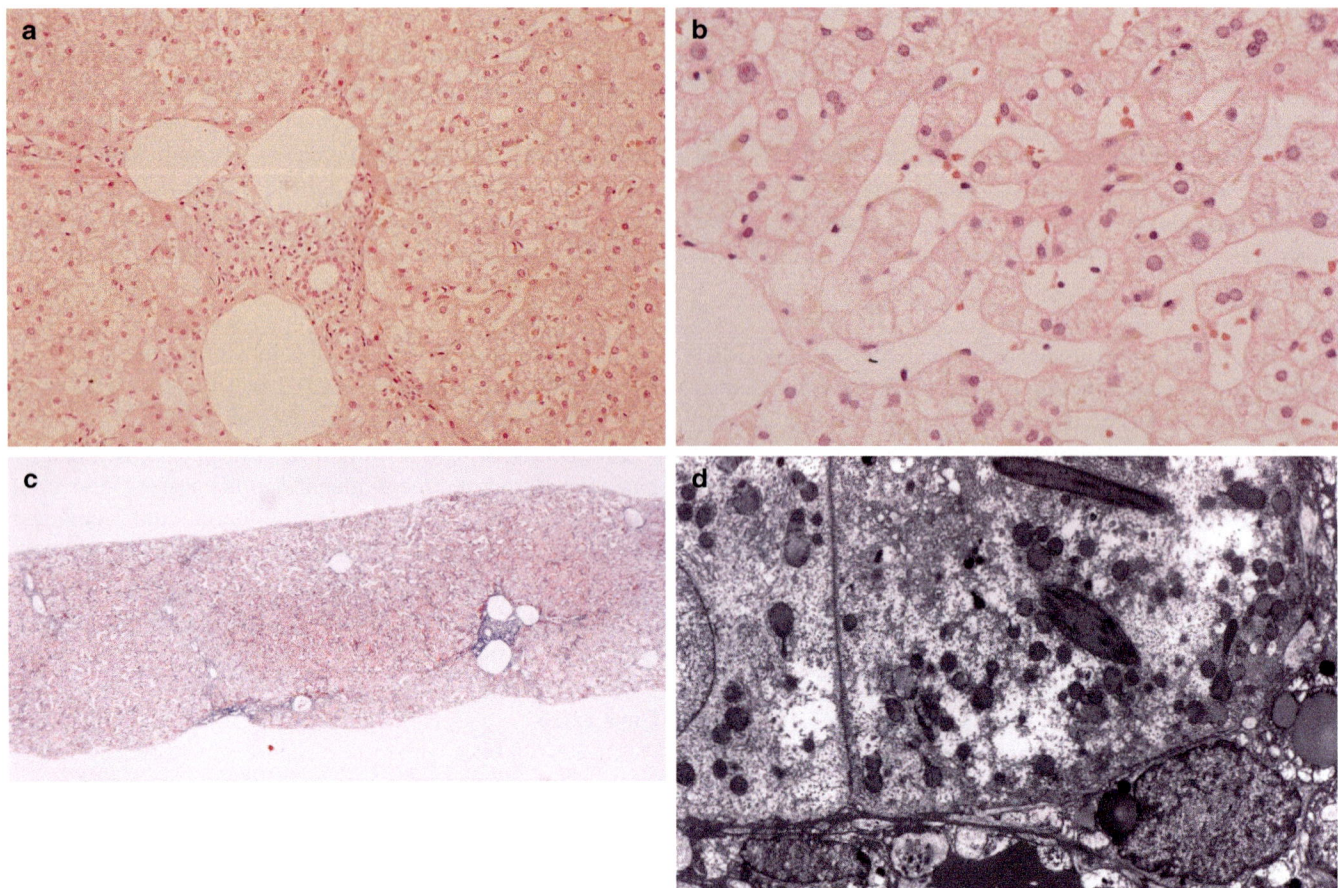

Fig. 12.18 Histological findings of liver with anorexia nervosa and electron microscopic findings of hepatocytes. (**a**) Trabecular structure is disarrayed in portal tract and hepatic cytoplasm is clear and sinusoids are dilated. (**b**) Sinusoids are dilated with retention of red blood cells in pericentral area and hepatic cytoplasm is clear. (**c**) Fibrosis is seen in portal tract and slightly detected in perisinusoidal space. Mallory-Azan staining. (**d**) Electron microscopy shows low density in cytoplasm and presence of giant mitochondria. Cristae in mitochondria are unclear, and rough endoplasmic reticulum and Golgi apparatus are not well preserved. Ito's cell with lipid is seen

vacuolated nuclei; sinusoids were compressed by swollen hepatocytes (Figs. 12.18 and 12.19).

Liver functional disturbance is seen in types I,III,IV,VI, and IX. Type III,IV,VI and IX are caused by deficiency of debrancher enzyme; amylo-alpha-1,6-glucosidase, branched enzyme; amylo-1,4 1,6-transglucosidase, liver phosphorylase E and liver phosphorylase kinase, and they are characterized by accumulation of glycogen not only in liver but also in heart, skeletal muscle, and kidney. The diagnosis is made by liver or muscle analysis for specific enzyme activity or genetic analysis or suggested by ultrastructure finding of glycogen structure.

For patients of types III and IV to maintain blood sugar, the diet used for type 1A patients is supplied by nocturnal nasogastric or gastrostomy tube.

12.9 Citrullinemia

Citrin is a liver-type mitochondrial aspartate-glutamate carrier [104]. Citrin deficiency is caused by a mutation of the SLC25A13 gene on the long arm of chromosome 7 [105] and is an autosomal recessive disorder and is prevalent in Japan and East Asia countries. Its disorder is classified into infantile (NICCD, neonatal intrahepatic cholestasis caused by citrin deficiency), child (FTTDCD, failure to thrive and dyslipidemia caused by citrin deficiency), and adult (CTLN2, citrullinemia type II) types, depending on onset.

The mutated gene disturbs the function of argininesuccinic acid synthetase, and hyperammonemia and citrullinemia occur. CTLN2 presents suddenly in older child or almost adulthood between ages 20 and 50 years. Disturbance

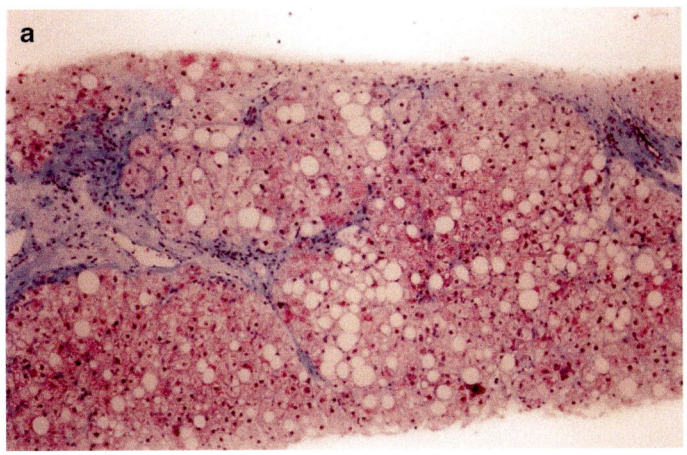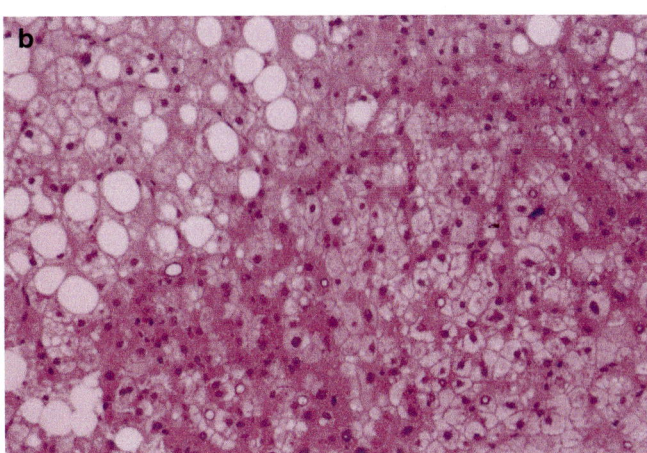

Fig. 12.19 von Gierke's disease. (**a**) Fibrosis is bridged from the portal tract, and fatty metamorphosis is seen. (**b**) Macrovesicular or microvesicular formation is seen in many hepatocytes, and nuclei are centrally localized. The cytoplasm is rarefied, and swollen hepatocytes compress sinusoids

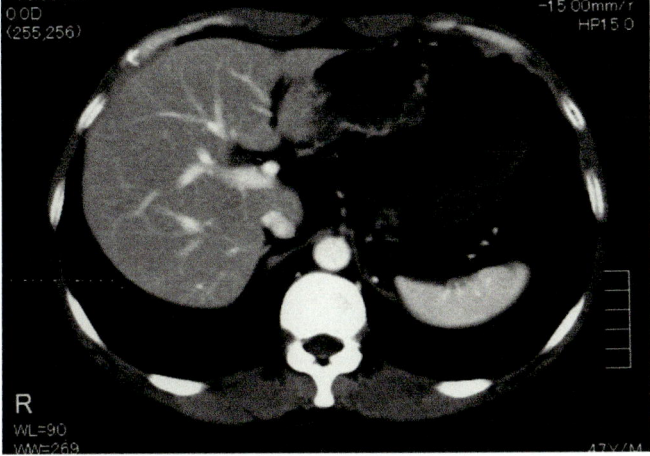

Fig. 12.20 Citrullinemia. CT with contrast medium shows smooth surface of normal-sized liver. CT density is lower in the liver than in the spleen. (Reuse of Fukumoto K, et al. A case of adult-onset type 2 citrullinemia having a liver histology of nonalcoholic steatohepatitis. Jpn J Gastroenterol 2008; 105: 244–51., with permission of Jpn Soc Gastroenterol)

of consciousness and abnormal behavior and seizures develop due to hepatic encephalopathy [106], and symptoms are provoked by alcohol, sugar intake, medication, and surgical treatment, and most individuals are fond of protein- and fat-rich foods such as beans and peanuts. Significant liver disease is evidenced by hepatomegaly and elevations of serum alanine transaminase, ammonia, citrulline, and arginine. Citrin deficiency causes excessive deposit of NADH, which induces overproduction of fatty acid in hepatocytes and inhibits its metabolism [107]. Steatosis is induced, and a second hit of oxidative stress develops nonalcoholic steatohepatitis. Liver histology shows fatty change [108], mild periportal fibrosis, nonalcoholic steatohepatitis [109], interface hepatitis, and cirrhotic change. To treat citrullinemia, low-carbohydrate, high-fat, and high-protein diet is recommended [110], and moderate amino acids including Asp, Asn, and Arg or an antioxidant derivative—as well as vitamin E—should be administered. Arginine should be infused to lessen hyperammonemia. To correct all the metabolic abnormalities or rescue hepatic encephalopathy, liver transplantation is considered [111].

Case 12.11

A 57-year-old male presented with liver functional disturbance for several years and dizziness for 2 months. He was hardly aroused when his name was called. His liver function test showed TBIL 1.5 mg/dL, ALT 55 IU/L, AST 40 IU/L, ALP 404 IU/L, GGT 192 IU/L, and NH3 132 μg/dL. Analysis of amino acids in serum showed citrulline 530 nmoL/mL, arginine 280 nmoL/mL, and cystine 63 nmoL/mL. A sequence of DNA extracted from white blood cells showed homozygotes of 851 del 14, and CTLN2 was diagnosed. Ultrasound examination showed blurred vision in the dorsal area of the liver. CT showed neither cirrhotic findings nor portosystemic shunts, and CT density was lower in the liver than in the spleen (Fig. 12.20). Liver histology showed fatty metamorphosis in zones 2 and 3, and mild fibrosis or pericellular fibrosis was seen around the central vein; macrovascular steatosis was observed around the central vein, and mild inflammatory cells were seen in the portal tracts; and neutrophilic leukocytes were concentrated in the necrotic area around the central vein (Fig. 12.21).

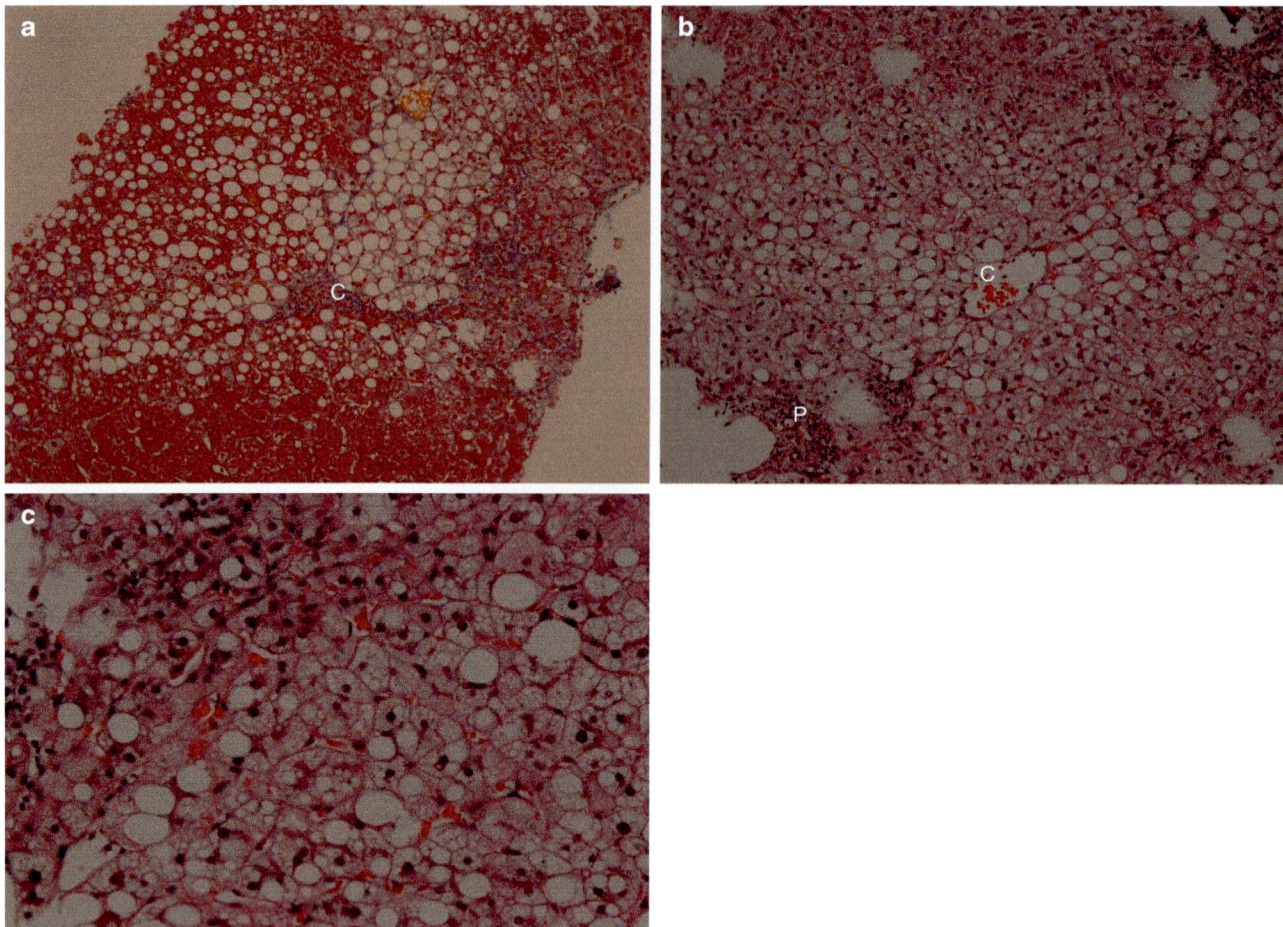

Fig. 12.21 Citrullinemia. (**a**) Mallory-Azan stain shows severe fatty metamorphosis in zones 2 and 3, and mild fibrosis is observed around the central vein. (**b**) Macrovesicular steatosis is seen around the central vein, and inflammatory cells are seen in the portal tracts. (**c**) Macrovesicular steatosis is seen around the central vein, and neutro-philic leukocytes are infiltrated. *C* central vein, *P* portal tract. (Reuse of Fukumoto K, et al. A case of adult-onset type 2 citrullinemia having a liver histology of nonalcoholic steatohepatitis. Jpn J Gastroenterol 2008; 105: 244–51., with permission of Jpn Soc Gastroenterol)

Acknowledgments Emeritus Professor Hisao Hayashi in Aichi Gakuin University School of Pharmacy and Dr. Hironori Mitsuyoshi in Kyoto Chubu Medical Center are acknowledged for their help in editing content of hemochromatosis and Wilson's or other copper-related diseases.

References

1. Powell LW, Kerr JF. The pathology of the liver in hemochromatosis. Pathobiol Anu. 1975;5:317–37.
2. Niederau C, Fischer R, Sonnenberg A, Stremmel W, Trampisch HJ, Strohmeyer G. Survival and causes of death in cirrhotic and non-cirrhotic patients with primary hemochromatosis. N Engl J Med. 1985;313:1256–62.
3. Feder JN, Gnirke A, Thomas W, et al. A novel MHC class I-like gene is mutated in patients with hereditary hemochromatosis. Nat Genet. 1996;13:399–408.
4. Pietrangelo A. Non-HFE hemochromatosis. Semin Liver Dis. 2005;25:450–60.
5. Létocart E, Le Gac G, Majore S, et al. A novel missense muta-tion in SLC40A1 results in resistance to hepcidin and confirms the existence of two ferroportin-associated iron overload diseases. Br J Haematol. 2009;147:379–85.
6. Pietrangelo A. Genetics, genetic testing, and management of hemo-chromatosis. Gastroenterology. 2015;149:1240–51.
7. Hussain SP, Raja K, Amstad PA, Sawyer M, Trudel LJ, Wogan GN, Hofseth LJ, Shields PG, Billiar TR, Trautwein C, Hohler T, Galle PR, Phillips DH, Markin R, Marrogi AJ, Harris CC. Increased p53 mutation load in nontumorous human liver of Wilson disease and hemochromatosis: oxyradical overload diseases. Proc Natl Acad Sci U S A. 2000;97:12770–5.
8. Tsui WM, Lam PW, Lee KC, Ma KF, Chan YK, Wong MW, et al. The C282Y mutation of the HFE gene is not found in Chinese haemochromatotic patients: multicentre retrospective study. Hong Kong Med J. 2000;6:153–8.
9. Wonke B, Hoffbrand AV, Brown D, Dusheiko G. Antibody to hepatitis C virus in multiply transfused patients with thalassaemia major. J Clin Pathol. 1990;43:638–40.
10. Kaji K, Nakanuma Y, Sasaki M, Unoura M, Kobayashi K, Nonomura A. Hemosiderin deposition in portal endothelial cells:

a novel hepatic hemosiderosis frequent in chronic viral hepatitis B and C. Human Pathol. 1995;26:1080–5.

11. Kothari T, Swamy AP, Lee JC, Mangla JC, Cestero RV. Hepatic hemosiderosis in maintenance hemodialysis (MHD) patients. Dig Dis Sci. 1980;25:363–8.

12. Schafer AI, Cheron RG, Dluhy R, Cooper B, Gleason RE, Soeldner JS, et al. Clinical consequences of acquired transfusional iron overload in adults. N Engl J Med. 1981;304:319–24.

13. Ali M, Fayemi AO, Rigolosi R, Frascino J, Marsden T, Malcolm D. Hemosiderosis in hemodialysis patients. An autopsy study of 50 cases. JAMA. 1980;244:343–5.

14. Carthew P, Dorman BM, Edwards RE, Francis JE, Smith AG. A unique rodent model for both the cardiotoxic and hepatotoxic effects of prolonged iron overload. Lab Investig. 1993;69: 217–22.

15. de Leeuw AM, McCarthy SP, Geerts A, Knook DL. Purified rat liver fat-storing cells in culture divide and contain collagen. Hepatology. 1984;4:392–403.

16. Ramm GA, Li SC, Li L, Britton RS, O'Neill R, Kobayashi Y, et al. Chronic iron overload causes activation of rat lipocytes in vivo. Am J Phys. 1995;268(3 Pt 1):G451–8.

17. Akalli O, Ropraz P, Trzeciak A, Benzonana G, Gillessen D, Gabbiani G. A monoclonal antibody against α-smooth muscle actin: a new probe for smooth muscle differentiation. J Cell Biol. 1986;103:2787–96.

18. Chezmar JL, Nelson RC, Malko JA, Bernardino ME. Hepatic iron overload: diagnosis and quantification by noninvasive imaging. Gastrointest Radiol. 1990;15:27–31.

19. Howard JM, Ghent CN, Valberg LS. Diagnostic efficacy of hepatic computed tomography in the detection of body iron overload. Gastroenterology. 1983;84:209–15.

20. Miller FH, Fisher MR, Soper W, Gore RM. MRI of hepatic iron deposition in patients with renal transplant. Gastrointest Radiol. 1991;16:229–33.

21. Stål P. Iron as a hepatotoxin. Dig Dis Sci. 1995;13:205–22.

22. Bacon BR, Britton RS. The pathology of hepatic iron overload: a free radical-mediated process? Hepatology. 1990;11:127–37.

23. Bacon BR, Tavill AS, Brittenham GM, Park CH, Recknagel RP. Hepatic lipid peroxidation in vivo in rats with chronic iron overload. J Clin Invest. 1983;71:429–39.

24. Yokoi Y, Namihisa T, Matsuzaki A, Yamaguchi Y. Distribution of Ito cells in experimental hepatic fibrosis. Liver. 1988;8:48–52.

25. Enzan H, Himeno H, Iwamura S, Saibara T, Ohnishi S, Yamamoto Y, et al. Sequential changes in human Ito cells and their relation to postnecrotic liver fibrosis in massive and submassive hepatic necrosis. Virchows Arch. 1995;426:95–101.

26. Schmitt-Graff A, Kruger S, Bochard F, Gabbiani G, Denk H. Modulation of alpha smooth muscle actin and desmin expression in perisinusoidal cells of normal and diseased human livers. Am J Pathol. 1991;138:1233–42.

27. Britton RS, Ramm GA, Olynyk J, Singh R, O'Neil R, Bacon BR. Pathophysiology of iron toxicity. Adv Exp Med Biol. 1994;356:239–53.

28. Ludwig JL, Hashimoto E, Porayko MK, Moyer TP, Baldus WP. Hemosiderosis in cirrhosis: a study of 447 native livers. Gastroenterology. 1997;112:882–8.

29. Grove J, Daly AK, Burt AD, Guzall M, James OF, Bassendine MF, et al. Heterozygotes for HFE mutations have no increased risk of advanced alcoholic liver diseases. Gut. 1998;43:262–6.

30. Bonkovsky HL, Jawaid Q, Tortorelli K, LeClair P, Cobb J, Lambrecht RW, et al. Non-alcoholic steatohepatitis and iron: increased prevalence of mutations of the HFE gene in non-alcoholic steatohepatitis. J Hepatol. 1999;31:421–9.

31. Bugianesi E, Manzini P, D'Antico S, Vanni E, Longo F, Leone N, et al. Relative contribution of iron burden, HFE mutations, and insulin resistance to fibrosis in nonalcoholic fatty liver. Hepatology. 2004;39:179–87.

32. Riordan SM, Williams R. The Wilson's disease gene and phenotypic diversity. J Hepatol. 2001;34:165–71.

33. Mehta R, Templeton D, O'Brien PJ. Mitochondrial involvement in genetically determined transition metal toxicity. II. Copper toxicity. Chem Biol Interact. 2006;163:77–85.

34. Roberts EA, Schilsky ML. A practice guideline on Wilson disease. Hepatology. 2003;37:1475–92.

35. Ala A, Walker AP, Ashkan K, et al. Wilson's disease. Lancet. 2007;369:397–408.

36. Roberts EA, Schilky ML. Diagnosis and treatment of Wilson disease: an update. Hepatology. 2008;47:2089–111.

37. Ferenci P, Caca K, Loudianos G, et al. Diagnosis and phenotypic classification of Wilson disease. Liver Int. 2003;23:139–42.

38. Nicastro E, Ranucci G, Vajro P, et al. Re-evaluation of the diagnostic criteria for Wilson disease in children with mild liver disease. Hepatology. 2010;52:1948–56.

39. Hayashi H, Tatsumi Y, Yahata S, et al. Acute hepatic phenotype of Wilson's disease: clinical features of acute episodes and chronic lesions remaining in survivors. J Clin Transl Hepatol. 2015;3:239–45.

40. Walshe JM. Diagnosis and treatment of presymptomatic Wilson's disease. Lancet. 1988;2:435–7.

41. Scheinberg IH, Sternlieb I. Wilson's disease. In: Smith Jr LH, editor. Major problems in internal medicine, vol. 23. Philadelphia, PA: WB Saunders; 1984. p. 25–35.

42. Strohmeyer FW, Ishak KG. Histology of the liver in Wilson's disease: a study of 34 cases. Am J Clin Pathol. 1980;73:12–24.

43. Sternlieb I. Evolution of the hepatic lesion in Wilson's disease (hepatolenticular degeneration). Prog Liver Dis. 1972;4: 511–25.

44. Strand S, Hofmann WJ, Grambihler A, et al. Hepatic failure and liver cell damage in acute Wilson's disease involve CD95 (APO-1/Fas) mediated apoptosis. Nat Med. 1998;4:588–93.

45. Korman JD, Volenberg I, Balko J, et al. Pediatric and adult acute liver failure study groups. Screening for Wilson disease in acute liver failure: a comparison of currently available diagnostic tests. Hepatology. 2008;48:1167–74.

46. Ala A, Walker AP, Ashkan K, Dooley JS, Schilsky ML. Wilson's disease. Lancet. 2007;369:397–408.

47. Davis W, Chowrimootoo GF, Seymour CA. Defective biliary copper excretion in Wilson's disease: the role of caeruloplasmin. Eur J Clin Investig. 1996;26:893–901.

48. Walshe JM. Treatment of Wilson's disease with trientine (triethylene tetramine) dihydrochloride. Lancet. 1982;1:643–7.

49. Dhawan A, Taylor RM, Cheeseman P, et al. Wilson's disease in children: 37-year experience and revised King's score for liver transplantation. Liver Transplant. 2005;11:441–8.

50. Bellary SV, Hassanein T, van Thiel DH. Liver transplantation for Wilson's disease. J Hepatol. 1995;23:373–81.

51. Rakela J, Kurtz SB, McCarthy JT, Ludwig J, Ascher NL, Bloomer JR, et al. Fulminant Wilson's disease treated with postdilution hemofiltration and orthotopic liver transplantation. Gastroenterology. 1986;90:2004–7.

52. Pankit AN, Bhave SA. Copper metabolic defects and liver disease: environmental aspect. J Gastroenterol Hepatol. 2002;17(Supp. 3):S403–7.

53. Adamson M, Reiner B, Olson JL, et al. Indian child cirrhosis in an American child. Gastroenterology. 1992;102:1771–7.

54. Joshi VV. Indian child cirrhosis. Perspect Pediatr Pathol. 1987;11:175–92.

55. Muller T, Langner C, Fuchsbichler A, et al. Immunohistochemical analysis of Mallory bodies in Wilsonian and non-Wilsonian hepatic copper toxicosis. Hepatology. 2004;39:963–9.

56. Bawdekar AR, Bhave SA, Pradham AM, et al. Long-term survival in Indian childhood cirrhosis treated with D-penicillamine. Arch Dis Child. 1996;74:32–5.

57. Muller T, Feichtinger H, Berger H, Muller W. Endemic Tyrolean infantile cirrhosis: an ecogenic disorder. Lancet. 1996;347:877–80.

58. Muller-Hocker J, Summer KH, Schramel P, Rodeck B. Different pathomorphologic patterns in exogenic infantile copper intoxication of the liver. Pathol Res Pract 1998; 194: HAHN MD.

59. Hayashi H, Shinohara T, Goto K, et al. Liver structures of a patient with idiopathic copper toxicosis. Med Mol Morphol. 2012;45:105–9.

60. Petris M, Mercer JFB, Culvenor JG, et al. Ligand-regulated transport of the Menkes copper P-type ATPase from the Golgi apparatus to the plasma membrane; a novel mechanism of regulated trafficking. ENBO J. 1996;15:6084–95.

61. Montgomery BD, Anderson KE, Bonkovsky HL. Porphyrias. N Engl J Med. 2017;377(9):862–72.

62. Anderson KE, Bloomer JR, Bonkovsky HL, et al. Recommendations for the diagnosis and treatment of the acute por-phyrias. Ann Intern Med. 2005;142:439–50.

63. Whatley SD, Badminton MN. Acute intermittent porphyria. In: Pagon RA, Adam MP, Ardinger HH, et al., editors. GeneReviews. Seattle: University of Washington; 2013.

64. Bissell DM, Lai JC, Meister RK, Blanc PD. Role of delta-aminolevulinic acid in the symptoms of acute porphyria. Am J Med. 2015;128:311–7.

65. Pischik E, Kauppinen R. An update of clinical management of acute intermittent porphyria. Appl Clin Genet. 2015;8:201–14.

66. Kappas A, Sassa S, Galbraith RA, Nordman Y. The porphyrias. In: Scriver CR, Beaaudet A, Sly WS, Valle D, editors. The metabolic basis of inherited disease. New York: McGraw-Hill; 1989. p. 1305–65.

67. Okano J, Horie Y, Kawasaki H, Kondo M. Interferon treatment of porphyria cutanea associated with chronic hepatitis C. Hepato-Gastroenterol. 1997;44:525–8.

68. Kondo M, Horie Y, Okano J, et al. High prevalence of hepatitis C virus infection in Japanese patients with porphyria cutanea tarda. Hepatology. 1997;26:246.

69. Ashwani K, Singal AK, Parker C, Bowden C, Thapar M, Liu L, McGuire BM. Liver transplantation in the Management of Porphyria. Hepatology. 2014;60:1082–9.

70. Kyle RA, Gertz MA. Primary systemic amyloidosis: clinical and laboratory features in 474 cases. Semin Hematol. 1995;32:45–59.

71. Gertz MA, Kyle RA. Hepatic amyloidosis (primary [AL], immunoglobulin light chain): the natural history in 80 patients. Am J Med. 1988;85:73–80.

72. Kyle RA, Greipp PR. Amyloidosis (AL). Clinical and laboratory features in 229 cases. Mayo Clin Proc. 1983;58:665–83.

73. Levy M, Fryd CH, Eliakim M. Intrahepatic obstructive jaundice due to amyloidosis of the liver. A case report and review of the literature. Gastroenterology. 1971;61:234–8.

74. Peters RA, Koukoulis G, Gimson A, Portman B, Westaby D, Williams R. Primary amyloidosis and severe intrahepatic cholestatic jaundice. Gut. 1994;35:1322–5.

75. Yamamoto T, Maeda N, Kawasaki H. Hepatic failure in a case of multiple myeloma-associated amyloidosis (kappa-AL). J Gastroenterol. 1995;30:393–7.

76. Dohmen K, Nagano M, Iwakiri M, Yamano Y, Kikuchi Y, Mizoguchi M, et al. A case of prominent hepatic cholestasis developing to hepatic failure in lambda-AL amyloidosis. Gastroenterol Jpn. 1991;26:376–81.

77. Zeijen RNM, Sels JPJE, Flendrig JA, Arends JW. Portal hypertension and intrahepatic cholestasis in hepatic amyloidosis. Netherland J Med. 1991;38:257–61.

78. Hormans Y, Brenard R, Ferrant A, Lagneaux G, Geubel AP. Long-term favorable outcome of portal hypertension complicating primary systemic amyloidosis. Liver. 1995;15:332–4.

79. Melato M, Manconi R, Magris D, Morassi P, Benussi DG, Tiribelli C. Different morphologic aspects and clinical features in massive hepatic amyloidosis. Digestion. 1984;29:138–45.

80. Mergo PJ, Ros PR, Buetow PC, Buck JL. Diffuse disease of the liver: radiologic-pathologic correlation. Radiographics. 1994;14:1291–307.

81. Itescu S. Hepatic amyloidosis. An unusual cause of ascites and portal hypertension. Arch Intern Med. 1984;144:2257–9.

82. Beck K, Dischler W, Helms M, Kiani B, Sickinger K, Tenner R. Atlas der Laparoskopie. F.K. Schattauer-Verlag: Stuttgart and New York; 1968.

83. Stauffer MH, Gross JB, Foulk WT, Dahlin DC. Amyloidosis: diagnosis with needle biopsy of the liver in eighteen patients. Gastroenterology. 1961;41:92–6.

84. Iwata T, Hoshii Y, Kawano H, Gondo T, Takahashi M, Ishihara T, et al. Hepatic amyloidosis in Japan: histological and morphometric analysis based on amyloid proteins. Hum Pathol. 1995;26:1148–53.

85. Skinner MS, Kattine AA, Spurlock BO. Electron microscope: Pico observations of early amyloidosis in human liver. Gastroenterology. 1966;50:243–7.

86. Livni N, Behar AJ, Lafair JS. Unusual amyloid bodies in human liver. Ultrastructural and freeze-etching studies. Isr J Med Sci. 1977;13:1163–70.

87. Finkelstein SD, Fornasier VL, Pruzanski W. Intrahepatic cholestasis with predominant pericentral deposition in systemic amyloidosis. Hum Pathol. 1981;12:470–2.

88. Mir-Madjlessi SH, Farmer RG, Hawk WA Jr. Cholestatic jaundice associated with primary amyloidosis. Cleve Clin Q. 1972;39:167–75.

89. Tsukada N, Ackerley CA, Phillips MJ. The structure and organization of bile canalicular cytoskeleton with special reference to actin and actin-binding proteins. Hepatology. 1995;21:1106–13.

90. Terada T, Hirata K, Hisada Y, Hoshii Y, Nakanuma Y. Obstructive jaundice caused by the deposition of amyloid-like substances in the extrahepatic and large intrahepatic bile ducts in a patient with multiple myeloma. Histopathology. 1994;24:485–7.

91. Kyle RA, Gerz MA, Greipp PR, et al. A trial of three regimens for primary amyloidosis: colchicine alone, melphalan, prednisone, and colchicine. N Engl J Med. 1997;336:1202–7.

92. Palladini G, Milani P, Foli A, et al. Oral melphalan and dexamethasone grants extended survival with minimal toxicity in AL amyloidosis: long term results of a risk-adapted approach. Hema. 2014;99:743–50.

93. Morie AG. Immunoglobulin light chain amyloidosis: 214 update on diagnosis, prognosis, and treatment. Am J Hematol. 2014;89:1133–40.

94. Gertz MA, Landau H, Comenzo RL, et al. First-in-human phase I/II study of NEOD001 in patients with light chain amyloidosis and persistent organ dysfunction. J Clin Oncol. 2016;34:1097–103.

95. Rosen E, Bakshi N, Watters A, Rosen HR, Mehler PS. Hepatic complications of anorexia nervosa. Dis Dis Sci. 2017;62:2977–81.

96. Rautou PE, Cazals-Hatem D, Moreau R, Francoz C, Feldmann G, Lebrec D, Ogier-Denis E, Bedossa P, Valla D, Durand F. Acute liver cell damage in patients with anorexia nervosa: a possible role of starvation-induced hepatocyte autophagy. Gastroenterology. 2008;135:840–8.

97. Komuta M, Harada M, Ueno T, Uchimura Y, Inada C, Mitsuyama K, Sakisaka S, Sata M, Tanakawa K. Unusual accumulation of glycogen in liver parenchymal cells in a patient with anorexia nervosa. Int Med. 1998;37:678–82.

98. Bridet L, Martin JJ, Nuno JL. Acute liver damage and anorexia nervosa: a case report. Turk J Gastroenterol. 2014;25:205–8.

99. von Gierke E. Liver and kidney in glycogen storage disease. Beitr Pathol Anat. 1929;82:497–513.

100. Labrune P, Trioche P, Duvaltier I, Chevalier P, Odièvre M. Hepatocellular adenomas in glycogen storage disease type I and III: a series of 43 patients and review of the literature. J Pediatr Gastroenterol Nutr. 1997;24:276–9.

101. Coire CI, Qizilbash AH, Castelli MF. Hepatic adenomata in type Ia glycogen storage disease. Arch Pathol Lab Med. 1987;111:166–9.

102. Limmer J, Fleig WE, Leupold D, Bittner R, Ditschuneit H, Beger HG. Hepatocellular carcinoma in type I glycogen storage disease. Hepatology. 1988;8:531–7.

103. Panaro F, Andorno E, Basile G, et al. Simultaneous liver-kidney transplantation for glycogen storage disease type 1A (von Girke's disease). Tranplant Proc. 2004;36:1483–4.

104. Parmieri L, Pardo B, Lasorsa FM, del Arco A, Kobayashi K, Iijima M, Runswick MJ, Walker JE, Saheki T, Satrustegui J, Palmieri F. Citrin and aralar1 are Ca2+−stimulated aspartate/glutamate transporters in mitochondria. EMBO J. 2001;20:5060–9.

105. Kobayashi K, Sinasac DS, Iijima M, Boright AP, Begum L, Lee JR, et al. The gene mutated in adult-onset type II citrullinaemia encodes a putative mitochondrial carrier protein. Nat Genet. 1999;22:159–63.

106. Kobayashi K, Saheki T. Aspartate glutamate carrier (Citrin) deficiency. In: Brorer S, Wagner CA, editors. Membrane transporter diseases. New York, NY: Kluwer Academic/Plenum Publishers; 2003. p. 147–60.

107. Saheki T, Kobayashi K. Mitochondrial aspartate glutamate carrier (citrin) deficiency as the cause of adult-onset type IIcitrullinemia (CTLN2) and idiopathic neonatal hepatitis (NICCD). J Hum Genet. 2002;47:333–41.

108. Saheki T, Kobayashi K, Iijima M, Horiuchi M, Begum L, Jalil MA, et al. Adult-onset type II citrullinemia and idiopathic neonatal hepatitis caused by citrin deficiency: involvement of the aspartate glutamate carrier for urea synthesis and maintenance of the urea cycle. Mol Genet Metab. 2004;81(Suppl 1):S20–6.

109. Takagi H, Hagiwara S, Hashizume H, Kanda D, Sato K, Sohara N, et al. Adult onset type II citrullinemia as a cause of non-alcoholic steatohepatitis. J Hepatol. 2006;44:236–9.

110. Nakamura M, Yazaki M, Kobayashi Y, Fukushima K, Ikeda S, Kobayashi K, Saheki T, Nakaya Y. The characteristics of food intake in patients with type II citrullinemia. J Nutr Sci Vitaminol. 2011;57:239–45.

111. Todo S, Starzl TE, Tzakis A, Benkov KJ, Kalousek F, Saheki T, et al. Orthotopic liver transplantation for urea cycle enzyme deficiency. Hepatology. 1992;15:419–22.

Hyperbilirubinemia

13

Toshinori Kamisako, Masaki Iwai, and Wilson M. S. Tsui

Contents

Abbreviations

ABC   ATP-binding cassette
BDG   Bilirubin diglucuronide
BMG   Bilirubin monoglucuronides
BRIC   Benign recurrent intrahepatic cholestasis
GST   Glutathione-S-transferase
ICP   Intrahepatic cholestasis of pregnancy
MRP2   Multidrug resistance-related protein 2
OATP   Organic anion transporting polypeptides
PFIC   Progressive familial intrahepatic cholestasis
TJP   Tight junction protein
UCB   Unconjugated bilirubin

T. Kamisako, MD, PhD (✉)
Osaka, Japan
e-mail: kamisako@med.kindai.ac.jp

M. Iwai, MD, PhD
Kyoto, Japan

W. M. S. Tsui, MD, FRCPath
Hong Kong, China

13.1 Bilirubin Metabolism Under Physiological Conditions

Approximately 250–300 mg bilirubin is formed in a normal adult in a day. Bilirubin, the final product of heme degradation, is catabolized by heme oxygenase-1 and biliverdin reductase, which are distributed in the liver, spleen, bone marrow, and reticuloendothelial systems [1]. Eighty percent of bilirubin is derived from hemoglobin in erythrocytes. The remaining 20% is derived from ineffective erythropoiesis in the bone marrow and from rapid hepatic metabolism of heme (shunt bilirubin) and hemoproteins, such as cytochrome P450 and myoglobin [2–4].

Under normal conditions, much of serum bilirubin exists as unconjugated bilirubin (UCB). The conjugated bilirubin con-

© Springer Nature Singapore Pte Ltd. 2019
E. Hashimoto et al. (eds.), *Diagnosis of Liver Disease*, https://doi.org/10.1007/978-981-13-6806-6_13

stitutes only less than 5% of total bilirubin in the serum of normal subjects [5]. Much of the serum UCB is bound mainly to albumin [6] or high-density lipoprotein [7], as UCB is poorly soluble in water. The bound UCB in the blood is transported to the liver. After transfer from the sinusoids into Disse's space, bilirubin is dissociated from albumin and is taken up into the hepatocyte across the sinusoidal membrane.

Uptake into the hepatocyte appears to be partly in a passive manner [8], and partly mediated by organic anion transporters [9]. Several proteins that transport organic anions, including bile acids and bilirubin, have been identified in the hepatocyte basolateral membrane. Organic anion transporting polypeptides (OATPs) are the sinusoidal organic anion transporters. OATP1B1, a member of the OATP family, is thought to be the most important bilirubin transporter protein that transports bilirubin from the blood to the hepatocyte [9]. However, the exact mechanism of UCB uptake has not been fully clarified [10].

After transport into the cytoplasm of hepatocyte, UCB is bound to glutathione-S-transferase (GST) A, also called ligandin [11], and is transported to the endoplasmic reticulum. After transfer into the endoplasmic reticulum, hydrophobic UCB undergoes glucuronidation to hydrophilic conjugated bilirubin. One or two sugar moieties are coupled to the –COOH of the propionic acid side chains of UCB in an ester linkage, resulting in bilirubin monoglucuronides (BMG), and then bilirubin diglucuronide (BDG), respectively [12]. The conjugation is catalyzed by bilirubin UDP-glucuronyltransferase, an enzyme encoded by the *UGT1A1* gene. UGT1A1 is a member of the UGT1 family in microsomal membranes.

Bilirubin becomes hydrophilic after conjugation for excretion into the bile. Conjugated bilirubin (BMG and BDG) is excreted into bile against the concentration gradient. It is transported by one of the canalicular ATP-binding cassette (ABC) transporters, multidrug resistance-related protein 2 (MRP2) [13]. In addition to the biliary excretion, conjugated bilirubin in hepatocyte is also secreted into sinusoidal blood flow by basolateral transporter MRP3 under physiological condition. The conjugated bilirubin in the sinusoidal blood flow is reuptaken by OATP1B1 and OATP1B3 subsequently for biliary excretion [14].

Biliary conjugated bilirubin is excreted to the intestine. In the intestinal lumen, bilirubin is converted to urobilinogens by bacterial enzymes. A minor part of bilirubin glucuronides undergoes deconjugation, mainly by bacterial enzymes, and the ensuing UCB undergo intestinal reabsorption.

13.2 Unconjugated Hyperbilirubinemia

The upper limit of normal serum UCB is 1.2 mg/dL (20 μM). Increases in serum UCB concentration can be due to an increase in the rate of the production of bilirubin, a decrease in uptake of bilirubin to hepatocytes, or a decrease in conjugation by UGT1A1.

13.2.1 Overproduction of Bilirubin

Overproduction of bilirubin is manifested by an increase in the serum UCB. The main source of bilirubin is hemoglobin in the erythrocytes. Hemolysis is one of the main causes of bilirubin overproduction. The increase in ineffective erythropoiesis—the increase in the destruction of developing erythrocytes in the bone marrow—is also an important disorder of bilirubin overproduction. It occurs in sideroblastic anemia, lead poisoning, erythropoietic porphyria, and primary shunt hyperbilirubinemia [15].

13.2.2 Constitutional Jaundice with Unconjugated Hyperbilirubinemia

Non-hemolytic unconjugated hyperbilirubinemia caused by the mutations in *UGT1A1* is classified into Crigler-Najjar syndrome type 1, Crigler-Najjar syndrome type 2, or Gilbert's syndrome. Crigler-Najjar syndrome type 1 is a severe unconjugated hyperbilirubinemia, characterized by complete loss of hepatic UGT1A1 activity [16]. Crigler-Najjar syndrome type 2 is a moderate unconjugated hyperbilirubinemia, characterized by a decrease of hepatic UGT1A1 activity to ≤10% of normal subjects [16, 17]. Gilbert's syndrome is a mild unconjugated hyperbilirubinemia in which the activity of UGT1A1 in liver homogenate drops to about 30% of normal [17]. In principle, the macroscopic findings and histology of

Table 13.1 Differential characteristics of constitutional jaundice with unconjugated hyperbilirubinemia

Variable	Crigler-Najjar syndrome type 1	Crigler-Najjar syndrome type 2	Gilbert's syndrome
Serum bilirubin	Increased: > 340 μM	Increased: between 103 μM and 339 μM	Increased: between 20 μM and 102 μM
Routine liver function	Normal	Normal	Normal
Hepatic UGT1A1 activity	Complete loss	10% or less of normal subjects	30% of normal
Molecular pathology	Mutation of UGT1A1 coding lesion	Mutation of UGT1A1 coding lesion, promoter lesion	Mutation of UGT1A1 coding lesion, promoter lesion
Pathology of liver	Normal	Normal	Normal; in some cases, lipofuscin pigment is deposited
Treatment	Phototherapy, plasmapheresis, liver transplantation	Phototherapy	None
Prognosis	Kernicterus in almost all patients	Usually benign	Benign

UGT1A1 uridine diphosphoglucuronyltransferase 1A1 gene

liver are normal in patients with non-hemolytic unconjugated hyperbilirubinemia (Table 13.1).

13.3 Gilbert's Syndrome

Gilbert's syndrome is a hereditary, chronic, and mild unconjugated hyperbilirubinemia resulting from impaired hepatic bilirubin clearance in humans [18]. The diagnosis of Gilbert's syndrome is based on:

- Normal liver function test with regular ultrasound findings.
- Fluctuating mild unconjugated hyperbilirubinemia.
- Lack of overt hemolysis or ineffective erythropoiesis.

Gilbert's syndrome is the most common constitutional jaundice with an incidence of about 2–7% in the general population. It is more common in men than in women. The serum bilirubin level is >1.2 mg/dL (20 μM), but <6.0 mg/dL (102 μM). Serum bilirubin is raised after fasting, physical exertion, and infections. UGT1A1 induction by phenobarbital is effective to reduce serum bilirubin concentration, but it provides no benefit other than a cosmetic reason [19]. The histological findings of liver biopsy are normal in most patients. However, it has been reported that lipofuscin pigment is deposited in higher amounts in some patients with Gilbert's syndrome [20]. Ultrastructurally, the hepatocytes reveal hypertrophy of smooth endoplasmic reticurum [21].

Case 13.1
A 65-year-old male presented with hyperbilirubinemia without any symptoms. His liver function test showed TBIL 4.54 mg/dL, DBIL 0.99 mg/dL, ALT 19 IU/L, AST 20 IU/L, ALP 211 IU/L, and GGT 21 IU/L. Ultrasound findings were normal. He had no overt hemolysis and was

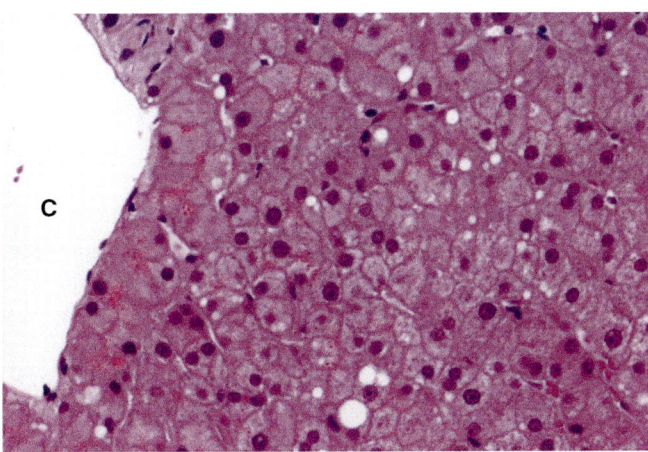

Fig. 13.1 Histological findings in patient with Gilbert's syndrome. Increased lipofuscin pigment is seen in hepatocytes of the pericentral area. (*C* central vein)

diagnosed with Gilbert's syndrome. His liver tissue showed small amounts of lipofuscin granules in pericentral hepatocytes (Fig. 13.1).

13.4 Crigler-Najjar Syndrome

Crigler-Najjar syndrome type 1 was first described by Crigler and Najjar in 1952 [22]. It is a rare disorder characterized by severe, inherited unconjugated hyperbilirubinemia. Until the introduction of phototherapy or plasmapheresis, most patients suffer from kernicterus in infancy and die in the first 18 months of life. Total serum bilirubin concentration is >20 mg/dL (340 μM) in this disorder. All serum bilirubin is UCB; no conjugated bilirubin is found in the serum using high-performance liquid chromatography, the most sensitive bilirubin measurement method. Treatment is aimed at reduction of serum bilirubin level to prevent kernicterus. Phenobarbital, which induces hepatic UGT1A1 in patients with Crigler-Najjar syndrome type 2 and Gilbert's syndrome, is ineffective in Crigler-Najjar syndrome type 1. Phototherapy [23] or plasmapheresis [24] is effective to reduce the risk of kernicterus. However, phototherapy in older children with Crigler-Najjar syndrome type 1 is less effective because of thickening of the skin, skin pigmentation, and decreased body surface compared with body weight. Liver transplantation is indicated [25].

Crigler-Najjar syndrome type 2, described by Arias in 1962, is characterized by moderate levels of hyperbilirubinemia [26]. In patients with this disorder, the total serum bilirubin level is >6 mg/dL (103 μM), but <20 mg/dL (340 μM). Unlike in Crigler-Najjar syndrome type 1, kernicterus is rare, and phenobarbital administration induces residual UGT1A1 activity with a reduction in serum bilirubin levels. In Crigler-Najjar syndrome type 2 patients, the bile contains significant amounts of bilirubin glucuronides [27]. Histological findings of liver biopsy are normal in Crigler-Najjar syndrome types 1 and 2.

13.5 UGT1A1 in Hereditary Unconjugated Hyperbilirubinemia

To date, more than 100 variant allelic genotypes have been identified in the human UGT1A1 gene [28]. In Gilbert's syndrome, two types of UGT1A1 mutations are described. The first phenotype can be described by a dinucleotide polymorphism in the TATA box promoter of the UGT1A1 gene, most frequently A(TA)₇TAA (*UGT1A1*28*) instead of A(TA)₆TAA (*UGT1A1*1*) [29]. Homozygosity for the A(TA)₇TAA is observed in most cases of Gilbert's syndrome in Caucasians and Africans, the frequency of UGT1A1*28 allele being 35–40% [30]. But the frequency is lower in Asians at 11–16% [31, 32]. The second phenotype is a missense mutation in the coding region of the UGT1A1, most commonly Gly71Arg in exon 1 (*UGT1A1*6*). This mutation is rare in Caucasians, but common in Asians [33–36].

Crigler-Najjar syndrome type 1 is characterized by a complete loss of bilirubin glucuronidation and provides evidence for coding region mutations within exons 1–5 of the UGT1A1 gene locus [37–40]. Mutations that cause a stop codon or shift the reading frame—thereby altering or deleting a large number of amino acid residues—always abolish UGT1A1 activity. The truncated protein loses one or more of its critical functional domains.

In patients with Crigler-Najjar syndrome type 2, molecular genetic studies have demonstrated presence of mutations in the coding regions of UGT1A1 [41–44]. Furthermore, unlike Crigler-Najjar syndrome type 1, nucleotide polymorphism in the TATA box promoter of the UGT1A1 gene has been reported [45]. From these findings on UGT1A1, it is important to recognize that Gilbert's syndrome represents one end of a spectrum of UGT1A1 activity that continuously extends to Crigler-Najjar syndrome type 1, which is a complete lack of UGT1A1 activity.

13.6 Conjugated Hyperbilirubinemia

Most conjugated hyperbilirubinemia syndromes are caused by hepatobiliary disease, and the rest are caused by rare constitutional jaundice (Dubin-Johnson syndrome or Rotor syndrome).

13.6.1 Hyperbilirubinemia Caused by Hepatobiliary Diseases

Disturbance in bilirubin secretion due to an acquired hepatobiliary disease (such as acute hepatitis, cirrhosis, alcohol-related liver disease, and cholestatic diseases) typically causes conjugated hyperbilirubinemia. Acquired hepatobiliary diseases are described in detail in other chapters of this book. In this section, cholestasis associated with genetic abnormalities of ABC transporters is described.

13.6.2 Cholestasis with Genetic Abnormalities of ABC Transporters

The hereditary defects of three ABC transporters have been linked to several hepatobiliary disorders, ranging from the severe form of progressive familial intrahepatic cholestasis (PFIC) to the mild form of benign recurrent intrahepatic cholestasis (BRIC) and intrahepatic cholestasis of pregnancy (ICP). In severe hereditary cholestasis, there are three types of PFIC caused by ABC transporters. These are the result of mutations in the ATP8B1 (PFIC type 1) [46], ABCB11 (PFIC type 2) [47, 48], and ABCB4 (PFIC type 3) [49] genes.

ATP8B1 is an inward flippase for phosphatidylserine, which is crucial to maintaining cell membrane asymmetry. Mutations in the ATP8B1 gene cause PFIC type 1 (also known as Byler's disease), presenting in the neonatal period and characterized by elevated levels of serum bile acids, bilirubin and transaminases, low serum GGT activity, and low biliary bile acid concentrations. Diarrhea and growth failure are major complications, sensorineural deafness develops in 30% of patients, and progression to liver cirrhosis is slow. Mutations in the BSEP gene result in PFIC type 2. In this disease, liver damage is relatively restricted to hepatocytes, since bile acids do not reach the bile canaliculi and bile ducts; this explains the normal GGT levels in these patients. Accumulation of bile acids in hepatocytes causes giant cell hepatitis and progressive liver damage. A complete loss of this protein is associated with development of neoplasm in the liver including hepatocellular carcinoma [50] and cholangiocarcinoma [51]. PFIC type 3 is caused by mutations in the encoding MDR3. This protein is essential for entry of the main phospholipid, phosphatidylcholine, into bile. This disease is characterized by high GGT levels, bile duct disease, and progressive cholestasis in infants, leading to end-stage liver disease.

Liver biopsy from patients with PFIC types 1, 2, and 3 shows canalicular cholestasis with abnormal bile duct epithelium in the early stages of the diseases and biliary cirrhosis in later phase. In PFIC type 1, canalicular cholestasis is seen (Fig. 13.2a), and coarse bile juice is ultrastructurally visible in the dilated bile canaliculus with the loss of microvilli (Fig. 13.2b), and bile is coarsely granular. In PFIC type 2, hepatocellular necrosis, moderate inflammatory infiltrate, and portal bridging fibrosis are seen (Fig. 13.3a). Inflammation is more pronounced than in PFIC type 1 [52], and focal giant cell transformation is evident (Fig. 13.3b), and bile is ultrastructurally filamentous. Liver biopsy of PFIC type 3 shows nonspecific portal inflammation (Fig. 13.4a) [49], and ductular reaction and subsequent fibrosis are seen in the first year of life (Fig. 13.4b).

These three liver diseases can progress rapidly and cause patients to require liver transplantation at an early age. Ursodeoxycholic acid may ameliorate symptoms and normalize hepatic biochemical tests in up to 60% of PFIC type 3 patients. Liver transplantation is required in 50% of patients.

Mild variants of PFIC types 1 and 2 are thought to be forms of BRIC [53, 54]. MDR3 heterozygous mutations may also play an important role in ICP [55–57]. Patients with ICP are healthy under nonpregnant conditions, though they may develop symptoms with exposure to high levels of estrogens.

In addition to these three PFICs, another type of PFIC, PFIC type 4, is described in 2014. PFIC type 4 is not caused by ABC transporter mutation but is attributed to

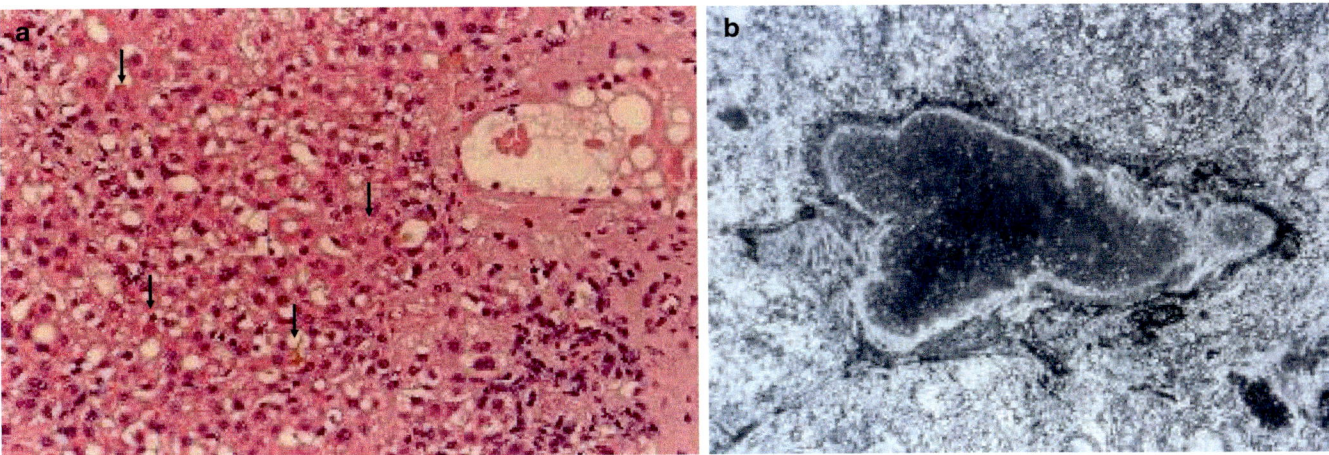

Fig. 13.2 Histological and electron microscopic findings in PFIC type 1 (Byler's disease). (**a**) Bland cholestasis is seen in dilated canaliculi (arrows), and there is little inflammatory activity. (**b**) Dilated canaliculus with loss of microvilli is filled with loose, coarsely granular bile

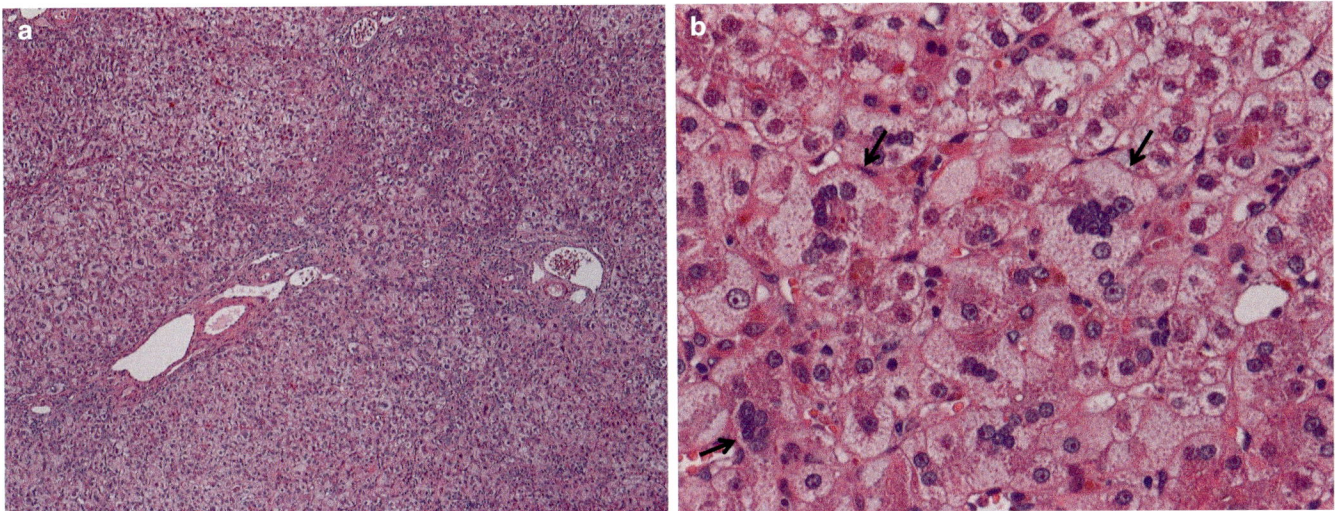

Fig. 13.3 Histological findings in PFIC type 2. (**a**) Liver biopsy shows chronic hepatitic picture with portal-to-portal fibrous bridging, moderate inflammatory infiltrate, intact interlobular bile ducts, and swollen hepatocytes. (**b**) Cholestasis is prominent, hepatocytes are swollen, and focal giant cell transformation (arrows) is evident

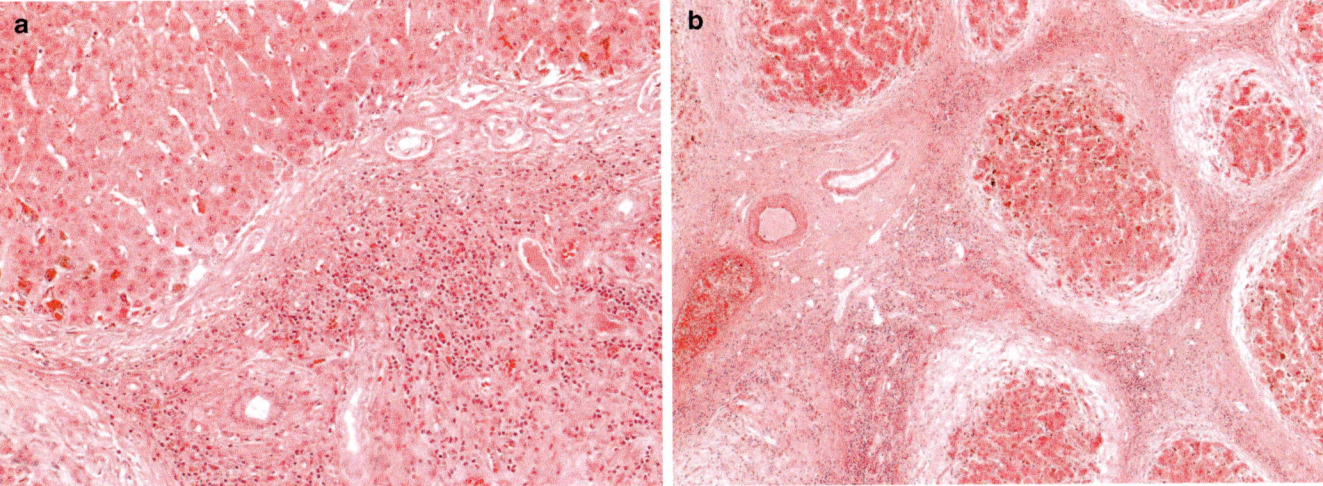

Fig. 13.4 Histological findings in PFIC type 3. (**a**) There is nonspecific inflammation in portal area with ductular reaction. (**b**) There is progressive fibrosis leading to cirrhosis

Table 13.2 Differential characteristics of constitutional jaundice with conjugated hyperbilirubinemia

Variable	Dubin-Johnson syndrome	Rotor syndrome
Serum bilirubin	Increased: between 34 and 85 µM (occasionally as high as 340 µM)	Increased: between 34 and 85 µM (occasionally as high as 340 µM)
Routine liver function	Normal (except for bilirubin)	Normal (except for bilirubin)
BSP administration		
– 45-min serum retention	Normal or slightly increased	Markedly increased
	Secondary rise at 90–120 min	No secondary rise
Urinary coproporphyrin excretion	Normal	Markedly increased
Proportion of coproporphyrin I (normal: ~ 25%)	Markedly increased (> 80%)	Increase (~ 60%)
Prognosis	Good	Good
Treatment	None	None
Pathology of liver	Black or greenish liver; dark brown pigment in hepatocyte (predominantly in centrilobular region)	Normal
Molecular pathology	Defect of MRP2 in canalicular membrane	Defect of OATP1B1/1B3 in sinusoidal membrane

BSP bromosulfthalein, *MRP2* multidrug resistance-associated protein 2

mutations in gene encoding the tight junction protein (TJP) 2 [58].

13.6.3 Constitutional Jaundice with Conjugated Hyperbilirubinemia

Constitutional jaundice with conjugated hyperbilirubinemia is classified into Dubin-Johnson syndrome or Rotor syndrome. Biliary bilirubin excretion is disturbed in both syndromes (Table 13.2).

13.7 Dubin-Johnson Syndrome

Dubin-Johnson syndrome is a rare hereditary hyperbilirubinemia characterized by fluctuating low levels of conjugated hyperbilirubinemia [59]. The clinical picture is chronic or intermittent hyperbilirubinemia, with serum bilirubin concentration between 2 and 5 mg/dL (34 and 85 µM) [60]. The bilirubin concentration occasionally elevates to 20 mg/dL (340 µM), which may be caused by several stress factors. The serum bilirubin is predominantly conjugated (60% of total), and two-thirds of conjugated bilirubin is BDG. Other laboratory tests, including serum activities of transaminase, alkaline phosphatase, and serum bile acid concentration, are normal.

Immunofluorescence and laser scanning microscopy have indicated the absence of MRP2 protein from the hepatocyte canalicular membrane in Dubin-Johnson syndrome [61]. Mutations in the MRP2 gene have been reported [62, 63]. After intravenous injection of bromosulfthalein (BSP), serum BSP decreases at near-normal rate for 45 min; however, the concentration increases afterward in Dubin-Johnson syndrome. The characteristic second serum BSP peak was identified after 90 min. Glutathione-conjugated BSP is also a

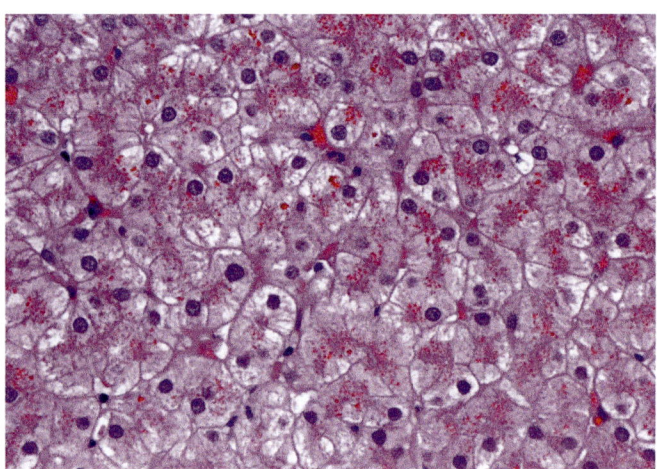

Fig. 13.5 Histological findings of Dubin-Johnson syndrome. Liver biopsy shows brown pigmentation in hepatocytes, and coarsely granular pigment in the perivenular area

substrate for MRP2 [64]. The defect in biliary excretion caused by MRP2 mutation produces the secondary BSP rise resulting from reflux of conjugated BSP from hepatocyte into blood.

The excretion of coproporphyrins in urine is normal; however, the amount of urinary coproporphyrin I is elevated and that of coproporphyrin III is reduced. The excretion pattern is also useful in the diagnosis of Dubin-Johnson syndrome. However, the relationship between porphyrin abnormalities and organic anion transport defect is not known.

Laparoscopic findings of livers of patients with Dubin-Johnson syndrome show the organ to be greenish black in color. This is due to the presence of pigment within hepatocyte lysosome that is more concentrated in the pericanalicular region and more prominent in centrilobular hepatocytes (Fig. 13.5). The pigment is thought to be a by-product of

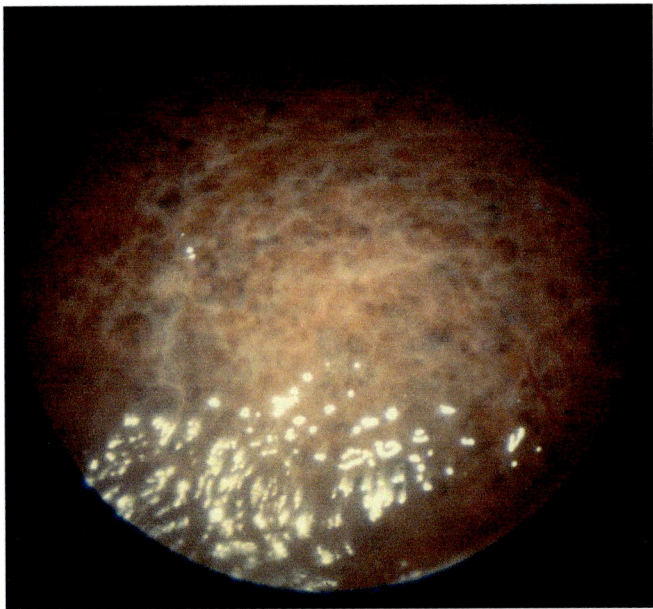

Fig. 13.6 Laparoscopic findings in patient with Dubin-Johnson syndrome and acute hepatitis. Scattered black maculae are seen on green liver surface

polymerization of catecholamine. It is reported to have disappeared in a patient who suffered from acute hepatitis. The prognosis is good, and no therapy is required. However, one should remain cautious over the metabolic delay of anionic drugs.

Case 13.2

A 45-year-old female complained of general malaise and brown urine, and her liver function test showed TBIL 5.6 mg/dL, ALT 1018 IU/L, AST 889 IU/L, ALP 468 IU/L, and positive IgM HAV antibody. After 1 month, the liver function test returned to normal values, but total and direct bilirubin remained elevated. Laparoscopy showed scattering black maculae on the green liver surface (Fig. 13.6).

13.8 Rotor Syndrome

Rotor syndrome is a disorder of chronic conjugated hyperbilirubinemia. It was first described by A.B. Rotor in 1948 [65]. The serum bilirubin concentration is between 2 and 5 mg/dL (34 and 85 μM) and is elevated by various stress factors as in Dubin-Johnson syndrome. The disappearance of serum BSP and indocyanine green (ICG) is delayed, and there is no secondary rise in BSP seen in the Dubin-Johnson syndrome. Biliary BSP and ICG transport is greatly delayed. Unlike in Dubin-Johnson syndrome, total coproporphyrins in urine are markedly elevated. Recently, homozygous mutation in both *SLCO1B1* and *SLCO1B3* genes resulting in complete and simultaneous deficiency of OATP1B1 and OATP1B3 has been identified as the molecular mechanism of Rotor syndrome [14].

The laparoscopic findings and histology of the livers of patients with Rotor syndrome are normal. As with Dubin-Johnson syndrome, the prognosis is good, and no therapy is required.

References

1. Maines MD. Heme oxygenase: function, multiplicity, regulatory mechanisms, and clinical applications. FASEB J. 1988;2:2557–68.
2. Berk PD, Howe RB, Bloomer JR, Berlin NI. Studies of bilirubin kinetics in normal adults. J Clin Invest. 1969;48:2176–90.
3. Israels LG, Yamamoto T, Skanderberg J, Zipursky A. Shunt bilirubin: evidence for two components. Science. 1963;139:1054–5.
4. Yamamoto T, Skanderberg J, Zipurskay A, Israels LG. The early appearing bilirubin: evidence for two components. J Clin Invest. 1965;44:31–41.
5. Adachi Y, Inufusa H, Yamashita M, Kambe A, Yamazaki K, Sawada Y, et al. Human serum bilirubin fractionation in various hepatobiliary diseases by the newly developed high performance liquid chromatography. Gastroenterol Jpn. 1988;23:268–72.
6. Brodersen R. Aqueous solubility, albumin binding, and tissue distribution of bilirubin. In: Ostrow JD, editor. Bile pigments and jaundice. New York, NY: Marcel Dekker Inc; 1986. p. 157–81.
7. Suzuki N, Yamaguchi T, Nakajima H. Role of high-density lipoprotein in transport of circulating bilirubin in rats. J Biol Chem. 1988;263:5037–43.
8. Zucker SD, Goessling W, Hoppin AG. Unconjugated bilirubin exhibits spontaneous diffusion through model lipid bilayers and native hepatocyte membranes. J Biol Chem. 1999;274:10852–62.
9. Cui Y, König J, Leier I, Buchholz U, Keppler D. Hepatic uptake of bilirubin and its conjugates by the human organic anion transporter SLC21A6. J Biol Chem. 2001;276:9626–30.
10. Wang P, Kim RB, Chowdhury JR, Wolkoff AW. The human organic anion transport protein SLC21A6 is not sufficient for bilirubin transport. J Biol Chem. 2003;278:20695–9.
11. Mannervik B. The isoenzymes of glutathione transferase. Adv Enzymol Relat Areas Mol Biol. 1985;57:357–417.
12. Jansen PL, Chowdhury JR, Fischberg EB, Arias IM. Enzymatic conversion of bilirubin monoglucuronide to diglucuronide by rat liver plasma membranes. J Biol Chem. 1977;252:2710–6.
13. Kamisako T, Leier I, Cui Y, König J, Buchholz U, Hummel-Eisenbeiss J, et al. Transport of monoglucuronosyl and bisglucuronosyl bilirubin by recombinant human and rat multidrug resistance protein 2. Hepatology. 1999;30:485–90.
14. van de Steeg E, Stránecký V, Hartmannová H, Nosková L, Hřebíček M, Wagenaar E, van Esch A, de Waart DR, Oude Elferink RP, Kenworthy KE, Sticová E, al-Edreesi M, Knisely AS, Kmoch S, Jirsa M, Schinkel AH. Complete OATP1B1 and OATP1B3 deficiency causes human Rotor syndrome by interrupting conjugated bilirubin reuptake into the liver. J Clin Invest. 2012;122:519–28.
15. Berlin NI. Overproduction of bilirubin. In: Ostrow JD, editor. Bile Pigments and Jaundice. New York, NY: Marcel Dekker Inc; 1986. p. 271–7.
16. Arias IM, Gartner LM, Cohen M, Ezzer JB, Levi AJ. Chronic non-hemolytic unconjugated hyperbilirubinemia with glucuronyl transferase deficiency. Clinical, biochemical, pharmacologic and genetic evidence for heterogeneity. Am J Med. 1969;47:395–409.
17. Black M, Billing BH. Hepatic bilirubin UDP-glucuronyl transferase activity in liver disease and Gilbert's syndrome. New Engl J Med. 1969;280:1266–71.

18. Powell LW, Hemingway E, Billing BH, Sherlock S. Idiopathic unconjugated hyperbilirubinemia (Gilbert's syndrome). A study of 42 families. N Engl J Med. 1967;277:1108–12.

19. Black MM, Sherlock S. Treatment of Gilbert's syndrome with phenobarbitone. Lancet. 1970;295:1359–61.

20. Barth RF, Grimely PM, Berk PD, Bloomer JR, Howe PB. Excess lipofuscin accumulation in constitutional hepatic dysfunction (Gilbert's syndrome). Arch Pathol. 1971;91:41–7.

21. Dawson J, Seymour CA, Peters TJ. Gilbert's syndrome: analytical subcellular fractionation of liver biopsy specimens. Enzyme activities, organelle pathology and evidence for subpopulations of the syndrome. Clin Sci (Lond). 1979;57:491–7.

22. Crigler JF, Najjar VA. Congenital familial nonhemolytic jaundice with kernicterus. Pediatrics. 1952;10:169–80.

23. Shevell MI, Bernard B, Adelson JW, Doody DP, Laberge JM, Guttman FM. Crigler-Najjar syndrome type I: treatment by home phototherapy followed by orthotopic hepatic transplantation. J Pediatr. 1987;110:429–31.

24. Berk PD, Martin JF, Blaschke TF, Scharschmidt BF, Plotz PH. Unconjugated hyperbilirubinemia. Physiologic evaluation and experimental approaches to therapy. Ann Intern Med. 1975;82:552–70.

25. Fox IJ, Chowdhury JR, Kaufman SS, Goertzen TC, Chowdhury NR, Warkentin PI, et al. Treatment of the Crigler-Najjar syndrome type I with hepatocyte transplantation. New Engl J Med. 1998;338:1422–6.

26. Arias IM. Chronic familial nonhemolytic jaundice with conjugated bilirubin in the serum. Gastroenterology. 1962;43:588–90.

27. Sinaasappel M, Jansen PL. The differential diagnosis of Crigler-Najjar disease, types 1 and 2, by bile pigment analysis. Gastroenterology. 1991;100:783–9.

28. Strassburg CP, Lankisch TO, Manns MP, Ehmer U. Family 1 uridine-5'-diphosphate glucuronosyltransferases (UGT1A): from Gilbert's syndrome to genetic organization and variability. Arch Toxicol. 2008;82:415–33.

29. Bosma PJ, Chowdhury JR, Bakker C, Gantle S, de Boer A, Oostra BA, et al. The genetic basis of the reduced expression of bilirubin UDP-glucuronosyltransferase 1 in Gilbert's syndrome. N Engl J Med. 1995;333:1171–5.

30. Beutler E, Gelbart T, Demina A. Racial variability in the UDP-glucuronosyltransferase 1 (UGT1A1) promoter: a balanced polymorphism for regulation of bilirubin metabolism? Proc Natl Acad Sci U S A. 1998;95:8170–4.

31. Ando Y, Chida M, Nakayama K, Saka H, Kamataki T. The UGT1A1*28 allele is relatively rare in a Japanese population. Pharmacogenetics. 1998;8:357–60.

32. Ki CS, Lee KA, Lee SY, Kim HJ, Cho SS, Park JH, Cho S, Sohn KM, Kim JW. Haplotype structure of the UDP-glucuronosyltransferase 1A1 (UGT1A1) gene and its relationship to serum total bilirubin concentration in a male Korean population. Clin Chem. 2003;49:2078–81.

33. Aono S, Adachi Y, Uyama E, Yamada Y, Keino H, Nanno T, et al. Analysis of genes for bilirubin UDP-glucuronosyltransferase in Gilbert's syndrome. Lancet. 1995;345:958–9.

34. Koiwai O, Nishizawa M, Hasada K, Aono S, Adachi Y, Mamiya N, et al. Gilbert's syndrome is caused by a heterozygous missense mutation in the gene for bilirubin UDP-glucuronosyltransferase. Hum Mol Genet. 1995;4:1183–6.

35. Kamisako T, Soeda Y, Yamamoto K, Sato H, Adachi Y. Multiplicity of mutation in UDP-glucuronosyltransferase 1*1 gene in Gilbert's syndrome. Int Hepatol Commun. 1997;6:249–52.

36. Takeuchi K, Kobayashi Y, Tamaki S, Ishihara T, Maruo Y, Araki J, et al. Genetic polymorphisms of bilirubin uridine diphosphate-glucuronosyltransferase gene in Japanese patients with Crigler-

37. Najjar syndrome or Gilbert's syndrome as well as in healthy Japanese subjects. J Gastroenterol Hepatol. 2004;19:1023–8.

37. Bosma PJ, Chowdhury JR, Huang TJ, Lahiri P, Elferink RP, Van Es HH, et al. Mechanisms of inherited deficiencies of multiple UDP-glucuronosyltransferase isoforms in two patients with Crigler-Najjar syndrome, type I. FASEB J. 1992;6:2859–63.

38. Labrune P, Myara A, Hadchouel M, Ronchi F, Bernard O, Trivin F, et al. Genetic heterogeneity of Crigler-Najjar syndrome type I: a study of 14 cases. Hum Genet. 1994;94:693–7.

39. Koiwai O, Yasui Y, Hasada K, Aono S, Sato H, Fujikake M, et al. Three Japanese patients with Crigler-Najjar syndrome type I carry an identical nonsense mutation in the gene for UDP-glucuronosyltransferase. Jpn J Hum Genet. 1995;40:253–7.

40. Kadakol A, Ghosh SS, Sappal BS, Sharma G, Chowdhury JR, Chowdhury NR. Genetic lesions of bilirubin uridine-diphosphoglucuronate glucuronosyltransferase (UGT1A1) causing Crigler-Najjar and Gilbert syndromes: correlation of genotype to phenotype. Hum Mutat. 2000;16:297–306.

41. Bosma PJ, Goldhoorn B, Oude Elferink RP, Sinaasappel M, Oostra BA, Jansen PL. A mutation in bilirubin uridine 5'-diphosphate-glucuronosyltransferase isoform 1 causing Crigler-Najjar syndrome type II. Gastroenterology. 1993;105:216–20.

42. Aono S, Yamada Y, Keino H, Sasaoka Y, Nakagawa T, Onishi S, et al. A new type of defect in the gene for bilirubin uridine 5'-diphosphate-glucuronosyltransferase in a patient with Crigler-Najjar syndrome type I. Pediatr Res. 1994;35:629–32.

43. Koiwai O, Aono S, Adachi Y, Kamisako T, Yasui Y, Nishizawa M, et al. Crigler-Najjar syndrome type II is inherited both as a dominant and as a recessive trait. Hum Mol Genet. 1996;5:645–7.

44. Yamamoto K, Soeda Y, Kamisako T, Hosaka H, Fukano M, Sato H, et al. Analysis of bilirubin uridine 5'-diphosphate (UDP)-glucuronosyltransferase gene mutations in seven patients with Crigler-Najjar syndrome type II. J Hum Genet. 1998;43:111–4.

45. Kadakol A, Sappal BS, Ghosh SS, Lowenheim M, Chowdhury A, Chowdhury S, et al. Interaction of coding region mutations and the Gilbert-type promoter abnormality of the UGT1A1 gene causes moderate degrees of unconjugated hyperbilirubinaemia and may lead to neonatal kernicterus. J Med Genet. 2001;38:244–9.

46. Klomp LW, Vargas JC, van Mil SW, Pawlikowska L, Strautnieks SS, van Eijk MJ, et al. Characterization of mutations in ATP8B1 associated with hereditary cholestasis. Hepatology. 2004;40:27–38.

47. Strautnieks SS, Bull LN, Knisely AS, Kocoshis SA, Dahl N, Arnell H, et al. A gene encoding a liver-specific ABC transporter is mutated in progressive familial intrahepatic cholestasis. Nat Genet. 1998;20:233–8.

48. Strautnieks SS, Byme JA, Pawlikowska L, et al. Severe bile salt export pump deficiency: 82 different ABCB11 mutations in 109 families. Gastroenterology. 2008;134:1203–14.

49. de Vree JM, Jacquemin E, Sturm E, Cresteil D, Bosma PJ, Aten J, et al. Mutations in the MDR3 gene cause progressive familial intrahepatic cholestasis. Proc Natl Acad Sci U S A. 1998;95:282–7.

50. Knisely AS, Strautnieks SS, Meier Y, Stieger B, Byrne JA, Portmann BC, et al. Hepatocellular carcinoma in ten children under five years of age with bile salt export pump deficiency. Hepatology. 2006;44:478–86.

51. Scheimann AO, Strautnieks SS, Knisely AS, Byrne JA, Thompson RJ, Finegold MJ. Mutations in bile salt export pump (ABCB11) in two children with progressive familial intrahepatic cholestasis and cholangiocarcinoma. J Pediatr. 2007;150:556–9.

52. Alonso EM, Snover DC, Montag A, Freese DK, Whitington PF. Histologic pathology of the liver in progressive familial intrahepatic cholestasis. J Pediatr Gastroenterol Nutr. 1994;18:128–33.

53. van Mil SW, van der Woerd WL, van der Brugge G, Sturm E, Jansen PL, Bull LN, et al. Benign recurrent intrahepatic cholesta-

sis type 2 is caused by mutations in ABCB11. Gastroenterology. 2004;127:379–84.

54. Tygstrup N, Steig BA, Juijn JA, Bull LN, Houwen RH. Recurrent familial intrahepatic cholestasis in the Faeroe Islands. Phenotypic heterogeneity but genetic homogeneity. Hepatology. 1999;29:506–8.

55. Painter JN, Savander M, Sistonen P, Lehesjoki AE, Aittomaki K. A known polymorphism in the bile salt export pump gene is not a risk allele for intrahepatic cholestasis of pregnancy. Scand J Gastroenterol. 2004;39:694–5.

56. Mullenbach R, Bennett A, Tetlow N, Patel N, Hamilton G, Cheng F, et al. ATP8B1 mutations in British cases with intrahepatic cholestasis of pregnancy. Gut. 2005;54:829–34.

57. Painter JN, Savander M, Ropponen A, Nupponen N, Riikonen S, Ylikorkala O, et al. Sequence variation in the ATP8B1 gene and intrahepatic cholestasis of pregnancy. Eur J Hum Genet. 2005;13:435–9.

58. Sambrotta M, Strautnieks S, Papouli E, Rushton P, Clark BE, Parry DA, et al. Mutations in TJP2 cause progressive cholestatic liver disease. Nat Genet. 2014;46:326–8.

59. Dubin IN, Johnson FB. Chronic idiopathic jaundice with unidentified pigment in liver cells: a new clinicopathologic entity with a report of 12 cases. Medicine (Baltimore). 1954;33:155–97.

60. Dubin IN. Chronic idiopathic jaundice. A review of 50 cases. Am J Med. 1958;24:268–91.

61. Kartenbeck J, Leuschner U, Mayer R, Keppler D. Absence of the canalicular isoform of the MRP gene-encoded conjugate export pump from the hepatocytes in Dubin-Johnson syndrome. Hepatology. 1996;23:1061–6.

62. Wada M, Toh S, Taniguchi K, Nakamura T, Uchiumi T, Kohno K, et al. Mutations in the canalicular multispecific organic anion transporter (cMOAT) gene, a novel ABC transporter, in patients with hyperbilirubinemia II/Dubin-Johnson syndrome. Hum Mol Genet. 1998;7:203–7.

63. Tsujii H, König J, Rost D, Stockel B, Leuschner U, Keppler D. Exon-intron organization of the human multidrug-resistance protein 2 (MRP2) gene mutated in Dubin-Johnson syndrome. Gastroenterology. 1999;117:653–60.

64. König J, Nies AT, Cui Y, Leier I, Keppler D. Conjugate export pumps of the multidrug resistance protein (MRP) family: localization, substrate specificity, and MRP2-mediated drug resistance. Biochim Biophys Acta. 1999;1461:377–94.

65. Rotor AB, Manahan L, Florentin A. Familial non-hemolytic jaundice with direct van den Bergh reaction. Acta Med Philipp. 1948;5:37–49.

Granulomatous Liver Diseases

14

Masako Mishima, Masahiko Koda, and Wilson M. S. Tsui

Contents

Abbreviations

BCG   Bacillus Calmette-Guerin
HIV   Human immunodeficiency virus
PBC   Primary biliary cholangitis

M. Mishima, MD
Kyoto, Japan

M. Koda, MD, PhD (✉)
Tottori, Japan

W. M. S. Tsui, MD, FRCPath
Hong Kong, China

14.1 Introduction

The liver is the largest parenchymal organ in the body and a prime target for the formation of granulomas because of its large population of fixed macrophages, the Kupffer cells. Granulomas are defined as circumscribed collections of inflammatory cells, such as activated macrophages, lymphocytes, histiocytes, and plasma cells. The diagnosis of granulomatous liver diseases is made by histological examination of liver specimens. However, the presence of the disease cannot be predicted by clinical symptoms and signs or serological data. The clinical manifestations are due to cytokines released by activated macrophages and lymphocytes. Symptoms are pyrexia, anorexia, night sweats, weight loss, and nonspecific constitutional

© Springer Nature Singapore Pte Ltd. 2019
E. Hashimoto et al. (eds.), *Diagnosis of Liver Disease*, https://doi.org/10.1007/978-981-13-6806-6_14

symptoms. Liver manifestations are hepatomegaly and deranged liver function such as elevated alkaline phosphatase. It is often asymptomatic and discovered as an incidental finding.

14.2 Etiology

Granuloma formation is due to bacterial, mycobacterial, rickettsial, chlamydial, fungal, viral, or parasitic infection, immunological disease, hypersensitivity, foreign materials, neoplasm, and other miscellaneous factors (Table 14.1). Sarcoidosis, infection, drug reactions, and primary biliary cholangitis are the four most common causes, accounting for >80% of cases. The incidence of the different etiologies, however, varies according to geographic region, characteristics of the patient population, and biopsy habits of clinicians. Diagnosis of granulomatous liver diseases is determined by its histological findings of caseous or non-caseous necrosis, location in acini, and bile duct injury. Thus the importance of hepatic granulomas lies in the opportunity to diagnose the underlying disease, which dictates prognosis and treatment. [1–3]

14.3 Diagnostic Evaluation

Hepatic granulomas have been classified into four morphologic types [4]. The first type is foreign body granuloma. The second one is lipogranuloma, which forms when histiocytes

Table 14.1 Etiology of hepatic granuloma

Infectious		Mycobacteria
		Tuberculosis
		Mycobacterium leprae
		Mycobacterium avium-intracellulare
		BCG immunotherapy
		Brucellosis
		Systemic mycoses
		Candidiasis
		Histoplasmosis
		Parasitic infections
		Schistosomiasis
		Toxoplasmosis
		Rickettsial infections
		Viral infections
		Hepatitis C
		EBV
		CMV
Noninfectious	Immunology disorder	Sarcoidosis
		Primary biliary cholangitis
		Common variable immunodeficiency
	Drugs and chemicals	Beryllium, thorotrast, allopurinol, sulfonamides, phenytoin, carbamazepine, chlorpropamide, quinidine, methyldopa, nitrofurantoin, isoniazid, amiodarone, diazepam
	Malignancy	Lymphoma
		Renal cell carcinoma
	Other cause	Foreign materials

ingest fat droplets released by ruptured steatotic hepatocytes or in mineral oil lipidosis. The third is an epithelioid type which consists of activated macrophages. These macrophages secreted a large amount of cytokines and are often multinucleated and surrounded by lymphocytes and plasma cells. The fourth is an inflammatory (lymphohistiocytic) type, composed of lymphocytes, plasma cells, and occasionally eosinophils and neutrophils without epithelioid cells.

Pathologically significant granulomas involve the formation of epithelioid cells. However, if the host is immunocompromised, the reaction may take the form of aggregates of foamy macrophages, without the formation of epithelioid cells and with little inflammatory response. Examples include lepromatous leprosy and Mycobacterium avium-intracellulare infection in AIDS patients. Besides epithelioid granulomas, other types of granulomas may not be clinically significant. Kupffer cell granulomas (or microgranulomas) are small and round clusters of unmodified histiocytes and are usual nonspecific findings resulting from the cleanup of necrotic hepatocytes or other debris by Kupffer cells. Bile granulomas, resulting from small clusters of bile-laden and foamy histiocytes, are often associated with surrounding extracellular bile or evidence of cholestasis [5].

The pathologist plays a key role in etiological diagnosis. Infections may often be identified morphologically, even before culture results are available. In suspected drug reactions, the finding of granulomatous hepatitis may serve to confirm the diagnosis. Thus, careful and systematic examination of the pathological specimen is important. This includes assessment of the features described below [6–8].

14.4 Distinctive Features of Granulomas

Sarcoid granulomas are characteristically large and noncaseating. They contain Schaumann bodies, asteroid bodies, or calcium oxalate crystals. They often coalesce to form conglomerates and undergo fibrosis. Epithelioid granulomas with a caseous or necrotic center are suggestive of an infective etiology, such as tuberculosis (Fig. 14.1). Associated

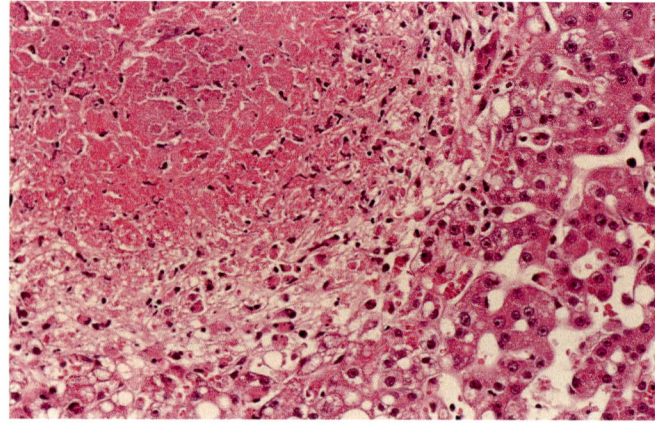

Fig. 14.1 Tuberculosis. Caseous necrosis is commonly present in tuberculous granuloma, and epithelioid cells and lymphocytes are present in the surrounding area

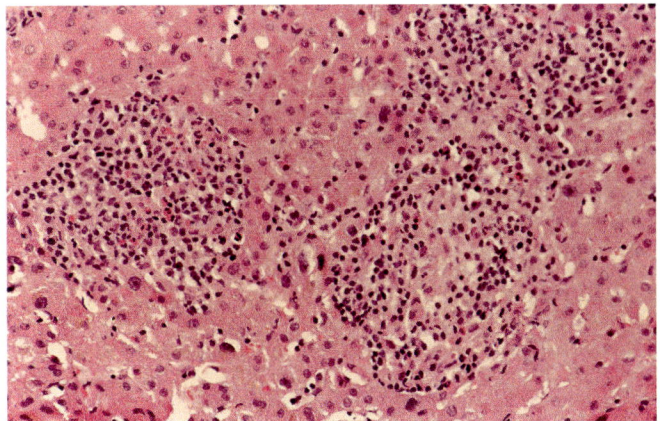

Fig. 14.2 Chlorpropamide-induced liver injury. Abundant eosinophils are seen in granulomas induced by chlorpropamide administration

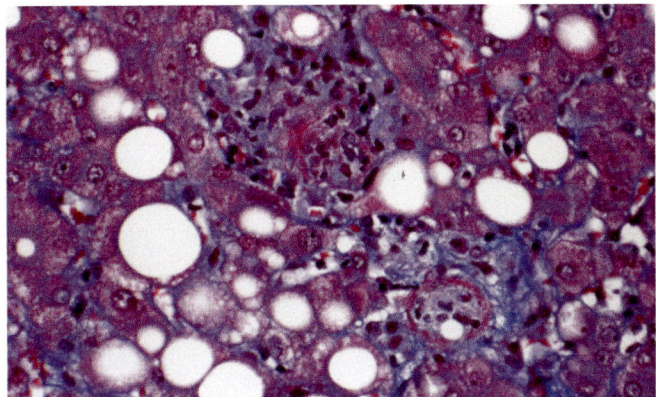

Fig. 14.3 Allopurinol-induced liver injury. Biopsied specimen of liver stained by Masson-Trichrome shows an eosinophilic ring of fibrin in granuloma

suppurative inflammation is commonly due to fungal infection or chronic granulomatous disease. Abundant eosinophils within or at the periphery of the granulomas are observed in acute drug reactions (Fig. 14.2) or parasitic infestation. The presence of fibrin-ring granulomas is characteristic of Q fever [9], but it is also reported in allopurinol-induced injury (Figure 14.3) [10], Epstein-Barr virus [11], cytomegalovirus [12], toxoplasmosis [13], leishmaniasis [14], and Hodgkin's disease [13].

14.5 Acinar Distribution

Sarcoid granulomas are diffusely distributed, though often portal or periportal in location. Granulomas in primary biliary cholangitis and schistosomiasis are mostly portal-based and are related to damaged bile ducts in the former (Figure 14.4) and obliterated portal venous branches in the latter. Granulomas caused by tuberculosis and drug reactions are randomly present in the parenchyma.

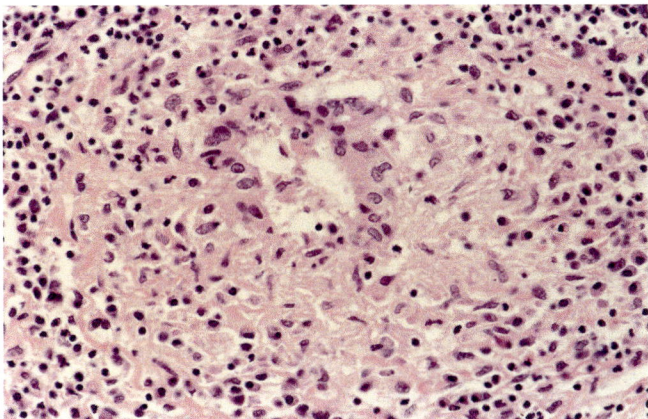

Fig. 14.4 Primary biliary cholangitis. An epithelioid granuloma surrounds damaged bile duct and is accompanied by lymphocytes, plasma cells, and neutrophils in the periphery

14.6 Associated Parenchymal Changes

Infective and drug-induced granulomas may be associated with a true hepatitis-like background. Fungal infection with angioinvasion can cause confluent necrosis or infarction. Bile duct damage and destruction are noted in primary biliary cirrhosis, sarcoidosis, and some drug reactions (Table 14.2).

14.7 Identifiable Etiological Agents

Apart from careful investigation at multiple levels, special histochemical and immunohistochemical stains for microorganisms are invaluable in the evaluation of granulomas. Polarization microscopy should be used to detect foreign bodies. **Polymerase chain reaction** can also be performed on liver specimens for infectious agents.

In many cases of granulomas, however, there are no morphological clues to the diagnosis. Hence, a complete workup needs to be done. Culture should be taken from suitable specimens from the patient, and a detailed drug history must always be taken. Other investigations, such as skin tests and serology, are performed as a diagnostic tool. In spite of these measures, the cause cannot be established in 10–25% of patients.

14.8 Immunological Disease

14.8.1 Sarcoidosis

Sarcoidosis is an inflammatory disorder of unknown etiology characterized by noncaseating granulomas [15]. There is usually no subjective complaint, and in the acute stage, high fever is generally found. Lung and intrathoracic lymph nodes are always affected, and extrathoracic organs are frequently involved. The

Table 14.2 Pathological features of granuloma and liver injury

		Non-necrotizing	Caseating	Location	Giant cell	Bile duct injury	Remarks
Infectious cause	Tuberculosis		+	Randomly present	+		HIV coinfections, drug abuser, multidrug resistance, and immunocompromised host
	Fungal infection		+		± (candidiasis)		Candidiasis - suppurative central necrosis and giant cells
							Aspergillosis - neutrophilic infiltration in granuloma
							Cryptococcosis - inflammatory reaction or granuloma
Sarcoidosis		+		Portal or periportal	+	±	Portal hypertension (±)
PBC		+		Portal		+	Anti-mitochondrial antibody(+) chronic nonsuppurative destructive cholangitis
Drugs and chemicals		+		Randomly present		±	Liver injury(+); hepatocellular, cholestatic, or mixed type
Malignancy		+					

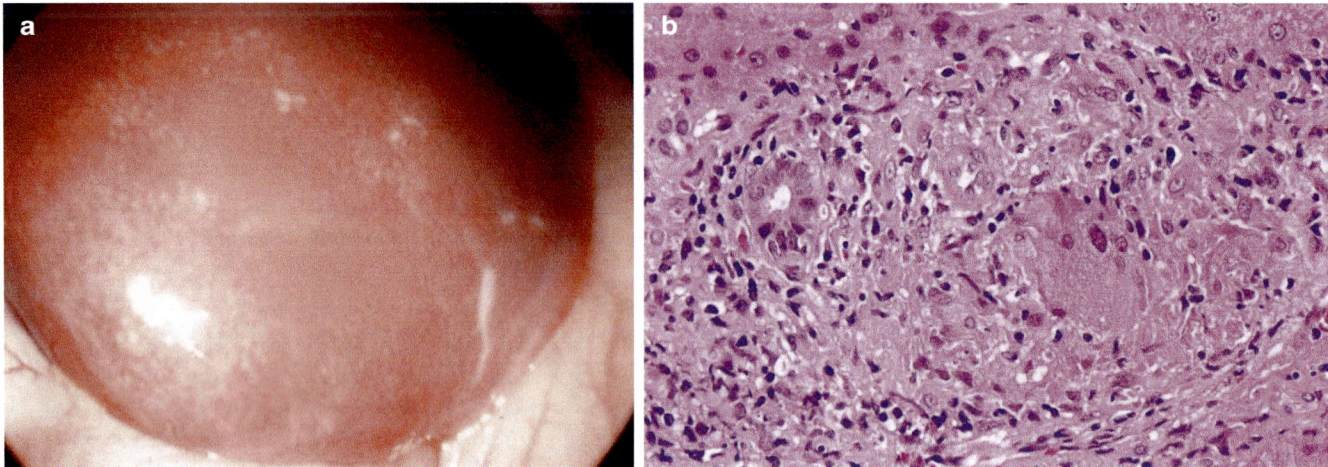

Fig. 14.5 Sarcoidosis. (**a**) Peritoneoscopy shows enlarged liver with granular formations. (**b**) Granuloma is seen in portal tract, and a giant cell is visible in the center, and lymphocytes and histiocytic cells are observed

incidence of hepatic involvement is reported to be 17–90%. Sarcoidosis is often associated with serum elevation of angiotensin-converting enzyme and calcium levels [16], and its diagnosis is frequently established by peritoneoscopy or liver biopsy [17, 18]. Sarcoid granulomas are epithelioid type and are diffusely distributed and tend to be more frequent in portal tracts or periportal area. They consist of aggregated epithelioid cells with multinucleated giant cells surrounded by lymphocytes and macrophages [18]. They often coalesce to form conglomerates, undergo fibrosis, and may be complicated by portal hypertension in 6–8% of patients and primary biliary cholangitis-like lesions. Cirrhotic change can occur by portal inflammation and fibrosis, associated with phlebitis and thrombosis of portal or hepatic veins [19], though it is uncommon [20]. It is necessary to make a diagnosis of hepatic sarcoidosis in the early phase by biopsy. Evidence for the treatment of hepatic sarcoidosis is lacking. Sarcoidosis does not respond well to therapeutic drugs, and corticosteroid administration does not prevent the development of liver lesions; however, it is recommended to treat hepatic sar-

coidosis in symptomatic patients by its administration [21]. Liver transplantation is done in some cases complicated with liver cirrhosis, but the disease may recur in the allograft.

Case 14.1

A 26-year-old male complained of high fever. Chest radiograph revealed swelling of bilateral hilar lymph nodes. Uveitis was present. Serum angiotensin-converting enzyme was 33.7 mU/mL. Peritoneoscopy showed white granulomas on the liver surface, while liver biopsy showed granulomas in portal tract; giant cells were surrounded by fibrous tissues with epithelioid cells and rimmed by lymphocytes and macrophages (Figure 14.5).

Case 14.2

Granular shadow in the lower field of bilateral lung was detected in a 28-year-old male by chest CT several years ago (Fig. 14.6a), and his laboratory data showed AST 18 IU/L, ALT 14 IU/L, CRP 0.1 mg/dL, WBC 6100/μL, PLT 27 × 10⁴/μL, KL-6425 U/mL, Quantiferon (−), and ACE 15.6 U/L. CD4/

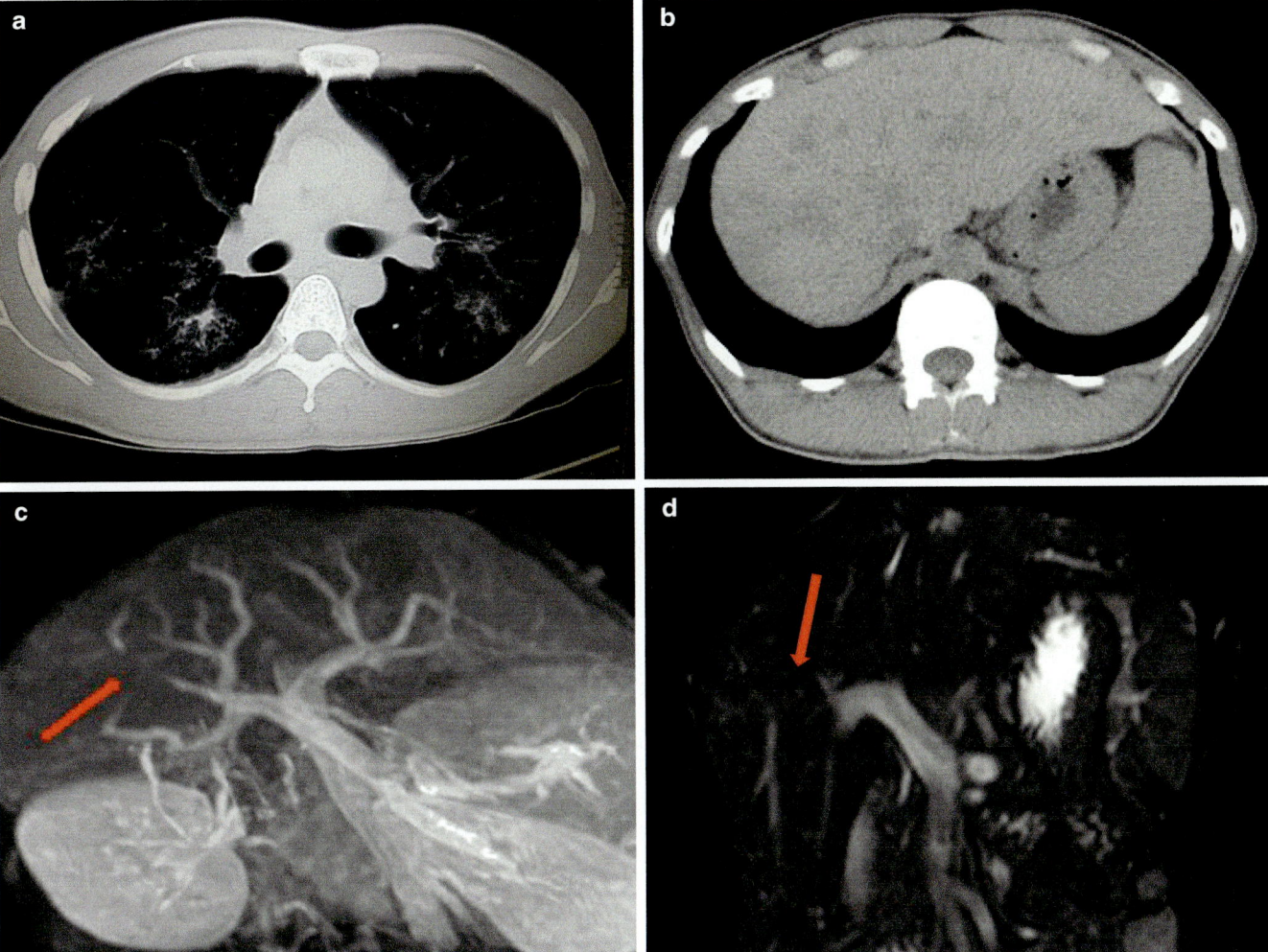

Fig. 14.6 Sarcoidosis. (**a**) Chest CT shows high-density area in lower field of bilateral lung, and granular shadows are detected. (**b**) Abdominal CT without contrast medium shows presence of multiple low-density area in the right lobe. (**c**) MRI with contrast medium shows stenotic area in S8-branch of the portal vein (arrow). (**d**) MRI shows partial interruption of the right hepatic vein (arrow)

CD8 was proved to be high in aspiration tissue taken by bronchofiberscope. Abdominal CT without contrast medium showed presence of multiple low-density area in right lobe (Fig. 14.6b), and low-density area was faintly enhanced by contrast medium in early phase, and enhancement was remained in late phase, and low-density area was seen in enlarged spleen. MRI with contrast medium showed stenotic area in S8-branch of portal vein (Fig. 14.6c), and right hepatic vein is partly interrupted with presence of developing collateral vein (Fig. 14.6d). Liver biopsy under US guidance showed granulomatous lesions with central non-caseous necrosis with giant cells surrounded by mononuclear cells (Fig. 14.7a), and pseudolobular formation was established (Fig. 14.7b).

14.9 Primary Biliary Cholangitis (PBC)

PBC targets the small intrahepatic bile ducts. Chronic nonsuppurative destructive cholangitis is histologically characteristic of PBC. Noncaseating granuloma is seen in about 25% of patient with PBC and is a requisite component of the florid duct lesion in the early stage [22]. Granuloma involves damaged interlobular or septal bile duct in the center surrounded by infiltration of epithelioid cells, plasma cells, lymphocytes, and eosinophils (Fig. 14.4).

14.10 Infectious Cause

14.10.1 Hepatic Tuberculosis

The liver involvement in tuberculosis is histologically classified into miliary, nodule (tuberculoma), and abscess. Miliary pattern is the most common form in the liver and part of generalized or localized disease. Patients with chronic liver diseases due to hepatitis B or C virus, HIV, or alcohol and with a past history of tuberculosis should be examined by biochemical test including albumin/globulin ratio and alkaline phosphatase. Granulomas in hepatic tuberculosis are due to

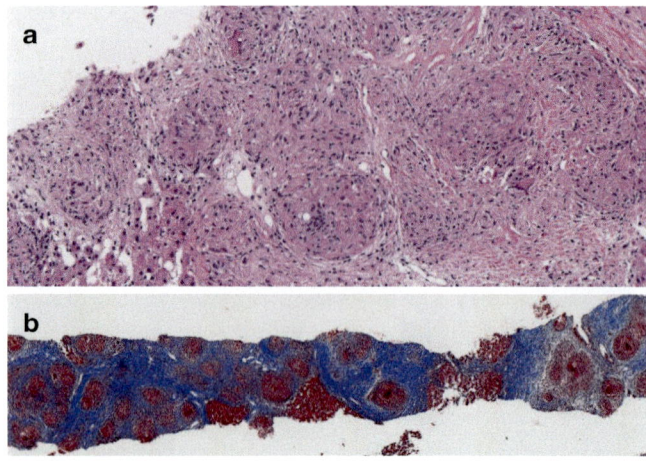

Fig. 14.7 Sarcoidosis. (**a**) Liver biopsy shows multiple non-necrotizing granulomas with giant cells and intermixed mononuclear cells, and granulomatous lesions are cohesive and associated with fibrosis. (**b**) Serial section stained with Masson-Trichrome shows pseudolobular formation

cell-mediated immunological response to tuberculosis antigens; they are well-demarcated and composed of epithelioid cells, lymphocytes (Fig. 14.5), and multinucleated Langhans giant cells. Central caseous necrosis may be observed in large granulomas. Granulomas in AIDS patients are typically absent or poorly formed and lack necrosis due to a dysfunctional immune system. Liver specimen for the diagnosis of hepatic tuberculosis should be stained for acid-fast bacilli or examined by PCR for mycobacterial DNA. Combination of isoniazid, rifampicin, pyrazinamide, and ethambutol is used for the treatment of hepatic tuberculosis. [23–26]

14.10.2 Immunotherapy in Bacillus Calmette-Guerin

Local immunotherapy using an attenuated live strain of *Mycobacterium bovis*, Bacillus Calmette-Guerin (BCG), is effective for bladder cancer. However, intravesical BCG administration sometimes induces granulomatous hepatitis with high value of serum alkaline phosphatase or gamma-glutamyl transpeptidase as a rare and serious systemic side effect, as well as sepsis and pneumonitis after its hematogenous dissemination [27–29]. Formation of granulomas in the liver is considered to be due to hematogenous infection of *Mycobacterium bovis* or its hypersensitive reaction. Granulomatous hepatitis should be treated by combination of isoniazid, rifampicin, and ethambutol. Corticosteroid should be administered when interstitial pneumonia is complicated [30].

Case 14.3

A 65-year-old male suffered from superficial bladder cancer. He was administered bladder instillations with BCG.

At the second administration, fever and general malaise developed, and his liver function tests showed TBIL 2.38 mg/dL, AST 195 IU/L, ALT 235 IU/L, ALP 813 IU/L, GGT 340 IU/L, CRP 0.8 mg/dL, and WBC 5900/μL. CT showed hepatomegaly, but neither low-density areas nor dilatation of intrahepatic bile ducts could be detected. Peritoneoscopy showed small, white macular patches on liver surface, with white capsule; liver biopsy showed proliferation of Kupffer cells in sinusoids, a few microvesicular fat vacuoles in hepatocytes and scattered granulomas; and granulomas were noncaseating and comprised epithelioid cells and giant cells, surrounded by lymphocytes or macrophages (Fig. 14.8). A 6-month course of isoniazid plus rifampin was recommended, with administration of pyrazinamide for the first 2 months [31]. His liver function tests returned to normal values, and fever disappeared.

Case 14.4

A 66-year-old male received BCG immunotherapy for early cancer of urinary bladder 13 times for 3 years, and he was admitted because of high fever and general malaise. Liver function test showed AST 46 U/L, ALT 52 U/L, ALP 558 U/L, γ-GTP 148 U/L, and CRP 12.7 mg/dL, and abdominal US and CT showed hepatosplenomegaly (Fig. 14.9a). Liver biopsy showed non-caseous granuloma with presence of giant cells (Fig. 14.9b), and BCG immunotherapy was considered to induce granulomatous hepatitis. INH, EB, and RFP were administered, and liver function test gradually reverted to normal value with alleviation of fever. However, dyspnea developed and CT of chest showed interstitial pneumonia (Fig. 14.9c). Lung biopsy under guidance of bronchofiberscope showed non-caseous granuloma with giant cells (Fig. 14.9d). Thereafter, PSL pulse therapy improved his dyspnea.

14.11 Syphilis Infection

Hematogenous dissemination of the pathogen, *Treponema pallidum*, which causes syphilis takes place in the primary and secondary stages of the disease. Syphilitic hepatitis is found in 10% of those infected.

In secondary syphilis, there is focal liver cell necrosis infiltrated with lymphocytes, eosinophils, and granulocytes, portal inflammation with numerous neutrophils around bile ductules, and epithelioid granulomatous formation. Vasculitis is sometimes seen in portal tract [32].

In the tertiary stage, lesions are gumma-necrotizing granulomas accompanied by plasma cells and endarteritis obliterans leading to fibrous scarring and hepar lobatum. Diagnosis is derived from serological tests for specific antigens, and administration of penicillin is recommended for treatment.

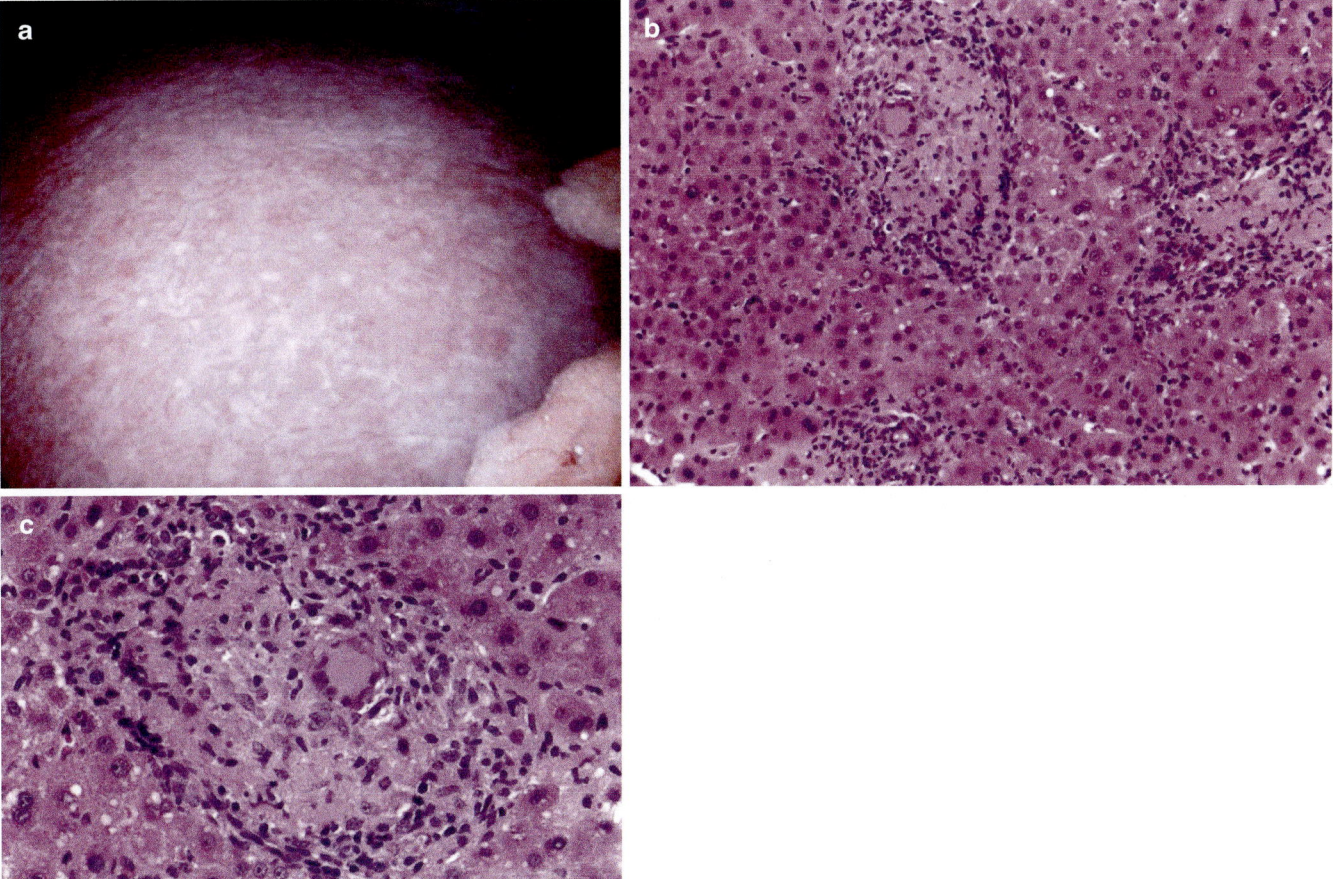

Fig. 14.8 Bacillus Calmette-Guerin immunotherapy-induced liver injury. (**a**) Peritoneoscopy shows diffuse presence of granules on liver surface. (**b**) Granulomatous lesions are visible in the liver. (**c**) Giant cells and epithelioid cells are seen in the center, and lymphohistiocytic infiltrates are observed in peripheral area of granuloma

Case 14.5

An 18-year-old female complained of general malaise, and jaundice was seen. Physical examination showed tonsillitis and erythematous lesions on the foot. Liver function test showed TBIL 5.3 mg/dL, AST 744 IU/L, ALT 678 IU/L, LDH 694 IU/L, ALP 659 IU/L, and GGT 260 IU/L. Rapid plasma reagin and *Treponema pallidum* haemagglutination tests were positive with a titer of 1:16 and 1:1280, respectively. Liver histology showed many inflammatory cells and vasculitis in portal tract, with numerous neutrophils and lymphocytes (Fig. 14.10).

14.12 Schistosomiasis

The great majority of schistosomal liver diseases are caused by *Schistosoma mansoni* in Africa and South America, by *S. japonicum* in Asia, and by *S. mekongi* in Laos and Cambodia [33]. Other species mainly involve bladder or bowel and cause minor non-symptomatic hepatic lesions [34]. Fever, chills, headaches, arthralgia, pain in the right epigastrium, diarrhea, protein-losing enteropathy, weight loss, lymphadenopathy, and urticaria may rarely be manifested in acute infection, due to hypersensitivity [35].

However, the cardinal characteristic manifestations of advanced hepatic disease are related to the development of presinusoidal portal hypertension. Eggs are produced by mature worms in the mesenteric veins, carried to the liver, and trapped in the small portal venules, eliciting a granulomatous reaction. The granulomas consist of lymphocytes, histiocytes, eosinophils, and multinucleated giant cells with ova. The end result is marked portal and periportal fibrosis, described as "clay pipestem fibrosis," and occasionally leads to distortion and scarring simulating hepar lobatum [36]. The obstruction of portal venules due to eggs and portal fibrosis leads to presinusoidal portal hypertension. Egg-laying worms are sometimes present in the intestinal microvasculature of the inferior mesenteric venous plexus, and deposition of eggs in the large intestine induces exudative granuloma resulting in formation of inflammatory polyps, and fibrosis and wall thickening cause stenosis [37]. Clinical features are bloody diarrhea, anemia, and protein-losing enteropathy [35]. Praziquantel or oxamniquine should be administered to prevent schistosomiasis [38, 39].

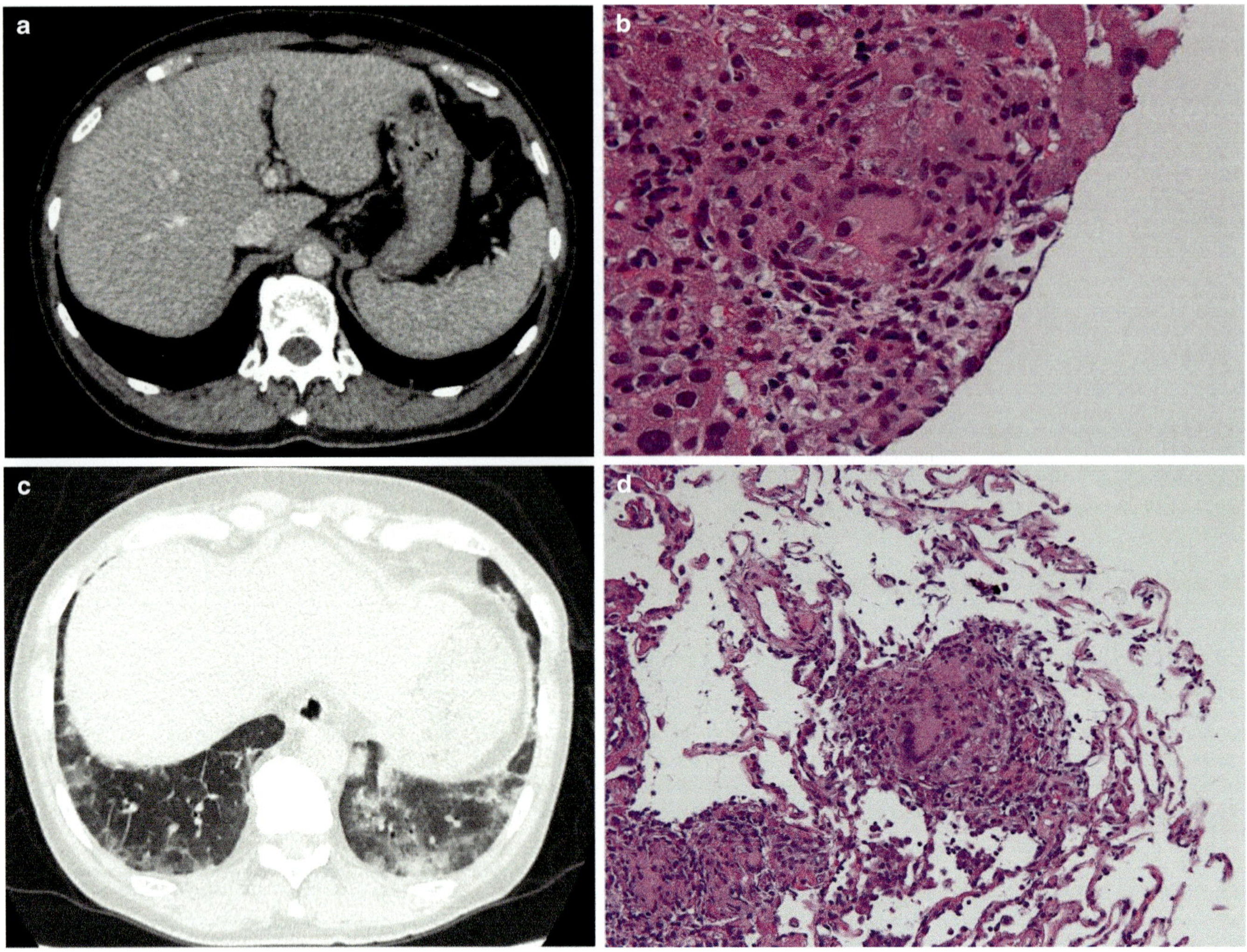

Fig. 14.9 Bacillus Calmette-Guerin immunotherapy-induced liver injury. (**a**) Abdominal CT with contrast medium shows hepatosplenomegaly. (**b**) Liver specimen shows a granulomatous lesion with giant cell. (**c**) Chest CT shows high-density shadows in lower field of both lungs. (**d**) Lung specimen shows a non-caseating granuloma with giant cell

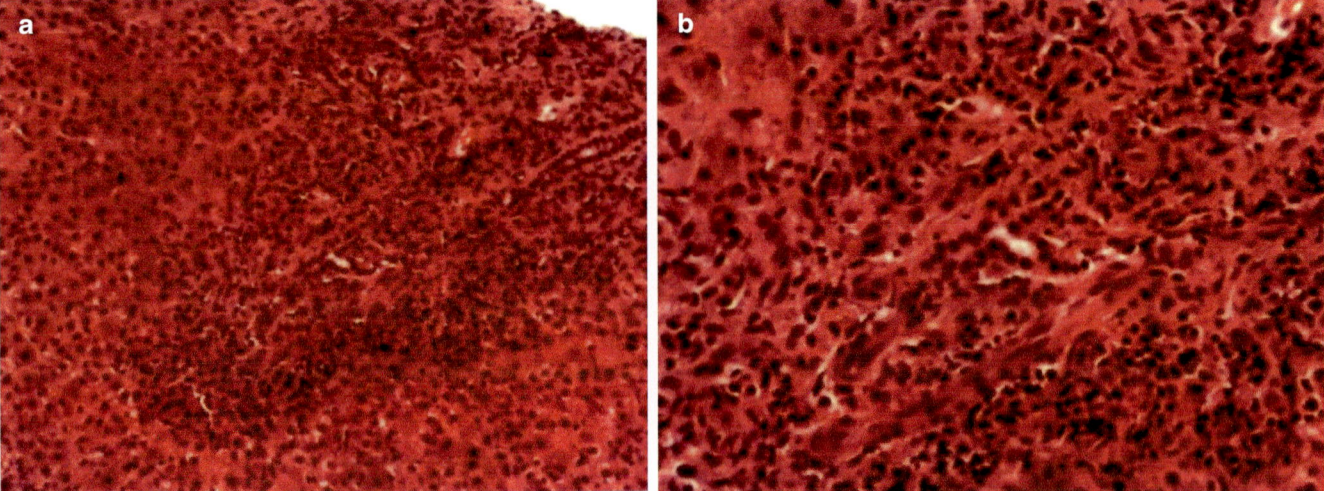

Fig. 14.10 Syphilis. (**a**) Inflammatory cells are present in portal tract, clustering around bile ductules. (**b**) Portal tract is infiltrated by polymorphs and lymphocytes, and vasculitis is seen

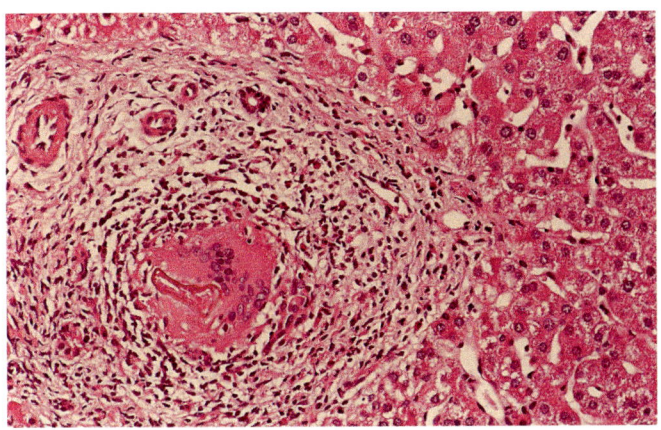

Fig. 14.11 Schistosomiasis. Granuloma is seen in portal tract, and a schistosome egg is ingested by multinucleated giant cell

Case 14.6

A 76-year-old man presented with repeated hematemesis. His liver function was normal. Endoscopy showed bleeding from abnormal vessels in gastric fundus. CT showed splenomegaly and normal-sized liver with no mass lesion. Laparotomy was required to control repeated bleeding from gastric varices. Splenectomy was also performed, and wedge liver biopsy was undertaken to find the underlying cause of portal hypertension. Biopsy showed normal architecture with no evidence of cirrhosis. Portal tracts were enlarged and fibrotic, and many portal venous branches were obliterated. Clusters of schistosome ova were deposited in region of obliterated veins, and an occasional foreign body-type granuloma was noted (Fig. 14.11).

Case 14.7

A 37-year-old female who had stayed in Southeast Asia when she was 18 years old was admitted because of right hypochondriac pain. Liver function test showed AST 123 U/L, ALT 84 U/L, ALP 113 U/L, γ-GTP 50 U/L, and CRP 0.6 mg/dL. Abdominal US showed hyperechoic edges of large or peripheral portal vein (Fig. 14.12a). Liver biopsy showed eggs in portal vein surrounded by fibrosis, and lobular structure is disarrayed (Fig. 14.12b). Colonoscopy showed atrophic mucosa, irregular yellow fleck, and telangiectatic spots (Fig. 14.12c). Colon mucosa showed the presence of eggs in venules, and mucosa was infiltrated by lymphocytes and eosinophils (Fig. 14.12d).

14.13 Drugs

Many drugs and chemicals induce hepatic granuloma with infiltration of eosinophils, and hepatitis, cholestasis, steatosis, ballooning of hepatocyte, and apoptosis are often seen in liver injury. Granulomas usually are small and present within hepatic lobule accompanied by a portal and lobular inflammation. Chemical materials of beryllium and thorotrast and phenylbutazone, allopurinol (Fig. 14.3), phenytoin, carbamazepine, chlorpromazine (Fig. 14.2), methyldopa, isoniazid, amiodarone, and diazepam are known to cause formation of hepatic granulomas [3]. It may be difficult to diagnose a relationship between drug usage and hepatic granuloma formation. However, the resolution of granulomas after discontinuation of the drug is helpful in establishing the diagnosis.

14.14 Lymphomas

Hepatic noncaseating epithelioid granuloma has been reported to occur in patients with Hodgkin's lymphoma and non-Hodgkin's lymphoma [40, 41]. Hepatic lesions are difficult to detect in image analysis. Liver biopsy sometimes demonstrates lymphoid aggregates with atypical cells or Reed-Sternberg cells and sinusoidal dilatation with or without infiltration of atypical cells. Macroscopic findings in the livers of non-Hodgkin's lymphoma patients are classified into disseminated infiltrate in sinusoids, multiple granulomas in the portal tract, multiple macronodules, and solitary tumor mass. The relationship between malignant lesions and the development of hepatic granuloma is not clear. Hepatic granuloma in lymphoma is non-necrotic, and atypical cells are almost present in granulomas and rarely not seen, and the presence of granuloma does not affect the prognosis of lymphoma [3].

Clinical manifestations of patients with malignant lymphomas include high fever, night sweats, weight loss, hepatosplenomegaly, and swelling of lymph nodes. Serum values of alkaline phosphatase and C-reactive protein are high, and lactate dehydrogenase is sometimes elevated. Liver biopsy is recommended for differential diagnosis and staging, and guidance under peritoneoscopy is essential to prevent bleeding. The diagnostic process is described in greater detail in Chap. 15.

Case 14.8

A 93-year-old man complained of unknown fever and had anemia. His liver function test showed AST 11 IU/L, ALT 7 IU/L, ALP 280 IU/L, TP 4.8 g/dL, and CRP 8.3 mg/dL. Peripheral blood examination showed Hb 6.5 g/dL, WBC 3800/μL, RBC 249 × 10⁴/μL, and PLT 30.1 × 10⁴/μL. Spike in fever remained, and serum test 2 weeks later revealed AST 58 IU/L, ALT 34 IU/L, ALP 3782 IU/L, GGT 110 IU/L, and CRP 17 mg/dL. Liver biopsy showed dilatation of sinusoids filled with red blood cells in middle zone to central area. Granulomas were seen in portal tract (Fig. 14.13), and many atypical lymphocytes were present in clusters. He was diagnosed with lymphoma.

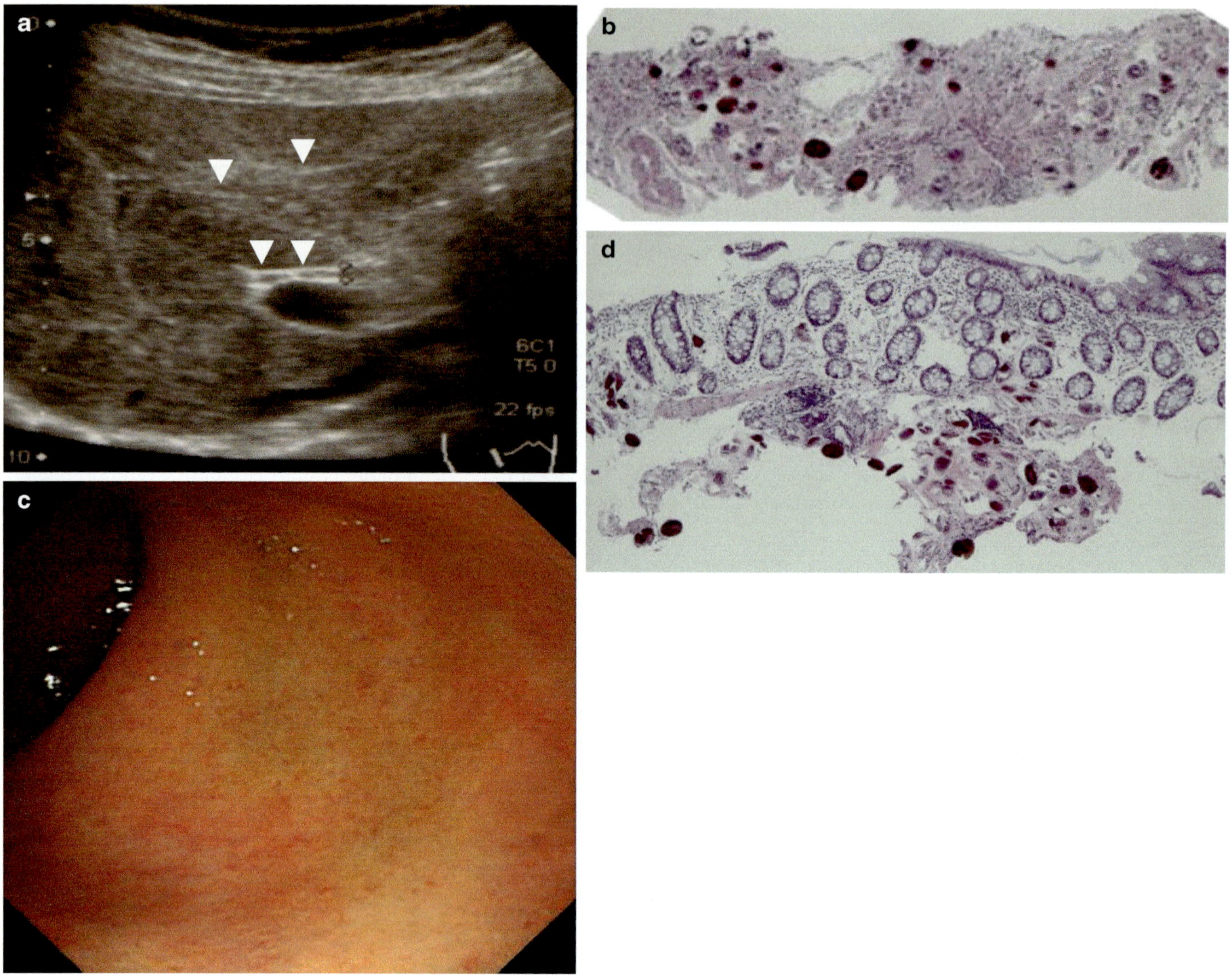

Fig. 14.12 Schistosomiasis. (**a**) Abdominal US shows hyperechoic edges (arrow) of portal vein. (**b**) Liver biopsy shows eggs in portal veins surrounded by fibrosis and infiltrated by inflammatory cells, and lobular structure is in disarray. (**c**) Colonoscopy reveals atrophic mucosa, irreg-ular flecks, and telangiectatic spots. (**d**) Large intestinal biopsy shows presence of eggs in venules and infiltrate of lymphocytes and eosino-phils in mucosa and submucosa

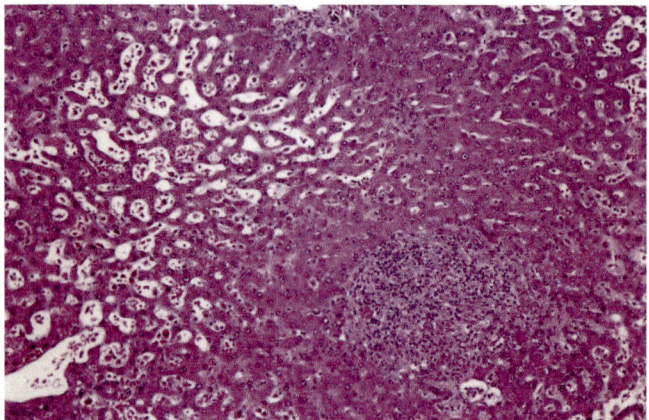

Fig. 14.13 Malignant lymphoma. Liver biopsy shows dilatation of sinusoids filled with red blood cells and atypical lymphocytes in mid-zonal to centrilobular areas and granuloma in portal tract

References

1. Turhan N, Kurt M. Hepatic granulomas: a clinicopathologic analy-sis of 86 cases. Pathol Res Pract. 2011;207:359–65.
2. Gaya DR, Thorburn D, Oien KA, Morris AJ, Stanley AJ. Hepatic granulomas: a 10 year single Centre experience. J Clin Pathol. 2003;56:850–3.
3. Coash M, Porouhar F, Wu CH, Wu GY. Granulomatous liver dis-ease: a review. J Formosan Med Assoc. 2012;111:3–13.
4. Dincsoy HP, Weesner RE, MacGee J. Lipogranulomas in non-fatty human livers. A mineral oil induced environmental disease. Am J Clin Pathol. 1982;78:35–41.
5. Ferrell LD. Hepatic granulomas: a morphologic approach to diag-nosis. Surg Pathol. 1990;3:87–106.
6. Denk H, Scheuer PJ, Baptista A, Bianchi L, Callea F, De Groote J, et al. Guidelines for the diagnosis and interpretation of hepatic granulomas. Histopathology. 1994;25:209–18.
7. Lefkowitch JH. Hepatic granulomas. J Hepatol. 1999;30(Suppl 1):40–5.

8. Kleiner DE. Granulomas of the liver. Sem Diag Pathol. 2006;23:161–9.
9. Hofmann CE, Heaton JW Jr. Q fever hepatitis: clinical manifestations and pathological findings. Gastroenterology. 1982;83:474–9.
10. Vanderstigel M, Zafrani ES, Lejonc JL, Schaeffer A, Portos JL. Allopurinol hypersensitivity syndrome as a cause of hepatic fibrin-ring granulomas. Gastroenterology. 1986;90:188–90.
11. Nenert M, Mavier P, Dubuc N, Deforges L, Zafrani ES. Epstein-Barr virus infection and hepatic fibrin-ring granulomas. Hum Pathol. 1988;19:608–10.
12. Lobdell DH. "Ring" granulomas in cytomegalovirus hepatitis. Arch Pathol Lab Med. 1987;111:881–2.
13. Marazuela M, Moreno A, Yebra M, Cerezo E, Gomez-Gesto C, Vargas JA. Hepatic fibrin-ring granulomas. A clinicopathologic study of 23 patients. Hum Pathol. 1991;22:607–13.
14. Moreno A, Marazuela M, Yebra M, Hernández MJ, Hellín T, Montalbán C, et al. Hepatic fibrin-ring granulomas in visceral leishmaniasis. Gastroenterology. 1988;95:1123–6.
15. Zumla A, James DG. Granulomatous infections: etiology and classification. Clin Infect Dis. 1996;23:146–58.
16. Iannuzzi MC, Rybicki BA, Teirstein AS. Sarcoidosis. N Engl J Med. 2007;357:2153–65.
17. Devaney K, Goodman ZD, Epstein MS, Zimmerman HJ, Ishak KG. Hepatic sarcoidosis. Clinical features in 100 patients. Am J Surg Pathol. 1993;17:1272–80.
18. Ishak KG. Sarcoidosis of the liver and bile ducts. Mayo Clin Proc. 1998;73:467–72.
19. Moreno-Merlo F, Wanless IR, Shimamatsu K, Sherman M, Greig P, Chiasson D. The role of granulomatous phlebitis and thrombosis in the pathogenesis of cirrhosis and portal hypertension in sarcoidosis. Hepatology. 1997;26:554–60.
20. Blich M, Edoute Y. Clinical manifestations of sarcoid liver disease. J Gastroenterol Hepatol. 2004;19:732–7.
21. Cremers JP, Drent M, Bauqhman RP, Wijnen PA, Koek GH. Therapeutic approach of hepatic sarcoidosis. Curr Opin Pulm Med. 2012;18:472–82.
22. Gaspar R, Andrade P, Silva M, Peixoto A, Lopes J, Carneiro F, Liberal R, Macedo G. Hepatic granulomas: a 17-year single tertiary Centre experience. Histopathology. 2018;73:240. https://doi.org/10.1111/his.13521.. [Epub ahead of print].
23. Hickey AJ, Gounder L, Moosa MYS, Drain PK. A systematic review of hepatic tuberculosis with considerations in human immunodeficiency virus co-infection. BMC Infect Dis. 2015;15:209.
24. Chaudhary P. Hepatobiliary tuberculosis. Ann Gastroenterol. 2014;27:207–11.
25. Saukkonen JJ, Cohn DL, Jasmer RM. An official ATS statement: hepatotoxicity of antituberculous therapy. Am J Respir Crit Care Med. 2006;174:935–52.
26. Chandan K, Ashwin MP. Hepatic Tuberculosis: a multimodality imaging review. Insights Imaging. 2015;6:647–58.
27. Proctor DD, Chopra S, Rubenstein SC, Jokela JA, Uhl L. Mycobacteremia and granulomatous hepatitis following initial intravesical bacillus Calmette-Guerin instillation for bladder carcinoma. Am J Gastroenterol. 1993;88:1112–5.
28. Leebeek FW, Ouwendijk RJ, Kolk AH, Dees A, Meek JC, Nienhuis JE, et al. Granulomatous hepatitis caused by Bacillus Calmette-Guerin (BCG) infection after BCG bladder instillation. Gut. 1996;38:616–8.
29. Larsen BT, Smith ML, Grys TE, Colby TV. Histopathology of disseminated mycobacterium bovis infection complicating intravesical BCG immunotherapy for orolithelial carcinoma. Int J Surg Pathol. 2015;23:189–95.
30. Khaled D, Ihab S, Osama AA. Acute hepatitis and pneumonitis caused by disseminated Bacillus Calmette-Guérin infection. ACG Case Reports J. 2016;3:130–2.
31. Graziano DA, Jacobs D, Lozano RG, Buck RL. A case of granulomatous hepatitis after intravesical bacillus calmette-guerin administration. J Urol. 1991;146:1118–9.
32. Romeu J, Rybak B, Dave P, Coven R. Spirochetal vasculitis and bile ductular damage in early hepatic syphilis. Am J Gastroenterol. 1980;74:352–4.
33. WHO. The control of schistosomiasis. Second report of the WHO expert committee. Geneva: WHO; 1993.
34. Van Wijk HB, Elias EA. Hepatic and rectal pathology in Schistosoma intercalatum infection. Trop Geog Med. 1975;27:237–48.
35. Manzella A, Ohmoto K, Monzawa S, Lim JH. Schistosomiasis of the liver. Abdom Imaging. 2008;33:144–50.
36. Tsui WM, Chow LT. Advanced schistosomiasis as a cause of hepar lobatum. Histopathology. 1993;23:495–7.
37. Elbaz T, Esmat G. Hepatic and intestinal schistosomiasis: review. J Adv Res. 2013;4:445–52.
38. Utzinger J, Raso G, Brooker S, De Savigny D, Tanner M, Ornbjerg N, et al. Schistosomiasis and neglected tropical diseases: towards integrated and sustainable control and a word of caution. Parasitology. 2009;136:1859–74.
39. Bica I, Hamer DH, Stadecker MJ. Hepatic schistosomiasis. Infect Dis Clin N Am. 2000;14:583–604.
40. Kim H, Dorfman RF. Morphological studies of 84 untreated patients subjected to laparotomy for the staging of non-Hodgkin's lymphomas. Cancer. 1974;33:657–74.
41. Abt AB, Kirschner RH, Belliveau RE, O'Connell MJ, Sklansky BD, Greene WH, et al. Hepatic pathology associated with Hodgkin's disease. Cancer. 1974;33:1564–71.

Liver Disorders in Systemic Diseases

15

Masaki Iwai, Kenichi Miyoshi, Masahiko Koda,
and Wilson M. S. Tsui

Contents

Abbreviations

AIDS	Acquired immunodeficiency syndrome
ANC	Absolute neutrophil count
C-MOPP-ABVD	Combination chemotherapy-Mustargen, oncovin, procarbazine, prednisone-Adriamycin, bleomycin, vinblastine, dacarbazine
CREST	Calcinosis cutis, Raynaud's phenomenon, esophageal dysfunction, sclerodactyly, and telangiectasia
DIC	Disseminated intravascular coagulopathy
EMH	Extramedullary hemopoiesis
HELLP	Hemolysis, elevated liver tests, and low platelets
IBD	Inflammatory bowel disease
MALT	Mucosa-associated lymphoid tissue
MDR3	Multidrug resistance protein 3

M. Iwai, MD, PhD
Kyoto, Japan

K. Miyoshi, MD, PhD · M. Koda, MD, PhD
Tottori, Japan

W. M. S. Tsui, MD, FRCPath (✉)
Hong Kong, China
e-mail: mstsui@ha.org.hk

Liver disease may occur in association with various systemic diseases. These primary diseases are predominantly extrahepatic, but associated hepatic dysfunction may develop and often is of clinical significance and diagnostic importance. In some cases, liver disease simply represents a manifestation of the systemic disease process involving the liver, as in disseminated malignancy, systemic infection, and some metabolic diseases. Rarely, it may constitute a relatively unique manifestation of a systemic disease, as in primary sclerosing cholangitis associated with ulcerative colitis.

© Springer Nature Singapore Pte Ltd. 2019
E. Hashimoto et al. (eds.), *Diagnosis of Liver Disease*, https://doi.org/10.1007/978-981-13-6806-6_15

15.1 Liver in Hematolymphoid Diseases

15.1.1 Malignant Hematological Disorders

The liver is an extranodal organ where lesions are seen frequently in malignant hematological disorders and also may be the primary site in a small number of cases [1, 2]. Diagnosis of malignant hematological disorders and evaluation of their staging are important to establish appropriate therapy, and demonstrating hepatic involvement is vital because it can lead to restaging of the disease and altering treatment strategy. Serum alkaline phosphatase and lactic dehydrogenase are often elevated in patients with malignant hematological disorders [1], but scintigraphy, ultrasonography (US), computed tomography (CT), and magnetic resonance imaging (MRI) may not always reveal involvement of the liver [3, 4]. Sinusoidal infiltration and granuloma formation as well as nodular formation are reported in the liver in malignant lymphoma [5–7]; therefore, peritoneoscopy may be required to detect liver involvement in malignant hematological disorders. We have demonstrated peritoneoscopic findings of the liver surface characteristic of malignant hematological disorders, thereby reflecting the histological features of liver.

Case 15.1

A 66-year-old, asymptomatic male carrier of hepatitis B complained of minimal fever of 1 month. He had intermittent high fever. His conjunctiva was neither pale nor icteric. The liver was palpable 3 cm beneath the right costal margin, but the spleen was not enlarged. On admission, the laboratory data showed WBC 2480/μL, Hb 12.8 g/dL, PLT 16 × 10⁴/μL, ESR 59 mm/h, CRP 13.2 mg/dL, AST 59 IU/L, and ALP 666 IU/L. CT and US revealed neither nodules nor tumors in the liver. Various antibiotics and antituberculosis drugs were administered, but fever persisted. Peritoneoscopy was carried out with liver biopsy. It revealed diffuse white maculae with or without fusion on liver surface, and peripheral portal veins were dilated; histology

showed granulomas in portal tract and sinusoidal congestion in lobule, but few lymphoma cells were seen in granulomas (Fig. 15.1). Malignant lymphoma was suggested based on peritoneoscopic findings. A lymph node 1.5 cm in diameter seen in the submandibular area became palpable after 1 month, and the incised node showed non-Hodgkin's lymphoma. Combined chemotherapy was administered with adriamycin, cyclophosphamide, vincristine sulfate, and prednisolone. Liver function tests returned to normal values, and enlarged liver reduced in size. He lived for 12 years, while combined therapy was effective.

Case 15.2

A 72-year-old male patient complained of general malaise and high fever. His conjunctiva was neither anemic nor icteric. The liver was palpable 2 cm beneath the right costal margin. His laboratory data showed WBC 6900/μL, Hb 12.3 g/dL, PLT 7.0 × 10⁴/μL, CRP 8.5 mg/dL, ESR 112 mm/h, LDH 449 IU/L, ALT 25 IU/L, and ALP 1281 IU/L. A submandibular lymph node 1.8 cm in diameter was palpable. Neither US nor CT showed tumors. Peritoneoscopy showed enlarged liver with peliosis hepatis, scattered white maculae, and dilated peripheral portal veins; fibrin was deposited on thick liver capsule; there were portal fibrosis, congestion, and granulomas in the portal tract; and magnified view showed cluster of lymphoma cells with Reed-Sternberg cells (Fig. 15.2). Submandibular lymph node biopsy revealed Hodgkin's cells. C-MOPP-ABVD was given. His liver function tests returned to normal values, and liver was reduced in size. He survived for 3 years and 8 months.

Case 15.3

A 19-year-old female complained of polydypsia and general malaise due to diabetes insipidus. Nausea, vomiting, and right hypochondriac pain developed, along with high fever. Her conjunctiva was anemic and icteric, and the liver was elastic and palpable 5 cm beneath the right costal margin. Laboratory data revealed WBC 13,510/μL, Hb 7.0 g/dL, PLT 39.8 × 10⁴/

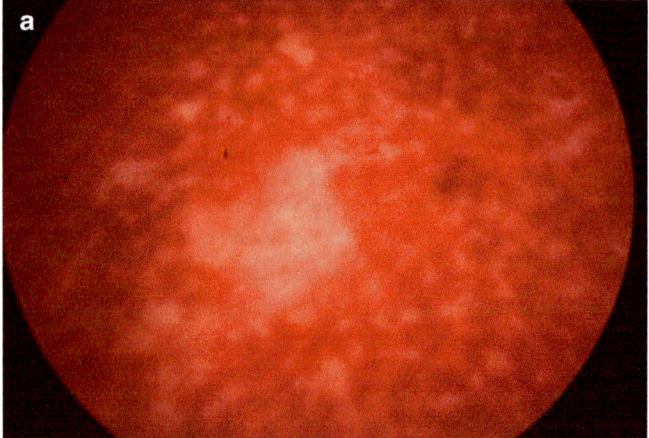
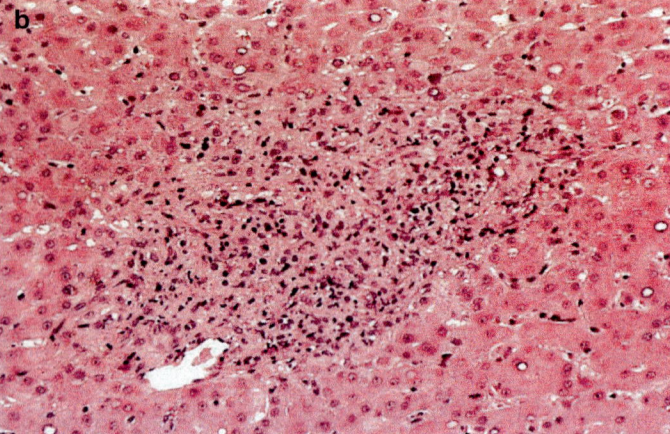

Fig. 15.1 Malignant lymphoma. (**a**) Peritoneoscopy shows maculae or white spots on liver surface, which are cohesive. (**b**) Granulomatous lesions are observed in portal tracts, and malignant cells are absent in granulomas. (Reuse of Iwai M, et al. Macroscopic and microscopic findings of livers in malignant hematologic disorders, biopsied under peritoneoscopy. J Clin Gastroenterol 2002; 35: 262–5, with permission of Wolters Kluwer Health, Inc.)

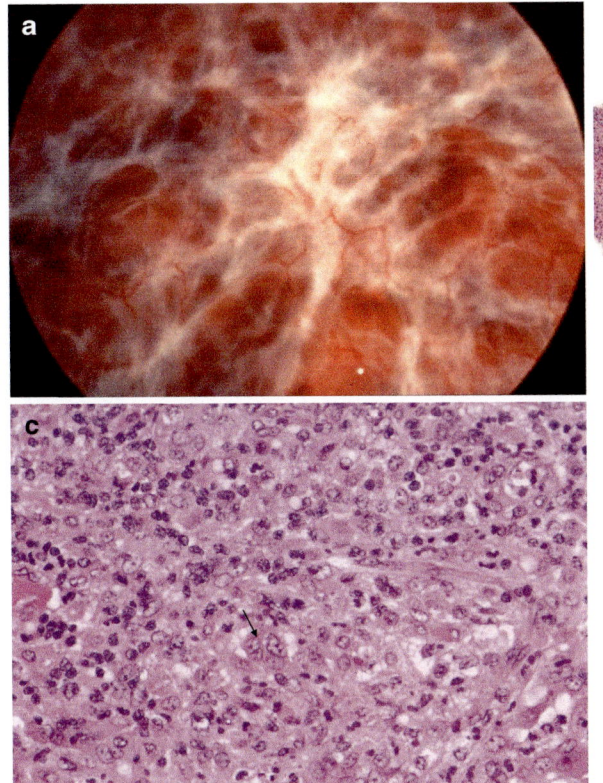

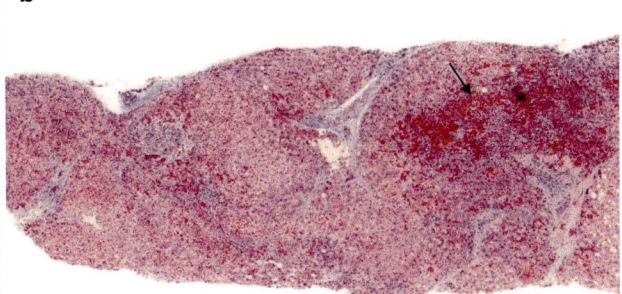

Fig. 15.2 Hodgkin's lymphoma. (**a**) Peritoneoscopic findings show peliosis hepatis with dilatation of peripheral portal veins. Liver capsule is thick, and fibrin is deposited. (Reuse of Iwai M, et al. Macroscopic and microscopic findings of livers in malignant hematologic disorders, biopsied under peritoneoscopy. J Clin Gastroenterol 2002; 35: 262–5, with permission of Wolters Kluwer Health, Inc.) (**b**) Granulomatous formation (arrowhead), congestion (arrow), and portal fibrosis are visible. (**c**) Magnified view shows Reed-Sternberg cell with mirror imaged nucleus (arrow)

μL, fibrinogen 816 mg/dL, ESR 148 mm/h, positive CRP 6, TBIL 6.7 mg/dL, AST 63 IU/L, ALT 38 IU/L, LDH 478 IU/L, ALP 1731 IU/L, and GGT 661 IU/L. US showed multiple small, high-echoic lesions in the liver. Conventional CT showed multiple low-density areas. Endoscopic retrograde cholangiopancreatography revealed stenotic area in the lower portion of the common bile duct, and cystic or irregular dilatation was observed in the main pancreatic duct (Fig. 15.3). Peritoneoscopy showed the enlarged liver with uneven surface and white maculae. Some maculae were cohesive, lymph vessels were dilated on the surface, and peliosis hepatis was scattered; liver biopsy showed clusters of foam cells in portal tract that tested positive for S100 protein and contained Birbeck granules (Fig. 15.4). She was diagnosed with Langerhans cell granulomatosis, and vinblastine was administered. Diabetes insipidus improved greatly, liver function tests returned to normal levels, and the liver reduced in size. After 3 years, hepatic lesions became resistant to vinblastine, and jaundice appeared. She died 4 years later from liver failure due to cirrhotic change, with bleeding of esophageal varices (Fig. 15.5).

Enlargement of the liver is often seen in patients with malignant hematological disorders [8, 9]. On physical examination, the liver is elastic in patients with malignant lym-

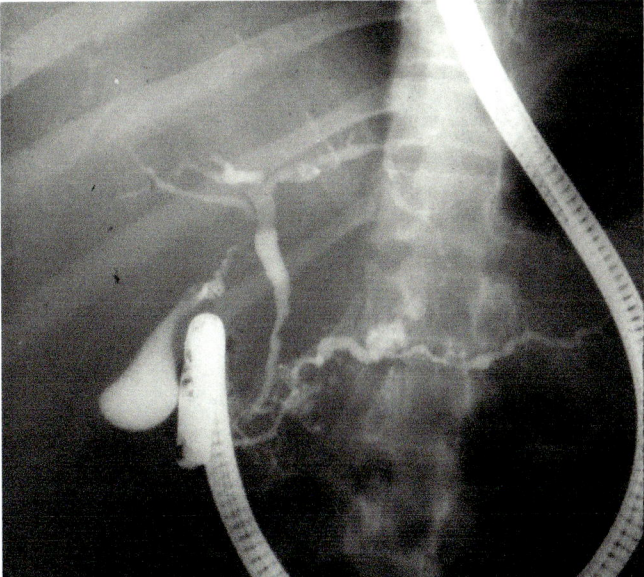

Fig. 15.3 Langerhans cell histiocytosis. Endoscopic retrograde cholangiopancreatography shows stenotic area in lower portion of common bile duct and cystic and irregular dilatation of the main pancreatic duct. (Reuse of Iwai M, et al. Cholestatic liver disease in a 20-yr-old woman with histiocytosis X. Am J Gastroenterol 1988; 83: 164–8, with permission of Springer Nature)

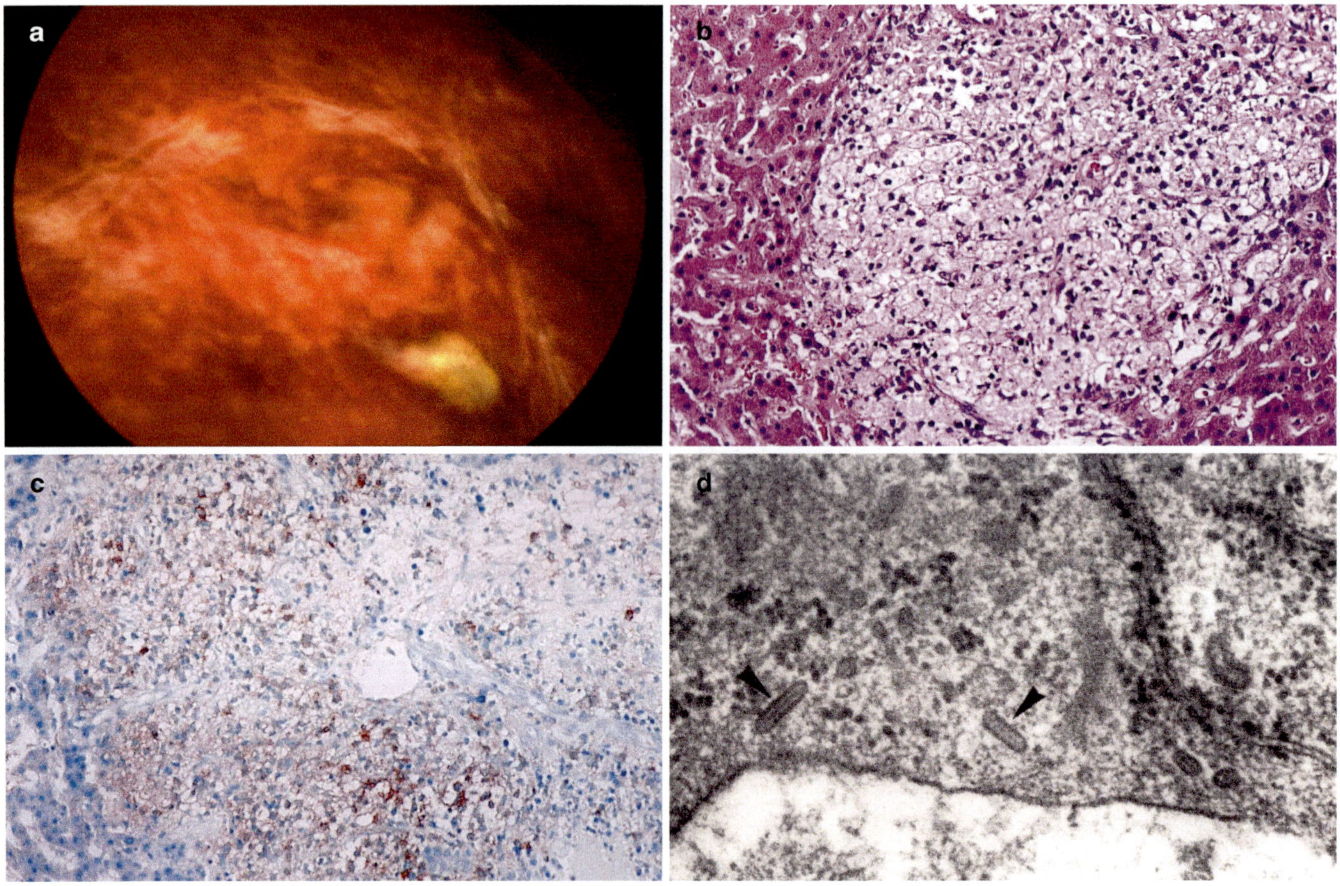

Fig. 15.4 Langerhans cell histiocytosis. (**a**) Peritoneoscopic findings show diffuse maculae on liver surface, which are cohesive. The lymph vessels are dilated. (**b**) Clusters of foamy cells are seen in granuloma around portal tract. (**c**) Immunocytochemical investigation shows S-100 protein immunoreactivity in foamy cells. (**d**) Electron microscopy shows Birbeck granules (arrowheads) in foamy cells. ((**a**) and (**d**); reuse of Iwai M, et al. Cholestatic liver disease in a 20-yr-old woman with histiocytosis X. Am J Gastroenterol 1988; 83: 164–8, with permission of Springer Nature)

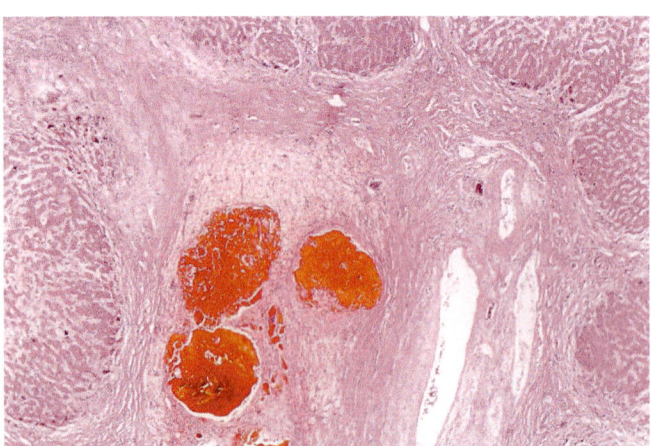

Fig. 15.5 Langerhans cell histiocytosis. Cholestasis is seen in the large bile ducts of the portal tract, and portal fibrosis has developed, establishing pseudolobular formation

phoma and Langerhans cell histiocytosis. Serum ALP and LDH show high values, while ALT and AST remain in the normal range or slightly elevated. In Case 15.3, serum CRP was positive, and ESR was elevated.

Patients with enlarged liver and high serum value of ALP or LDH and CRP or ESR are considered to have liver involvement in malignant hematological disorders [10, 11]. However, image analysis does not always show an abnormal space-occupying lesion, except for enlargement of the liver. Therefore, peritoneoscopy with liver biopsy is necessary and important to assess the involvement of the liver in patients suspected of malignant hematological disorders.

Liver tissues can be obtained by CT-guided or open biopsy for diagnosis of hematological disorders. CT can also show low-density areas in the liver of malignant hematological disorders [3], but small lesions cannot be detected. Macroscopic findings of the liver surface can be observed during open biopsy or under peritoneoscopy and are diagnostic in malignant hematological disorders. Therefore, open biopsy and biopsy under peritoneoscopy have greater specificity and sensitivity than CT-guided biopsy. Open biopsy is carried out under general anesthesia [12], and peritoneoscopy is done under local or lumbar anesthesia [13, 14]. Hence, peritoneoscopy with liver biopsy is superior to open biopsy to preserve the general condition and shorten hospital stay [15].

In our patients, peritoneoscopy showed white maculae on liver surface, and some of these were fused. White maculae can be seen on the liver surface not only in malignant hematological disorders but also in tuberculosis and sarcoidosis. Maculae are cheesy or chalky in tuberculosis [16, 17] and are geographically scattered in sarcoidosis [18]. The maculae in our patients were flattened, irregular in size, and present diffusely on the liver surface. Moreover, they were fused and so large that image analysis showed a space-occupying lesion by US or low-density area by CT after diagnosis or therapy. Maculae in lymphoma are histologically equivalent to granulomatous lesions with or without malignant cells, and granulomas without lymphoma cells are indicative of positive host response [19]. Biopsied tissues are used not only to observe microscopic and ultrastructural features of malignant cells but also to identify expression of surface markers or specific proteins by immunohistochemistry and flow cytometry. In our patients, lymphoma cells were mixed with those of the Reed-Sternberg type in granulomas, and foamy cells were found to be histiocytes. These findings were diagnostic of Hodgkin's lymphoma and Langerhans cell histiocytosis. Peritoneoscopy with liver biopsy is necessary not only to detect liver involvement in malignant hematological disorders early but also to make an accurate diagnosis.

Portal-based hematolymphoid neoplasms are typically of lymphoid histogenesis, mostly low-grade lymphomas. These correspond to the "white maculae" seen under peritoneoscopy and the so-called granulomas in clinical terms. The interpretation of a significant subset of these cases can be quite subtle, mimicking quiescent hepatitis or chronic biliary disease. Examples include mast cell disease, classical Hodgkin's lymphoma, chronic lymphocytic leukemia, and extranodal marginal zone lymphoma of MALT-type (MALToma). Damage to bile duct epithelium may even be seen. Recognition of the difference in cell content from inflammatory diseases in terms of cell count, monotonous appearance of cellular infiltrate, expansile and sometimes destructive nature of the infiltrate, and low threshold for suspicion should elicit an immunophenotypic workup and molecular study.

Case 15.4

A 68-year-old female complained of high fever, and her laboratory data showed LDH 1980 IU/L, AST 34 IU/L, ALT 23 IU/L, ALP 27.7 KAU, CRP 4.2 mg/dL, and ESR 31 mm/h. CT and US revealed no definite low-density area, and diffuse uptake was seen in gallium scintigraphy. Liver biopsy under echo guidance showed lymphoma cells in dilated sinusoids of middle zone to central area and congestion; lymphoma cells and phagocytosing red blood cells were seen scattered in dilated sinusoids (Fig. 15.6).

Hepatic sinusoidal dilatation has been reported in lymphoma, and it may be a consequence of an alteration in the sinusoidal barrier [20] and infiltration of lymphoma cells with phagocytosis of red blood cells along the sinusoids [21]. Peliosis hepatis could be seen on the liver surface in our cases of malignant lymphomas and Langerhans cell histiocytosis. Granulomatous lesions may compress sinusoids and cause hepatic sinusoidal dilatation. Infiltration of malignant cells causes alteration of the sinusoidal barrier and congestion. Therefore, retention of sinusoidal flow or peliosis hepatis can be observed by peritoneoscopy. Liver biopsy under peritoneoscopy can be carried out to make an accurate diagnosis of malignant hematological disorders, and bleeding from biopsied area can be prevented simultaneously.

A different pattern of lymphomatous involvement of the liver is seen in sinusoidal lymphocytosis. In general, this pattern is characterized by increased mononuclear cells throughout sinusoids, with no zonal predilection, giving the appearance of a string of pearls. This may be associated with sinusoidal dilatation. Sinusoidal lymphocytosis can be seen in chronic hepatitis C, systemic infectious diseases such as Epstein-Barr virus infection (infectious mononucleosis), cytomegalovirus infection, and toxoplasmosis. Mild infiltrates can occur with "hepatic involvement by systemic inflammatory conditions," such as collagen vascular diseases. Almost any hematolymphoid neoplasm can present with this pattern, although the most characteristic diagnoses are leukemias (acute or chronic), hairy cell leukemia, hepatosplenic T-cell lymphoma, and peripheral T-cell lymphoma unspecified.

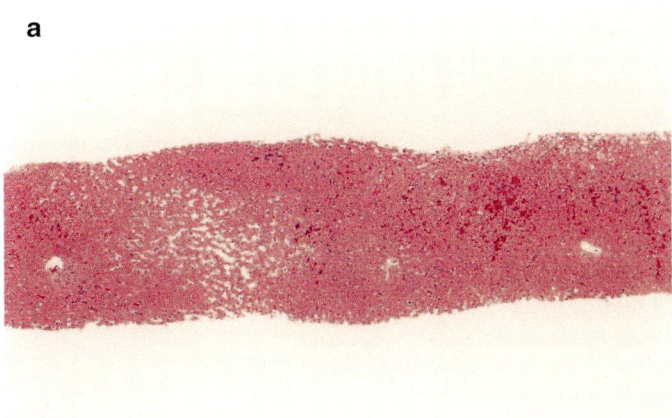
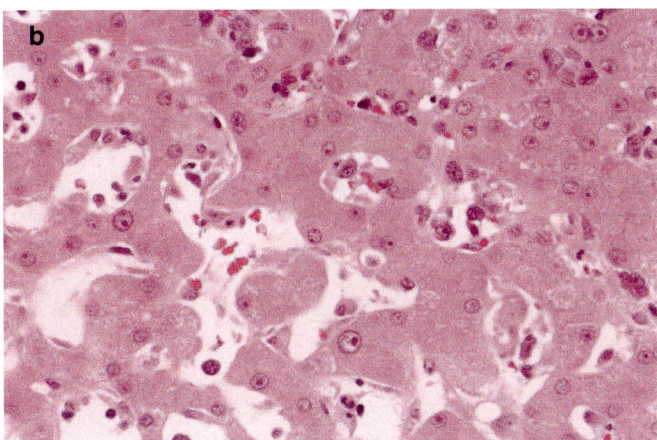

Fig. 15.6 Malignant lymphoma. (**a**) Sinusoids are dilated, and there is congestion in lobules. (**b**) Sinusoids are dilated and permeated by lymphoma cells

Awareness of this pattern, and correlation with clinical and serological data, should allow for appropriate workup for the possibility of lymphoma and leukemia. In our patients with malignant lymphoma and Langerhans cell histiocytosis, white maculae and peliosis hepatis were observed on the liver surface. Peritoneoscopy with liver biopsy is useful not only for staging of malignant hematological disorders but also for early diagnosis.

Hematolymphoid malignancy involving the liver can manifest several different patterns that should alert the pathologist to the possibility of lymphoma, leukemia, or other malignant disorders, despite significant morphologic overlap with nonneoplastic inflammatory liver diseases [22]. The most straightforward situation is a solitary tumor mass, most often seen in intermediate- and high-grade lymphomas, and rarely observed in plasmacytoma and histiocytosis. This is an uncommon presentation, but biopsy is clearly indicative of neoplastic cells that require only immunophenotypic confirmation for a final diagnosis.

Multiple myeloma affects the liver, and diffuse (sinusoidal), granular (portal), or mixed and nodular patterns have been described, and diffuse disease is the predominant pattern of liver involvement [23]. Hepatic plasmacytoma is defined as a single mass of clonal plasma cells, with no or minimal bone marrow plasmacytosis and with no other symptoms than those derived from the primary lesion. At diagnosis, ultrasonography shows hypoechoic space-occupying lesion [24], and the sensitivity and specificity of PET/CT is higher than that of MRI. While radiotherapy or chemotherapy remains the recommended treatment, extra-medullary plasmacytoma of the liver after treatment sometimes progresses to multiple myeloma [25, 26].

Case 15.5

A 75-year-old male was diagnosed with multiple myeloma 4 years ago, and complete remission was obtained by treatment. PET-CT revealed multiple FDG accumulation in the liver after the re-elevation of serum M protein. The results for blood routines and liver function were within normal ranges. Enhanced CT showed multiple hypervascular tumors in the liver (Fig. 15.7). B-mode ultrasonography showed hypoechoic tumors with mosaic pattern in part. Sonazoid-enhanced ultrasonography demonstrated whole tumor staining in vascular phase (Fig. 15.8a) and complete defect in post vascular phase (Fig. 15.8b). Needle biopsy revealed the invasion of heterotypic cells showing differentiation into plasma cells (Fig. 15.9). After additional treatment, all liver tumors disappeared.

Case 15.6

A 58-year-old male presented with multiple histiocytic tumors in the liver and spleen. Laboratory data showed WBC

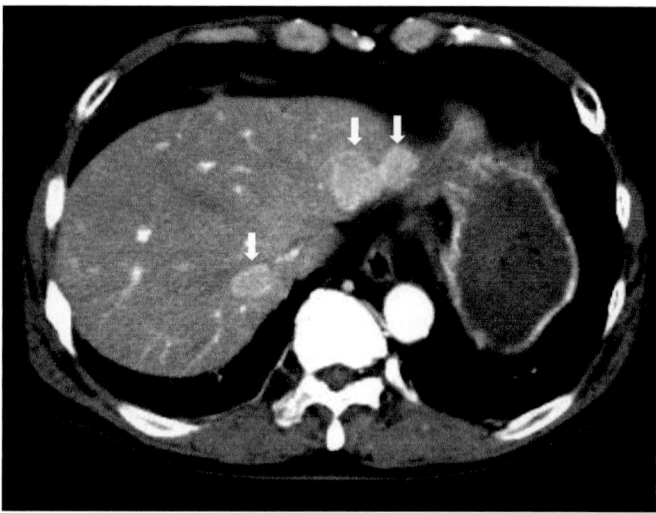

Fig. 15.7 Hepatic plasmacytoma. Contrast-enhanced CT showed multiple hypervascular tumors (arrows) in the liver

9500/μL, CRP 6.9 mg/L, ESR 77 mm/h, and soluble interleukin-2 receptor 1255 ng/mL. CT showed space-occupying lesions in the liver and spleen; MRI revealed high-intensity area in the liver and spleen, and it was more intense at the edge and in the center (Fig. 15.10). Diagnostic splenectomy showed large splenic tumor with small nodule and enlarged lymph node in the hilus. Histopathological examination of tumor in the spleen revealed proliferation of histiocytic cells with abundant clear cytoplasm and horseshoe-shaped nucleus (Fig. 15.11). Immunohistochemical studies revealed S-100 protein and CD1a antigen in the tumor cells (Fig. 15.12). No lymphocytic markers or lysozymes were detected. Ultrastructural findings showed clear cytoplasm and an invaginated nucleus; rough endoplasmic reticulum was swollen, but no definite Birbeck granules were seen (Fig. 15.13). Tumor cells could be classified into Langerhans cell type without Birbeck granules. Administration of adriamycin, vincristine, cyclophosphamide, and prednisolone reduced size and number of the liver tumors. Histiocytic cells could not be detected in tissues biopsied repeatedly from the liver.

15.1.2 Extramedullary Hemopoiesis

Extramedullary hemopoiesis (EMH) of the liver is a physiological process in the fetal and neonatal periods, but EMH is regarded as a pathological condition in adults. It occurs mainly in aplastic anemia and marrow replacement syndromes, including myeloproliferative disease, osteomyelofibrosis, myelomatosis, bone marrow carcinomatosis, and osteopetrosis. Hepatomegaly and massive splenomegaly are often seen, and portal hypertension may develop with ascites. Both diffuse microscopic infiltration and focal mass-like lesions in the liver have been reported with EMH [26].

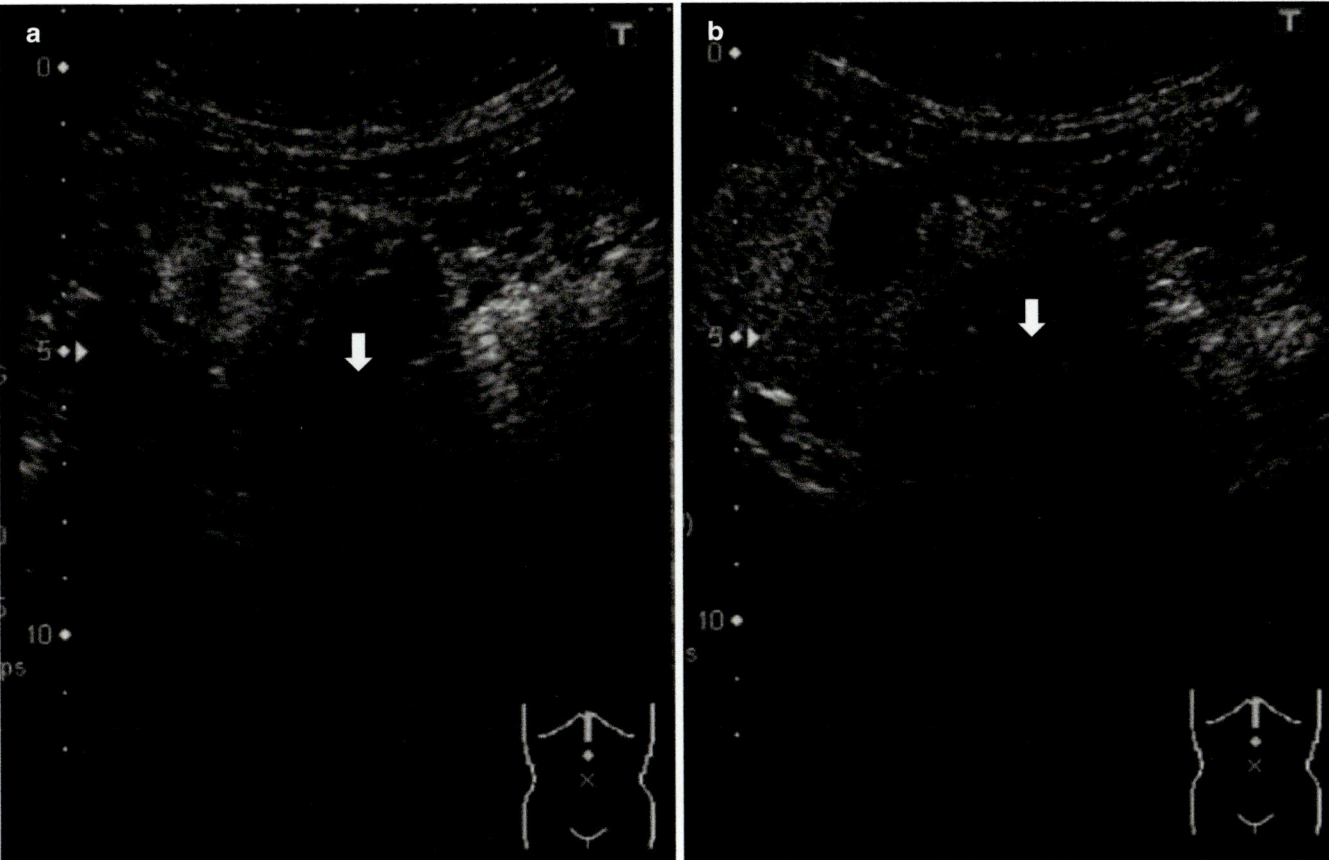

Fig. 15.8 Hepatic plasmacytoma. (**a**) Contrast-enhanced ultrasonography showed whole tumor stained in vascular phase (arrow). (**b**) Contrast-enhanced ultrasonography showed complete defect in post vascular phase (arrow)

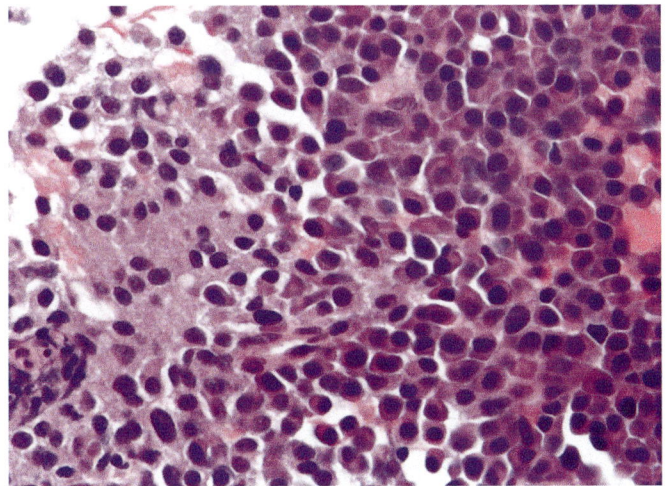

Fig. 15.9 Hepatic plasmacytoma. Pathological findings showed the invasion of heterotypic cells differentiating into plasma cells

Case 15.7

A 78-year-old female suffered from polycythemia vera for 30 years, and myelofibrosis developed. Abdominal fullness and diarrhea were present for 1 year, and abdominal CT showed ascites, hepatomegaly, and splenomegaly. The ascites increased gradually. Her laboratory data showed WBC 16,000/μL (myelocyte 8%, band 19%, segment 55%, basophil 4%, eosinophil 5%, lymphocyte 7%, and monocyte 2%), RBC 353 × 10⁴/μL and PLT 30.7 × 10⁴/μL. Liver tests revealed TBIL 1.5 mg/dL, LDH 749 IU/L, AST 95 IU/L, ALT 98 IU/L, ALP 784 IU/L, and GGT 62 IU/L. CT with or without contrast medium showed splenomegaly and ascites, and dilatation of splenic and superior mesenteric vein was detected by CT with contrast medium. Liver biopsy under US guidance showed intrasinusoidal megakaryocytes and erythropoietic precursors, which are the key cells to be identified and distinguished from sinusoidal infiltrate of hematolymphoid malignancy (Fig. 15.14).

15.1.3 Hemophagocytic Syndrome

Hemophagocytic syndrome (hemophagocytic lymphohistiocytosis) is characterized by fever, anorexia, and irritability. Blood cytopenia is present; jaundice and hepatosplenomegaly may develop later [27]. The syndrome, which was reported initially in patients with viral infection, occurs in

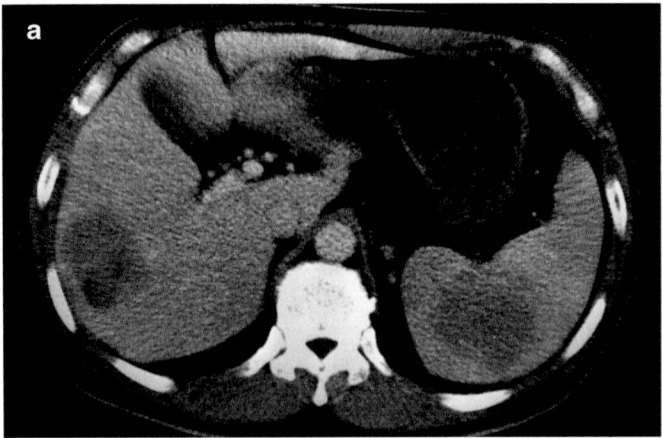 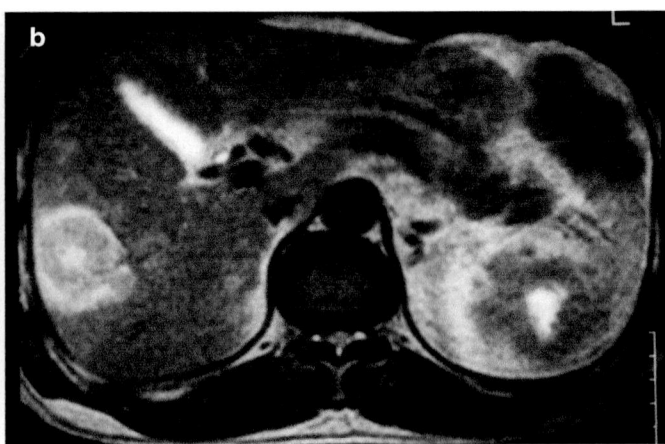

Fig. 15.10 Histiocytic tumor. (**a**) CT with contrast medium shows low-density area in the liver and spleen. (**b**) T2-weighted magnetic resonance image reveals high-intensity area in the liver and spleen and is more intensified at the edge and in the center. (Redrawn from Iwai M, et al. Langerhans cell histiocytosis of an adult with tumors in liver and spleen. Hepato-Gastroenterol 2001; 48: 581–4)

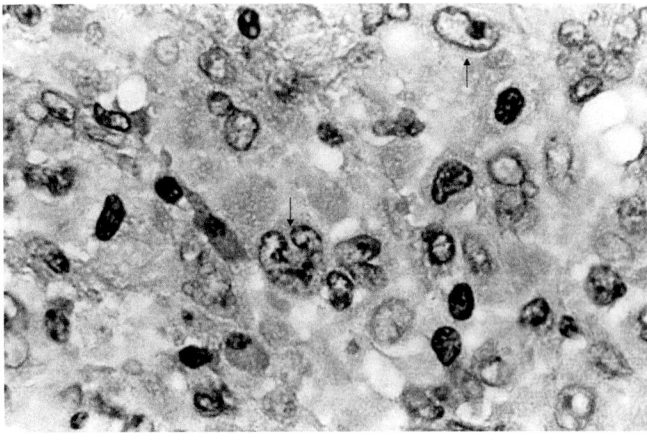

Fig. 15.11 Histiocytic tumor. Histiocytic cells with abundant clear cytoplasm and horseshoe-shaped nucleus (arrows) have proliferated in the spleen. (Redrawn from Iwai M, et al. Langerhans cell histiocytosis of an adult with tumors in liver and spleen. Hepato-Gastroenterol 2001; 48: 581–4)

association with various lymphoproliferative disorders, bacterial infections, acquired immunodeficiency syndrome, systemic lupus erythematosus, immunosuppressive therapy, and neoplastic diseases. Many autopsied series have shown hemophagocytosis in the spleen, lymph nodes, and bone marrow; hepatic involvement is characterized by diffuse hyperplasia of Kupffer cells and prominent hemophagocytosis [27, 28]. In a substantial number of cases, the liver is involved by the underlying conditions triggering hemophagocytosis, especially when liver derangement is profound [28, 29]. Hemophagocytic phenomenon is also seen in familial hemophagocytic reticulosis, familial erythrophagocytic lymphohistiocytosis, histiocytic medullary reticulosis, and malignant histiocytosis, which constitute the differential diagnosis. Early diagnosis is essential to initiate appropriate

treatment and improve the quality of life and survival of patients with various infection, collagen vascular diseases, and malignant disorders [30].

Case 15.8

A 62-year-old man complained of general malaise and high fever and had lost 5 kg of body weight in 6 months. Physical examination revealed icteric skin and hepatomegaly of two fingers' breadth in epigastrium. Laboratory data showed WBC 1700/μL, RBC 314 × 10⁴/μL, PLT 13.4 × 10⁴/μL, PT 18.4 s (control, 11.4 s), fibrinogen 45 mg/dL, FDP 2.5 g/mL, ESR 4 mm/h, TBIL 21.35 mg/dL, DBIL 14.51 mg/dL, ALP 1300 IU/L, LDH 1341 IU/L, and CRP 4.2 mg/dL. Bone marrow showed ANC 65,000/μL, and no atypical cells were seen. Liver biopsy showed sinusoidal dilatation, and steatosis was seen in the hepatocytes; foamy cells phagocytosing red blood cells in the sinusoids were also seen (Fig. 15.15). Disseminated intravascular coagulopathy (DIC) developed while chemotherapy was carried out without immunosuppressive agents, and hemorrhagic diathesis was apparent. He died of multiple organ failure 1 month after chemotherapy.

15.2 Liver in Systemic Sepsis and Infection

15.2.1 Liver in Sepsis

In sepsis, the liver may be affected directly by infection, injury induced by circulatory toxins, inflammatory and immunological response, ischemic effect of septic shock, or a combination of these factors. The hepatic changes may be very complex.

The range of infective lesions includes abscess, cholangitis, pylephlebitis, vasculitis, granulomas, and tissue necrosis. Various organisms may induce specific changes of diagnostic

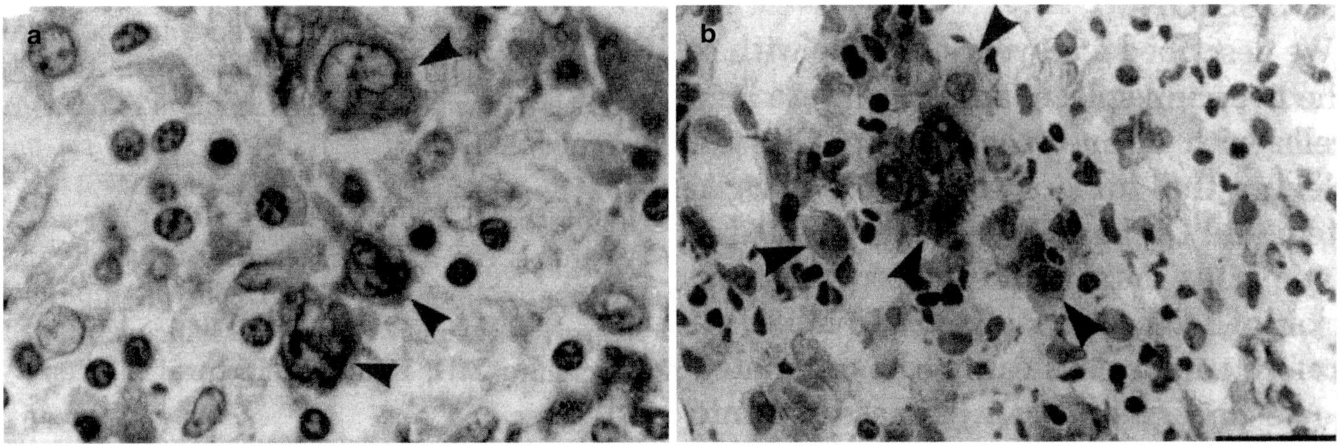

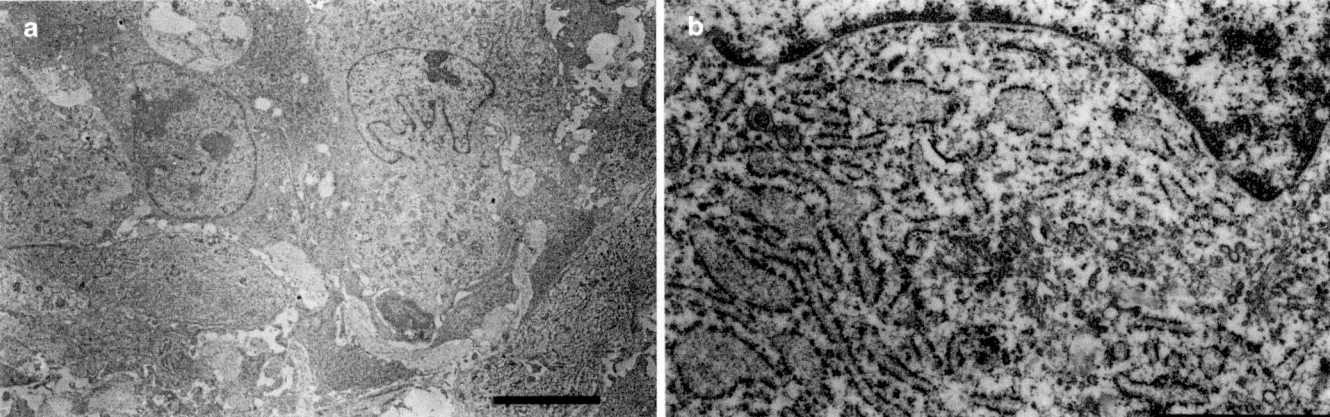

Fig. 15.12 Histiocytic tumor. (**a**) Histiocytic cells contain S-100 protein immunoreactivity (arrowheads). (**b**) Histiocytic cells contain CD1a antigen (arrowheads). (Redrawn from Iwai M, et al. Langerhans cell histiocytosis of an adult with tumors in liver and spleen. Hepato-Gastroenterol 2001; 48: 581–4)

Fig. 15.13 Histiocytic tumor. (**a**) Ultrastructural findings show clear cytoplasm and invaginated nucleus. Bar = 10 μm. (**b**) Rough endoplasmic reticulum is swollen, and no definite Birbeck granules are seen

importance. Other than direct involvement, reactive changes are common. The condition may be complicated by infection-associated hemophagocytic syndrome, in which liver function derangement may be profound [28].

Case 15.9

A 50-year-old man was admitted for abdominal pain and distension in poor condition. He died shortly after hospitalization. Blood culture grew *Escherichia coli*. Postmortem examination revealed fecal peritonitis as the cause of death. The biliary tree was patent. Liver section showed ductular proliferation at the margins of the portal tracts, with dilated ductules filled with inspissated bile along with neutrophilic infiltrate (Fig. 15.16).

Jaundice is common in patients with extrahepatic sepsis, especially due to gram-negative organisms. Three histological patterns have been described in such patients. The most common is perivenular canalicular cholestasis, associated variably with mild steatosis, Kupffer cell hyperplasia, and portal inflammatory infiltrate. Periportal ductular cholestasis with inflammation ("cholangitis lenta," as in Case 15.9) is common in the terminal stages of fatal sepsis, especially those complicating acute or chronic liver diseases. The rarest lesion is seen in toxic shock syndrome (mostly associated with the use of tampons), in which there is cholangitis with neutrophils in interlobular bile ducts (similar to bacterial cholangitis) attributed to a circulating staphylococcal toxin rather than to bacteremia.

15.2.2 Acquired Immunodeficiency Syndrome

In acquired immunodeficiency syndrome (AIDS), the liver is the target of a number of disease processes: opportunistic infections, AIDS-related tumors (Kaposi's sarcoma and lymphoma), concurrent infection with hepatitis viruses, and drug reactions [31].

Common opportunistic infections include atypical mycobacterium, cytomegalovirus, various fungi (such as histoplasma and cryptococcus with strong geographic variations), and protozoa (such as toxoplasma and pneumocystis). The pathology of these infections is no different from that seen in an immunocompetent host, except that there is generally less inflammation and poor granuloma formation. More distinctive lesions associated with human immunodeficiency virus (HIV) infection are bacillary angiomatosis and AIDS

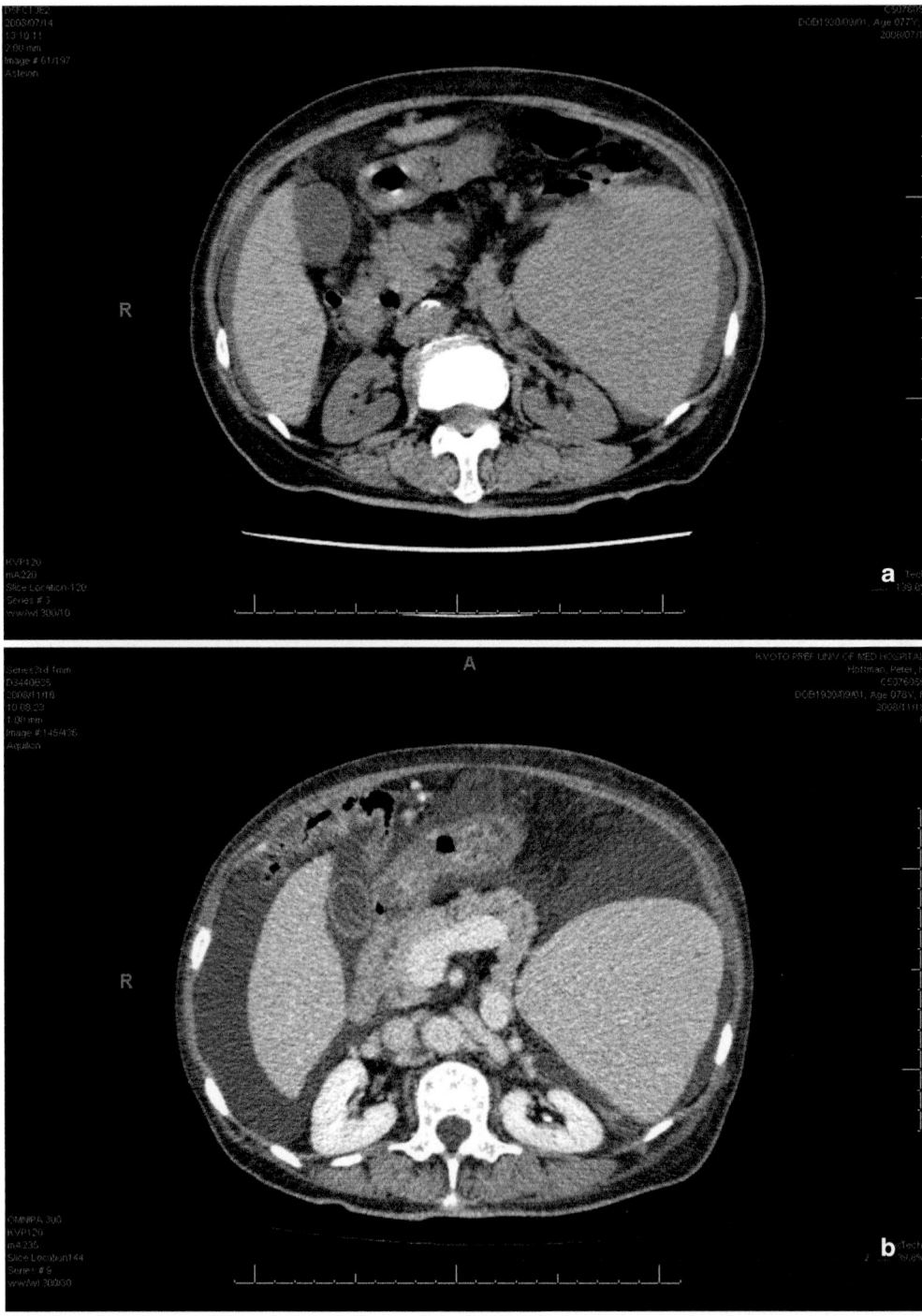

Fig. 15.14 Extramedullary hemotopoiesis. (**a**) CT without contrast medium shows splenomegaly with ascites. (**b**) CT with contrast medium shows dilated splenic and superior mesenteric vein. (**c**) Megakaryocytes and erythropoietic precursors are visible in sinusoids

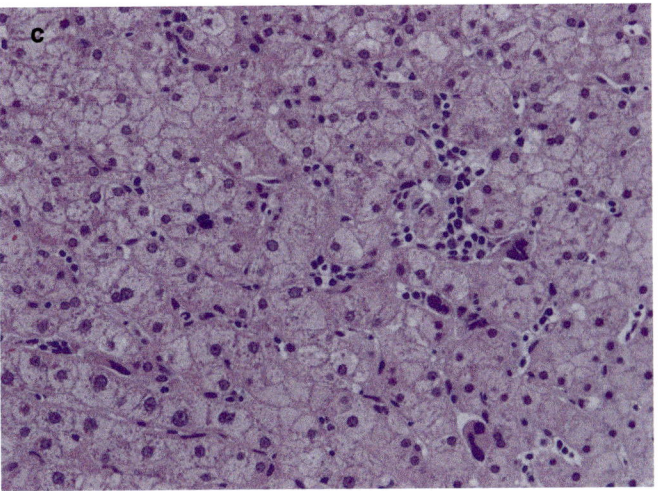

Fig. 15.14 (continued)

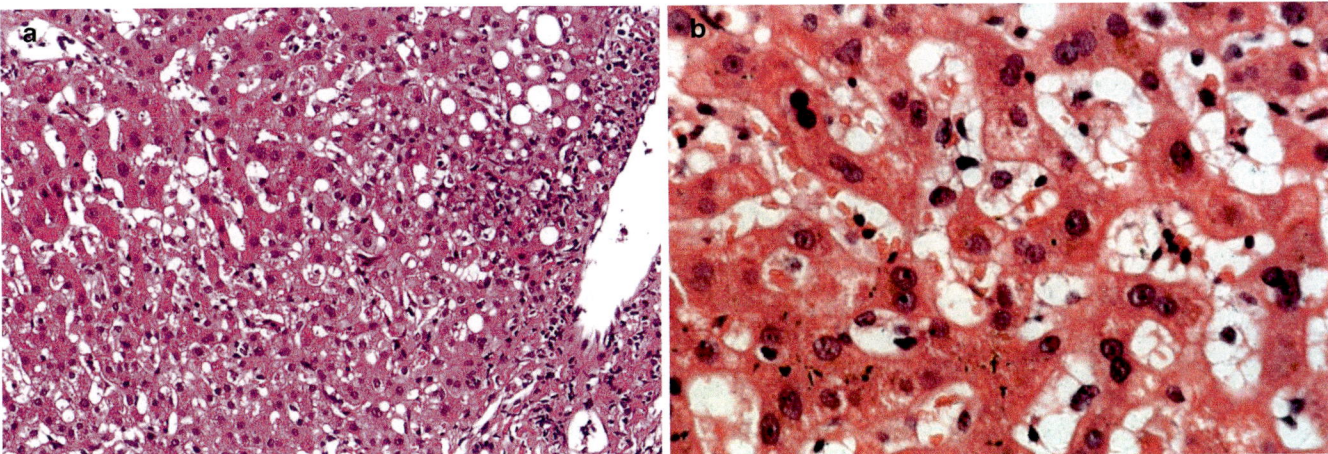

Fig. 15.15 Hemophagocytosis. (**a**) Sinusoidal dilatation and steatosis in hepatocytes. (**b**) There are foamy cells phagocytosing red blood cells in dilated sinusoids

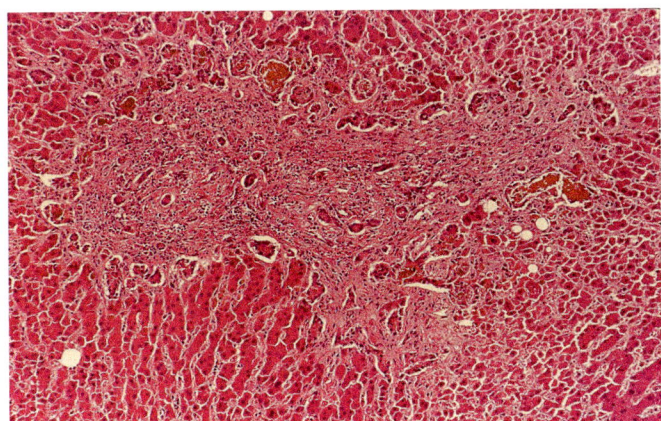

Fig. 15.16 Liver in sepsis. Ductular proliferation is seen at margins of portal tracts, and dilated ductules are filled with inspissated bile and infiltrated with neutrophilic leukocytes

cholangiopathy. The former shows peliotic blood spaces, fibromyxoid stroma alternating with angioproliferative spindle cells, and clumps of granular purple material shown to be rod-shaped bacilli (*Rochalimea henselae*) [32]. Cholangiopathy exhibits bile duct damage resembling that of graft-versus-host disease; sometimes, periductal fibrosis is indistinguishable from primary sclerosing cholangitis. These changes are seen with cryptosporidium or cytomegalovirus infection of the biliary tree [33].

Case 15.10
A 61-year-old-man presented with low-grade fever and nonproductive cough for 1 month. He was treated empirically with antibiotics. However, there was no improvement, and he developed high fever and diarrhea. Hepatomegaly and supraclavicular lymph nodes were detected, and fine-needle aspiration of

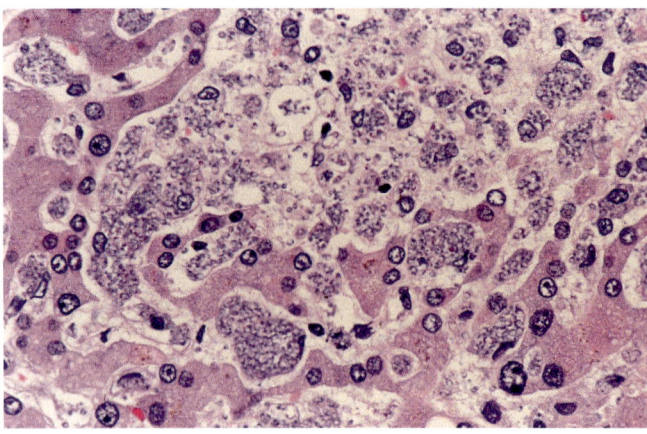

Fig. 15.17 Liver in AIDS. Histiocytes infiltrate with numerous intracellular yeast cells that are 2–4 μm in diameter (*Penicillium marneffei*)

the lymph node showed infection by a yeast organism, which was confirmed to be *Penicillium marneffei* on culture. HIV antibody was then found to be positive. Despite treatment with amphotericin B, his condition deteriorated and he died. Postmortem liver biopsy showed diffuse histiocytic infiltrates with numerous intracellular yeast cells 2–4 μm in diameter (Fig. 15.17). There was no evidence of pneumocystis or cytomegalovirus infection. It is known that the incidence and types of opportunistic, systemic fungal infection in AIDS patients vary widely according to geographic regions. *Penicillium marneffei* turns out to be the indicator organism for AIDS in Southeast Asia [34].

15.3 Liver in Pregnancy

Intercurrent liver diseases can occur in pregnancy and are the most common causes of jaundice: viral hepatitis (40%), drug reactions (10%), and large duct obstruction (6%). Several liver diseases are relatively unique to pregnancy. These include acute fatty liver of pregnancy, preeclampsia/eclampsia, HELLP syndrome, and intrahepatic cholestasis of pregnancy.

15.3.1 Acute Fatty Liver of Pregnancy

Acute fatty liver of pregnancy is the most serious of pregnancy-related liver diseases [35]. Without treatment, the maternal and fetal mortality rate may be as high as 80%. With increasing recognition, earlier diagnosis, and recognition of more mild forms of the disease, the mortality rate for both mother and fetus has decreased to between 5 and 50%. Prompt termination of pregnancy and improvements in supportive care for acute liver failure are thought to contribute to the improved outlook. It is caused by defects in mitochon-

drial fatty acid beta-oxidation and associated with a deficiency of long-chain 3-hydroxyacyl-CoA dehydrogenase [36]. The most common clinical presentation is a prodromal illness characterized by pruritus, severe vomiting, and jaundice in the final 4–10 weeks of gestation in a primigravid female. Acute liver failure ensues, with modest elevations of transaminases and bilirubin and doubling of prothrombin time. Many patients have hypertension and proteinuria.

Jaundice may develop following delivery. Grossly, the liver is yellow and usually small. Microscopically, hepatocytes are swollen, and the cytoplasm is transformed by tiny fat vacuoles [37]. The vesicles in microvesicular steatosis may be too small to appreciate, and the hepatocytes may simply appear ballooned; in this case, fat stains or electron microscopy may be necessary. Steatosis, which usually involves zones 2 and 3, is most prominent in zone 3 and is not infrequently panacinar. Macrovesicular steatosis can appear and is thought to result from coalescence of microvesicles over time.

While hepatocellular necrosis is not generally prominent, hepatocellular loss can be demonstrated on reticulin staining and, indirectly, by Kupffer cell hypertrophy and reduced organ weight. Other less specific features include canalicular and hepatocellular cholestasis, and mild mixed portal infiltrates with lymphocytes, eosinophils, and plasma cells. Serial biopsies of patients who have survived have demonstrated rapid resolution of microvesicular steatosis within days of delivery, with zone 3 hepatocytes being the last to resolve.

Case 15.11
A 30-year-old female was admitted with 3 weeks of jaundice prior to delivery of her third child, with meconium staining. She developed nausea and vomiting with lower abdominal and back pain and dark urine. Her liver biopsy showed microvesicular steatosis and brown-pigmented hepatocytes in zones 2 and 3 (Fig. 15.18). After delivery, her liver function tests returned to normal values, and she recovered completely.

15.3.2 Intrahepatic Cholestasis of Pregnancy

Intrahepatic cholestasis of pregnancy is characterized histologically by perivenular, canalicular cholestasis without steatosis, inflammation, or hepatocellular damage. Patients have pruritus and/or jaundice with elevated serum bile acid levels in late pregnancy. The disease regresses spontaneously following delivery, but frequently recurs during subsequent pregnancies or on administration of oral contraceptives. It is now associated with a canalicular phospholipid transporter defect, and heterozygous MDR3 gene mutation is identified [38].

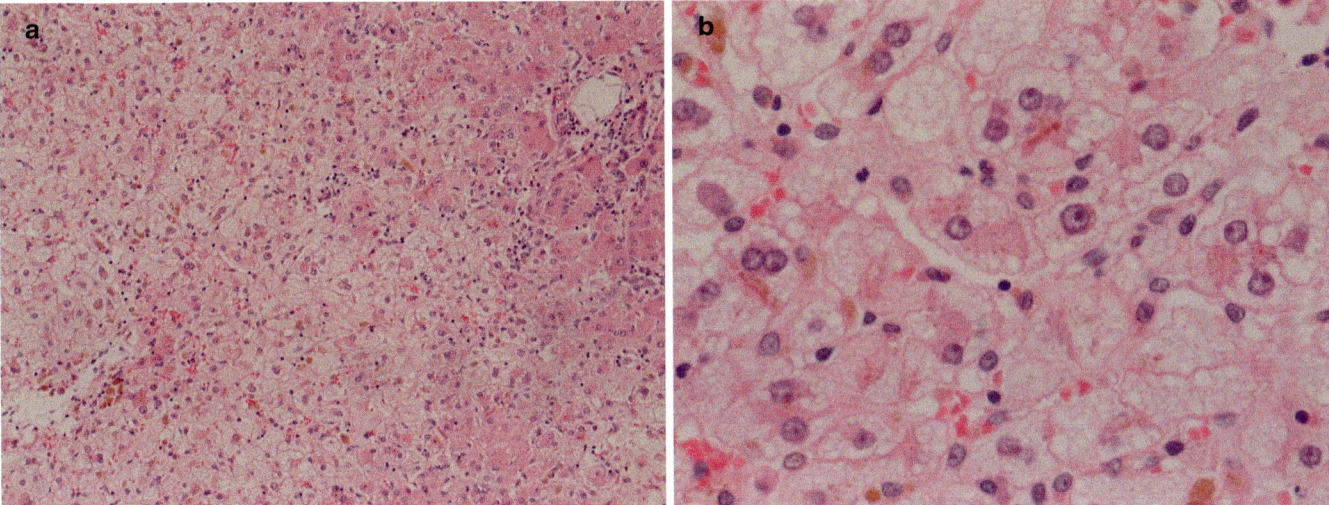

Fig. 15.18 Acute fatty liver of pregnancy. (**a**) Swollen, pale-staining hepatocytes are seen in zones 2 and 3, in contrast to rim of normal periportal hepatocytes. (**b**) Microvesicular steatosis is evident in pale hepatocytes, and canalicular cholestasis is also seen

15.3.3 Toxemia of Pregnancy

Toxemia of pregnancy includes preeclampsia and eclampsia and is characterized by hypertension, proteinuria, and edema (preeclampsia). In more severe cases, DIC is seen [39]. Fewer than 50% of patients have clinical evidence of liver disease, and many of them have normal biopsies. When jaundice occurs in the early stages of toxemia, it is usually not due to liver involvement but, rather, to hemolysis. In severe cases, the most characteristic findings are DIC with deposition of fibrin in sinusoids and focal hepatocellular necrosis of varying degrees, often—but not always—periportal. Portal areas have minimal infiltrates, and arterioles may have evidence of DIC with swollen endothelial cells and plasmatic vasculosis.

Case 15.12
A 32-year-old woman presented at 32 weeks of gestation with malaise, headache, and pain in the right hypochondrium. She was found to be hypertensive and proteinuric. Her laboratory data showed Hb 10.8 g/dL, PLT 57 × 10⁴/μL, PT 29 s (control, 15 s), and AST 400 IU/L. Her condition deteriorated, and she lapsed into a terminal coma with clinical features of a cerebral vascular accident. At autopsy, there was massive subarachnoid and cerebral hemorrhage. The 1.9-kg liver showed patchy congestion, yellow discoloration, and some areas of hemorrhage. Histology showed areas of liver cell necrosis, hemorrhage, and fibrin deposition around some portal tracts (Fig. 15.19).

HELLP syndrome (or hemolysis, elevated liver tests, and low platelets) is a multisystemic disorder of pregnancy and seen in a small percentage of patients with preeclampsia/eclampsia. It is characterized by hypertension, proteinuria,

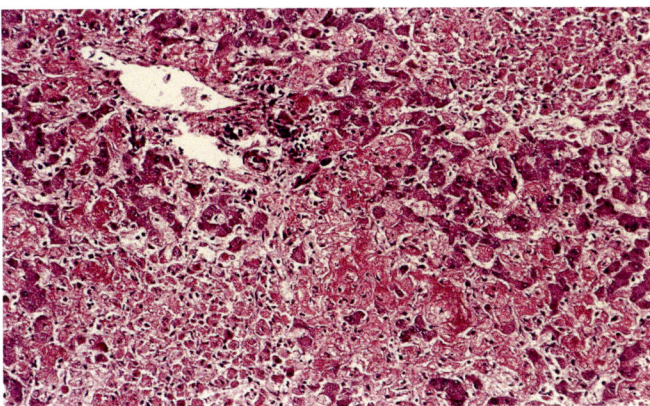

Fig. 15.19 Toxemia of pregnancy. Areas of periportal necrosis with intrasinusoidal fibrin deposition are present

and edema or seizure and coma, as in Case 15.12 [40]. The liver is involved in 10–20% of patients.

The syndrome may occur a few days after delivery, and there is no consensus on whether HELLP is a mild form of DIC or a subtype of toxemia. The histology is variable, ranging from normal to mild portal and lobular hepatitis to periportal fibrin and focal necrosis seen in toxemia (Fig. 15.20). Hepatic infarction and rupture have been reported in fatal cases. Treatment is aimed at controlling hypertension. Prednisolone is indicated, and delivery is recommended.

15.4 Liver in Collagen Vascular Diseases

Clinically, overt liver disease is unusual in collagen vascular diseases, but minor abnormalities in liver function tests are quite common [41]. Nonspecific abnormalities, such as fat or nonspecific reactive hepatitis, are also seen regularly

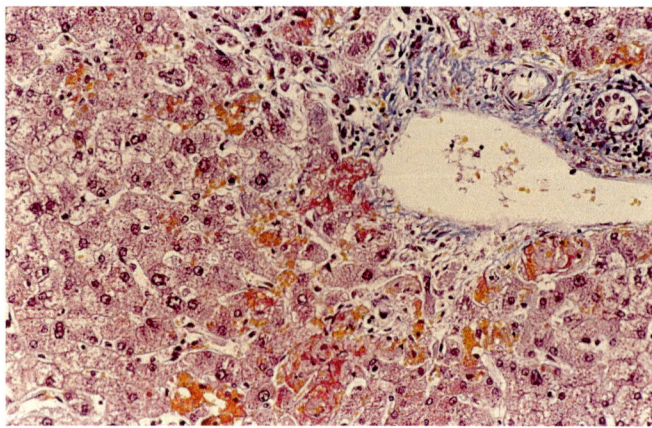

Fig. 15.20 Liver in HELLP. Martius scarlet blue stain shows red-stained fibrin in periportal sinusoids

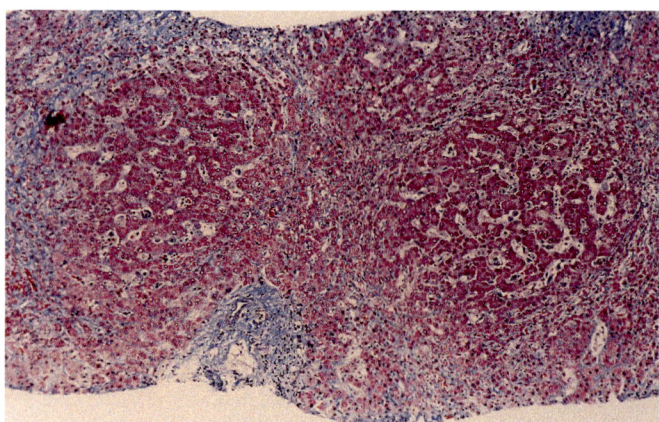

Fig. 15.21 Nodular regenerative hyperplasia. Masson's trichrome stain shows regenerative nodules delimited by rim of atrophic hepatocytes, without significant fibrosis

in liver biopsies. However, it may be difficult or impossible to distinguish changes due directly to the primary disease from those merely secondary to therapy (such as antirheumatic drugs) [42].

Patients with rheumatoid arthritis and its variants (Still's disease and Felty's syndrome) often have abnormal liver function. Besides nonspecific changes, concomitant primary biliary cirrhosis, chronic hepatitis, nodular regenerative hyperplasia, necrotizing arteritis, or amyloidosis may be found. Even rheumatoid nodules have been reported in the liver.

In systemic lupus erythematosus, abnormal liver function tests are occasionally present (approximately 10%) without serious liver lesions. However, chronic hepatitis, cirrhosis, and hepatic granulomas have been reported [43]. Most cases of chronic hepatitis are probably related to viral infection or drugs and do not bear any relationship to lupoid or autoimmune hepatitis. Other reported lesions include steatosis, cholestasis, nodular regenerative hyperplasia, and necrotizing arteritis.

Patients with polyarteritis nodosa may have necrotizing arteritis involving the liver, leading to infarction. In polymyalgia rheumatica-giant cell arteritis syndrome, granulomatous arteritis may be found in the liver.

Case 15.13

A 64-year-old female had a long history of systemic lupus erythematosus complicated by diffuse glomerulonephritis. In recent months, the liver function was deranged: TBIL was 268 μmol/L, ALP was 142 IU/L, and ALT and AST were normal. Hepatitis virus serologies were negative. CT showed small liver with features of portal hypertension. She developed progressive jaundice and ascites and finally succumbed to variceal bleeding. Postmortem liver biopsy showed distorted architecture, monoacinar

nodular formation, and preserved portal-central relationship (Fig. 15.21). The nodules consisted of hyperplastic hepatocytes in twin-celled plates delimited by a rim of atrophic hepatocytes and collapsed reticulin framework. Portal venules in about half of the portal tracts were narrowed or totally obliterated.

Some specific liver lesions are encountered more commonly in connective tissue diseases. Nodular regenerative hyperplasia (as in Case 15.13) is one such lesion and is frequently associated with Felty's syndrome [44]. It is attributable to vasculitis or thrombotic occlusion diffusely involving small intrahepatic vessels, leading to differential hyperplastic and atrophic zones and reorganization of the architecture.

Primary biliary cirrhosis may be associated with other autoimmune diseases, such as scleroderma, CREST syndrome (calcinosis cutis, Raynaud's phenomenon, esophageal dysfunction, sclerodactyly, and telangiectasia), rheumatoid arthritis, and Sjogren's syndrome [45].

15.5 Liver in Chronic Inflammatory Bowel Disease

The association between liver dysfunction and chronic inflammatory bowel disease (IBD) is well known, and clinicopathological reviews show fatty liver, primary sclerosing cholangitis, chronic hepatitis, cirrhosis, and hepatobiliary disease [46, 47]. Steatosis is the most common histological abnormality (up to 50%) in the liver. Severe steatosis is caused by malnutrition, anemia, and toxemia in IBD and may persist after colectomy [48].

Fatty metamorphosis is often seen in the livers of patients with IBD and is also detected in patients with ileostomy. Fatty change is more developed during intravenous infusion

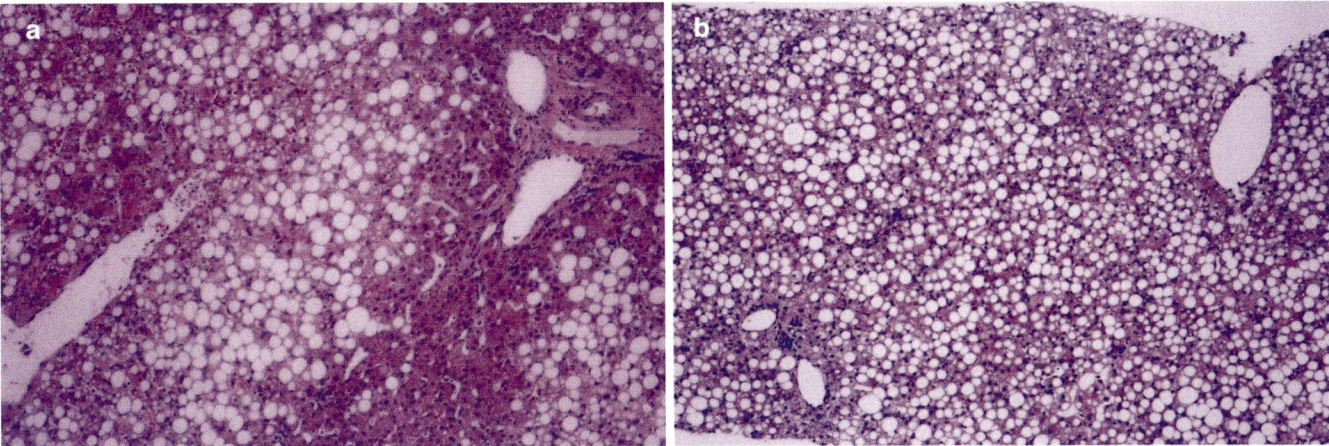

Fig. 15.22 Fatty liver in Crohn's disease. (**a**) Macrovesicular steatosis is seen in hepatocytes in zones 2 and 3. (**b**) Steatosis is distributed in all hepatocytes of lobule after intravenous infusion of high-calorie nutrients

of high-calorie nutrients. Therefore, long-term intravenous infusion of high-calorie nutrients and intake of a high-fat diet should be avoided.

Case 15.14

A 30-year-old man had suffered from Crohn's disease for 10 years. His liver function test showed TBIL 0.36 mg/dL, ALT 437 IU/L, AST 115 IU/L, ALP 409 IU/L, and GGT 30 IU/L. Liver biopsy revealed macrovesicular steatosis in the hepatocytes from perivenular area to middle zone. To prevent stimulation of the intestinal tract in Crohn's disease, high-calorie infusion was administered through intravenous hyperalimentation. Repeat liver tests showed TBIL 1.37 mg/dL, ALT 577 IU/L, AST 246 IU/L, ALP 1278 IU/L, and GGT 624 IU/L. Repeat biopsy demonstrated severe steatosis in hepatocytes compared to the first biopsy, and macrovesicular steatosis was seen in entire acinus (Fig. 15.22).

References

1. Cervantes F, Carreras E. Liver involvement in Hodgkin's disease: specific versus non-specific manifestations. Hematol Rev. 1994;8:305–11.
2. Greene FL. Laparoscopy in malignant disease. Surg Clin North Am. 1992;72:1125–37.
3. Hoane BR, Shields AF, Porter BA, Borrow JW. Comparison of initial lymphoma staging using computed tomography and magnetic resonance imaging. Am J Hematol. 1994;47:100–5.
4. Negendank WG, al-Katib AM, Karanes C, Smith MR. Lymphomas: MR imaging contrast characteristics with clinical-pathologic correlations. Radiology. 1990;177:209–16.
5. Ginaldi S, Bernardino ME, Jing BS, Green B. Ultrasonographic patterns of hepatic lymphoma. Radiology. 1980;136:427–31.
6. Chabner BA, Fisher RI, Young RC, DeVita VT. Staging of non-Hodgkin's lymphoma. Semin Oncol. 1980;7:285–91.
7. Loddenkemper LT, Hummel M, Ernestus K, Anagnostopoulos I, Dienes H-P, Schirmacher P, Stein H. Frequency and diagnostic patterns of lymphomas in liver biopsies with respect to the WHO classification. Virchows Arch. 2007;450:493–502.
8. Sans M, Andreu V, Bordas JM, Llach J, López-Guillermo A, Cevantes F, et al. Usefulness of laparoscopy with liver biopsy in the assessment of liver involvement at diagnosis of Hodgkin's and non-Hodgkin's lymphomas. Gastrointest Endosc. 1998;47:391–5.
9. Bain BJ, Chong KC, Coghlan SJ, Roberts SJ. Hepatic sinusoidal ectasia in association with Hodgkin's disease. Postgrad Med J. 1982;58:182–4.
10. Birrer MJ, Young RC. Differential diagnosis of jaundice in lymphoma patients. Semin Liver Dis. 1987;7:269–77.
11. Belliveau RE, Wiernik PH, Abt AB. Liver enzymes and pathology in Hodgkin's disease. Cancer. 1974;34:300–5.
12. Hirota K, Shiga T, Kimura K, Matsuki A, Oyama T. An anesthetic experience with a patient with ornithine transcarbamylase deficiency. Masui. 1989;38:98–101.
13. Hasaniya NW, Zayed FF, Faiz H, Severino R. Preinsertion local anesthesia at the trocar site improves perioperative pain and decreases costs of laparoscopic cholecystectomy. Surg Endosc. 2001;15:962–4.
14. Vaghadia H, Collins L, Sun H, Mitchell GW. Selective spinal anesthesia for outpatient laparoscopy. IV: population pharmacodynamic modelling. Can J Anaesth. 2001;48:273–8.
15. Lefor AT. Laparoscopic interventions in lymphoma management. Semin Laparosc Surg. 2000;7:129–39.
16. Alzalez SZ. Hepatobiliary tuberculosis. J Gastroenterol Hepatol. 1998;13:833–9.
17. Bhargava DK, Verma K, Malaviya AH. Solitary tuberculoma of the liver. Laparoscopic, histologic and etiologic diagnosis. Gastrointest Endosc. 1983;29:329–30.
18. Kataoka M, Nakata Y, Hiramatsu J, Okazaki K, Fujimori Y, Ueno Y, et al. Hepatic and splenic sarcoidosis evaluated by multiple imaging modalities. Intern Med. 1998;37:449–53.
19. Kanbay M, Altundag K, Gur G, Boyacioglu S. Non-Hodgkin's lymphoma presenting with granulomatous hepatitis and hemophagocytosis. Leuk Lymphoma. 2006;47:767–9.
20. Bruguera M, Caballero T, Carreras E, Aymerich M, Rodés J, Rozman C. Hepatic sinusoidal dilatation in Hodgkin's disease. Liver. 1987;7:76–80.
21. Jaffe ES. Malignant lymphomas: pathology of hepatic involvement. Semin Liver Dis. 1987;7:257–68.
22. Koto A, Moreki R, Santorineou M. Congenital hemophagocytic reticulosis. Am J Clin Pathol. 1976;65:495–503.

23. Thomas FB, Clausen KP, Greenberger NJ. Liver disease in multiple myeloma. Arch Intern Med. 1973;132:195–202.

24. Kelekis NL, Semelka RC, Warshauer DM, Sallah S. Nodular liver involvement in light chain multiple myeloma: appearance on US and MRI. Clin Imaging. 1997;21:207–9.

25. Caers J, Paiva B, Zamagni E, et al. Diagnosis, treatment, and response assessment in solitary plasmacytoma: updated recommendations from a European Expert Panel. J Hematol Oncol. 2018;11:10–9.

26. Dewar G, Leung NW, Ng HK, Bradley M, Li AK. Massive, solitary, intrahepatic, extramedullary hematopoietic tumor in thalassemia. Surgery. 1990;107:704–7.

27. Hsu TS, Kemp DM. Clinical features of familial histiocytosis. Am J Pediatr Hematol Oncol. 1981;3:61–5.

28. Tsui WM, Wong KF, Tse CC. Liver changes in reactive haemophagocytic syndrome. Liver. 1992;12:363–7.

29. de Kerguenec C, Hillaire S, Molinié V, Gardin C, Degott C, Erlinger S, et al. Hepatic manifestations of hemophagocytic syndrome: a study of 30 cases. Am J Gastroenterol. 2001;96:852–7.

30. Ramos-Casals M, Brito-Zerón P, López-Guillermo A, Khamashta MA, Bosch X. Adult haemophagocytic syndrome. Lancet. 2014;383:1503–16.

31. Lebovics E, Thung SN, Schaffner F, Radensky PW. The liver in the acquired immunodeficiency syndrome: a clinical and histologic study. Hepatology. 1985;5:293–8.

32. Slater LN, Welch DF, Min KW. Rochalimaea henselae causes bacillary angiomatosis and peliosis hepatis. Arch Intern Med. 1992;152:602–6.

33. Cello J. Human immunodeficiency virus-associated biliary tract diseases. Semin Liver Dis. 1992;12:213–8.

34. Tsui WMS, Ma KF, Tsang DNC. Disseminated *Penicillium marneffei* infection in HIV-infected subject. Histopathology. 1992;20:287–93.

35. Sherlock S. Acute fatty liver of pregnancy and microvesicular fat diseases. Gut. 1983;24:265–9.

36. Ibdah JA. Acute fatty liver of pregnancy: an update on pathogenesis and clinical implications. World J Gastroenterol. 2006;12:7397–404.

37. Rolfes DB, Ishak KG. Acute fatty liver of pregnancy: a clinico-pathologic study of 35 cases. Hepatology. 1985;5:1149–58.

38. Lucena JF, Herrero JI, Quiroga J, Sangro B, Garcia-Foncillas J, Zabalegui N, et al. A multidrug resistance 3 gene mutation causing cholelithiasis, cholestasis of pregnancy, and adulthood biliary cirrhosis. Gastroenterology. 2003;124:1037–42.

39. Rolfes DB, Ishak KG. Liver disease in pregnancy. Histopathology. 1986;10:555–70.

40. Sibai BM, Taslimi MM, el-Nazer A, Amon E, Mabie BC, Ryan GM. Maternal-perinatal outcome associated with the syndrome of hemolysis, elevated liver enzymes, and low platelets in severe preeclampsia-eclampsia. Am J Obstet Gynecol. 1986;155:501–9.

41. Walker NJ, Zurier RB. Liver abnormalities in rheumatic diseases. Clin Liver Dis. 2002;6:933–46.

42. Suissa S, Ernst P, Hudson M, Bitton A, Kezouh A. Newer disease-modifying antirheumatic drugs and the risk of serious hepatic adverse events in patients with rheumatoid arthritis. Am J Med. 2004;117:87–92.

43. Runyon BA, LaBrecque RD, Anuras S. The spectrum of liver disease in systemic lupus erythematosus: report of 33 histologically proven cases and review of the literature. Am J Med. 1980;69:187–94.

44. Blendis LM, Parkinson MC, Shilkin KB, Williams R. Nodular regenerative hyperplasia of the liver in Felty's syndrome. Q J Med. 1974;43:25–32.

45. Reynolds TB, Denison EK, Frankl HD, Lieberman FL, Peters RL. Primary biliary cirrhosis with scleroderma, Raynaud's phenomenon and telangiectasia. New syndrome. Am J Med. 1971;50:302–12.

46. Balistreri WF. Hepatobiliary complications of inflammatory bowel disease: overview of the issues. Inflamm Bowel Dis. 1998;4:220–4.

47. Bargiggia S, Maconi G, Elli M, Molteni P, Ardizzone S, Parente F, et al. Sonographic prevalence of liver steatosis and biliary tract stones in patients with inflammatory bowel disease: study of 511 subjects at a single center. J Clin Gastroenterol. 2003;36:417–20.

48. Eade MN. Liver disease in ulcerative colitis. I. Analysis of operative liver biopsy in 138 consecutive patients having colectomy. Ann Intern Med. 1970;72:475–87.

Liver Tumor I: Benign Tumors and Tumor-Like Lesions

16

Wilson M. S. Tsui, Takahiro Mori, and Masaki Iwai

Contents

Abbreviations

AFP	Alpha-fetoprotein
AML	Angiomyolipoma
BDA	Bile duct adenoma
CEA	Carcinoembryonic antigen
c-myc	Cancer-myelocytomatosis
ELISA	Enzyme-linked immunosorbent assay
FNH	Focal nodular hyperplasia
HCA	Hepatocellular adenoma
HCC	Hepatocellular carcinoma
HMB45	Human melanoma black 45
HNF-1	Hepatocyte nuclear factor 1
IL6ST	Interleukin 6 signal transducer
IPN	Intraductal papillary neoplasm
IPT	Inflammatory pseudotumor
L-FABP	Liver fatty acid binding protein
LMS	Larva migrans syndrome
MCN	Mucinous cystic neoplasm
p53	53-kilodalton protein
PECOMA	Perivascular epithelioid cell tumors
PIVKA2	Protein induced by vitamin K absence or antagonist-2

W. M. S. Tsui, MD, FRCPath (✉)
Hong Kong, China
e-mail: mstsui@ha.org.hk

T. Mori, MD, PhD
Hyogo, Japan

M. Iwai, MD, PhD
Kyoto, Japan

Compared to malignant tumors, benign tumors of the liver are encountered rarely in daily practice, although their true incidence is probably not low [1]. This is because they are either asymptomatic and not discovered or they are not biopsied and

© Springer Nature Singapore Pte Ltd. 2019
E. Hashimoto et al. (eds.), *Diagnosis of Liver Disease*, https://doi.org/10.1007/978-981-13-6806-6_16

left unresected. However, ultrasonographic imaging often may show benign tumors in the liver. Some of these tumors are true neoplasms, while others are tumor-like masses (Table 16.1) [2].

16.1 Hemangioma

Hemangioma is the most common benign tumor of the liver, being noted in 0.4–20% of cases in autopsy studies. The asymptomatic lesions are usually solitary and are typically <5 cm in diameter. Patients sometimes present with abdominal pain or discomfort and a palpable mass. Large tumors may rarely be

Table 16.1 Benign neoplasms and tumor-like lesions of the liver

Tumor	Lesion
Hepatocellular tumors	Focal nodular hyperplasia
	Hepatocellular adenoma
Biliary tumors	Biliary microhamartoma (von Meyenburg complex)
	Bile duct adenoma
	Biliary adenofibroma
	Mucinous cystic neoplasm (biliary cystadenoma)
	Intraductal papillary neoplasm (biliary papillomatosis)
	Other pancreatic type tumors
Vascular tumors	Hemangioma
	Infantile hemangioma
	Lymphangioma and lymphangiomatosis
Miscellaneous tumors	Angiomyolipoma and lipomatous tumors
	Leiomyoma
	Solitary fibrous tumor
	Mesenchymal hamartoma
	Benign teratoma
Miscellaneous lesions	Inflammatory pseudotumor
	Fibrosing necrotic nodule
	Parasitic granuloma
	Nodular transformation
	Pseudolipoma
	Heterotopia (adrenal, pancreas, spleen)
	Gauzeoma

complicated by rupture, thrombocytopenia, and consumptive coagulopathy (Kasabach-Merritt syndrome) [3]. A large or ruptured hemangioma requires immediate surgical intervention.

Histologically, liver hemangioma is mainly cavernous type. Complications such as thrombosis, infarction, sclerosis, and calcification may occur, leading to possible confusion with a more aggressive tumor. Although hemangiomas are grossly well circumscribed, microscopic extension of dilated vascular spaces into adjacent hepatic parenchyma may be observed [4]. Though extremely rare, diffuse and multiple lesions occur with progressive development [5], and some cases are associated with bone and lung involvement (diffuse systemic hemangiomatosis). Multiple or diffuse lesions must also be differentiated from peliosis hepatis and hereditary hemorrhagic telangiectasia. Recently a rare small vessel-type hemangioma with infiltrative border is recognized and has to be distinguished from angiosarcoma by immunohistochemical staining for p53, c-myc, and Ki-67 [6].

Hemangiomas are usually asymptomatic. The diagnosis is based on imaging studies. Abdominal ultrasonography (US) shows a hyperechoic structure with smooth margin; CT reveals hypodense tumor; and CT with contrast medium shows enhanced tumor in a peripheral-central direction with focal globular pattern. MRI displays low-signal T1 time and hyperintensity in the T2-weighted image. Sclerosed hemangioma has atypical imaging features and may be confused with hepatocellular carcinoma, cholangiocarcinoma, and metastatic tumor [7].

Case 16.1

A 51-year-old female complained of persistent right flank pain, and her ultrasonographic diagnosis was liver hemangioma. Her liver function test showed TBIL 0.92 mg/dL, AST 12 IU/L, ALT 12 IU/L, LDH 197 IU/L, and AFP 1.6 ng/mL. HBsAg and anti-HCV were negative. Computed tomography (CT) showed a low-density signal in the S6 area and enhancement on the edge of the tumor in the arterial phase (Fig. 16.1). The tumor had a larger circumference in the venous phase, and low density remained in the center. T1 image on magnetic resonance imaging (MRI) showed a low-intensity area in S6, MRI with

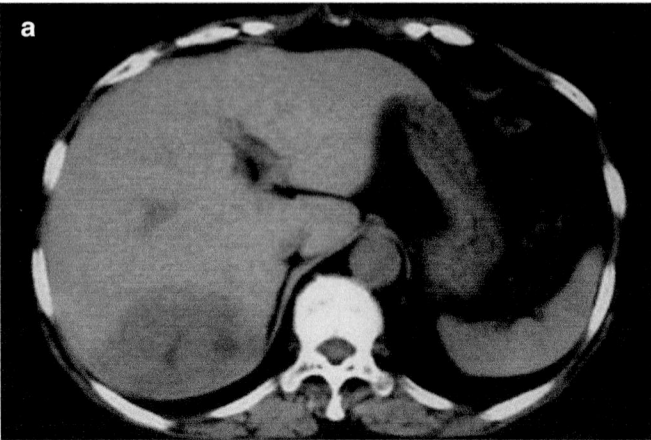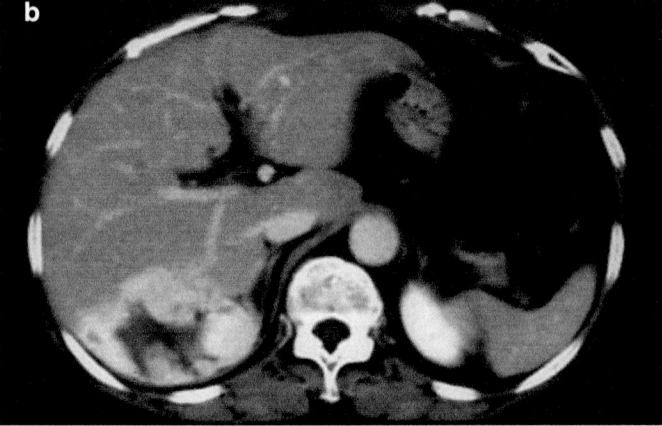

Fig. 16.1 Hemangioma. (**a**) CT without contrast medium shows low-density area in S6. (**b**) Contrast medium is retained from the edge to the center

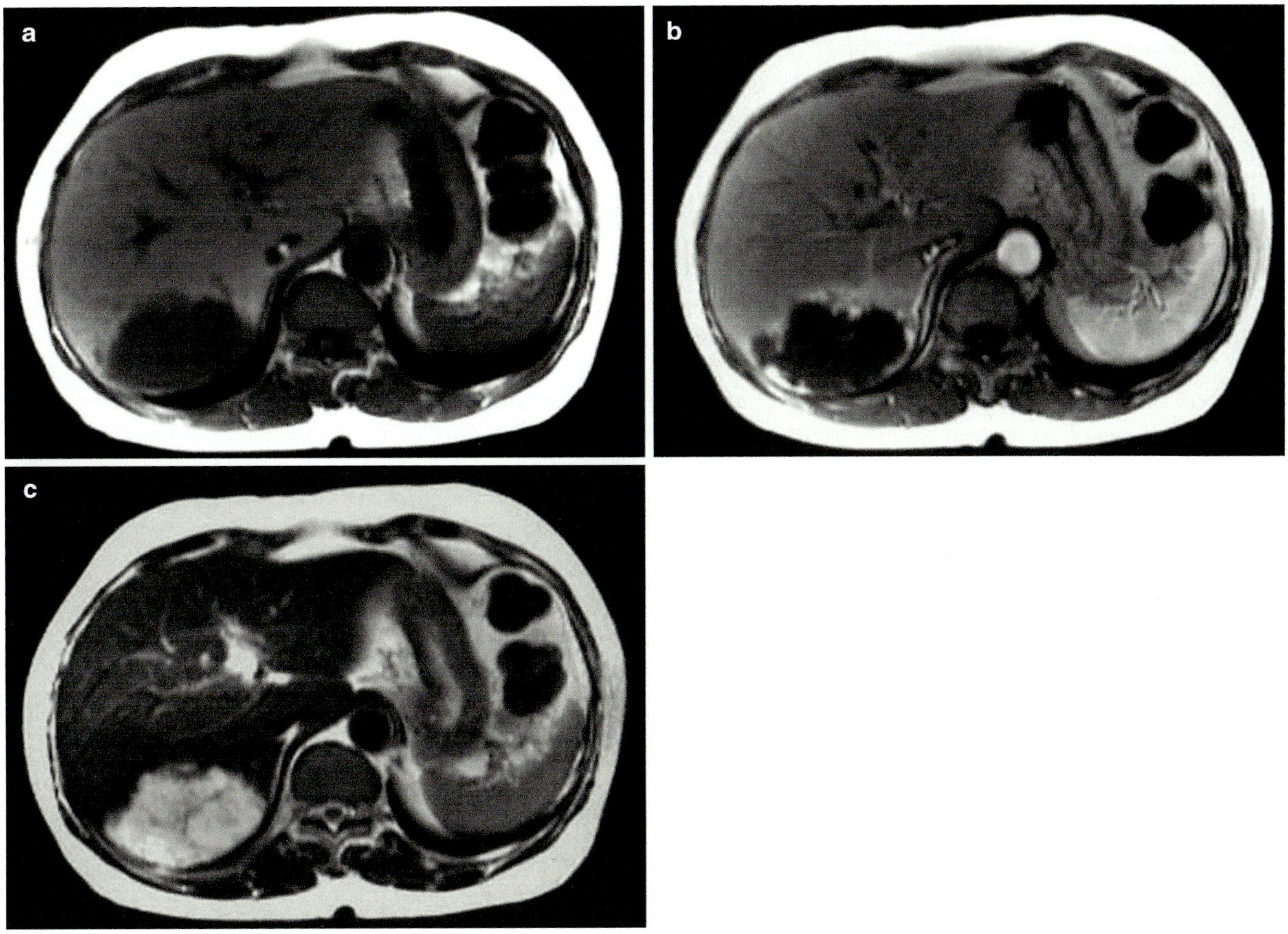

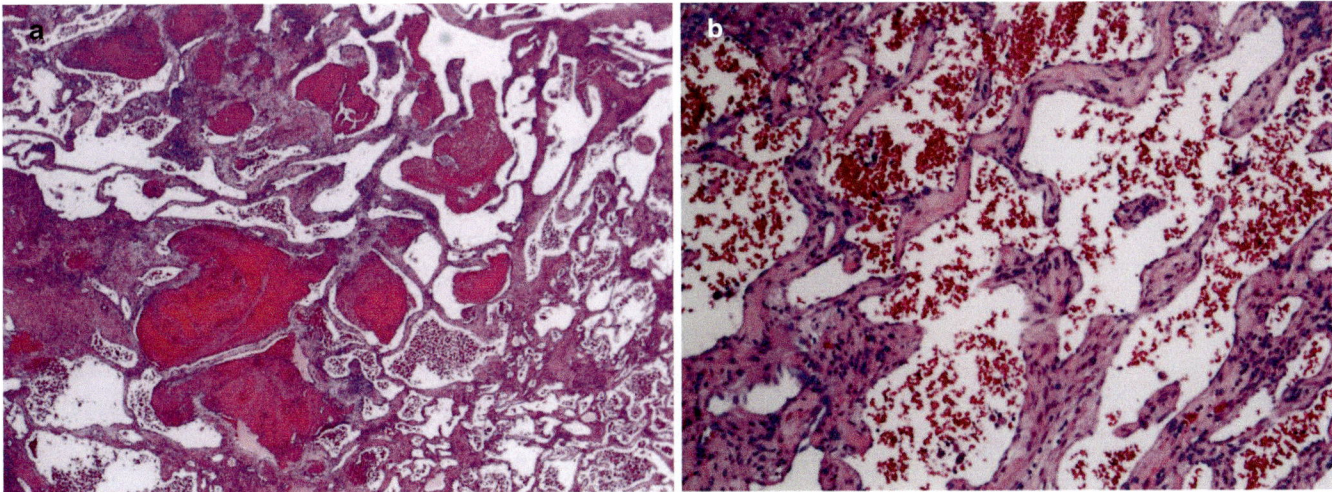

Fig. 16.2 Hemangioma. (**a**) T1-weighted image on MRI shows low intensity in S6. (**b**) MRI with contrast medium shows high-intensity area on the edge of tumor in early phase. (**c**) MRI with contrast medium reveals high intensity in tumor

Fig. 16.3 Hemangioma. (**a**) Histology shows cavernous spaces filled with blood cells. (**b**) Vascular spaces are lined by flattened endothelial cells and filled with blood cells

contrast medium revealed high-intensity area on the edge, and T2 revealed high intensity in the tumor (Fig. 16.2). Surgically resected tissues showed cavernous vascular spaces filled with blood cells or amorphous materials, and the cavernous spaces were separated by delicate fibrous strands and lined by flattened endothelial cells without atypia (Fig. 16.3).

Case 16.2

An obese female aged 76 years suffered from diabetes mellitus, and her abdominal CT showed low-density area (25 mm on diameter) in S4, and faint staining was detected in the center of tumor during early and late phase of enhanced CT (Fig. 16.4). All liver function tests were normal, and tumor markers of AFP, PIVKA2, CEA, and CA19-9 were within normal limit. MRI showed low intensity in the tumor by T1 and slightly high intensity by T2, and dynamic MRI revealed low intensity in tumor as well as non-tumor area in early and late phase and

slight retention of contrast medium in the center during the late phase (Fig. 16.5). Tumor biopsy under echo guidance revealed small- and variously sized vessels surrounded by thick myxoid walls and lined with flattened endothelial cells. Cavernous formation was not well developed, and red blood cells were scanty in the lumen (Fig. 16.6). The histological features are consistent with sclerosing cavernous hemangioma.

In this rare sclerosing cavernous hemangioma, the lesion cannot be detected as cavernous hemangioma by CT and MR imaging. There have been only a few studies to report radiological findings of sclerosed hemangiomas, and the majority is reported to present as a perfusion defect on enhanced CT [8]. In addition sclerosed hemangiomas exhibit mild to moderate hyperintensity on T2-weighted MR images, hypointensity on T1-weighted images, patchy enhancement during the arterial phase, and gradual enhancement during the delayed phases [9]. Hemorrhage, thrombosis, or infarction within a

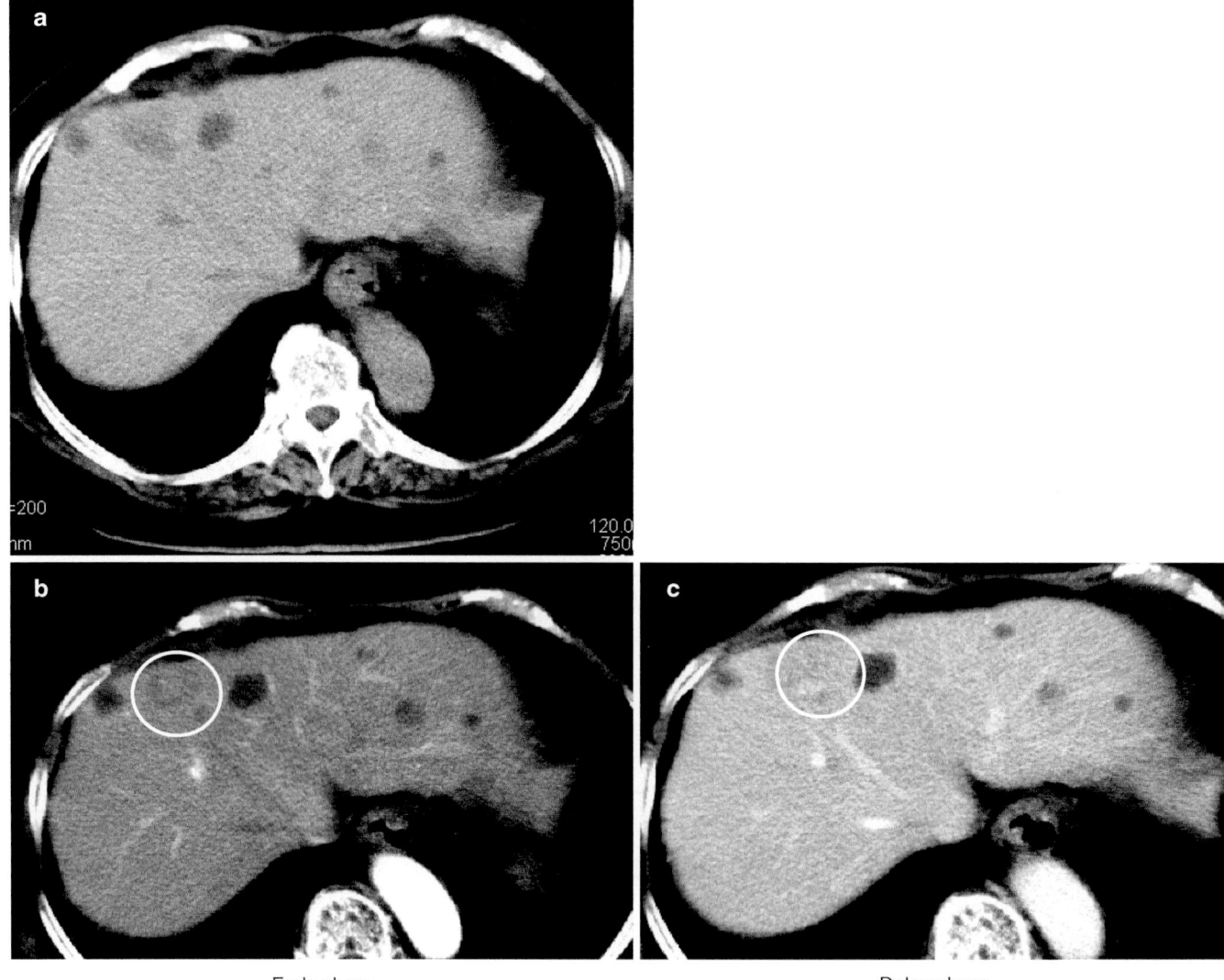

Early phase   Delay phase

Fig. 16.4 Sclerosing cavernous hemangioma. (**a**) Low-density area (LDA) (about 2.5 cm in diameter) is seen in S4, and several cystic lesions are seen in both lobes. (**b**) LDA is slightly enhanced from center by contrast medium in early phase. (**c**) Enhancement in center of LDA is retained in late phase

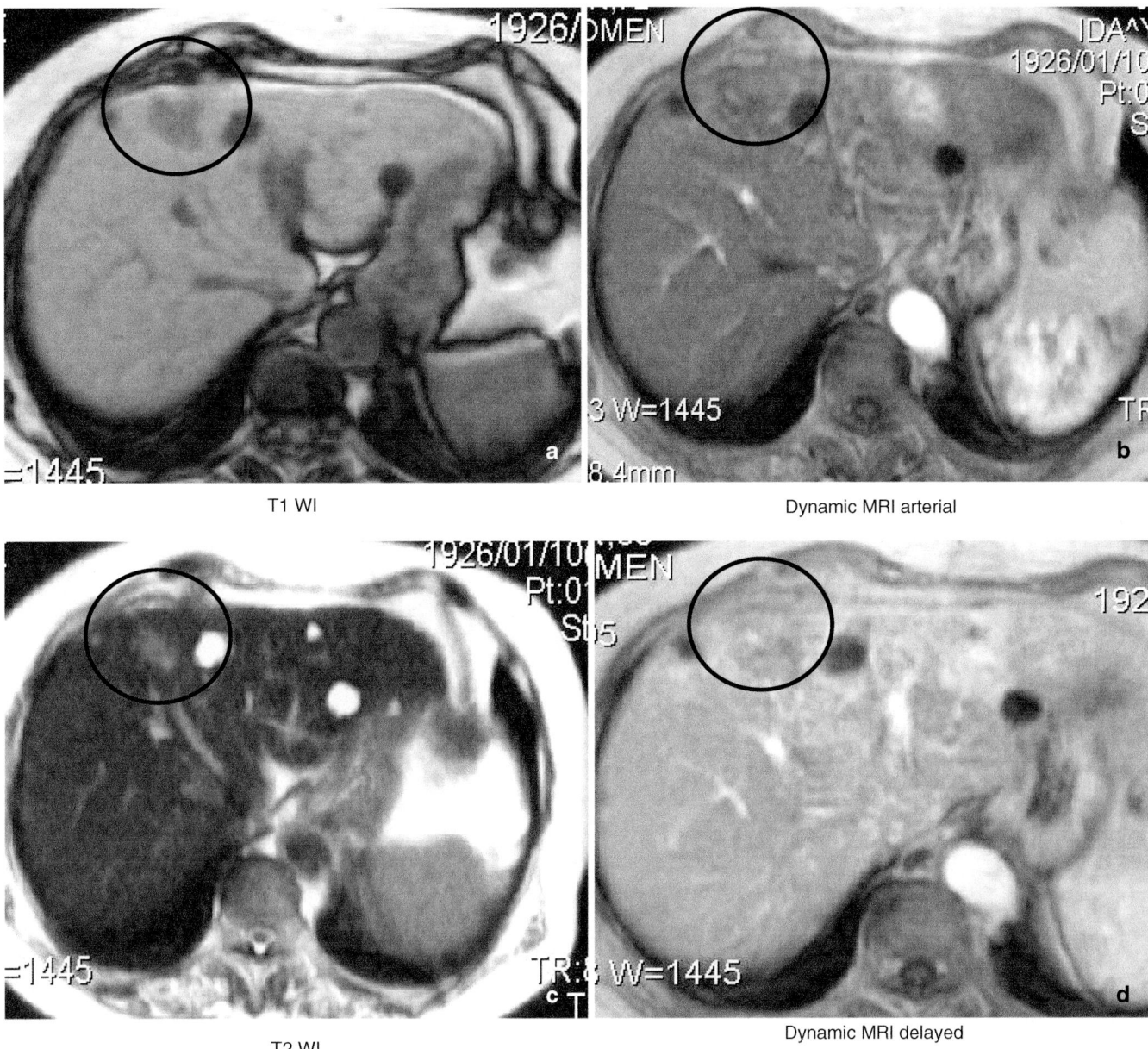

T1 WI   Dynamic MRI arterial

T2 WI   Dynamic MRI delayed

Fig. 16.5 Sclerosing cavernous hemangioma. (**a**) MRI intensified by T1 shows low intensity in tumor and (**b**) by T2 shows weakly high intensity in tumor. (**c**) Dynamic MRI shows iso-intensity in circumfer-ence of tumor in arterial and delayed phase, and low intensity is seen in center, and (**d**) enhancement is seen in center during delayed phase

cavernous hemangioma may instigate progression to a scle-rosed hemangioma, as a result of fibrosis and hyalinization of thick-walled blood vessels. Mast cells have been impli-cated in the development of this process [10].

16.2   Focal Nodular Hyperplasia

Focal nodular hyperplasia (FNH) is the second most com-mon benign liver process. It occurs in both sexes and across all ages, but most commonly in young adult women [11]. It is usually solitary but can be multiple in 20–30% of cases. It

is usually <5 cm in diameter and discovered incidentally on physical examination or by imaging, but it may also present with complications attributed to large size (or, rarely, due to hemorrhage or pain). Some patients with the so-called mul-tiple FNH syndrome have at least two FNHs associated with one or more lesions, such as hepatic hemangioma, arterial vascular malformations, meningioma, and astrocytoma.

FNH is a polyclonal nonneoplastic lesion [12]. The cur-rently favored hypothesis of its tumorigenesis is that it repre-sents a hyperplastic and altered growth response to changes in blood flow in the parenchyma surrounding a preexisting arterial malformation [13]. The ductular proliferation, once

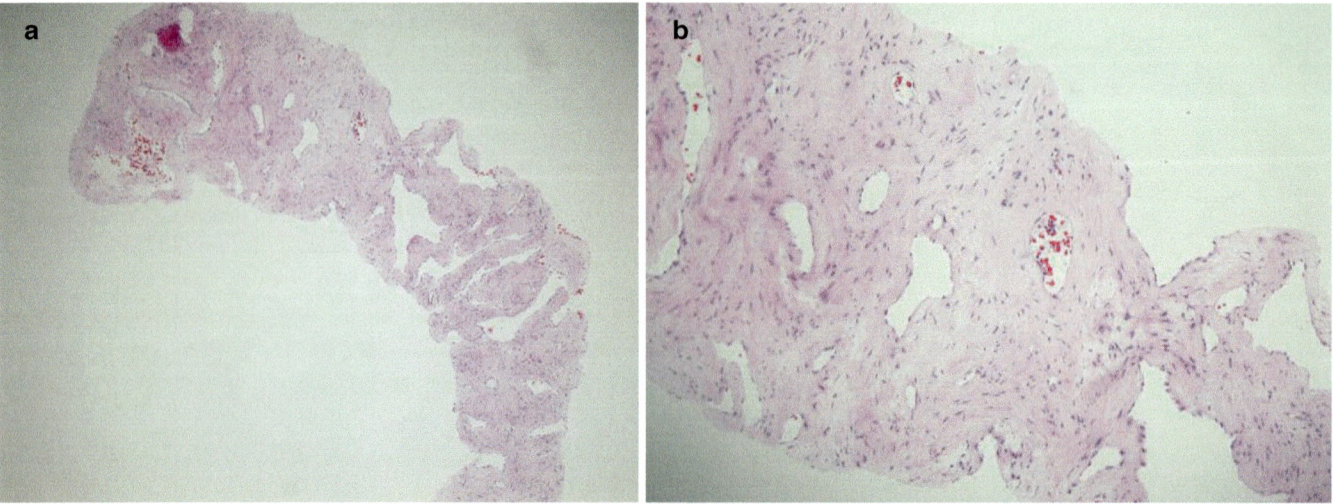

Fig. 16.6 Sclerosing cavernous hemangioma. (**a**) Blood spaces are separated by broad fibrotic septa. Vessels are generally small in size, and a few of them are dilated. (**b**) Small irregular vessels are lined by flattened endothelium, with small amount of red blood cells in lumen. Fibrotic septa area is broad and myxoid

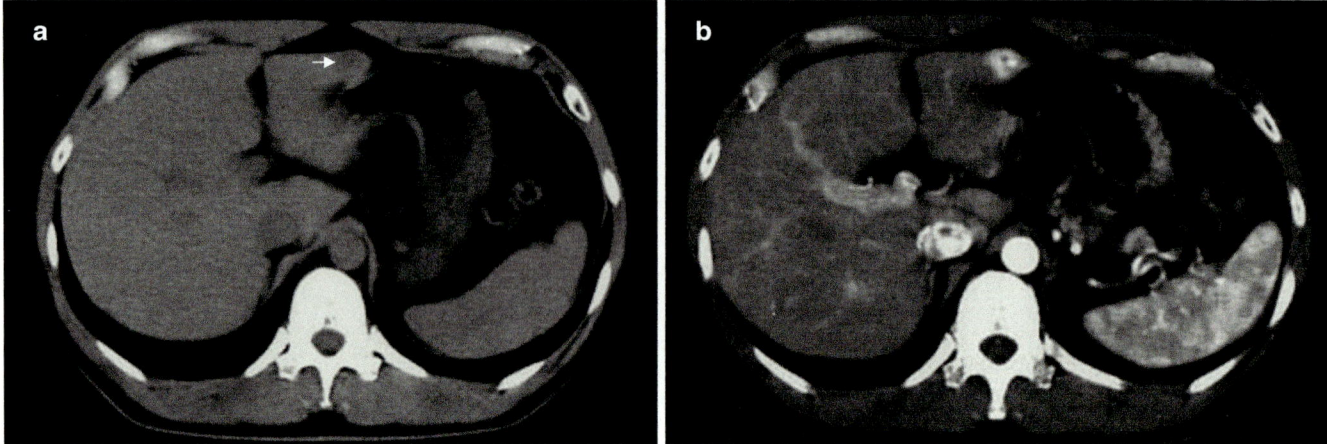

Fig. 16.7 Focal nodular hyperplasia. (**a**) CT without contrast medium shows small, low-density area (arrow) in S3. (**b**) CT with contrast medium shows enhanced area in the tumor. Its center is more enhanced, mixed with low-density area

thought to arise from biliary metaplasia of hepatocytes, appears to be an attempt to establish biliary drainage, as normal bile ducts are absent and features of chronic cholestasis (pseudoxanthomatous change, copper accumulation) are often present.

FNH is difficult to diagnose on biopsy if the central scar and abnormal vessels are not included in the samples and is frequently mistaken for hepatic adenoma, cirrhosis, or ductopenic syndrome (such as primary biliary cirrhosis). The demonstration of map-like immunostaining pattern of glutamine synthetase overexpression is very helpful for histological diagnosis. A rare variant of FNH, the telangiectatic type, which does not have the central fibrous scar and contains dilated blood-filled vascular spaces, is now regarded as the inflammatory subtype of hepatic adenoma [14, 15].

Case 16.3

A 38-year-old man was found to have a liver tumor by abdominal US during a medical examination. His liver function test revealed TBIL 1.1 mg/dL, ALT 27 IU/L, AST 22 IU/L, ALP 227 IU/L, CEA 1.4 ng/mL, and negative AFP. Both HBsAg and anti-HCV were negative. CT without contrast medium showed low-density area in S3, and CT in the arterial phase showed enhanced tumor in S3 with a densely stained center (Fig. 16.7). MRI T2-weighted image showed high-intensity area in S3 (Fig. 16.8). Angiography revealed tumor stain with radiating artery in the center in arterial phase, and it remained in the late venous phase (Fig. 16.9). Resected liver tumor showed well-demarcated, unencapsulated lesion with nodular appearance (simulating cirrhosis), pale color, and central fibrous scar. Microscopy revealed central scar formation with abnormal thick-walled muscular vessels and radiating fibrous septa; there were proliferating bile ductules, infiltration of inflammatory cells, and dilated vessels between septal fibrosis and nodule formation (Fig. 16.10). Hepatocytes were arranged in liver plates of normal or slightly increased thickness. No cirrhotic change was seen in non-nodular area.

16.3 Hepatocellular Adenoma

Hepatocellular adenoma (HCA) is a rare tumor seen almost exclusively in young women during their reproductive years and rarely in men or children. It can be single or multifocal;

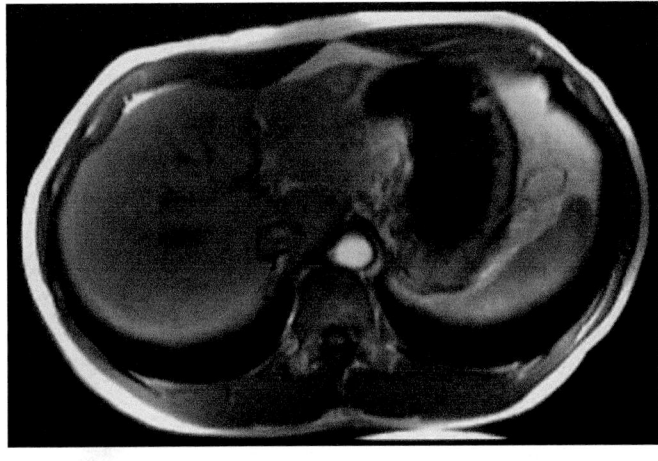

Fig. 16.8 Focal nodular hyperplasia. T2-weighted image on MRI shows high-intensity area in S3

the latter condition is known as multiple hepatocellular adenomatosis. The general clinical presentation is an abdominal mass, but some patients also complain of abdominal pain, discomfort, or nausea, and a significant number present with hemoperitoneum. Serum alkaline phosphatase may be elevated, but serum alpha-fetoprotein levels are generally normal or minimally elevated. On radiography, the lesions show increased vascular pattern.

HCA is strongly associated with oral contraceptive use and androgen steroid therapy, and occurs in a liver that is histologically normal or nearly normal. It can also occur spontaneously or be associated with underlying metabolic diseases, including type I glycogen storage disease, galactosemia, tyrosinemia, and familial diabetes mellitus. There is a significant risk of serious complications, such as hemorrhage and rupture. HCC is rarely found to arise from HCA, and this risk is higher in males and with large adenomas. Surgical resection is recommended if there is no tumor regression after the cessation of oral contraceptive use.

It has been observed recently that HCAs are heterogeneous with regard to their phenotypes and genotypes [16], based on which a new pathomolecular classification was proposed [17]. At least four subtypes are described:

1. HNF1-alpha-mutated adenomas, which account for 40% of adenomas, are characterized by prominent steatosis and negative expression of liver fatty acid binding protein (L-FABP).
2. Beta-catenin-mutated adenomas, which are preferentially encountered in male patients, are morphologically characterized by the presence of cellular atypia, association

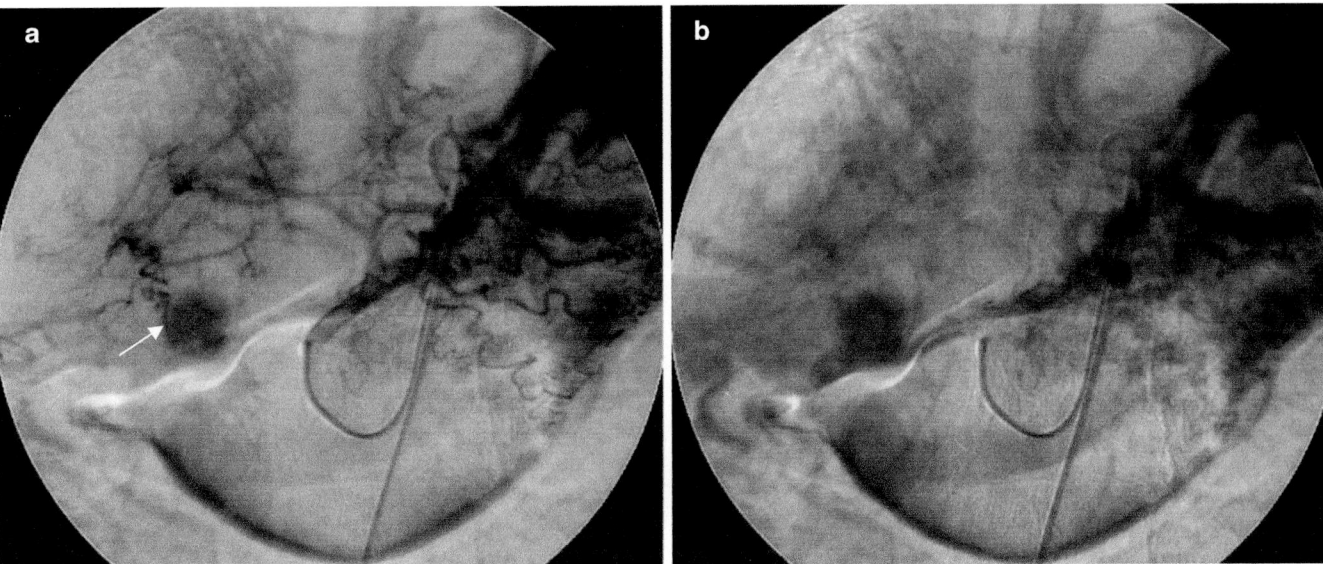

Fig. 16.9 Focal nodular hyperplasia. (**a**) Angiography shows stain with radiating vessels in tumor (arrow). (**b**) Tumor stain is retained in the late stage of venous phase

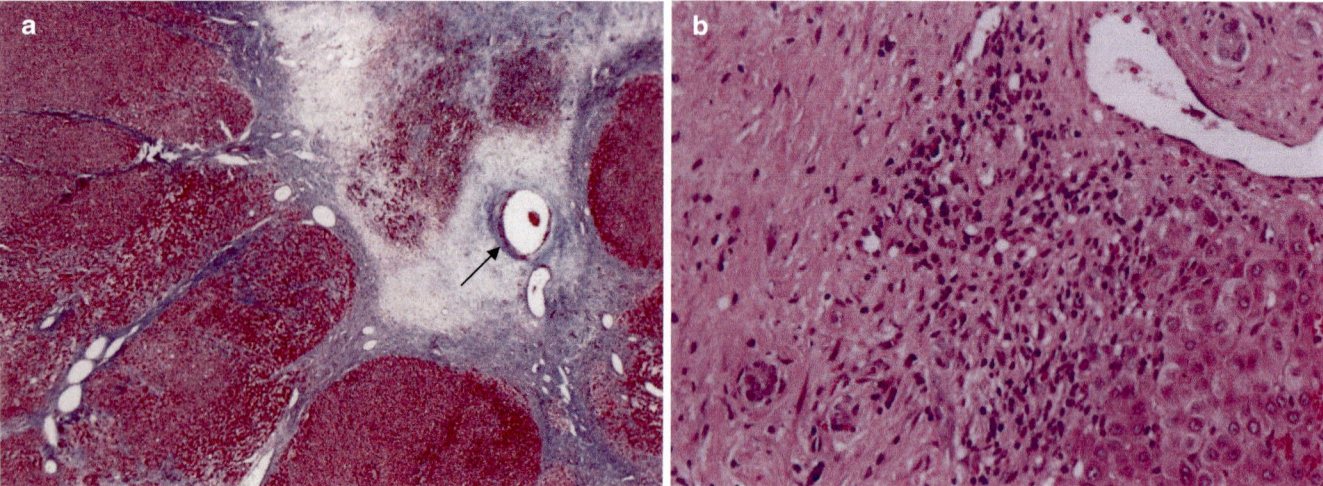

Fig. 16.10 Focal nodular hyperplasia. (**a**) Masson trichrome stain shows central stellate fibrous scar extending to the periphery and separating nodules. Arterial vessel (arrow) is seen in center of scar. (**b**) Infiltration of lymphocytes, proliferating bile ductules, and dilated vessels between radiating fibrosis and nodule formation are seen

with a higher risk of malignant transformation, and nuclear expression of β-catenin and overexpression of glutamine synthetase.
3. Inflammatory adenomas, which are related to mutations in the IL6ST gene, frequently display telangiectasia and inflammatory infiltrates and characteristically show positive immunostaining with markers of the acute-phase inflammatory proteins such as serum amyloid A (SAA) and C-reactive protein (CRP).
4. Unclassifiable adenomas without any specific clinical, morphological, or genetic characteristics.

Diagnostic problems arise most often in the differentiation of HCA from FNH or well-differentiated HCC, especially when hybrid features are present. Immunohistochemistry is now able to distinguish HA from either of these two lesions.

Case 16.4

A 36-year-old lady was found to have liver tumor by US during investigation for dysphagia. She was on oral contraceptives for several years and was also an HBsAg carrier. Her AFP level was not elevated, and liver function was normal. CT with contrast medium showed an isodense poorly enhancing 2.5-cm mass in the right lobe of the liver. Angiography revealed a hypervascular mass with lipiodol uptake and was demonstrated on subsequent CT. With a preoperative diagnosis of HCC, the tumor was resected, and a benign diagnosis was established from frozen section. The specimen showed a subcapsular, ill-defined, and yellowish-brown nodule. It comprised a relatively uniform population of larger and paler hepatocytes arranged in plates one to three cells thick, without free-floating trabecular formation; no capsule was seen between the nodule and non-nodular tissue. Reticulin

framework of the cell plates was either intact or only focally decreased. Thick-walled arterial vessels occurred in clusters, and thin-walled venous vessels were scattered throughout (Fig. 16.11). No portal tracts were detected.

16.4 Bile Duct Adenoma

Usually an incidental finding at surgery or autopsy, bile duct adenoma (BDA) presents as a solitary subcapsular nodule in 90% of patients. Its main clinical significance resides in its possible confusion with adenocarcinoma at laparoscopy or laparotomy.

BDA consists of a small (≤1 cm) disordered collection of ductules in connective tissue stroma showing varying degrees of chronic inflammation and collagenization, with occasional portal tracts enclosed in the nodule. Mucinous metaplasia, alpha-1 antitrypsin droplets, and neuroendocrine differentiation may be seen in the tubular lining cells.

The origin and pathogenesis of BDA are controversial. In early literature, it was regarded as a true neoplasm [18], but this view has been rejected. Researchers have proposed that it is a localized ductular proliferation following a focal injury or a form of peribiliary gland hamartoma [19, 20].

Case 16.5

A 43-year-old man was on follow-up for hepatitis B cirrhosis when he was found to have a 2.5-cm HCC during cancer screening. During surgery, another small 8-mm subcapsular nodule was detected and submitted for frozen section. Microscopy revealed tubular or curvilinear ductules lined by cuboidal epithelium, embedded in a fibrous stroma with patchy inflammatory infiltrate and some residual portal tracts (Fig. 16.12).

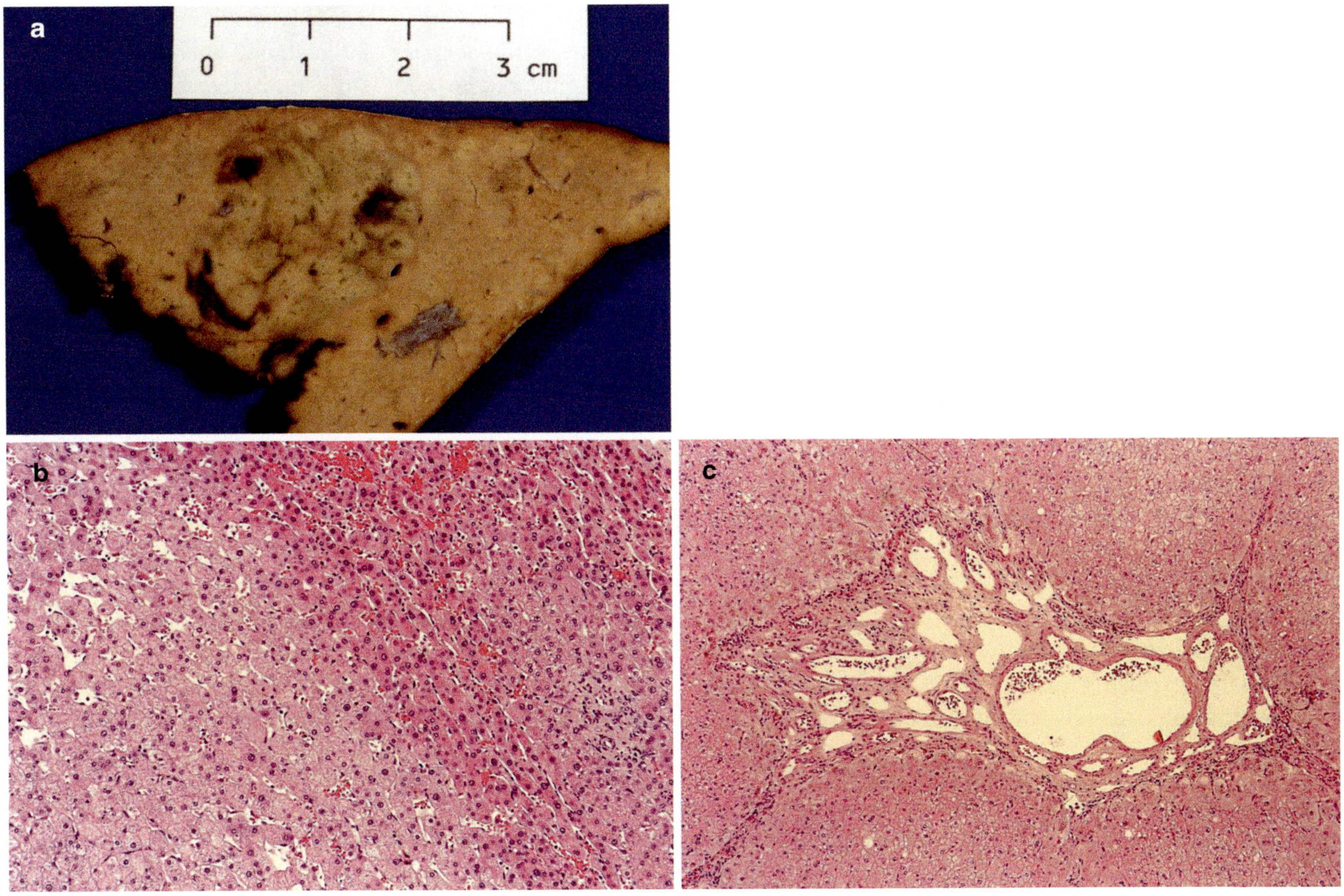

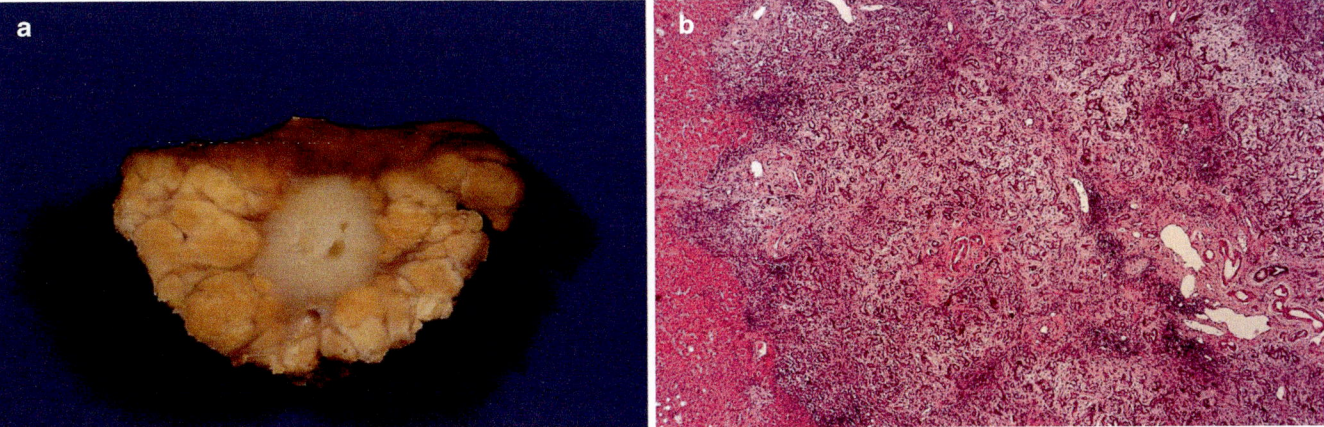

Fig. 16.11 Hepatic adenoma. (**a**) Resected tumor shows a subcapsular, ill-defined, and yellowish brown nodule. (**b**) Tumor comprises relatively uniform population of larger and paler hepatocytes arranged in cell plates that are one to three cells thick, and no capsular formation is seen in boundary between nodule and normal liver tissue. (**c**) Thick-walled arterial vessels occur in clusters

Fig. 16.12 Bile duct adenoma. (**a**) Resected specimen shows a subcapsular 8-mm whitish nodule against background of yellowish brown cirrhosis. (**b**) Nodule comprises many small ductules in fibrous stroma with patchy inflammatory infiltrate and trapped residual portal tracts

16.5 Biliary Adenofibroma

Biliary adenofibroma appears to be an extremely rare type of benign bile duct tumors. Only a few cases have been reported in the literature [21–23]. It is characterized by microcystic and tubuloacinar glandular structures lined by biliary epithelium and supported by fibroblastic stromal scaffolding.

There is evidence that this tumor might originate from preexisting biliary microhamartoma (von Meyenburg complex) based on similar morphological architecture and epithelial expression of D10, but not 1F6 [23]. Due to its size, proliferative activity, and p53 positivity, it is a potentially premalignant lesion [24]. Indeed, cases of malignant transformation are coming up [25, 26]. Another possibly neoplastic form of BDA, "atypical clear cell bile duct adenoma," has also been described [27].

Case 16.6

A 74-year-old woman presented with right upper abdominal pain, and US revealed gallstones and round liver mass with homogeneous echogenicity and lobulated border. CT showed hypodense lesion with heterogeneous contrast enhancement due to vessels in portions of the tumor. Laparotomy revealed a 7-cm tumor protruding from the inferior surface of the right lobe. Resected tumor showed honeycomb cut surface with thin fibrous septa delineating small cysts. Microscopically, it comprised acinar, microcystic, and tubuloglandular elements separated in most areas by thin fibrous bands. The lining epithelium consisted of a single layer of non-mucin-secreting flat to cuboidal to columnar cells, with occasional mitoses (Fig. 16.13).

16.6 Mucinous Cystic Neoplasm

Mucinous cystic tumor (MCN), previously referred to as biliary cystadenoma, is a solitary and multilocular cystic tumor that arises principally within the liver but may occur in the extrahepatic biliary tree including the gallbladder [28–30]. It has striking similarities to mucinous cystic neoplasm of the pancreas. Both are tumors predominantly found in middle-aged women in >90% of cases. The most common presenting symptoms are upper abdominal mass, discomfort, and pain.

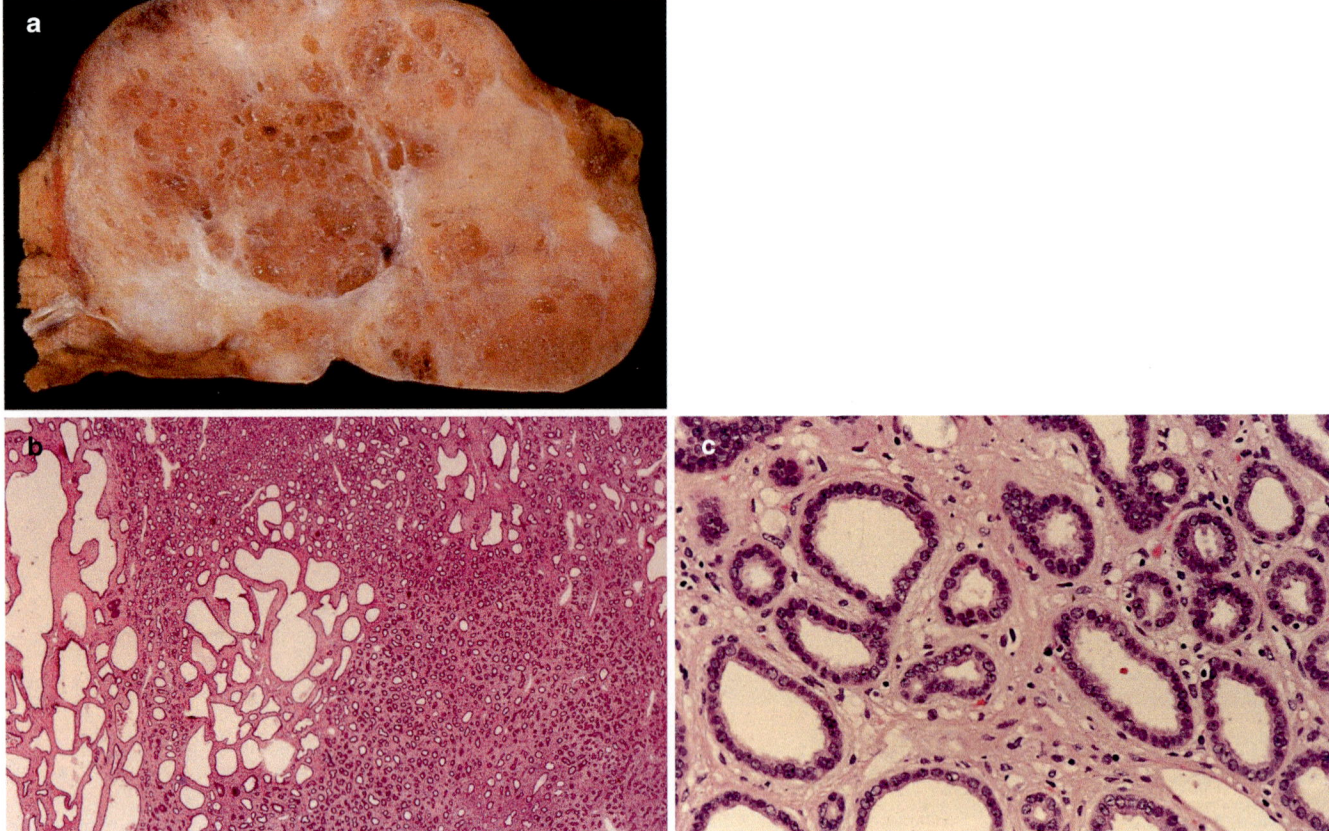

Fig. 16.13 Biliary adenofibroma. (**a**) Tumor is circumscribed with microcystic cut surface. (**b**) Tumor comprises tubules, acini, and microcysts in fibrotic stroma. (**c**) Lining epithelium has a single layer of cuboidal to columnar biliary-type cells, with occasional mitoses

A slow-growing tumor, MCN frequently reaches a large size and has a tendency to become malignant, usually over a period of many years. Foci of epithelial atypia indicate "borderline" or potentially malignant change. Recurrence is the rule following incomplete excision. Complete surgical removal is mandatory and usually curative.

The origin of MCN remains speculative. Embryonic foregut rests have been suggested as sources of the neoplasms [31]. Considering the site of occurrence, histological morphology, and frequent appearance of endocrine cells, it is likely that MCN originates from peribiliary glands with mucin secretion and cyst formation [32]. However, the female-specific mesenchymal stroma remains enigmatic.

Other pancreatic type tumors are occasionally found in the liver. Serous cystadenoma (microcystic adenoma) and papillary cystic tumor (solid pseudopapillary tumor) have been described [30, 33], and their occurrence has been attributed to pancreatic exocrine acini in peribiliary glands [34].

Case 16.7

A 48-year-old woman with a long history of intermittent abdominal pain had recently developed symptoms of indigestion and epigastric fullness. Upper endoscopy was negative for ulcer disease. CT and US of the abdomen revealed a 19-cm cyst in the left lobe of the liver compressing the hilum, gallbladder, and stomach. The resected specimen was a multilocular cyst. The locules were lined by a single layer of mucin-secreting columnar to cuboidal biliary type epithelium; the supporting stroma was compact and cellular, resembling ovarian stroma, and was immunoreactive with estrogen and progesterone receptors and inhibin (Fig. 16.14).

16.7 Intraductal Papillary Neoplasm

Intraductal papillary neoplasm (IPN), previously referred to as biliary papillomatosis, consists of multicentric papillary adenomas in the biliary tract, similar to intraductal papillary mucinous neoplasm of the pancreas, although not as commonly mucin secreting [35]. The gallbladder and major pancreatic ducts may also be involved. The adenomatous epithelium shows varying degrees of dysplasia and may mimic biliary epithelium and exhibit gastric or intestinal metaplasia. Based on morphologic characteristics and mucin expression, four subtypes of IPN are defined: pancreatobiliary, intestinal, gastric, and oncocytic. Patients usually present in middle to old age, with a male to female ratio of 2 to 1. The condition is characterized by recurrent bouts of cholangitis and obstructive jaundice. Occasional cases have been associated with ulcerative colitis, hepatolithiasis, Caroli's disease, choledochal cyst, and polyposis coli [36]. Preoperative diagnosis is difficult, but possible, by means of endoscopic retrograde cholangiopathy (ERCP) and endoscopic biopsy for extrahepatic cases and percutaneous transhepatic cholangioscopy (PTC) and fine needle aspiration cytology (FNAC) for intrahepatic tumors [37, 38].

Although histologically benign, its clinical behavior is regarded as having a borderline or low-grade malignant potential [39] due to its tendency to recur, multicentricity, susceptibility to malignant transformation, and significant morbidity and mortality arising from complications like recurrent bouts of cholangitis and obstructive jaundice, as well as episodes of sepsis and hemobilia. Management is difficult, and a cure is unlikely without liver transplantation [40]. Even then, the lesion may recur in the extrahepatic ducts.

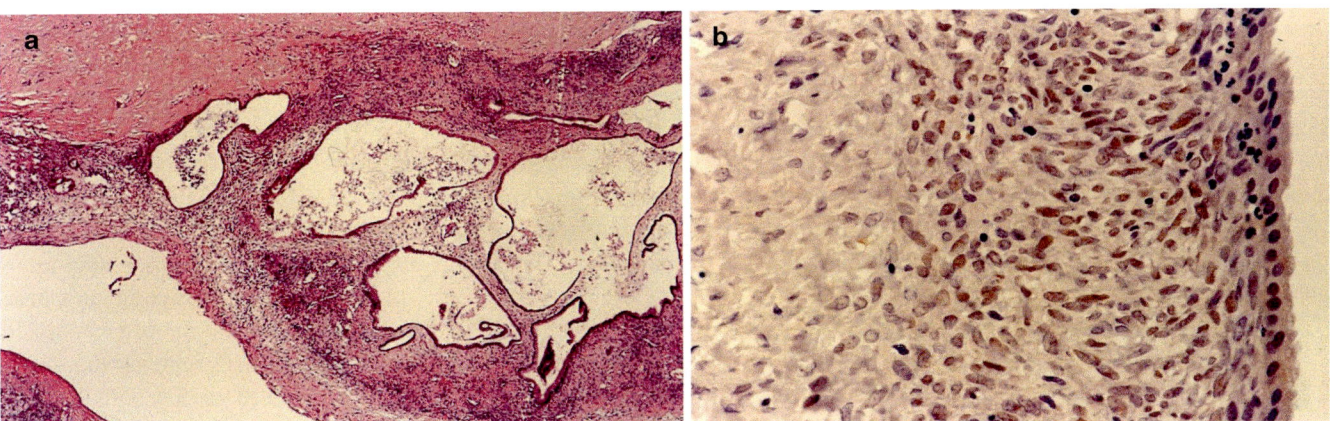

Fig. 16.14 Mucinous cystic neoplasm (biliary cystadenoma). (**a**) Multicystic locules are lined by a single layer of mucin-secreting epithelium. (**b**) Subepithelial mesenchymal stroma is ovarian-like and expressed estrogen receptor

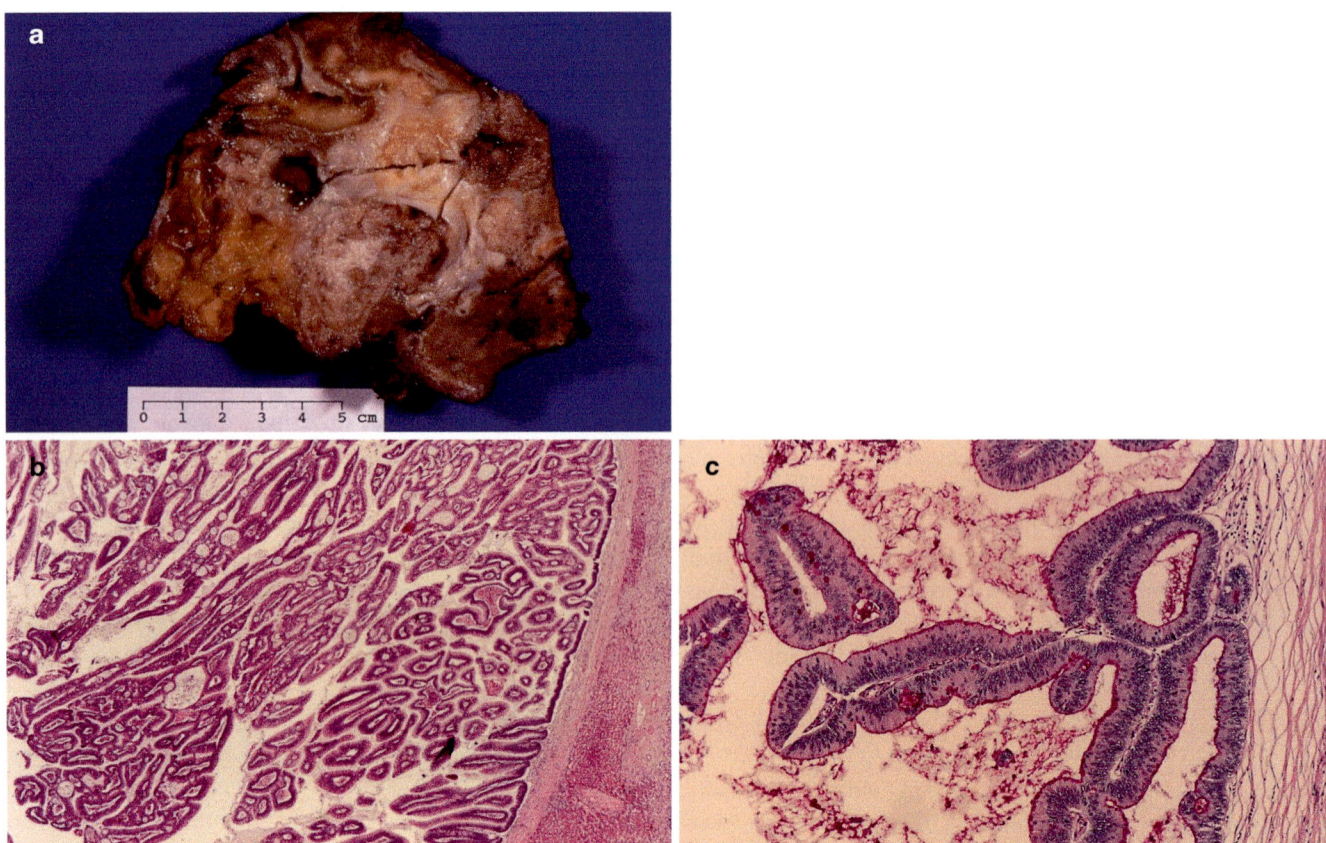

Fig. 16.15 Intraductal papillary neoplasm (biliary papillomatosis). (**a**) Left hemihepatectomy specimen shows dilated bile ducts filled with papillary tumors. (**b**) Long and branching papillae are lined by colum-nar cells and supported by delicate fibrovascular stroma. (**c**) The lining epithelium is mucin secreting and dysplastic

Case 16.8

A 70-year-old man was found to have liver lesions by US during investigation for epigastric pain. He has undergone biliary surgery 35 years ago. CT revealed markedly dilated intrahepatic bile ducts in atrophic left lobe. After failure of ERCP, left duct PTC was performed and revealed irregular left ducts and a long, irregular, and narrow segment in the proximal part, suggesting a malignant obstruction. FNAC of the left lobe diagnosed biliary papillomatosis, and left hemi-hepatectomy and right hepaticojejunostomy were performed. The resected specimen revealed papillary tumors filling up the dilated left intrahepatic bile ducts. The ducts contained papillary growth of columnar epithelial cells overlying fibro-vascular stalks; the epithelial layer was adenomatous with moderate degree of dysplasia, and apical mucin secretion was present (Fig. 16.15).

16.8   Angiomyolipoma and Lipomatous Tumors

A benign mesenchymal tumor, angiomyolipoma (AML) is rare in the liver [41–43]. It contains the same three components as the more commonly encountered renal AML,

namely, blood vessels, smooth muscle, and fat. This tumor occurs principally in adults, with a preponderance in females. Only about two-thirds of patients are symptomatic, most commonly with epigastric pain. Rupture with hemoperito-neum rarely occurs in large subcapsular tumors. An associa-tion with tuberous sclerosis is recognized in 5–10% of cases; these patients have coexisting renal AML and often have multiple liver tumors. Different ratios of the three compo-nents give this tumor its characteristic radiological features.

Case 16.9

Routine US in a 67-year-old man showed high-echoic area of 36 mm by 28 mm in S3 (Fig. 16.16). The liver function test was within normal limits, and HBsAg and anti-HCV were negative. Abdominal angiography showed tumor staining in early stage of the arterial phase, and it persisted in late phase (Fig. 16.17). Liver biopsy showed adipose cells admixed with epithelioid and spindle muscle cells and vascular com-ponents; fat droplets were also seen in the spindle cells (Fig. 16.18).

An important breakthrough in the understanding of this tumor comes from the documentation of HMB-45 and other melanoma-specific antibodies as reliable markers of AML (Fig. 16.19). Furthermore, recent molecular studies have

Fig. 16.16 Angiomyolipoma. US shows high-echoic area mixed with a small, low-echoic area in S3

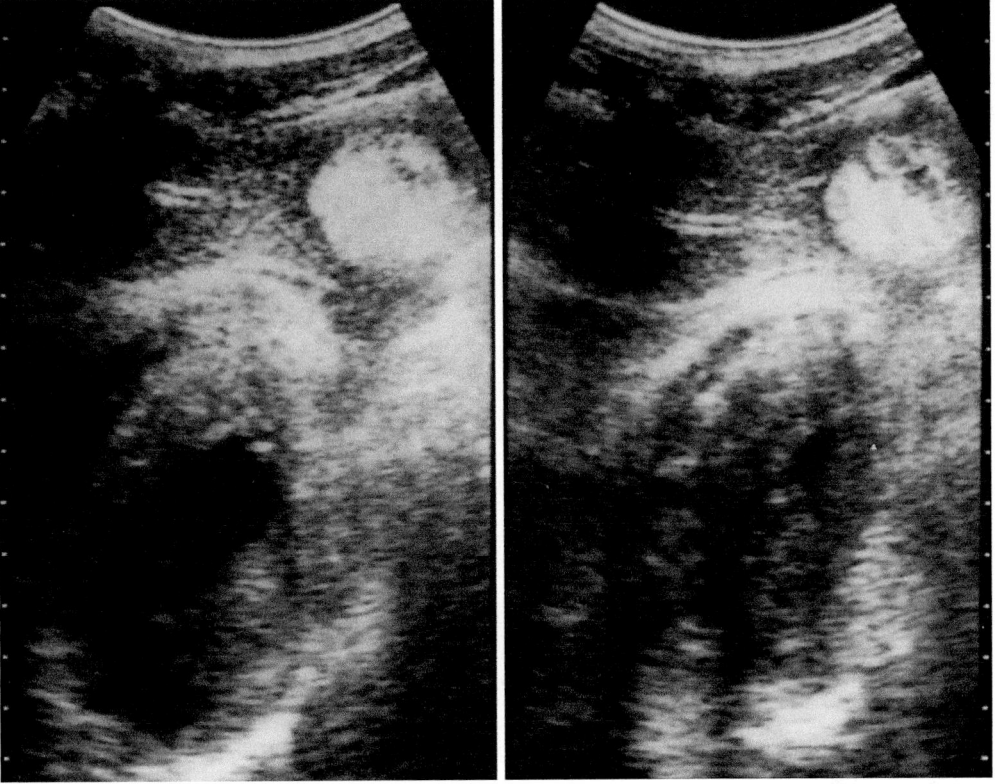

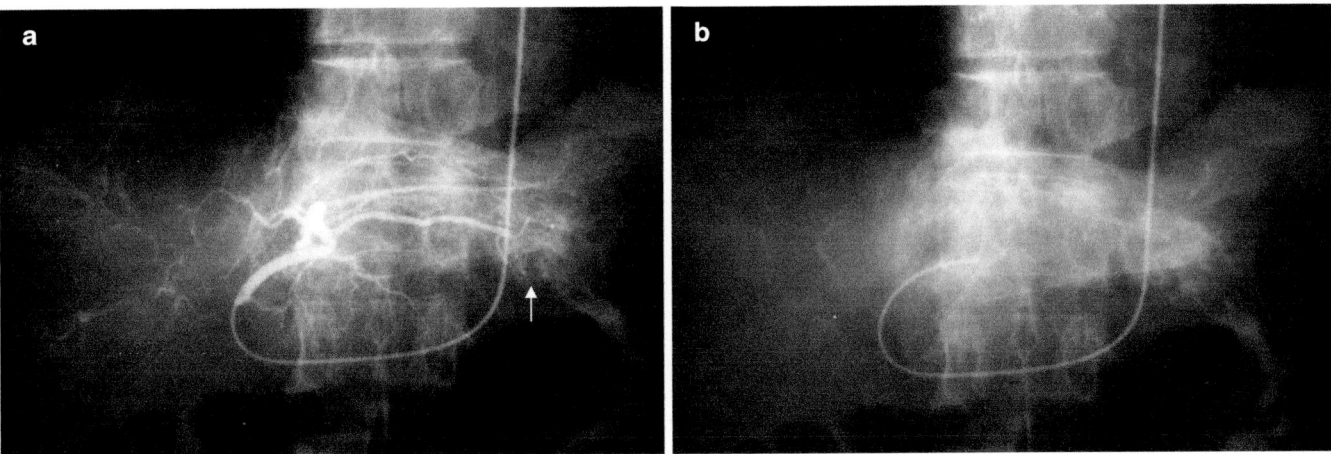

Fig. 16.17 Angiomyolipoma. (**a**) Angiography shows tumor stain (arrow) in early arterial phase. (**b**) Tumor stain is retained in late stage of arteriography

shown tumor clonality and loss of heterozygosity of tumor suppressor complex genes, indicating a neoplastic process. Once regarded as a hamartomatous lesion, AML is now regarded as a neoplasm belonging to the family of perivascular epithelioid cell tumors (PECOMA) and capable of dual myomatous and lipomatous differentiation and melanogenesis [44]. In most instances, it is a benign tumor, but rare sarcomatous transformation is well documented in renal and liver tumors [45].

AML contains varying proportions of smooth muscle, fat, and blood vessels. Extramedullary hemopoiesis is also frequently present in hepatic tumors, unlike their renal counterpart. According to the line of differentiation and predominance of tissue components, the tumors can be arbitrarily categorized into conventional mixed, lipomatous (>70% fat), myomatous (<10% fat), and angiomatous types [43]. Myomatous AMLs frequently exhibit unusual growth patterns: trabecular, pelioid, and inflammatory (Fig. 16.20).

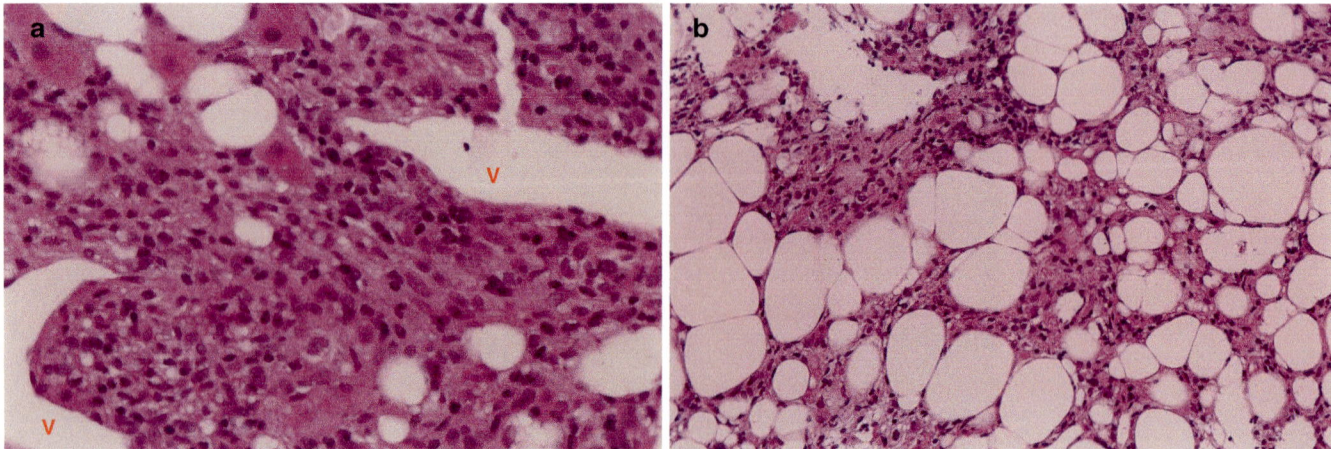

Fig. 16.18 Angiomyolipoma. (**a**) Adipose cells are admixed with epithelioid muscle cells and vascular components (V). (**b**) Besides adipose cells, fat droplets in spindle-shaped smooth muscle cells are visible

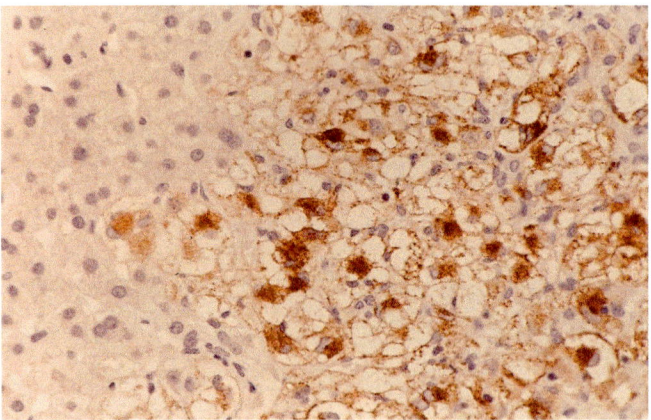

Fig. 16.19 Angiomyolipoma. Epithelioid cells express intense granular cytoplasmic staining of HMB-45, while hepatocytes are negative

The epithelioid cells may be clear (sugar cell with spiderweb appearance), oncocytic, or pleomorphic. Immunohistochemically, the myoid cells are consistently positive for HMB-45 and other melanogenesis markers; S-100 protein, actin, desmin, and vimentin expression is variable.

Unusual morphologic patterns and cellular features may lead to an erroneous diagnosis, especially of malignancy. Some of the lipomatous tumors reported under the various appellations of lipoma, hibernoma, myelolipoma, and even liposarcoma are all basically AMLs with varying proportions and/or unusual morphology of the different components. Lipomatous AML must be differentiated from focal fatty change, pseudolipoma, true lipoma, and liposarcoma. Myomatous tumors with epithelioid cells are mistaken most frequently for HCC (conventional, clear cell, fibrolamellar types), metastatic renal cell carcinoma, and epithelioid leiomyosarcoma. In AMLs with spindle cells and pleomorphic features, the most common misdiagnosis is some form of sarcoma. The radiological appearance of angiomatous tumors simulates vascular malformation. The diagnosis can be confirmed by a simple panel of immunomarkers, and conservative treatment can be adopted for small tumors after biopsy or FNAC.

16.9 Inflammatory Pseudotumor

Inflammatory pseudotumor (IPT) has been described as plasma cell granuloma, pseudolymphoma, fibroxanthoma, and histiocytoma, which reflects the variability of its appearance. Its occurrence in the lung is well known, and IPT is described in almost every other organ and body site. For liver lesions [46–48], there is a 3–1 male preponderance, and most cases occur in children, adolescents, and young adults. However, the age range varies from 10 months to 83 years. Most patients present with recurrent fever, weight loss, and abdominal pain; jaundice develops in a small number of cases. Laboratory investigations reveal neutrophil leukocytosis, a raised erythrocyte sedimentation rate, polyclonal hyperglobulinemia, and, less commonly, anemia, thrombocytopenia, and eosinophilia.

The lesion is solitary in 75% of cases and multiple in remaining cases; in 10% of cases, portal hepatis is involved. The diameter varies from 1 to 25 cm. The cellular composition of IPT varies, perhaps with the age of the lesion. Plump spindle cells with immunohistochemical and ultrastructural findings of myofibroblasts, admixed with polyclonal plasma cells, are consistent features. Lymphocytes, foamy macrophages, neutrophils, and eosinophils are variably present. The stroma is often very vascular and may exhibit a storiform pattern or show sclerosis. Giant-cell granulomas and endophlebitis are rarely observed.

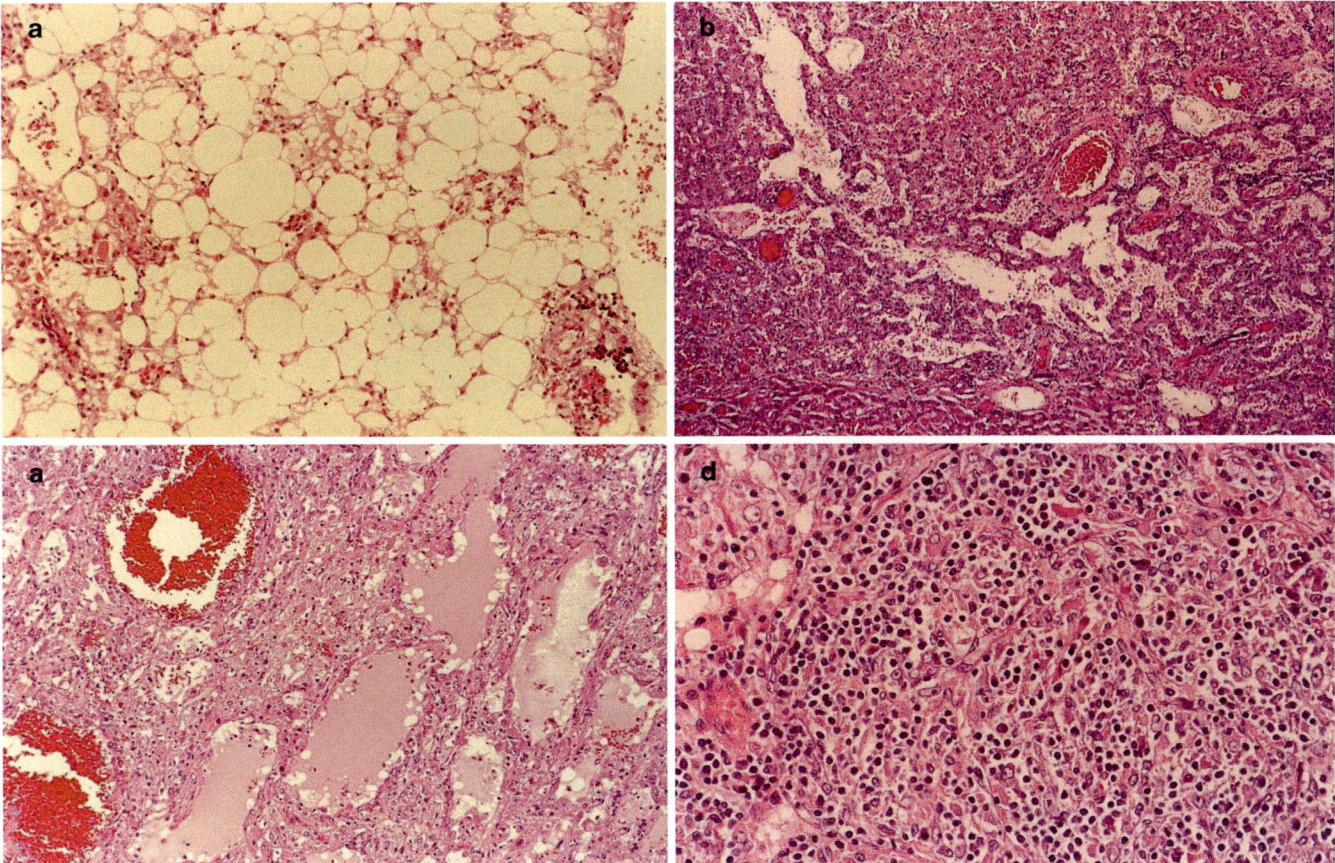

Fig. 16.20 Angiomyolipoma. (**a**) Lipomatous type AML shows diffuse sheets of adipocytes, with myoid cells webbed between fat cells. (**b**) Pure myomatous AML shows epithelioid cells arranged in trabeculae separated by sinusoids. (**c**) Myomatous AML shows formation of peliotic spaces that are not endothelium-lined. (**d**) AML with an inflammatory pseudotumor-like area, dense lymphoplasmacytic infiltrate, stromal sclerosis, and entrapped short spindle myoid cells

The etiology of IPT is unknown, although the myofibroblastic nature of spindle cells is well established. Very likely, it is a heterogeneous lesion, and various infectious or inflammatory causes have been proposed.

Complete recovery after surgery is the norm, except when major bile ducts are involved, in which case there may be persisting problems with obstructive jaundice, portal hypertension, or malabsorption. Spontaneous resolution, with or without treatment (steroids, antibiotics), is seen in 10% of cases.

Case 16.10

A 58-year-old man showed low-echoic space-occupying lesions mixed with isoechoic area in S5 (Fig. 16.21). CT with contrast medium showed low-density area; no staining was visible in late phase, and ambiguous low-density area remained (Fig. 16.22). T1-intensified image on MRI showed tumor with low intensity, and T2-intensified image revealed high intensity in tumor (Fig. 16.23). Angiography did not

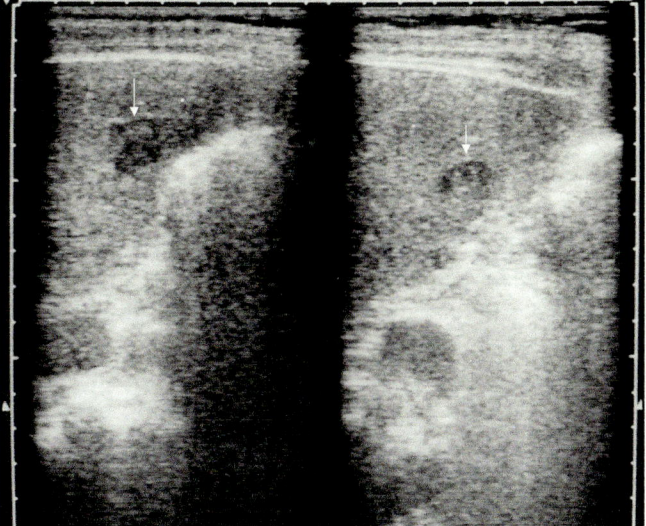

Fig. 16.21 Inflammatory pseudotumor. US shows low-echoic lesion (arrow) in S5; the edge is sharply defined

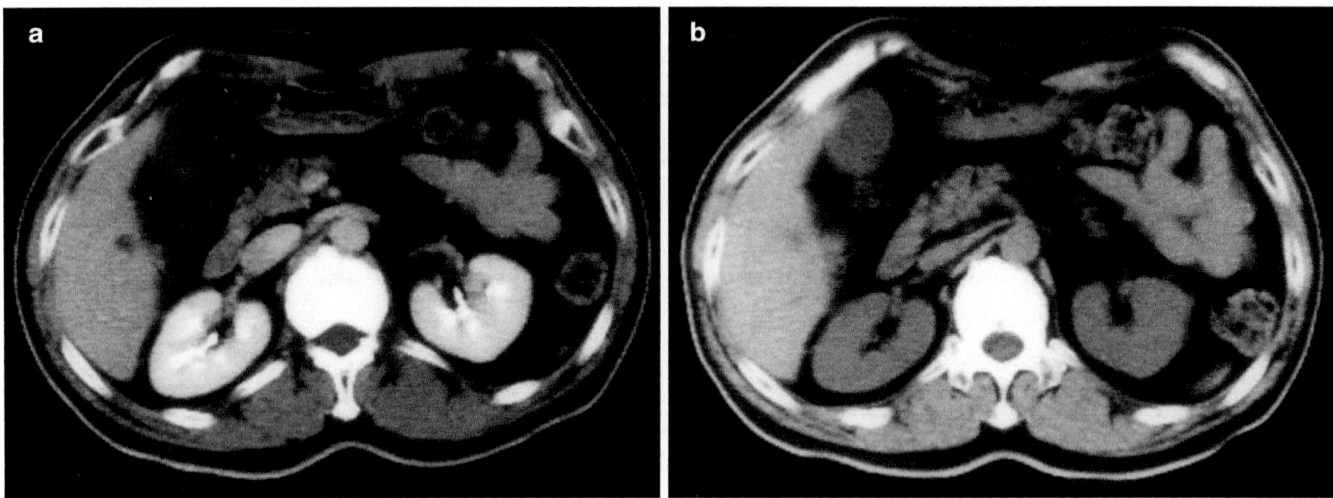

Fig. 16.22 Inflammatory pseudotumor. (**a**) CT with contrast medium shows sharp, low-density area. (**b**) CT without contrast medium shows ambiguous low-density area

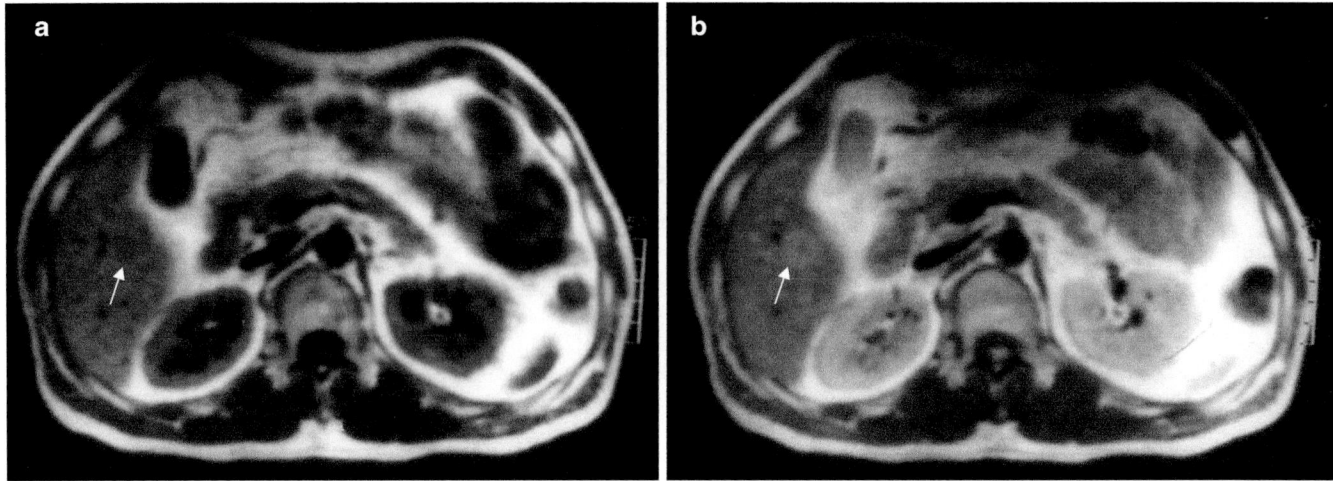

Fig. 16.23 Inflammatory pseudotumor. (**a**) T1-intensified image on MRI shows low-intensity area (arrow) in S5. (**b**) T2-intensified image on MRI shows high intensity in tumor (arrow)

reveal tumor staining in arterial stage; this was detected in venous phase (Fig. 16.24). Surgical resection of tumor revealed necrotic area surrounded by fibrous bands with a cluster of inflammatory cells; fibrous area showed small vessels, spindle fibroblasts, infiltrating macrophages, lymphocytes, and plasma cells (Fig. 16.25).

Lately, IgG4-related disease is found to form an important cause of IPT and responds to steroid therapy [49]. The lymphoplasmacytic type features perihilar fibroblastic mass with marked lymphoplasmacytic infiltration, prominent eosinophils, numerous IgG4-positive plasma cells, dense fibrosis of hilar and extrahepatic bile ducts (sclerosing cholangitis), and obliterative phlebitis (Fig. 16.26a). Fibrohistiocytic type is characterized by peripheral location, xanthogranulomatous inflammation, neutrophilic infiltration, and obliterated vessels (Fig. 16.26b) [50].

Clinical presentation and gross appearance of hepatic IPT may mimic malignant tumors, and these lesions may be mistaken for sarcoma if attention is not paid to the lack of nuclear atypia exhibited by the spindle cells. More commonly, other neoplasms with an inflammatory cell infiltrate are misdiagnosed as IPT. Examples include follicular dendritic tumor harboring Epstein-Barr virus [51], inflammatory myofibroblastic tumor or low-grade inflammatory fibrosarcoma [52], and inflammatory type of AML [41].

16.10 Gauzeoma

A retained foreign body is an uncommon, but not unknown, occurrence after surgical operation. Most patients are symptomatic, and the foreign body is detected by CT and US [53, 54].

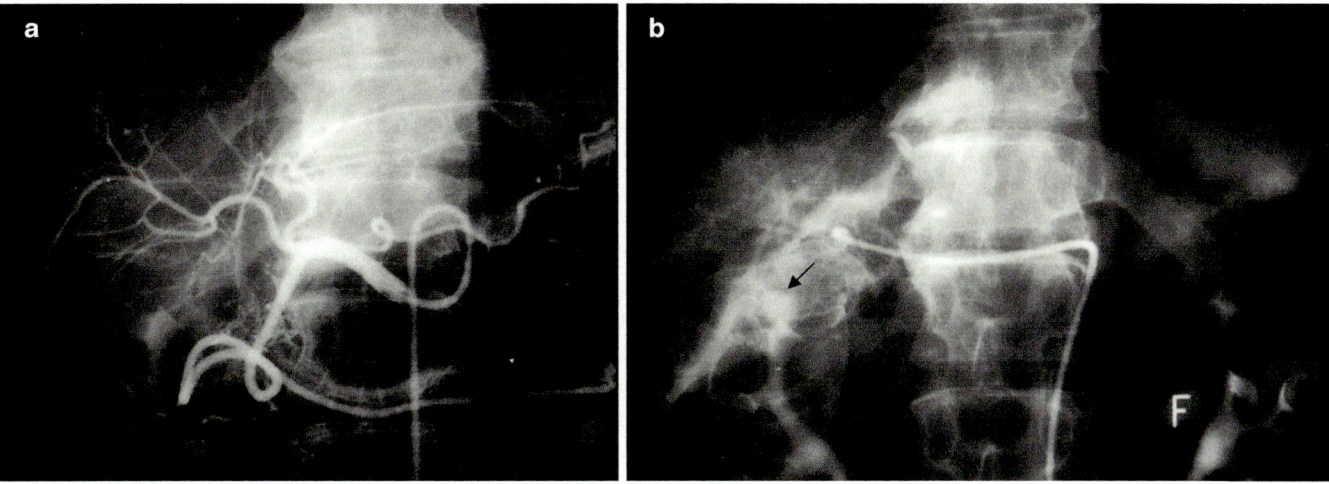

Fig. 16.24 Inflammatory pseudotumor. (**a**) Tumor cannot be detected in arterial phase of angiography. (**b**) Tumor stain (arrow) is seen in late phase of arteriography

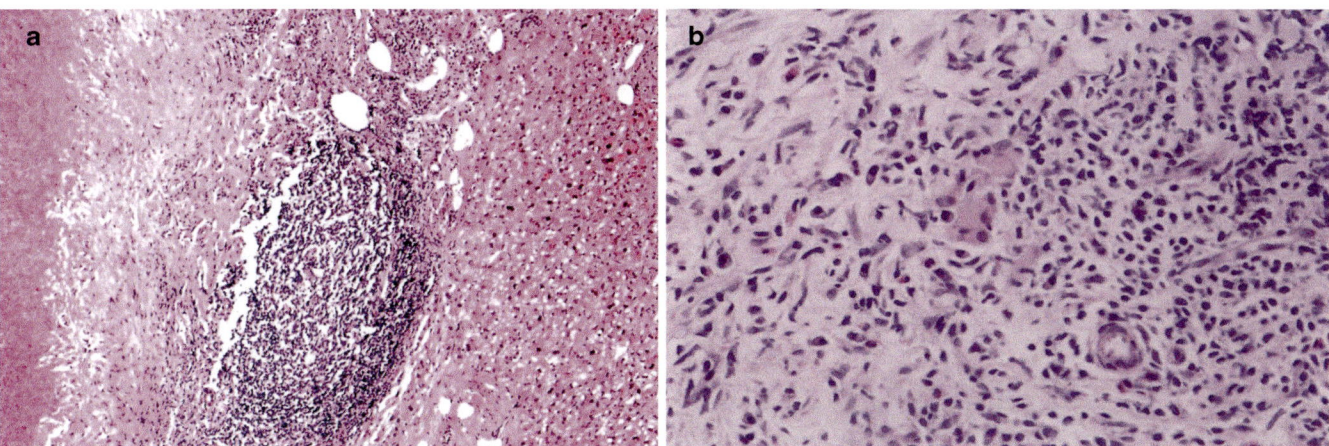

Fig. 16.25 Inflammatory pseudotumor. (**a**) Necrotic tissue is surrounded by fibrous tissue with clusters of inflammatory cells. Small vessels are seen in the outer fibrotic layer. (**b**) Infiltration of macro-phages, lymphocytes, and plasma cells mixed with small vessels are observed in inflammatory area

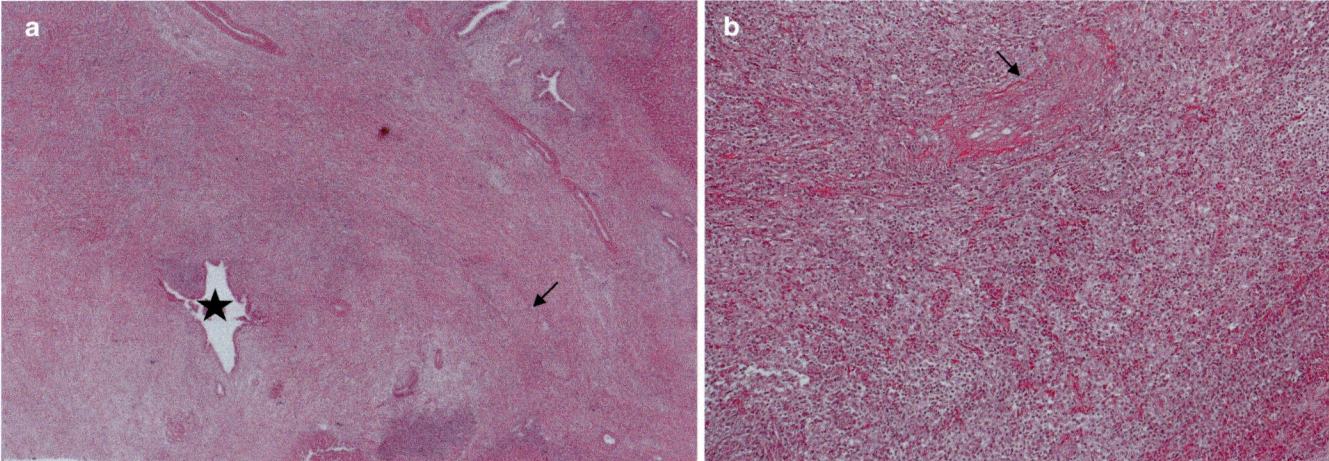

Fig. 16.26 Inflammatory pseudotumor. (**a**) Lymphoplasmacytic type features perihilar fibroblastic mass with marked lymphoplasmacytic infiltration, dense fibrosis of hilar bile ducts (asterisk), and obliterative phlebitis (arrow). (**b**) Fibrohistiocytic type is characterized by peripheral location, xanthogranulomatous inflammation, neutrophilic infiltration, and obliterated vessels (arrow)

Case 16.11

A patient presented with right hypochondralgia 7 years after cholecystectomy. US showed low-echoic lesion with high-echoic rim (Fig. 16.27). CT without contrast medium showed low-density area with high-density rim, and CT with contrast medium revealed high-density area on the rim and low-density area in the center (Fig. 16.28). The cut surface of the tumor revealed sponge-like formation with hemangiomatous structure, purple string-like material, and small vessels surrounded by fibrous bands. The

string-like material was found to be a retained gauze (Fig. 16.29).

16.11 Fibrosing Necrotic Nodule

Fibrosing or solitary necrotic nodule of the liver is an uncommon solid lesion. It comprises a central necrotic core enclosed by a hyalinized fibrotic capsule, which contains elastic fibers [55]. These are incidental findings at operation or autopsy.

The lesions are mainly solitary, subcapsular, small, well-demarcated, and round to oval. It has a firm, whitish rim and a core of yellowish white, cheese-like to solid material.

The entity is believed to be a burnt-out phase of a type of benign lesions, and not a lesion having a specific etiology. A small number of cases are claimed to be sclerosed hemangioma [56, 57], but a necrotic center would be unusual. A parasitic origin is documented in those nodules with shadows of degenerated cells, and partially preserved liver reticulin pattern is noted in the necrotic center [58].

Case 16.12

A 70-year-old man presented with acute pulmonary edema and a long history of hypertension. Subsequently, he developed left hemiplegia and died. At necropsy, apart from acute myocardial infarction and acute cerebral infarct, a single subcapsular nodule was found on the anterior surface of the left lobe of the liver; the wall of the nodule consisted of dense hyalinized fibrous tissue with elastic fibers and partially obliterated vessels on the outer portion and necrotic material toward the center (Fig. 16.30). There was no granulomatous inflammation or eosinophilic infiltrate.

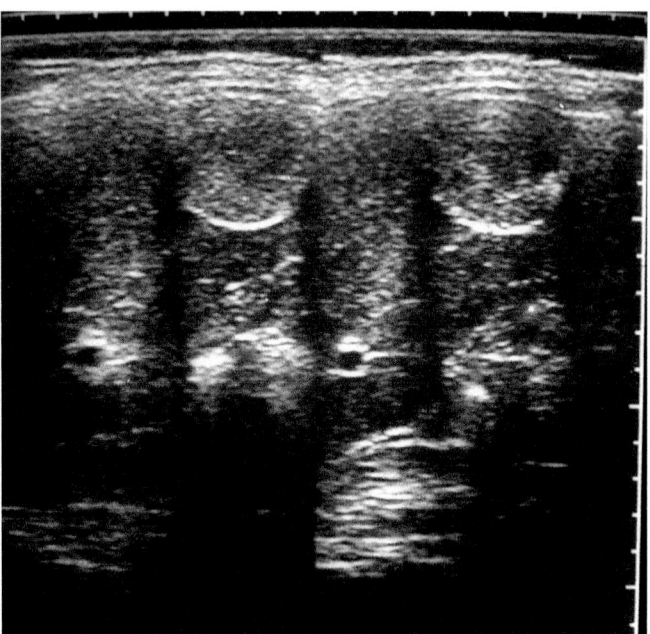

Fig. 16.27 Gauzeoma. US shows space-occupying lesions with high-echoic rim in S5

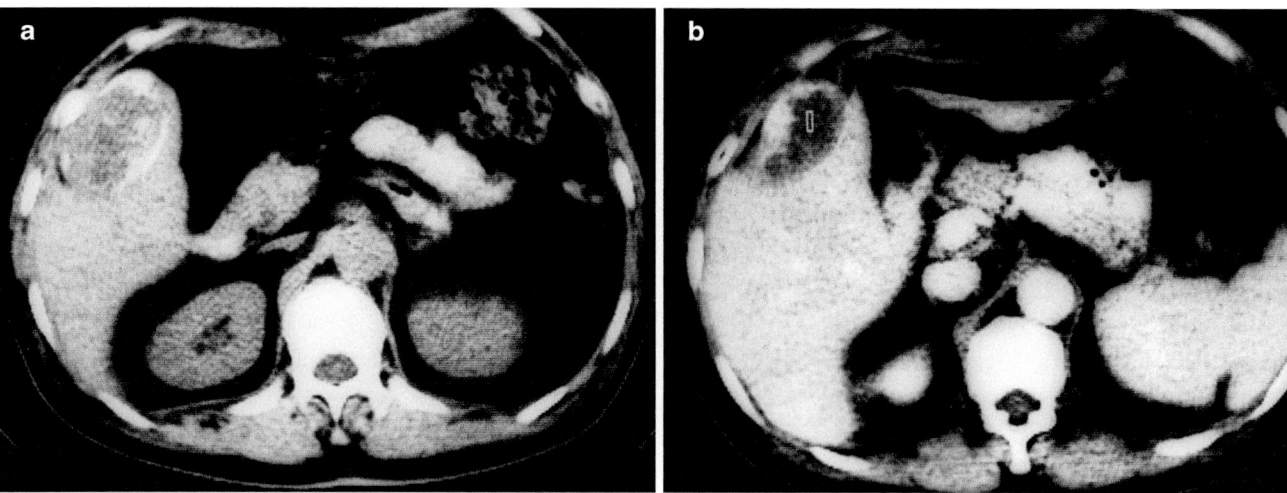

Fig. 16.28 Gauzeoma. (**a**) CT without contrast medium shows low-density area with high-density rim. (**b**) CT with contrast medium reveals low-density area, and rim is enhanced in scattered fashion

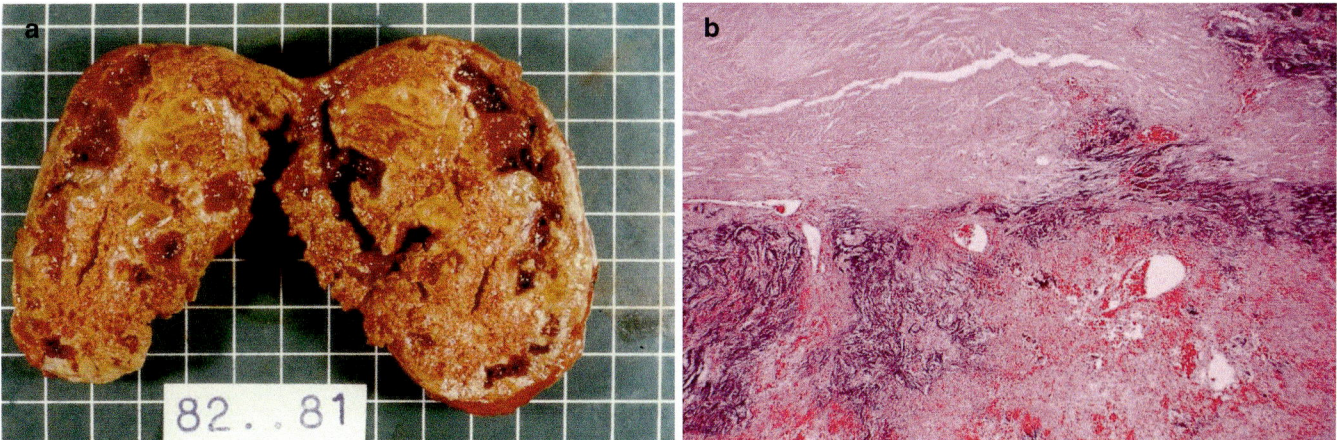

Fig. 16.29 Gauzeoma. (**a**) Tumor is encapsulated with sponge-like interior. (**b**) Outer surface of tumor comprises fibrous bands mixed with purple strings and small vessels. The inner part is mixed with small vessels, extravasated blood cells, and fibrous strands with purple strings

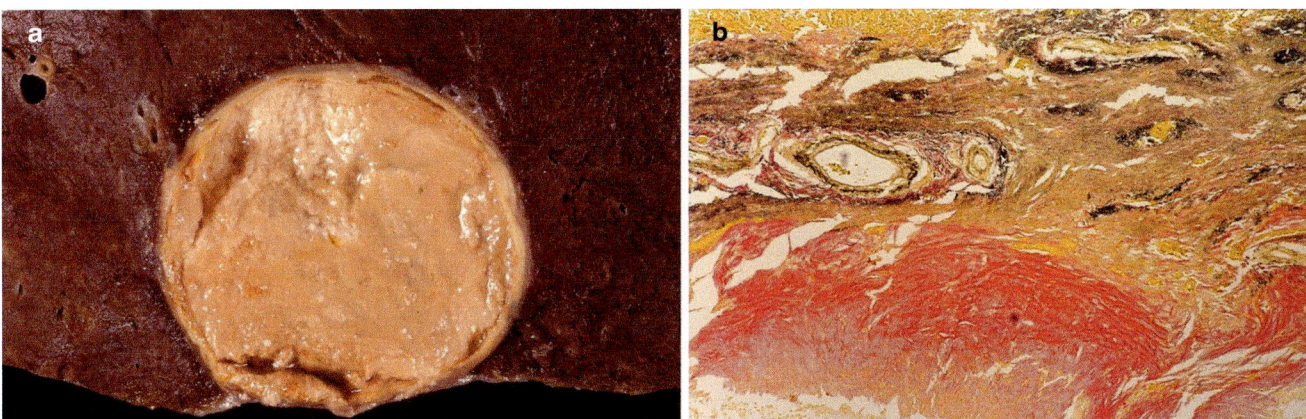

Fig. 16.30 Fibrosing necrotic nodule. (**a**) Postmortem liver shows well-circumscribed, subcapsular nodule with amorphous, yellowish center. (**b**) Elastic van Gieson stain shows densely fibrotic wall of nod-

ule with elastic fibers, partially obliterated vessels on the outer aspect, and necrotic material toward the center

16.12 Parasitic Granuloma

Various kinds of parasites can cause larva migrans syndrome (LMS) [59, 60], and *Toxocara* and *Ascaris* are the most popular culprits [61, 62]. LMS due to *Toxocara canis* or *Toxocara cati* is considered to be common in children of Europe and North America [63] but is reported to be more in number among adults of Japan [62]. After ingesting embryonated egg-contaminated vegetables and eating raw/undercooked paratenic host meat, such as chicken, pig, and beef, humans acquire the infection through intestinal mucosa. Larvae migrate to various tissues and organs through blood or lymph vessels, eliciting immune responses with eosinophilic inflammation. Typical target organs are the liver and lungs, and eyes, brain, and spinal cord may also be affected [63, 64]. Patients with LMS are sometimes asymptomatic or pres-

ent with fever, abdominal pain, probably due to hepato-splenomegaly, as well as coughing and asthma caused by parasitic pneumonia or bronchitis. Neural or ocular signs are sometimes detected. Hepatic lesions can be detected with various imaging techniques; US shows low echo of space-occupying lesions (about 1 cm in diameter) in the liver [65, 66]; CT reveals low-density area, of which the edge is enhanced by contrast medium; and MRI intensi-fied by T1 presents iso- or low intensity and high intensity by T2. Histopathological examination reveals tumor lesion or granulomas which mainly involve portal tracts. There is a central necrotic area or scar surrounded by eosinophils, lymphocytes, histiocytes, and plasma cells [67, 68]. The most commonly used diagnostic methods are serological techniques such as the enzyme-linked immunosorbent assay (ELISA) or Western blot [69, 70]. Albendazole, mebendazole, or ivermectin is administered

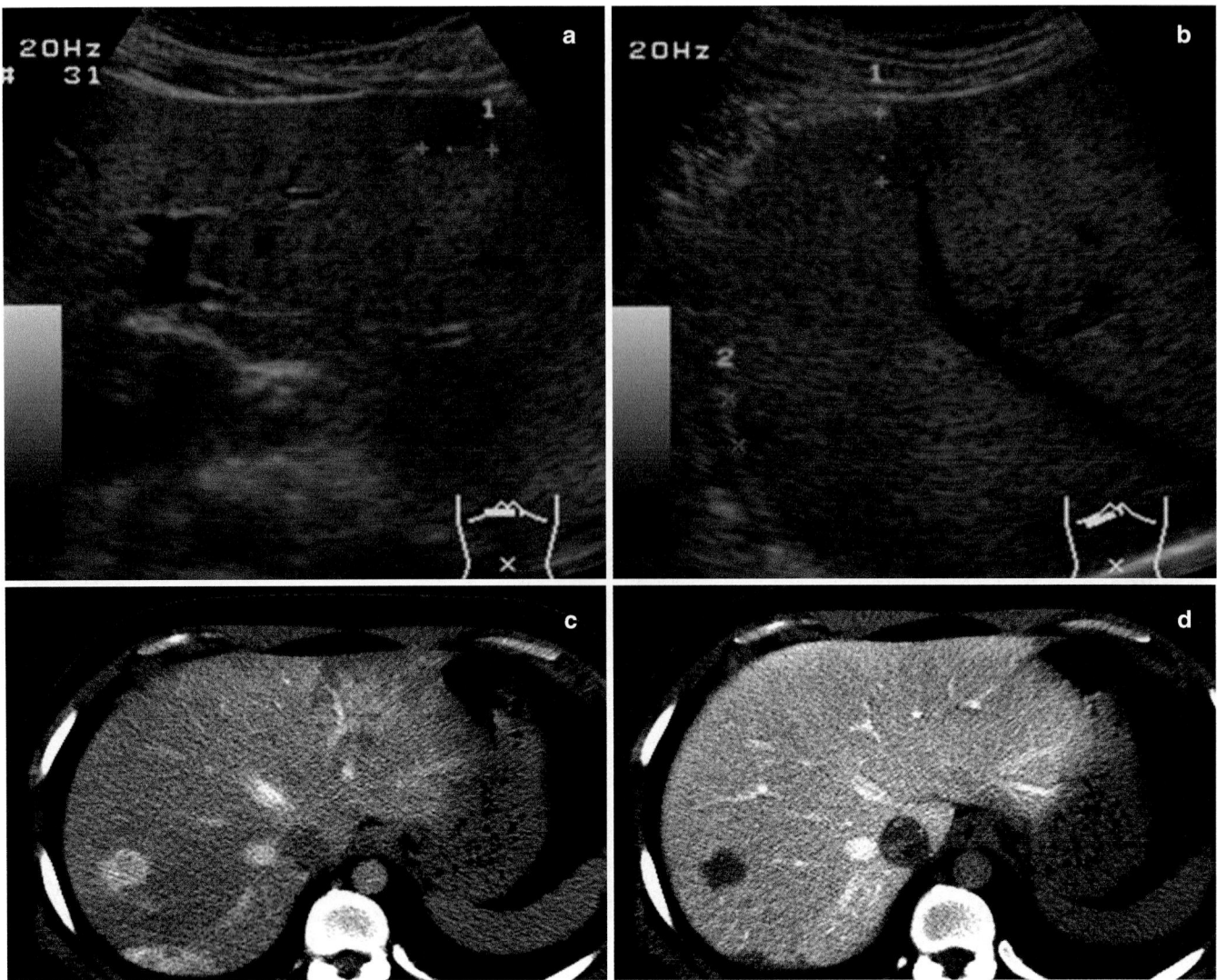

Fig. 16.31 Parasitic granuloma. (**a** and **b**) Many low-echoic areas (about 1 cm in diameter) are seen near liver surface. (**c**) CTA shows high density area in tumors. (**d**) CTAP shows low-density area in tumors

for treatment of ascariasis and toxocariasis, and piperazine can be used for intestinal obstruction due to their infection [71].

Case 16.13

A 34-year-old female was referred for investigation of anti-HCV-positive serum, and her laboratory test showed TBIL 0.4 mg/dL, AST 22 IU/L, ALP 180 IU/L, WBC 11,500/μL, eosinophilic leukocyte 28%, IgE 8200 IU/mL, and CA19-9 44 U/mL. Abdominal US showed multiple low-echoic areas (about 1 cm) near the liver surface (Fig. 16.31). CTA showed high density in tumor-like lesions detected by US, and CTAP showed low-density area. Surgical liver specimen revealed

multiple white lesions transparently seen from the surface. Microscopic examination showed nodular formation with central scar surrounded by proliferative bile ducts and infiltration of inflammatory cells and granulomatous formation in portal tracts with many inflammatory cells and proliferative bile ducts (Fig. 16.32). There were infiltration of eosinophilic and neutrophilic leukocytes along with lymphocytes and histiocytes and proliferative bile ducts accompanied by small arterial vessels. ELISA assay confirmed positive reaction for *Ascaris suis*.

Acknowledgment Prof. Alex Y. Chang was a coauthor of the first edition of this chapter.

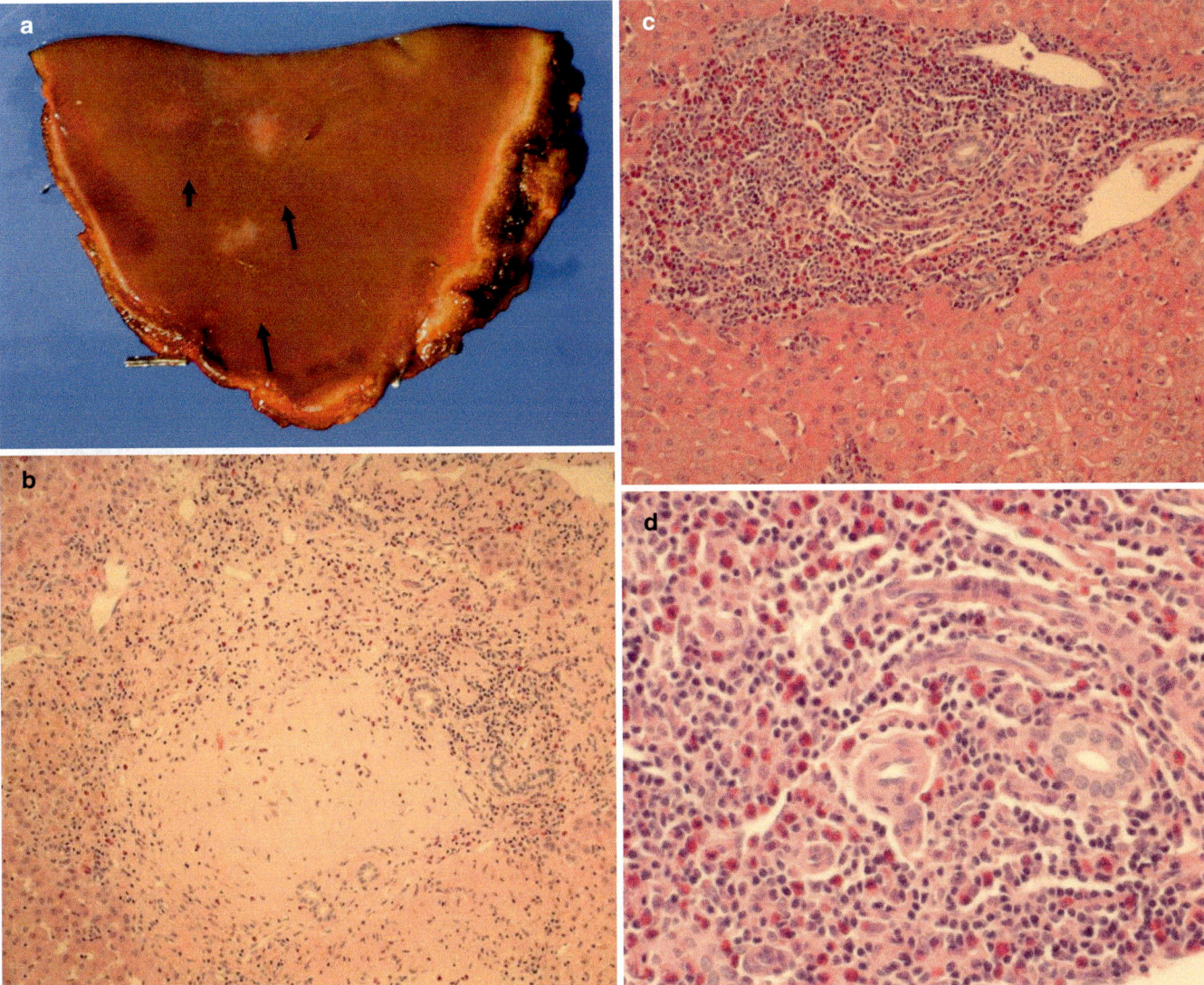

Fig. 16.32 Parasitic granuloma. (**a**) White-colored nodules are apparent from surface of resected liver. (**b**) Nodular lesion shows central scar surrounded by proliferated bile ductules and inflammatory infiltrate. (**c**) There is granuloma formation in portal tract with dense inflammatory infiltrate. (**d**) Many eosinophils, lymphocytes, and histiocytes are present in the granuloma, admixed with bile ductules and small arterioles

References

1. Goodman ZD. Benign tumors of the liver. In: Okuda K, Ishak KG, editors. Neoplasms of the liver. Berlin: Springer; 1988. p. 105–25.
2. Bosman FT, Carneiro F, Hruban RH, Theise ND, editors. WHO classification of tumours of the digestive system. 4th ed. Lyon: International Agency for Research on Cancer; 2010.
3. Shimizu M, Miura J, Itoh H, Saitoh Y. Hepatic giant cavernous hemangioma with microangiopathic hemolytic anemia and consumption coagulopathy. Am J Gastroenterol. 1990;85:1411–3.
4. Kim GE, Thung SN, Tsui WM, Ferrell LD. Hepatic cavernous hemangioma: underrecognized associated histologic features. Liver Int. 2006;26:334–8.
5. Lehmann FS, Beglinger C, Schnabel K, Terraciano L. Progressive development of diffuse liver angiomatosis. J Hepatol. 1999; 30:951–4.
6. Ryan RM, Buelow B, Mather C, et al. Hepatic small vessel neoplasm, a rare infiltrative vascular neoplasm of uncertain malignant potential. Hum Pathol. 2016;54:143–51.
7. Song JS, Kim YN, Moon WS. A sclerosing hemangioma of the liver. Clin Mol Hepatol. 2013;19:426–30.
8. Yamashita Y, Shimada M, Taguchi K, Gion T, Hasegawa H, Utsunomiya T, et al. Hepatic sclerosing hemangioma mimicking a metastatic liver tumor: report of a case. Surg Today. 2000;30:849–52.
9. Lee VT, Magnaye M, Tan HW, Thng CH, Ooi LL. Sclerosing haemangioma mimicking hepatocellular carcinoma. Singap Med J. 2005;46:140–3.
10. Makhlouf HR, Ishak KG. Sclerosed hemangioma and sclerosing cavernous hemangioma of the liver: a comparative clinicopathologic and immunohistochemical study with emphasis on the role of mast cells in their histogenesis. Liver. 2002;22: 70–8.

11. Stocker JT, Ishak KG. Focal nodular hyperplasia of the liver: a study of 21 pediatric cases. Cancer. 1981;48:336–45.

12. Paradis V, Laurent A, Flejou JF, Vidaud M, Bedossa P. Evidence for the polyclonal nature of focal nodular hyperplasia of the liver by the study of X chromosome inactivation. Hepatology. 1997;26:891–5.

13. Wanless I, Mawdsley C, Adams R. On the pathogenesis of focal nodular hyperplasia of the liver. Hepatology. 1985;5:1194–200.

14. Nguyen BN, Fléjou JF, Terris B, Belghiti J, Degott C. Focal nodular hyperplasia of the liver: a comprehensive pathologic study of 305 lesions and recognition of new histologic forms. Am J Surg Pathol. 1999;23:1441–54.

15. Paradis V, Benzekri A, Dargère D, Bièche I, Laurendeau I, Vilgrain V, et al. Telangiectatic focal nodular hyperplasia: a variant of hepatocellular adenoma. Gastroenterology. 2004;126:1323–9.

16. Zucman-Rossi J, Jeannot E, Nhieu JT, Scoazec JY, Guettier C, Rebouissou S, et al. Genotype-phenotype correlation in hepatocellular adenoma: new classification and relationship with HCC. Hepatology. 2006;43:515–24.

17. Bioulac-Sage P, Rebouissou S, Thomas C, Blanc JF, Sa Cunha A, Rullier A, et al. Hepatocellular adenoma subtype classification using molecular markers and immunohistochemistry. Hepatology. 2007;46:740–8.

18. Govindarajan S, Peters RL. The bile duct adenoma. A lesion distinct from Meyenburg complex. Arch Pathol Lab Med. 1984;108:922–4.

19. Allaire GS, Rabin L, Ishak KG, Sesterhenn IA. Bile duct adenoma: a study of 152 cases. Am J Surg Pathol. 1988;12:708–15.

20. Bhathal PS, Hughes NR, Goodman ZD. The so-called bile duct adenoma is a peribiliary gland hamartoma. Am J Surg Pathol. 1996;20:858–64.

21. Colombari R, Tsui WM. Biliary tumors of the liver. Semin Liver Dis. 1995;15:402–13.

22. Tsui WM, Loo KT, Chow LT, Tse CC. Biliary adenofibroma. A heretofore unrecognized benign biliary tumor of the liver. Am J Surg Pathol. 1993;17:186–92.

23. Varnholt H, Vauthey JN, Dal Cin P, Marsh Rde W, Bhathal PS, Hughes NR, et al. Biliary adenofibroma: a rare neoplasm of bile duct origin with an indolent behavior. Am J Surg Pathol. 2003;27:693–8.

24. Arnason T, Borger DR, Corless C, Hagen C, Iafrate AJ, Makhlouf H, Misdraji J, Sapp H, Tsui WM, Wanless IR, Zuluaga Toro T, Lauwers GY. Biliary adenofibroma of liver: morphology, tumor genetics, and outcomes in 6 cases. Am J Surg Pathol. 2017;41:499–505.

25. Thai E, Dalla Valle R, Evaristi F, Silini EM. A case of biliary adenofibroma with malignant transformation. Pathol Res Pract. 2016;212:468–70.

26. Thompson SM, Zendejas-Mummert B, Hartgers ML, Venkatesh SK, Smyrk TC, Mahipal A, Smoot RL. Malignant transformation of biliary adenofibroma: a rare biliary cystic tumor. J Gastrointest Oncol. 2016;7:E107–12.

27. Albores-Saavedra J, Hoang MP, Murakata LA, Sinkre P, Yaziji H. Atypical bile duct adenoma, clear cell type: a previously undescribed tumor of the liver. Am J Surg Pathol. 2001;25:956–60.

28. Ishak KG, Willis GW, Cummins SD, Bullock AA. Biliary cystadenoma and cystadenocarcinoma: report of 14 cases and review of the literature. Cancer. 1977;39:322–38.

29. Wheeler DA, Edmondson HA. Cystadenoma with mesenchymal stroma (CMS) in the liver and bile ducts. A clinicopathologic study of 17 cases, 4 with malignant change. Cancer. 1985;56:1434–45.

30. Devaney K, Goodman ZD, Ishak KG. Hepatobiliary cystadenoma and cystadenocarcinoma. A light microscopic and immunohistochemical study of 70 patients. Am J Surg Pathol. 1994;18:1078–91.

31. Subramony C, Herrera GA, Turbat-Herrera EA. Hepatobiliary cystadenoma. A study of five cases with reference to histogenesis. Arch Pathol Lab Med. 1993;117:1036–42.

32. Terada T, Kitamura Y, Ohta T, Nakanuma Y. Endocrine cells in hepatobiliary cystadenomas and cystadenocarcinomas. Virchows Arch. 1997;430:37–40.

33. Kim YI, Kim ST, Lee GK, Choi BI. Papillary cystic tumor of the liver. Cancer. 1990;65:2740–6.

34. Nakanuma Y, Sasaki M, Terada T, Harada K. Intrahepatic peribiliary glands of humans. II. Pathological spectrum. J Gastroenterol Hepatol. 1994;9:80–6.

35. Madden JJ Jr, Smith GW. Multiple biliary papillomatosis. Cancer. 1974;34:1316–20.

36. Chen TC, Nakanuma Y, Zen Y, Chen MF, Jan YY, Yeh TS, et al. Intraductal papillary neoplasia of the liver associated with hepatolithiasis. Hepatology. 2001;34:651–8.

37. Kim YS, Myung SJ, Kim SY, Kim HJ, Kim JS, Park ET, et al. Biliary papillomatosis: clinical, cholangiographic and cholangioscopic findings. Endoscopy. 1998;30:763–7.

38. Tsui WM, Lam PW, Mak CK, Pay KH. Fine-needle aspiration cytologic diagnosis of intrahepatic biliary papillomatosis (intraductal papillary tumor): report of three cases and comparative study with cholangiocarcinoma. Diagn Cytopathol. 2000;22:293–8.

39. Nakanuma Y, Sasaki M, Ishikawa A, Tsui W, Chen TC, Huang SF. Biliary papillary neoplasm of the liver. Histol Histopathol. 2002;17:851–61.

40. Rambaud S, Nores JM, Meeus F, Paolaggi JA. Malignant papillomatosis of the bile ducts: a new indication for liver transplantation? Am J Gastroenterol. 1989;84:448–9.

41. Goodman ZD, Ishak KG. Angiomyolipomas of the liver. Am J Surg Pathol. 1984;8:745–50.

42. Nonomura A, Mizukami Y, Kadoya M, Matsui O, Shimizu K, Izumi R. Angiomyolipoma of the liver: a collective review. J Gastroenterol. 1994;29:95–105.

43. Tsui WM, Colombari R, Portmann BC, Bonetti F, Thung SN, Ferrell LD, et al. Hepatic angiomyolipoma: a clinicopathologic study of 30 cases and delineation of unusual morphologic variants. Am J Surg Pathol. 1999;23:34–48.

44. Bonetti F, Pea M, Martignoni G, Zamboni G. The perivascular epithelioid cell and related lesions. Adv Anat Pathol. 1997;4:343–58.

45. Nguyen TT, Gormann B, Shileds D, Goodman Z. Malignant hepatic angiomyolipoma: report of case and review of literature. Am J Surg Pathol. 2008;32:793–8.

46. Anthony PP, Telesinghe PU. Inflammatory pseudotumour of the liver. J Clin Pathol. 1986;39:761–8.

47. Horiuchi R, Uchida T, Kojima T, Shikata T. Inflammatory pseudotumor of the liver. Clinicopathologic study and review of the literature. Cancer. 1990;65:1583–90.

48. Shek TW, Ng IO, Chan KW. Inflammatory pseudotumor of the liver. Report of four cases and review of the literature. Am J Surg Pathol. 1993;17:231–8.

49. Zen Y, Harada K, Sasaki M, Sato Y, Tsuneyama K, Haratake J, et al. IgG4-related sclerosing cholangitis with and without hepatic inflammatory pseudotumor, and sclerosing pancreatitis-associated sclerosing cholangitis: do they belong to a spectrum of sclerosing pancreatitis? Am J Surg Pathol. 2004;28:1193–203.

50. Zen Y, Fujii T, Sato Y, Masuda S, Nakanuma Y. Pathological classification of hepatic inflammatory pseudotumor, with respect to IgG4-related disease. Mod Pathol. 2007;20:884–94.

51. Selves J, Meggetto F, Brousset P, Voigt JJ, Pradère B, Grasset D, et al. Inflammatory pseudotumor of the liver. Evidence for follicular dendritic reticulum cell proliferation associated with clonal Epstein-Barr virus. Am J Surg Pathol. 1996;20:747–53.

52. Su LD, Atayde-Perez A, Sheldon S, Fletcher JA, Weiss SW. Inflammatory myofibroblastic tumor: cytogenetic evidence supporting clonal origin. Mod Pathol. 1998;11:364–8.

53. Gonzalez-Ojeda A, Rodriguez-Alcantar DA, Arenas-Marquez H, Sanchez Perez-Verdia E, Chavez-Perez R, Alvarez-Quintero R, et al. Retained foreign bodies following intra-abdominal surgery. Hepatogastroenterology. 1999;46:808–12.

54. Kalovidouris A, Kehagias D, Moulopoulos L, Gouliamos A, Pentea S, Vlahos L. Abdominal retained surgical sponges: CT appearance. Eur Radiol. 1999;9:1407–10.

55. Shepherd NA, Lee G. Solitary necrotic nodules of the liver simulating hepatic metastases. J Clin Pathol. 1983;36:1181–3.

56. Berry CL. Solitary "necrotic nodule" of the liver: a probable pathogenesis. J Clin Pathol. 1985;38:1278–80.

57. Sundaresan M, Lyons B, Akosa AB. "Solitary" necrotic nodules of the liver: an aetiology reaffirmed. Gut. 1991;32:1378–80.

58. Tsui WM, Yuen RW, Chow LT, Tse CC. Solitary necrotic nodule of the liver: parasitic origin? J Clin Pathol. 1992;45:975–8.

59. Feldmeier H, Schuster A. Mini review: hookworm-related cutaneous larva migrans. Eur J Clin Microbiol Infect Dis. 2012;31:915–8.

60. Liu Q, Li MW, Wang ZD, Zhao GH, Zhu XQ. Human sparganosis, a neglected food borne zoonosis. Lancet Infect Dis. 2015;15:1226–35.

61. Macpherson CN. The epidemiology and public health importance of toxocariasis: a zoonosis of global importance. Int J Parasitol. 2013;43:999–1008.

62. Maruyama H, Nawa Y, Noda S, Mimori T, Choi WY. An outbreak of visceral larva migrans due to *Ascaris suum* in Kyushu, Japan. Lancet. 1996;347:1766–7.

63. Despommier D. Toxocariasis: clinical aspects, epidemiology, medical ecology, and molecular aspects. Clin Microbiol Rev. 2003;16:265–72.

64. Pinelli E, Herremans T, Harms MG, Hoek D, Kortbeek LM. *Toxocara* and *Ascaris* seropositivity among patients suspected of visceral and ocular larva migrans in the Netherlands: trends from 1998 to 2009. Eur J Clin Microbiol Infect Dis. 2011;30:873–9.

65. Baldisserotto M, Conchin CF, Soares Mda G, Araujo MA, Kramer B. Ultrasound findings in children with toxocariasis: report on 18 cases. Pediatr Radiol. 1999;29:316–9.

66. Ishibashi H, Shimamura R, Hirata Y, Kudo J, Onizuka H. Hepatic granuloma in toxocaral infection: role of ultrasonography in hypereosinophilia. J Clin Ultrasound. 1992;20:204–10.

67. Parsons JC, Bowman DD, Grieve RB. Tissue localization of excretory-secretory antigens of larval Toxocara canis in acute and chronic murine toxocariasis. Am J Trop Med Hyg. 1986;27:492–8.

68. Kaplan KJ, Goodman ZD, Ishak KG. Eosinophilic granuloma of the liver: a characteristic lesion with relationship to visceral larva migrans. Am J Surg Pathol. 2001;25:1316–21.

69. de Savigny DH, Volle A, Woodruff AW. Toxocariasis: serological diagnosis by enzyme immunoassay. J Clin Pathol. 1979;32:284–8.

70. Magnaval JF, Fabre R, Maurieres P, Charlet JP, de Larrard B. Application of the western blotting procedure for the immunodiagnosis of human toxocariasis. Parasitol Res. 1991;77:697–702.

71. Khuroo MS. Ascariasis. Gastroenterol Clin North Am. 1996;25:553–77.

Liver Tumors II: Malignant Tumors of the Liver

17

Naoshi Nishida, Ryuichi Kita, Kenichi Miyoshi, Masahiko Koda, Masaki Iwai, and Arief A. Suriawinata

Contents

Abbreviations

AFP	α-Fetoprotein
ARID1	AT-rich interactive domain-containing protein 1A
BCLC	Barcelona clinic liver cancer
CCC	Cholangiocellular carcinoma
CEUS	Contract-enhanced US
CK	Cytokeratin
CoCC	Cholangiolocellular carcinoma
CT	Computed tomography
CTA	CT arteriography
CTAP	CT arterial portography
EZH2	Zeste homolog 2
Gd-EOB-DTPA	Gadolinium-ethoxybenzyl-diethylenetriamine pentaacetic acid
Gd-EOB-MRI	Gd-EOB-DTPA-enhanced MRI
HAIC	Hepatic arterial infusion chemotherapy
HBV	Hepatitis B virus
HCC	Hepatocellular carcinoma
HCV	Hepatitis C virus
MRI	Magnetic resonance imaging
NEC	Neuroendocrine cancer
NEN	Neuroendocrine neoplasm

N. Nishida, MD, PhD (✉)
Osaka, Japan
e-mail: naoshi@med.kindai.ac.jp

R. Kita, MD, PhD
Osaka, Japan

K. Miyoshi, MD, PhD · M. Koda, MD, PhD
Tottori, Japan

M. Iwai, MD, PhD
Kyoto, Japan

A. A. Suriawinata, MD
New Hampshire, USA

© Springer Nature Singapore Pte Ltd. 2019
E. Hashimoto et al. (eds.), *Diagnosis of Liver Disease*, https://doi.org/10.1007/978-981-13-6806-6_17

Table 17.1 Malignant tumor of the liver

Epithelial tumors	Hepatocellular	• Hepatocellular carcinoma
		• Hepatocellular carcinoma, fibrolamellar variants
		• Hepatoblastoma, epithelial variants
	Biliary	• Intrahepatic cholangiocarcinoma (cholangiocellular carcinoma)
		• Intraductal papillary neoplasm with an associated invasive carcinoma
		• Mucinous cystic neoplasm with an associated invasive carcinoma (mucinous cystadenocarcinoma)
	Mixed or uncertain origin	• Calcifying nested epithelial stromal tumor
		• Carcinosarcoma
		• Combined hepatocellular and cholangiocarcinoma
		• Hepatoblastoma, mixed epithelial-mesenchymal
		• Malignant rhabdoid tumor
Mesenchymal tumor	Vascular tumors	• Epithelioid hemangioendothelioma
		• Angiosarcoma
	Hematological tumor	• Malignant lymphoma
	Miscellaneous tumors	• Leiomyosarcoma
		• Rhabdomyosarcoma
		• Embryonal sarcoma (undifferentiated sarcoma)
		• Malignant fibrous histiocytoma
		• Malignant schwannoma
		• Hepatic liposarcoma
		• Kaposi sarcoma
		• Synovial sarcoma

Adapted from WHO classification of tumors of the liver and intrahepatic bile ducts (2010)

NET	Neuroendocrine tumor
OATP	Organic anion transporting polypeptide
PEI	Percutaneous ethanol injection
PIVKA-II	Prothrombin induced by vitamin K absence-II
PS	Performance status
PTC	Percutaneous transhepatic cholangiography
RFA	Radiofrequency ablation
SOL	Space-occupying lesion
TACE	Transarterial chemoembolization
TET1	Ten-eleven translocation methylcytosine dioxygenase 1
US	Ultrasonography

17.1 Definition and Classification

Primary liver tumors originate from hepatocytes, cholangiocytes, and mesenchymal cells (Table 17.1). Among liver tumors, hepatocellular carcinoma (HCC) is the most common; the majority of HCC develops as a result of chronic liver diseases that cause severe hepatocyte damage and regeneration. Chronic inflammation results in the formation of regenerative nodules as well as in the development of HCC through induction of many genetic/epigenetic alterations. Practitioners should attempt to differentiate HCC from benign and other malignant tumors and to treat it accordingly. Antiviral treatment for chronic hepatitis B (HBV) or C viruses (HCV) could reduce the risk of HCC emergence related to hepatitis virus [1, 2].

Cholangiocellular carcinoma (CCC) originates from intrahepatic or extrahepatic bile ducts and is the next most commonly encountered type of tumor after HCC. Recent whole-genome, epigenome, and transcriptome analysis revealed that there could be a molecular subtype in CCC that might reflect a difference of etiology. Cystadenocarcinoma is the malignant counterpart of bile duct cystadenoma. Hepatoblastoma is usually detected in children <2 years old, but a few cases in adolescents or young adults had been reported. Sarcomatous tumors are infrequently seen in the liver but angiosarcoma carries a grave prognosis.

17.2 Hepatocellular Carcinoma

HCC is a tumor with marked geographical variability in incidence, but both racial and genetic effects are of little importance in HCC. The relationship between HCC and chemicals, hormones, alcohol, nutrition, and the presence or absence of cirrhosis is complicated. Nevertheless, hepatitis B and C virus infection and aflatoxin exposure are significantly associated with the development of HCC [3, 4]. Therefore, it is important to follow patients chronically infected by HBV and HCV and exposed to aflatoxin by examining liver function tests, tumor markers, and image analysis. It is known that successful antiviral therapy could reduce the risk of HCC among patients with HBV and HCV infection [1, 2]. On the other hand, based on recent comprehensive genome and transcriptome analyses, a molecular classification of HCC that could relate to biological behavior of HCC has been proposed (Table 17.2).

Table 17.2 Classification of hepatocellular carcinoma based on transcriptome, genome, epigenome, and chromosomal alterations

Molecular feature	G1	G2	G3	G4	G5	G6
Alteration of cellular signaling based on the transcriptome analysis	Mitotic cell cycle				Wnt activation	
	AKT activation					
	Developmental and imprinting genes, IGF2		Cell cycle, nucleus pore		Stress and immune response	Amino acid metabolism, E-cadherin↓
Clinical feature	Woman. Africa, young, high AFP	Hemochromatosis				
	HBV-low copy number	HBV-high copy number				Satellite nodule
Methylation			CDKN2A		CHD1	
Mutation	AXIN1	TP53, AXIN1, PI3CA	TP53	HIF1A	CTNNB1	
Chromosomal status	Unstable				Stable	
Chromosomal alteration	4q, 16p, 16q	4q, 13q, 16p, 17p	4q, 5q, 16p, 17p, 21q, 22q			

Six HCC subgroups were determined through the unsupervised transcriptomic analysis by Boyault et al.; correspondence of the subgroups with their clinical characteristics as well as genetic, epigenetic, and chromosomal alterations were shown. (Boyault S et al. Transcriptome classification of HCC is related to gene alterations and to new therapeutic targets. Hepatology. 2007 Jan;45(1):42–52)

17.2.1 Etiology

Chronic HBV and HCV infections are the most frequent etiology of HCC. Other risk factors of HCC include alcoholic liver disease, nonalcoholic steatohepatitis, aflatoxin-B1 intake, diabetes, obesity, hereditary conditions, such as hemochromatosis, and metabolic disorders. Etiologies and risk factors of HCC vary by geographic locations.

17.2.2 Early HCC and Progressed HCC

It is well described that small HCC with less than 2 cm in diameter could be divided into two categories [5]: early and progressed HCCs. Early HCC is a small well-differentiated tumor with vaguely nodular appearance. On the other hand, progressed HCC is a mostly moderately differentiated tumor with distinct nodular appearance and microvascular invasion.

The histologic characteristics of early HCC include increased cell density more than two times of the surrounding liver, intratumoral portal tracts, pseudoglandular pattern, diffuse fatty change, and varying number of unpaired arteries. However, it is sometimes difficult to distinguish early HCC from high-grade dysplastic nodule, a premalignant lesion of HCC. The recognition of stromal invasion is the most important feature in differentiating early HCC from dysplastic nodule [5].

17.2.3 Diagnosis

The diagnosis of HCC is generally made by the increase of HCC-specific tumor markers, α-fetoprotein (AFP), AFP-L3, and prothrombin induced by vitamin K absence-II (PIVKA-II), and unique findings of diagnostic imaging [6–8]. Combination of measurement of serum AFP with PIVKA-II could increase the diagnostic accuracy of HCC.

During the development of HCC, several pathological changes are observed, such as increase of cellular density, decrease of portal vein flow, increase of arterial flow, and decrease of Kupffer cell. These pathological changes lead to the appearance of unique findings in imaging of HCC. Fibrous capsule and necrotic tissue are also detected in advanced tumor.

The findings of ultrasonography (US) image of HCC are as follows: mosaic pattern that reflects tumor heterogeneity, halo and lateral shadow that are associated with the presence of capsule, and nodule-in-nodule pattern that is attributed to multistep carcinogenesis of HCC [9, 10]. Portal vein and hepatic vein thromboses are also characteristic findings of HCC. Contract-enhanced US (CEUS) using perflubutane shows tumor stain at the early phase and defect in the Kupffer phase, because of the increase of arterial blood flow and decrease of Kupffer cell. Reperfusion defect in CEUS is one of the characteristic findings of HCC [11]. Dynamic computed tomography (CT) using multi-detector row CT is also used for the diagnosis of HCC; early vascular staining and washout of contrast agents at delayed phase are observed [12]. In advanced HCC, magnetic resonance imaging (MRI) is used to show low-intensity area and high-intensity area on T1-weighted image and T2-weighted image, respectively [13]. Gadolinium-ethoxybenzyl-diethylenetriamine pentaacetic acid (Gd-EOB-DTPA) is the most commonly used contrast medium for MRI diagnosis of HCC [14]. Gd-EOB-DTPA is incorporated into hepatocyte through the organic anion transporting polypeptide (OATP) transporter. Therefore, hepatobiliary phase of Gd-EOB-DTPA-enhanced MRI (Gd-EOB-MRI) shows defect in HCC because of the lack of OATP1B3 expression in the majority of HCC cells [15]. It is also known that a small subset of HCCs overexpressed OATP1B3 and showed increased uptake of Gd-EOB into tumor cells on hepato-

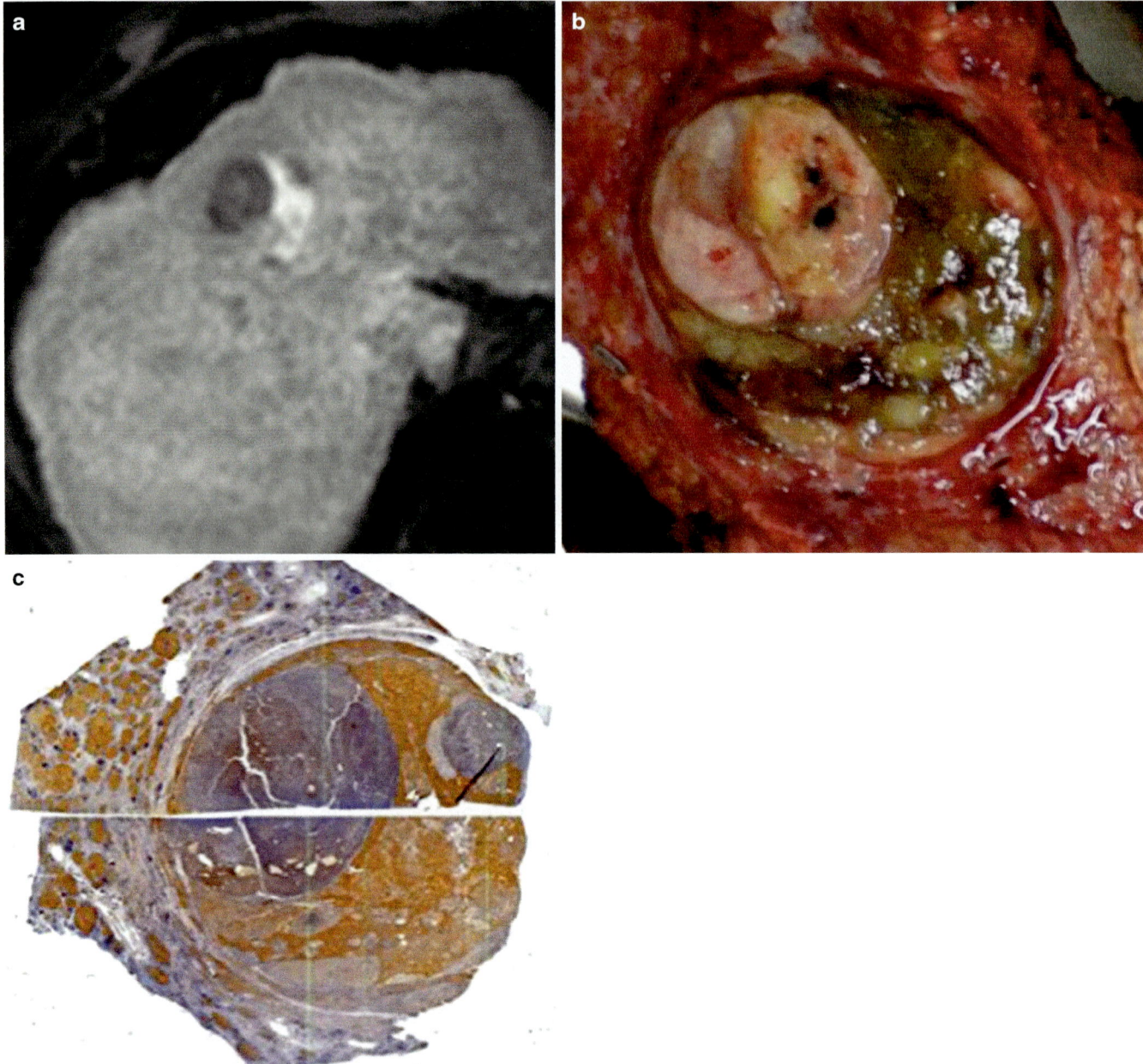

Fig. 17.1 Uptake of Gd-EOB-DTPA in the hepatobiliary phase of MRI in the tumor. The MRI image in the hepatobiliary phase of Gd-EOB-DTPA contract-enhanced MRI revealed high-intensity portion in the nodule (**a**). Macroscopic findings showed nodule-in-nodule pattern; the whitish nodule in green hepatoma with bile production abil-ity (**b**). The loupe image of the tumor with OATP1B3 immunostaining (**c**). The region expressing OATP1B3 in the tumor corresponded to the green portion in the loupe image and the high-intensity portion with Gd-EOB-DTPA uptake in the hepatobiliary phase MRI image

biliary phase image (Figs. 17.1 and 17.2). Angiography of HCC reveals hypervascular tumor.

Case 17.1 (HCC Nodule with Uptake of Gd-EOB-DTPA)
A 62-year-old male patient, who suffered from liver cirrhosis and hepatitis C virus infection, was referred to our hospital for further examination of the liver tumor. MRI examination revealed a 3 cm tumor in S4 with nodule-in-nodule pattern (Fig. 17.1). The region expressing OATP1B3 in the tumor corresponded to the portion with Gd-EOB-DTPA uptake in the hepatobiliary phase image (Figs. 17.1 and 17.2).

17.2.4 BCLC Staging System and Treatment of HCC

Barcelona Clinic Liver Cancer (BCLC) staging system is commonly applied for staging of HCC, which consists of five stages as follows [16]:

- Very early stage (0): tumor is less than 2 cm, performance status (PS) of the patient = 0, and Child-Pugh A.
- Early stage (A): a single tumor less than 5 cm or up to 3 tumors all less than 3 cm. PS 0 and Child-Pugh A or B.

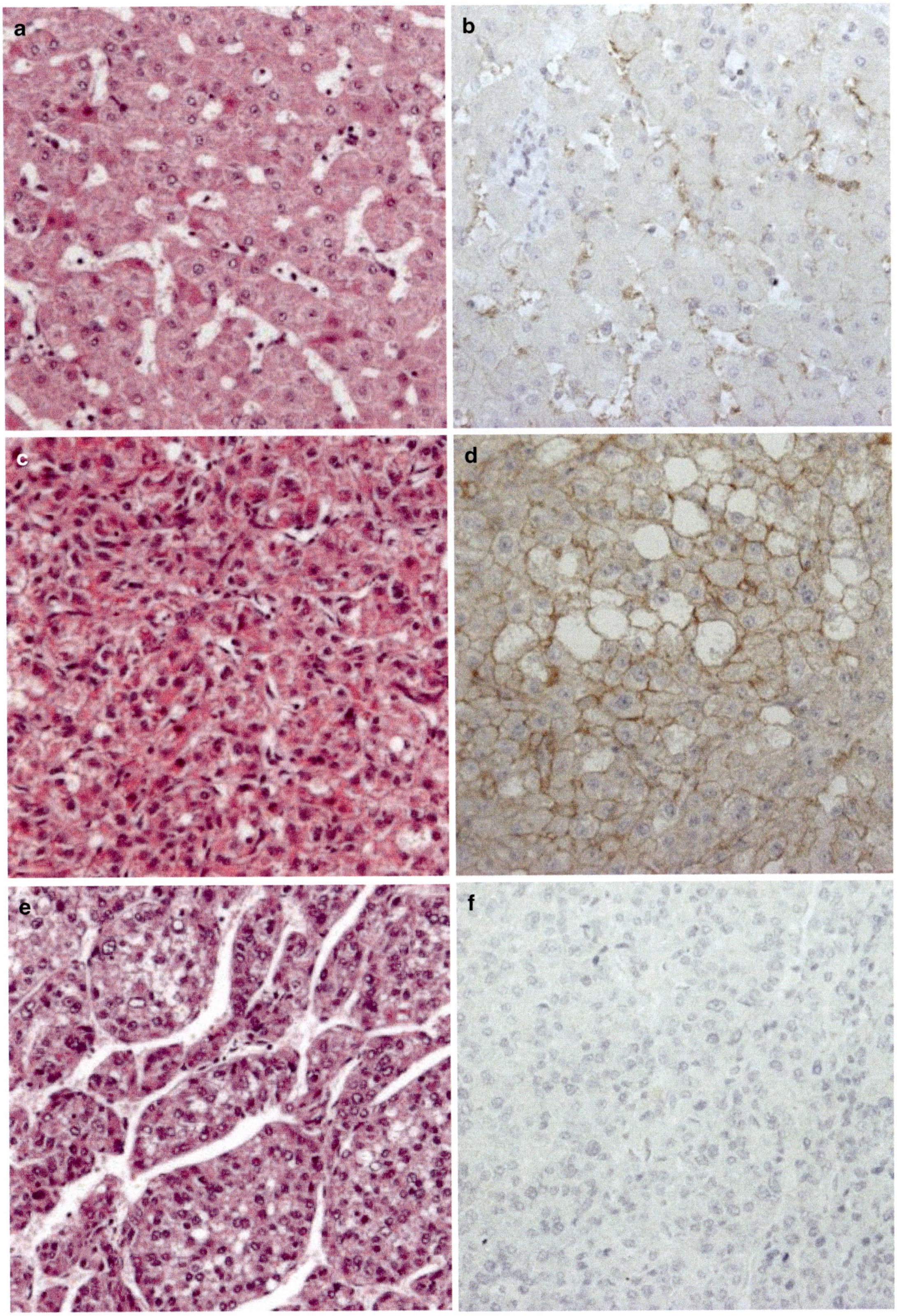

Fig. 17.2 Macroscopic images of surrounding noncancerous liver (**a**, **b**), the peripheral portion of HCC with Gd-EOB-DTPA uptake (**c**, **d**), and the central nodule without Gd-EOB-DTPA uptake (**e**, **f**). The images with HE staining (**a**, **c**, **e**) and immunohistochemical staining for OATP1B3 (**b**, **d**, **f**) are shown. Well- to moderately differentiated HCC in the peripheral portion of the tumor showed positive for mem-branous immunostaining of OATP1B3 on the cancer cells (**c**, **d**). Central tumor represents moderately differentiated HCC without expression of OATP8 (**e**, **f**). The surrounding noncancerous liver cells also showed expression of OATP1B8 (**b**), although the staining is weaker than that in the HCC cells in the peripheral region of the tumor (**d**)

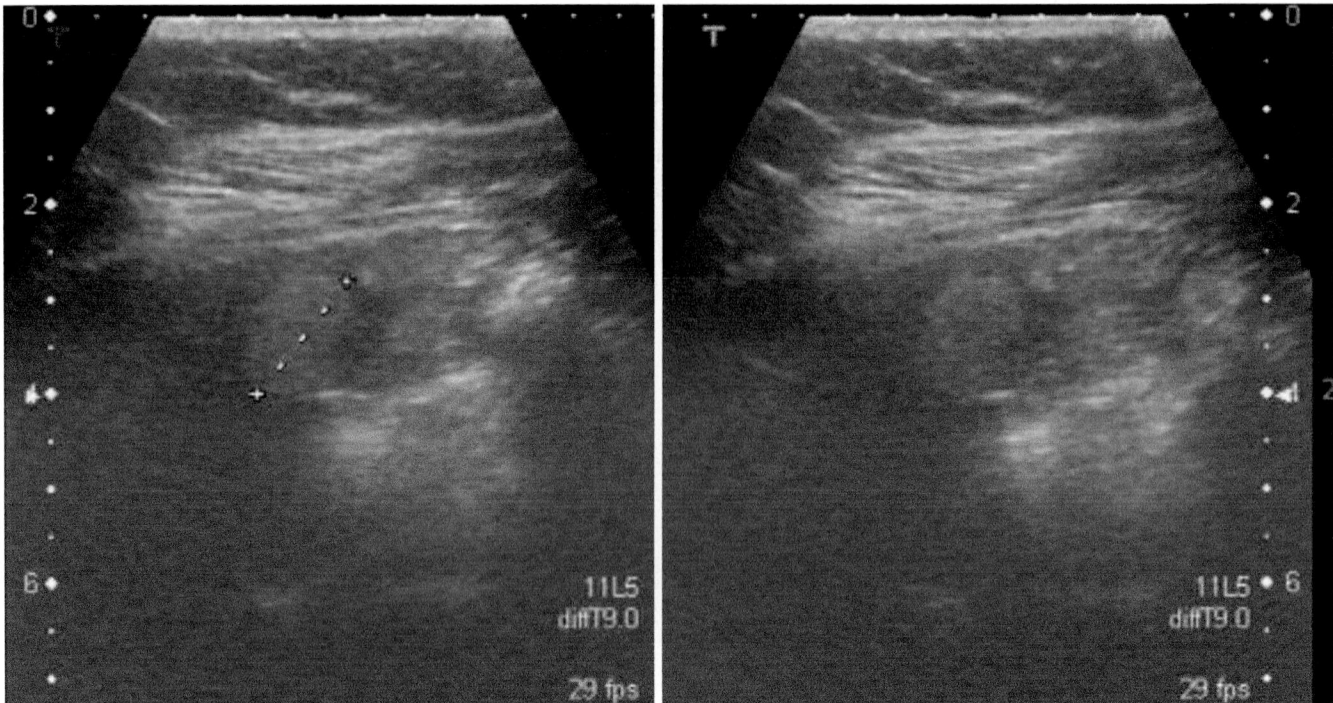

Fig. 17.3 US image of early HCC. The small high-echoic nodule (15 mm) is observed in the peripheral region of the right lobe

- Intermediate stage (B): multinodular tumors in the liver, PS 0, and Child-Pugh A or B.
- Advanced stage (C): HCC with vascular invasion and metastasis to lymph nodes or other body organs. PS 1 or 2. Child-Pugh A or B.
- Terminal stage (D): PS 3 or 4 or Child-Pugh C.

Based on this classification, patients with very-early- to early-stage HCC should be treated curatively, such as with resection, radiofrequency ablation (RFA), and liver transplantation. Transarterial chemoembolization (TACE) is recommended for intermediate-stage HCC cases. However, based on the recent advancement of molecular targeted therapies, intermediate stage of HCC could also be a target of molecular therapy if patients are refractory to TACE. Advanced-stage HCC is a candidate for molecular therapy, such as sorafenib, regorafenib, and lenvatinib [17–19]. HCC patients in terminal stage generally receive supportive care.

Case 17.2 (Early HCC)

An early HCC case in a patient with HCV-positive liver cirrhosis is presented herein. The patient underwent resection of a tumor emerging in the peripheral region of S6. B-mode US image represented a 1.5 cm highly echoic nodule (Fig. 17.3). Angio-CT showed a small low-density tumor before injecting contrast medium without significant enhancement in early and delayed phases, suggestive of a hypovascular tumor with fatty component (Fig. 17.4). The high-intensity tumor in in-phase T1-weighted image was depicted as low-intensity in out-of-phase image, indicating steatosis of the tumor. The

tumor was hypovascular in the early-phase image of contrast-enhanced MRI (Fig. 17.5). Macroscopically, tumor margin was unclear without fibrous capsule, and there were no findings of expansive growth. Diffuse fatty change and various numbers of portal tracts were observed within the tumor. Microscopically, increase of cell density, nuclear atypia, and stromal invasion are also observed (Fig. 17.6).

Case 17.3 (Progressed HCC)

A 44-year-old HBsAg-positive male, who underwent serological examinations a few times each year, was found to have an elevated alpha-fetoprotein (AFP) level of 56 ng/mL. Ultrasonography (US), computed tomography (CT), and angiography showed HCC with 1.5 cm in diameter in S8 (Fig. 17.7).

Case 17.4 (Hepatocellular Carcinoma)

A 64-year-old male with positive HCV RNA serum was referred for interferon therapy. His liver chemistry showed T-BIL 0.5 mg/dL, AST 49 IU/L, ALT 40 IU/L, ALP 301 IU/L, GGT 207 IU/L, hyarulonic acid 182 ng/mL, HCV genotype 1b, AFP 6.5 ng/mL, PIVKA-II 443 mAU/mL, PT 86%, PLT $17 \times 10^4/\mu L$, and $ICGR_{15}$ 12%. Abdominal US showed two neighboring space-occupying lesions in the S5 area. CEUS revealed large hypervascular and small hypovascular tumors in arterial phase. Defect of contrast medium was observed in both tumors in Kupffer phase (Fig. 17.8). CECT also showed large hypervascular and small hypovascular tumors in the early phase and defect on both tumors in the late phase; CT with angiography showed a hypervascular pattern in the larger

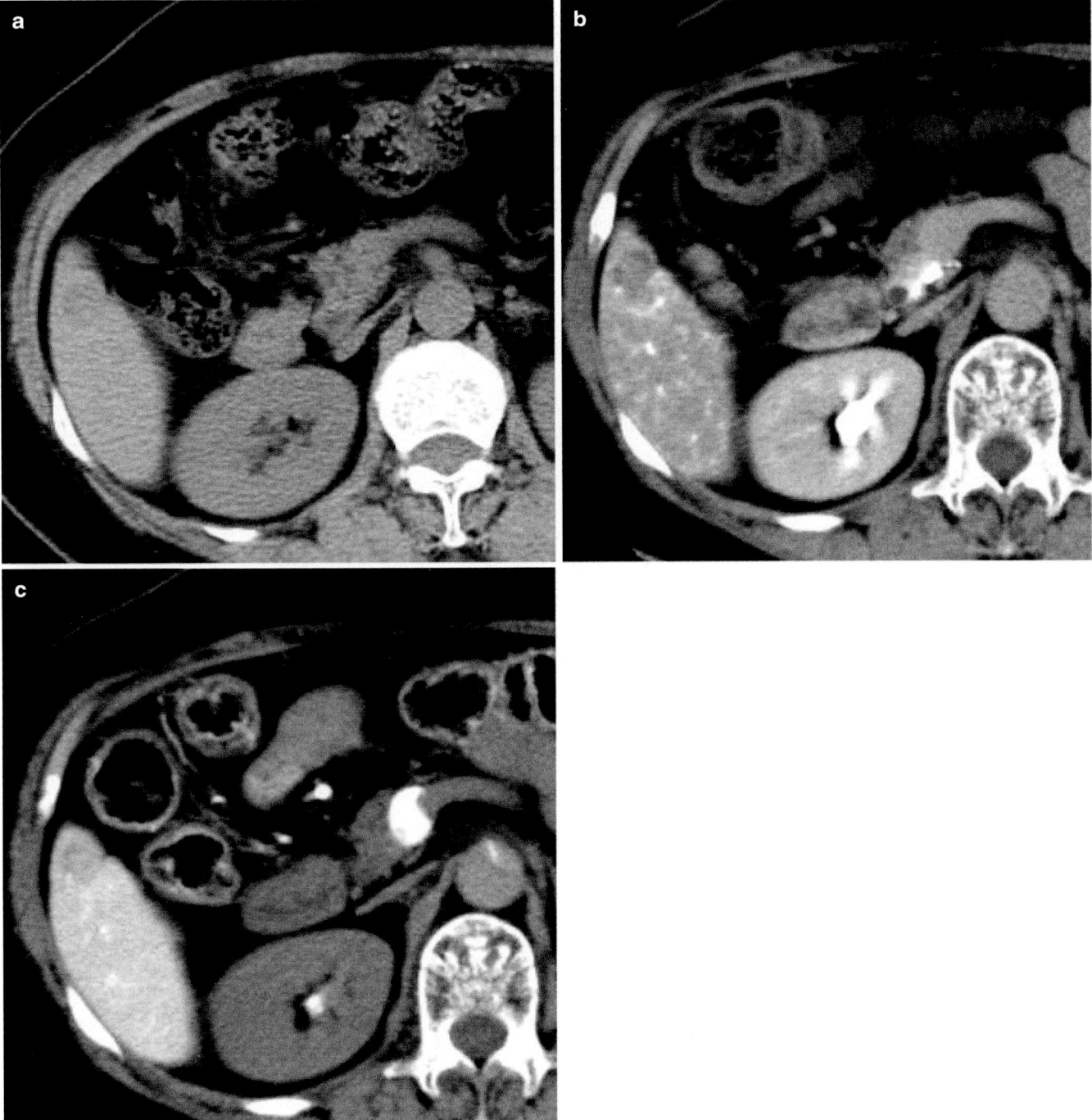

Fig. 17.4 Angio-CT for early HCC. The small low-density nodule is observed in S6 in plain CT image (**a**). CT arteriography (CTA) revealed the hypovascular tumor (**b**). CT arterial portography (CTAP) showed decrease of portal flow in the tumor (**c**)

tumor and a hypovascular pattern with partially enhanced area in the small tumors in the arterial phase; both tumors showed defect in the venous phase (Fig. 17.9). MRI showed low-intensity and high-intensity tumor in T1-weighted image and high intensity in both tumors in T2-weighted image; Gd-EOB-DTPA-enhanced MRI revealed enhancement in the former and defect in the latter in the vascular phase (Fig. 17.10). The resected large tumor was necrotic in the center. Both tumors

were surrounded by capsules. Neoplastic cells formed trabecular and partially glandular structures with canalicular and intracytoplasmic bile (Fig. 17.11). In the small tumor, necrosis with viable neoplastic cells was observed within the surrounding fibrosis (Fig. 17.12).

The treatment for HCC is either surgical or nonsurgical. Surgical interventions include resection or transplantation. Nonsurgical procedures include TACE or hepatic arterial

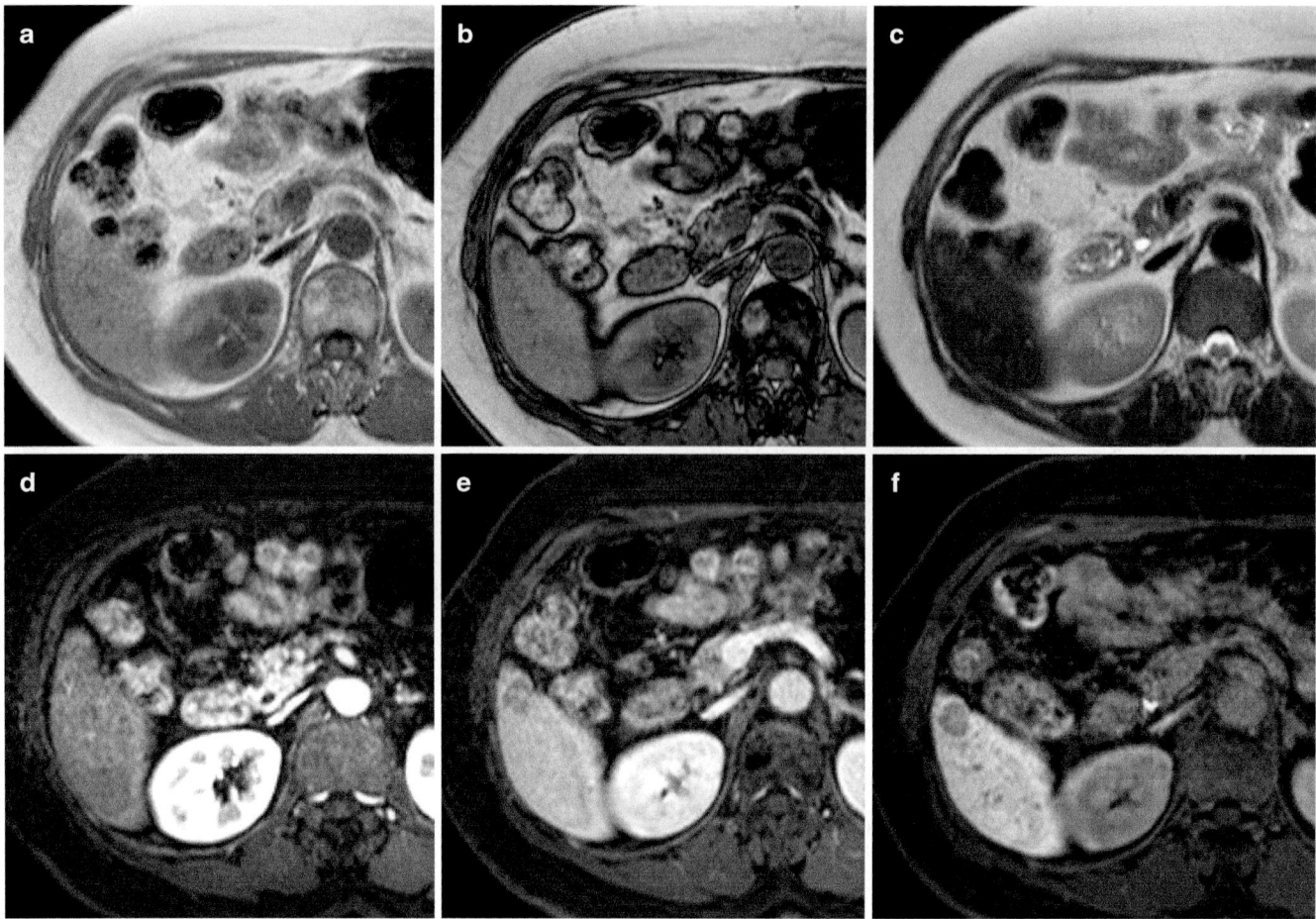

Fig. 17.5 MRI images of early HCC. In-phase T1-weighted image (**a**), out-of-phase T1-weighted image (**b**), T2-weighted image (**c**), arterial-phase image of Gd-EOB-DTPA contract-enhanced MRI (**d**), portal phase image of Gd-EOB-DTPA contract-enhanced MRI (**e**), and hepatobiliary phase image of Gd-EOB-DTPA contract-enhanced MRI for the tumor in S6. The high-intensity tumor in the in-phase T1-weighted image was depicted as low-intensity in out-of-phase image, suggesting the fatty change of the tumor. The tumor was revealed hypovascular in the contract-enhanced MRI images

infusion chemotherapy (HAIC), RFA [14], percutaneous ethanol injection (PEI) [20], or systemic therapy [21]. Figure 17.13 shows the HCC case treated with TACE. Resected tumor shows necrosis after embolization, and the internodular nonneoplastic liver parenchyma is hemorrhagic (Fig. 17.14).

The use of an anticancer drug doxorubicin or cisplatin with Lipiodol in HAIC resulted in specific retention in the tumor and induced complete necrosis surrounded by fibrous capsule (Fig. 17.15). Figure 17.16 shows the HCC case treated with PEI. US reveals the HCC with a halo; the lesion turned hyperechoic after PEI; and the resected tumor is encapsulated by a fibrous tissue with complete necrosis and hemorrhage (Fig. 17.16). Figure 17.17 shows the histology of HCC tissue after RFA with massive necrosis surrounded by fibrosis. After TACE, TAI, PEI, and RFA therapy, viable cells often remain inside or outside the fibrous capsule (Fig. 17.18). Sarcomatous change is sometimes observed in HCC after TACE or TAI treatment (Fig. 17.19).

Prognosis of HCC is dependent on its size, infiltrative growth, and metastatic spread, as well as the functional capacity of the non-tumorous part of the liver [14]. HCC may be complicated by arterioportal fistula formation, esophageal varices, and pulmonary hypertension with liver cirrhosis. In most cases, circulatory or renal failure occurs after retention of massive ascites, portal thrombosis of the tumor, and tumor rupture.

17.3 Intrahepatic Cholangiocarcinoma (Cholangiocellular Carcinoma)

Carcinoma of the biliary epithelium can arise anywhere in the intrahepatic or extrahepatic bile ducts. Tumors originating from the bile ducts are classified into three types according to the site. Depending on whether they arise in the liver, near the hilum, or from the extrahepatic ducts, they are called intrahepatic or peripheral cholangiocarci-

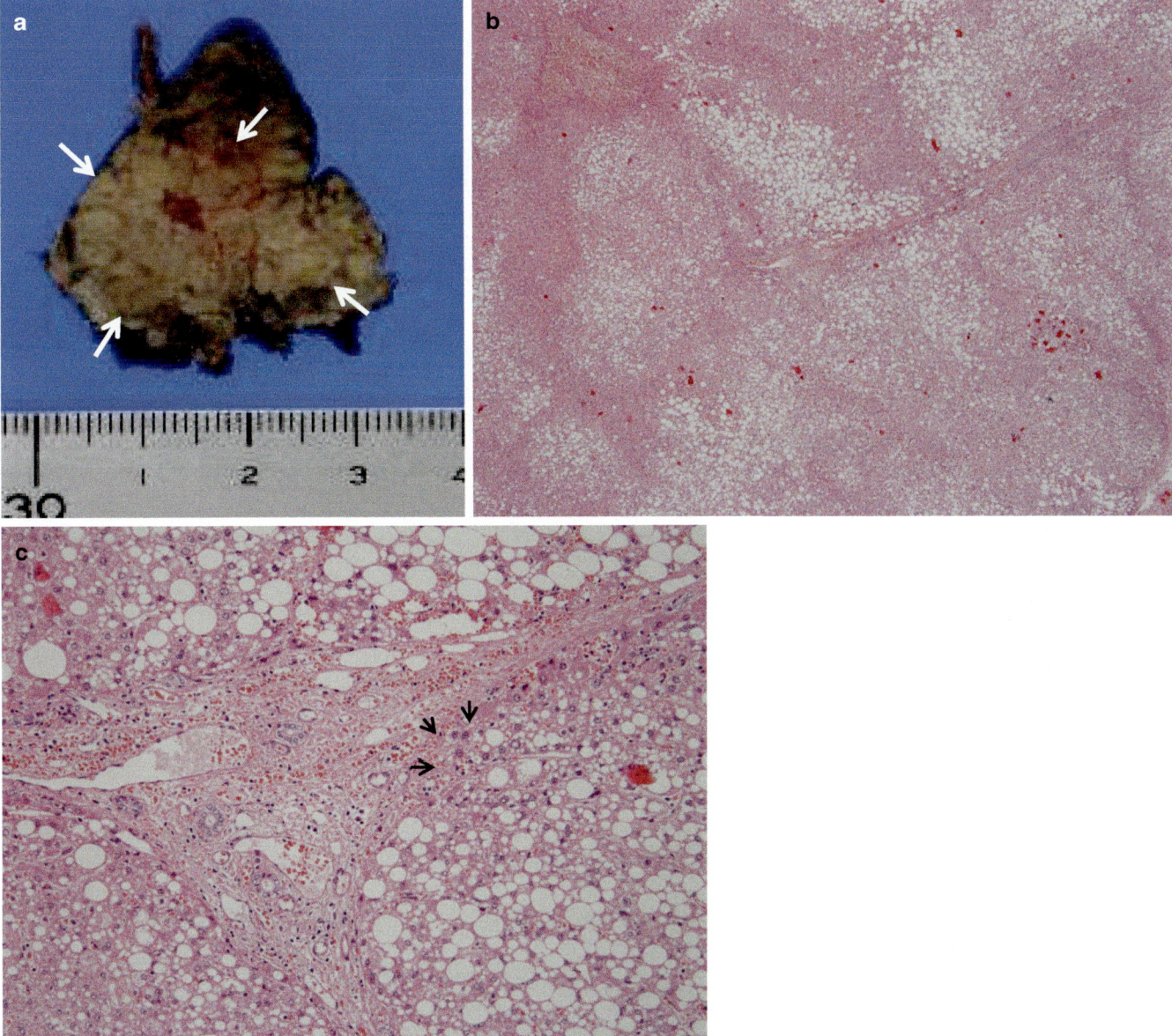

Fig. 17.6 Macroscopic and microscopic images of early HCC. Macroscopic view (**a**). Tumor with unclear margin and no fibrous capsule is observed (white arrow); tumor does not show an expansive growth pattern. Microscopic views (**b, c**). Diffuse fatty change and various numbers of portal tracts are observed within tumor. There is no fibrous capsule; tumor is distinguishable because of the steatosis (**b**: magnification, 40×). Increase of cell density and nuclear atypia are observed at magnification of 200× (**c**). Stromal invasion is observed (arrow)

noma, perihilar cholangiocarcinoma (including Klatskin tumor), and distal cholangiocarcinoma, respectively [22]. In addition, a subtype of CCC, morphologically similar to cholangioles, is known as cholangiolocellular carcinoma (CoCC), which is thought to arise in the canal of Hering (Fig. 17.20) [23]. It is reported that hepatic stem cells reside in the canal of Hering [24]. In addition, CoCC sometimes contains minor HCC components within the tumor, suggestive of hepatic stem cell origin. On the other hand, primary liver carcinomas with both hepatocytic and cholangiocytic differentiation have been referred to as "combined (or mixed) hepatocellular-cholangiocarcinoma" [25].

17.3.1 Etiology

Chronic inflammation of the bile duct could cause cholangiocarcinoma (CCC). The common predisposing factors are

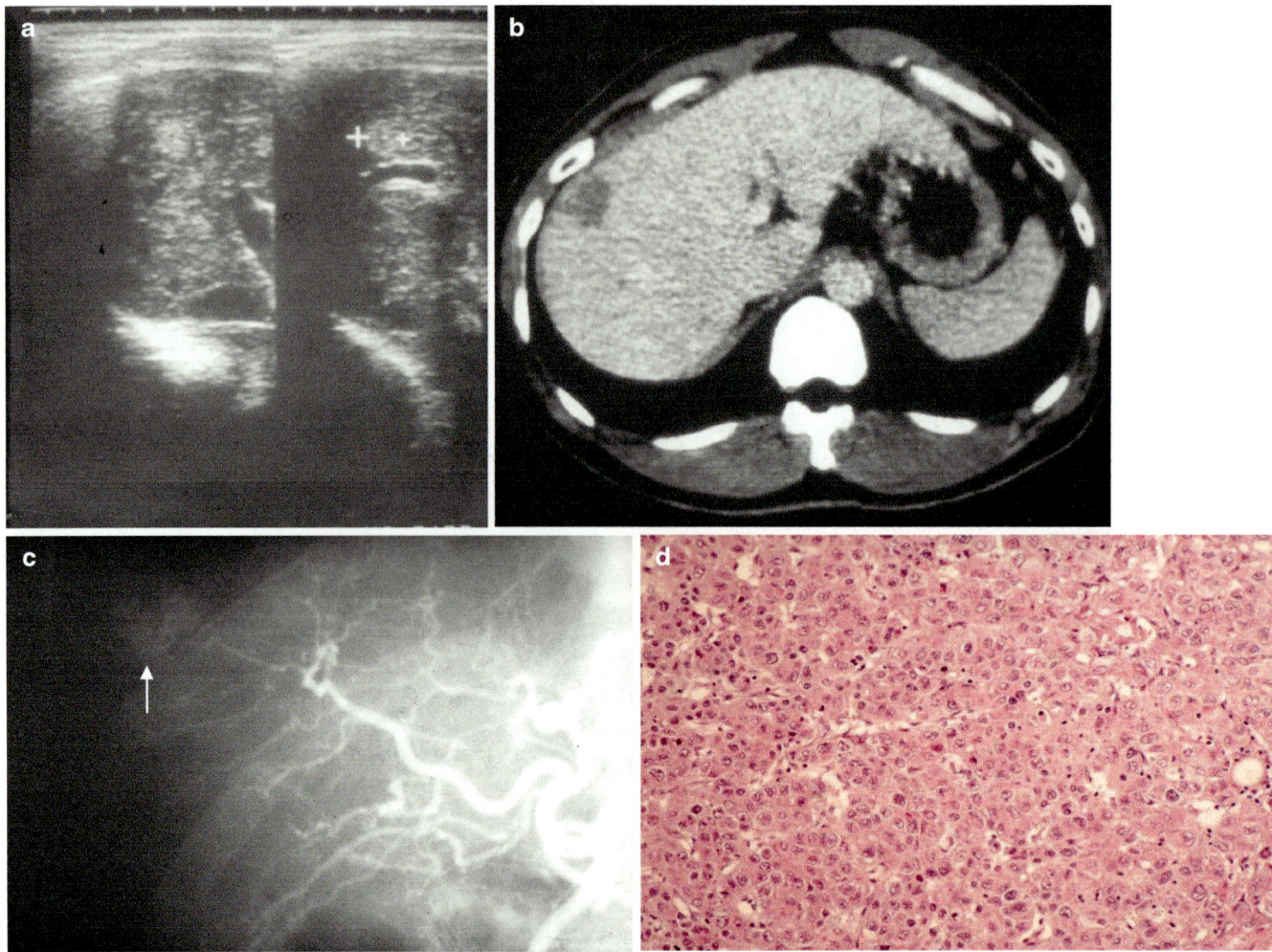

Fig. 17.7 Progressed hepatocellular carcinoma. US shows hyperechoic lesion of diameter 1.5 cm in S8 (**a**). CT with contrast medium shows the presence of a low-density area in the late phase (**b**). Common hepatic arteriography shows tumor staining (arrow) in S8 (**c**). The resected tumor tissue shows moderately differentiated type of hepatocellular carcinoma (**d**)

infestation with flukes [26], hepatolithiasis [27], primary sclerosing cholangitis, and congenital cystic diseases of the bile ducts [28]. Organic solvent, such as dichloromethane and 1,2-dichloropropane, and radioactive radiological contrast medium (Thorotrast) also induce CCC [29].

Interestingly, CCC is also divided into four subgroups based on the gene mutation and expression signature [30]. CCC caused by flukes infection is characterized by the hypermethylation on the promoter CpG, decrease of ten-eleven translocation methylcytosine dioxygenase 1 (TET1) expression, increase of histone methyltransferase enhancer of zeste homolog 2 (EZH2) expression, and frequent somatic mutation of AT-rich interactive domain-containing protein 1A (ARID1) gene, suggesting that epigenetic mechanism should be involved in carcinogenesis for this type of CCC. It is also reported the difference of mutation profile that should drive carcinogenesis among CCCs orig-

inated from different sites of bile tree [31]. These evidences suggested that difference of genetic and epigenetic alterations of CCC should be, at least partially, affected by its etiology. On the other hand, morphologically, the tumors are classified into mass-forming, periductal-infiltrating, and intraductal-growth types [32].

17.3.2 Diagnosis

Mass-forming CCC is a circumscribed tumor with lobular configuration and no capsule, while the periductal-infiltrating CCC is highly invasive and sometimes undetectable by US. Intraductal-growth CCC causes intraductal mass, obstruction, and dilatation of the bile duct. CEUS images of CCC generally show slightly hypervascular pattern. Ring enhancement of the tumor margin at early phase and delayed

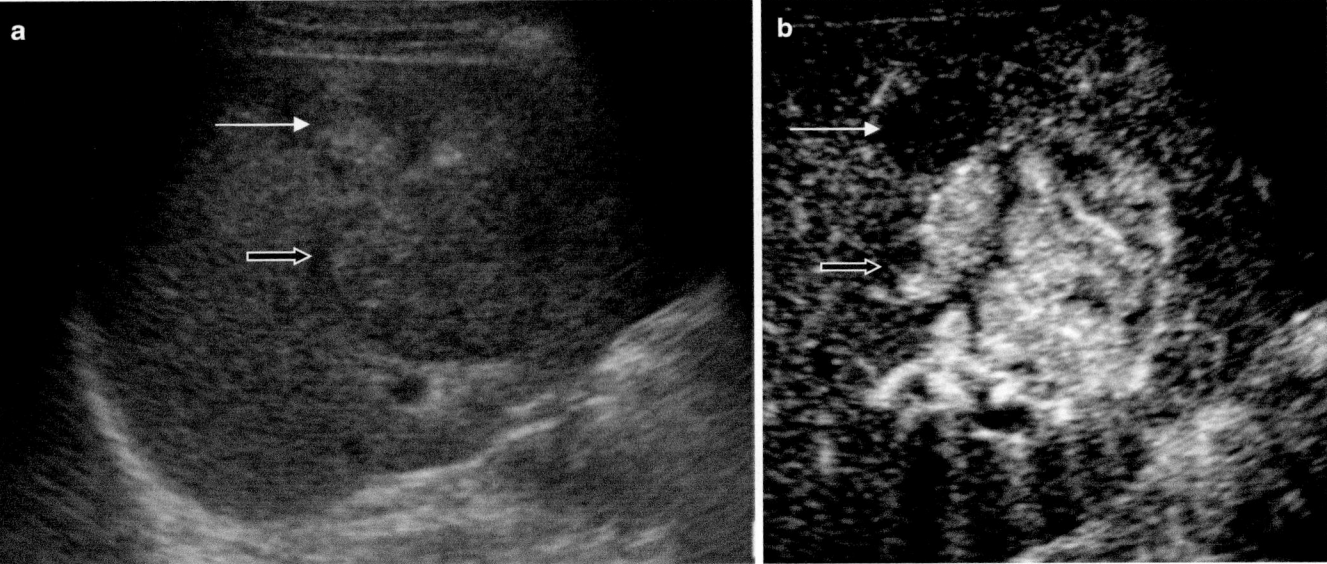

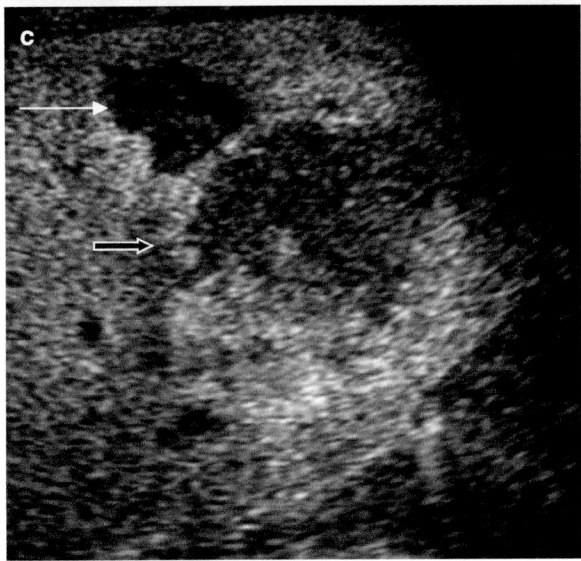

Fig. 17.8 Ultrasonographic findings with or without contrast medium in hepatocellular carcinoma. The isoechoic space-occupying lesion (SOL) (short arrow) with halo and a high-echoic SOL (long arrow) are mosaic in echo pattern (**a**). US image with contrast medium shows high echogenicity in the large SOL and low echogenicity in the small SOL in the vascular phase (**b**). A low-echoic pattern is seen in both SOLs in the Kupffer phase (**c**) (Courtesy of Dr. T. Mori)

enhancement can be detected in CCC cases, but these findings are also observed in metastatic tumors of the liver. MRI regularly shows low-intensity tumor on T1-weighted and high-intensity tumor on T2-weighted image [22].

17.3.3 Treatment

Surgical resection of tumor is the first line of the treatment; systemic chemotherapy using gemcitabine with/without cisplatin is generally the recommended treatment for unresectable cases. Radiation and chemotherapy are used for palliative treatment [33].

Case 17.5 (Cholangiocarcinoma, Mass-Forming Type)

A 66-year-old male presented with complaint of jaundice. US showed a large isoechoic tumor in S4 (Fig. 17.21). CT showed a tumor in S4 with delayed enhancement (Fig. 17.22). Percutaneous transhepatic cholangiogram showed dilatation of the right hepatic bile duct. US-guided tumor biopsy revealed glandular neoplastic structures with fibrosis (Fig. 17.23).

Case 17.6 (Cholangiocellular Carcinoma with Infection of *Clonorchis sinensis*)

A 72-year-old female presented with anorexia, general malaise, and jaundice. Her laboratory data showed T-BIL

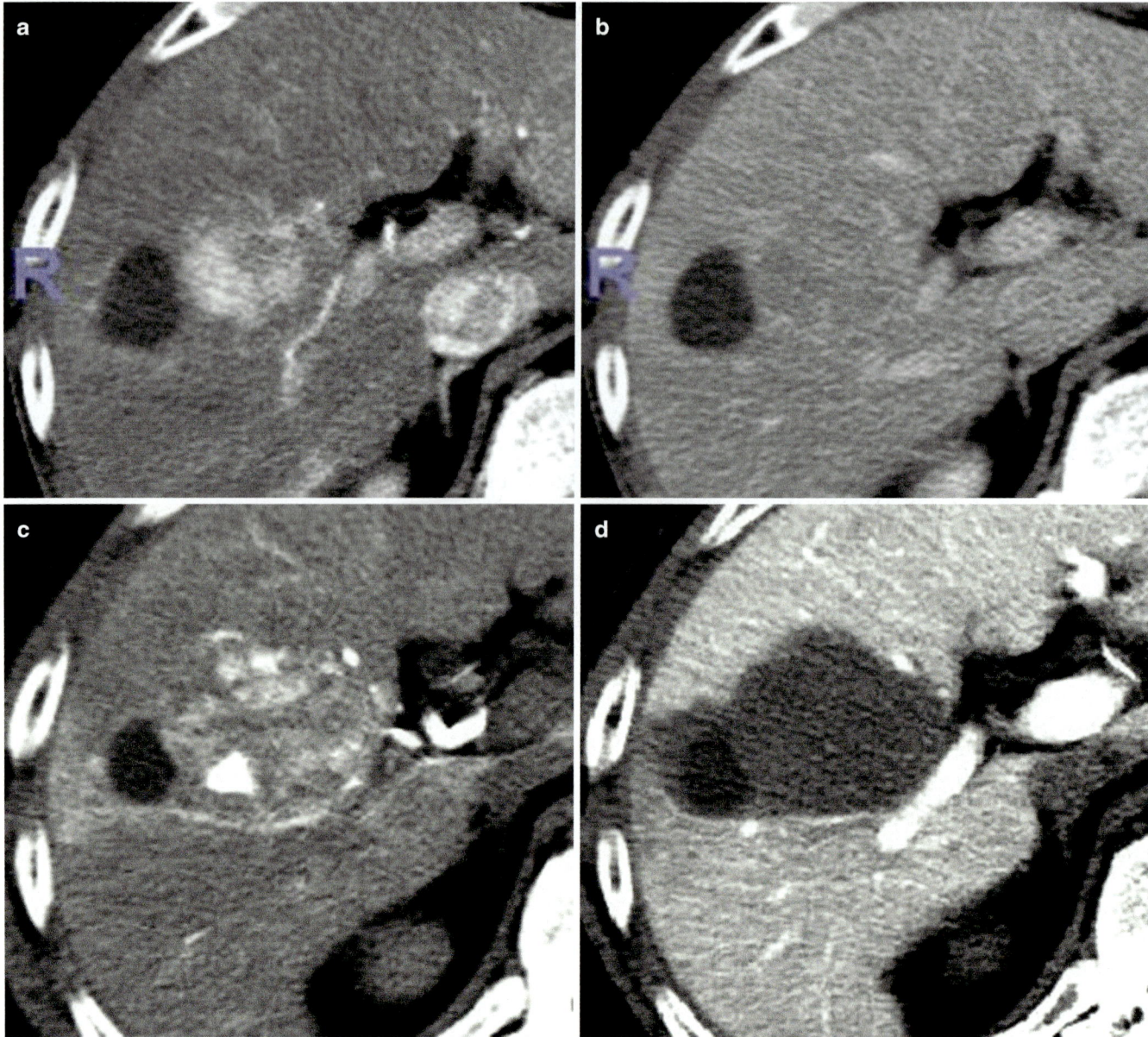

Fig. 17.9 CT with or without angiography in hepatocellular carcinoma. CECT shows high density in a large tumor and low density in a small tumor in the early phase (**a**), and iso- or low density is seen in both tumors in the late phase (**b**). Angio-CT revealed hypervascular in the former and in a partial area of the latter in the arterial phase (**c**). Angio-CT shows low density in both tumors in the venous phase (**d**) (Courtesy of Dr. T. Mori)

6.91 mg/dL, GOT 208 IU/L, GPT 315 IU/L, ALP 3952 IU/L, GGT 1194 IU/L, CRP 4.7 mg/dL, WBC 6400/mm³, eosinophils 9.6%, and CA19-9 9788 IU/L. Endoscopic nasal bile d**rainage** and percutaneous transhepatic cholangiodrainage were performed when bilirubin reached 23.36 mg/dL. The bile juice contained *Clonorchis sinensis* eggs. Endoscopic retrograde cholangiopancreatography showed obstruction at the junction of the left and right biliary ducts and peripheral ductal dilatation. CECT revealed low-density area in the portal trunk, swelling of the para-aortic lymph nodes, and small multiple low-density areas in the liver. The patient died of liver failure. Autopsy showed dysplastic glands in the portal tract with fibrosis and infiltration of neutrophilic leukocytes. Cholangiocarcinoma is commonly associated with fibrosis (Fig. 17.24).

Case 17.7 (Cholangiocarcinoma with a Component of Cholangiolocellular Carcinoma)

A 75-year-old female presented with liver cirrhosis type C and a liver nodule. Laboratory tests revealed HBsAg negative, positive for HCV Ab, AST = 58 IU/L, ALT = 33 IU/L,

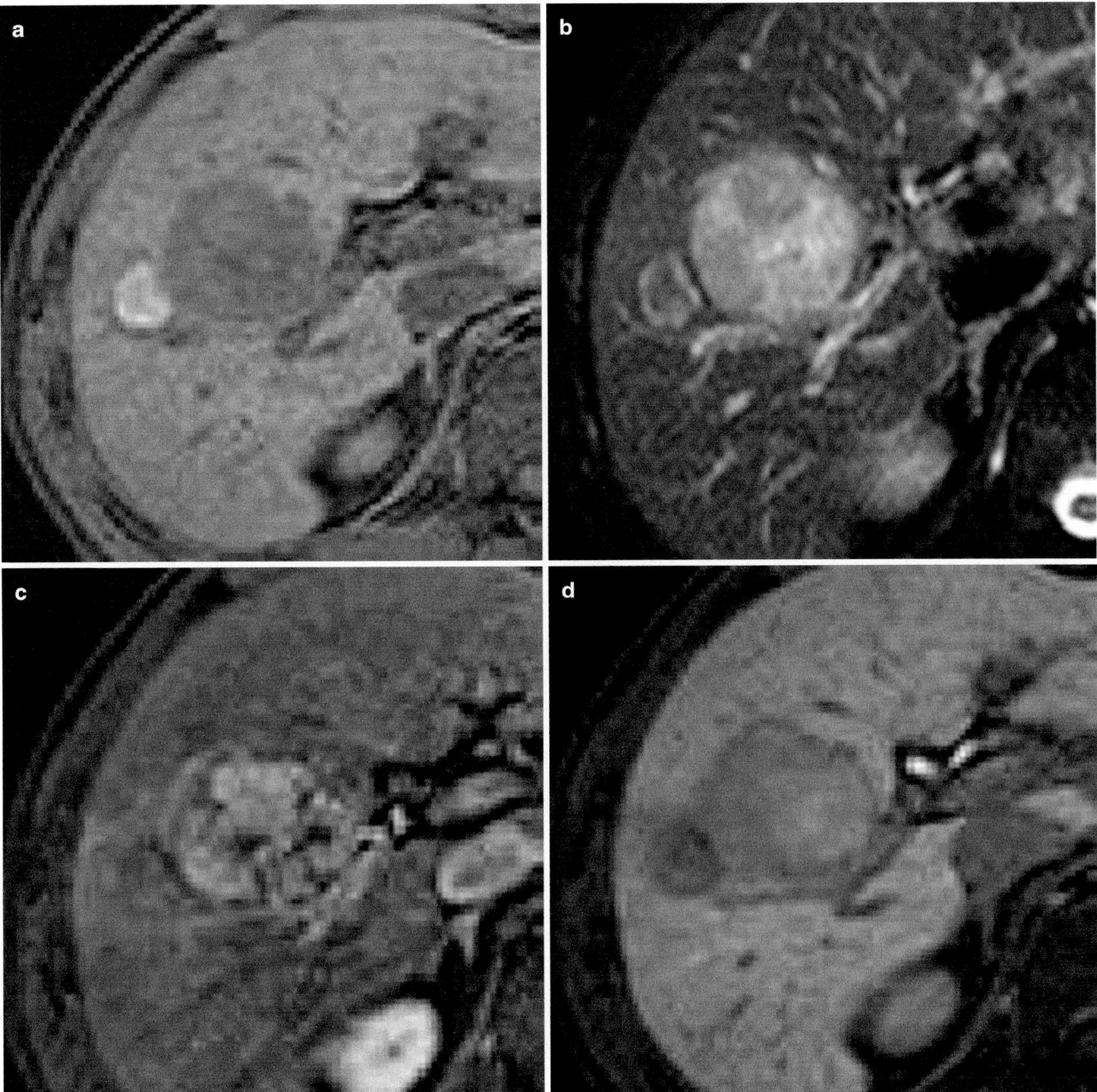

Fig. 17.10 Magnetic resonance image with Gd-EOB-DTPA in hepatocellular carcinoma. MRI with T1 intensification shows low density in a large tumor and high intensity in a small tumor (**a**). MRI with T2 intensification shows high intensity in the former and mixed intensity in the latter (**b**). Gd-EOB-DTPA-enhanced MRI image shows high intensity in a large tumor and iso-intensity in a small tumor in arterial phase (**c**); MRI with EOB shows low intensity in both tumors in hepatobiliary phase (**d**) (Courtesy of Dr. T. Mori)

ALP = 223 IU/L, AFP = 9.9 ng/mL, PIVKA-II = 25 mAU/mL, CEA = 3.7 ng/mL, and CA19-9 = 45.1 U/mL.

The B-mode image of US showed a low-echoic nodule in S4/8 (Fig. 17.25). The nodule showed slightly low density on plain CT, enhancement in the arterial phase, and partial defect in the central area (Fig. 17.26). The tumor revealed as defect in the hepatobiliary phase of the Gd-EOB-DTPA-enhanced image (Fig. 17.27). The tumor showed irregular margin and no capsule. Microscopic examination revealed the tumor consisted of CCC, CoCC, and poorly differentiated CCC components (Figs. 17.28 and 17.29).

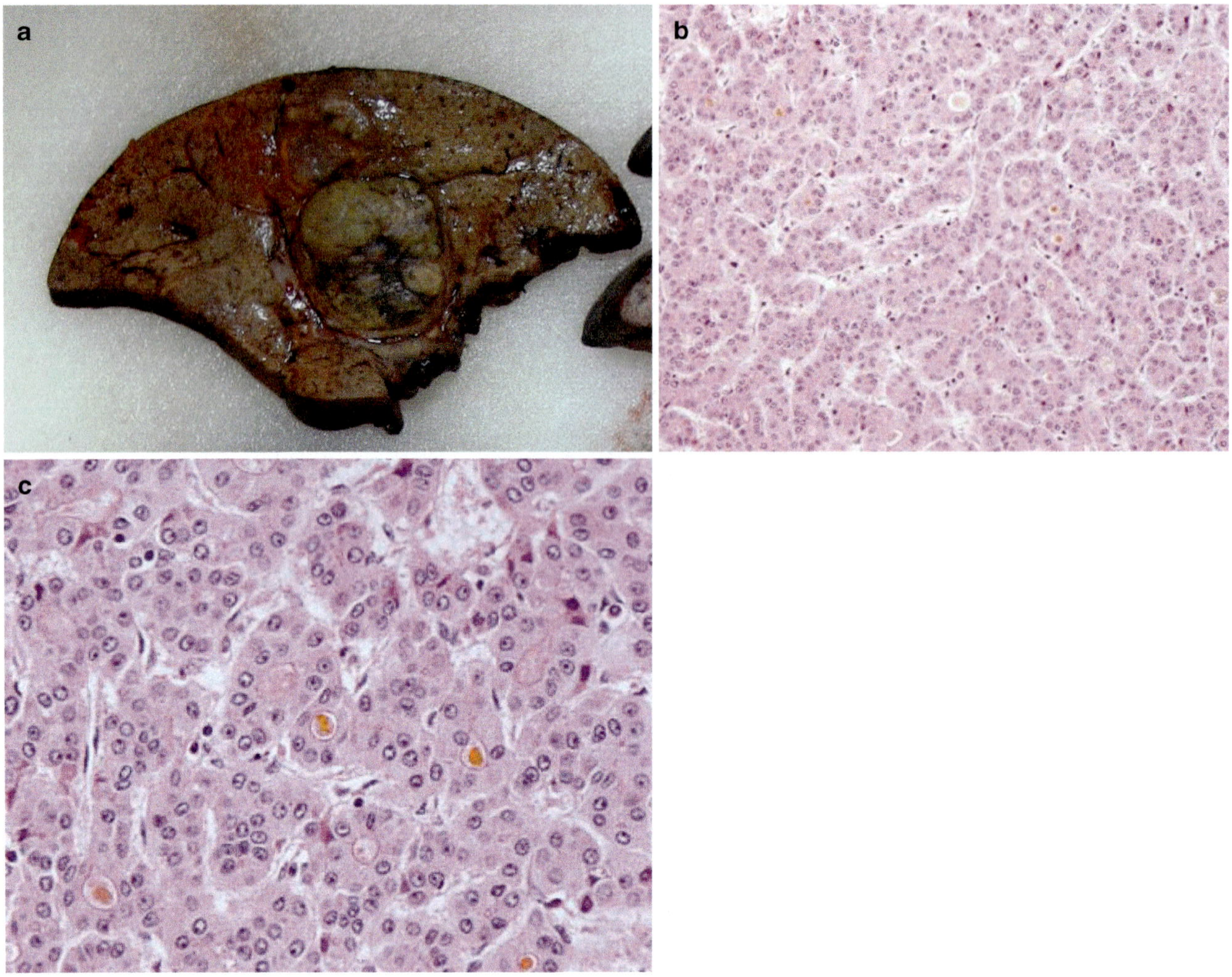

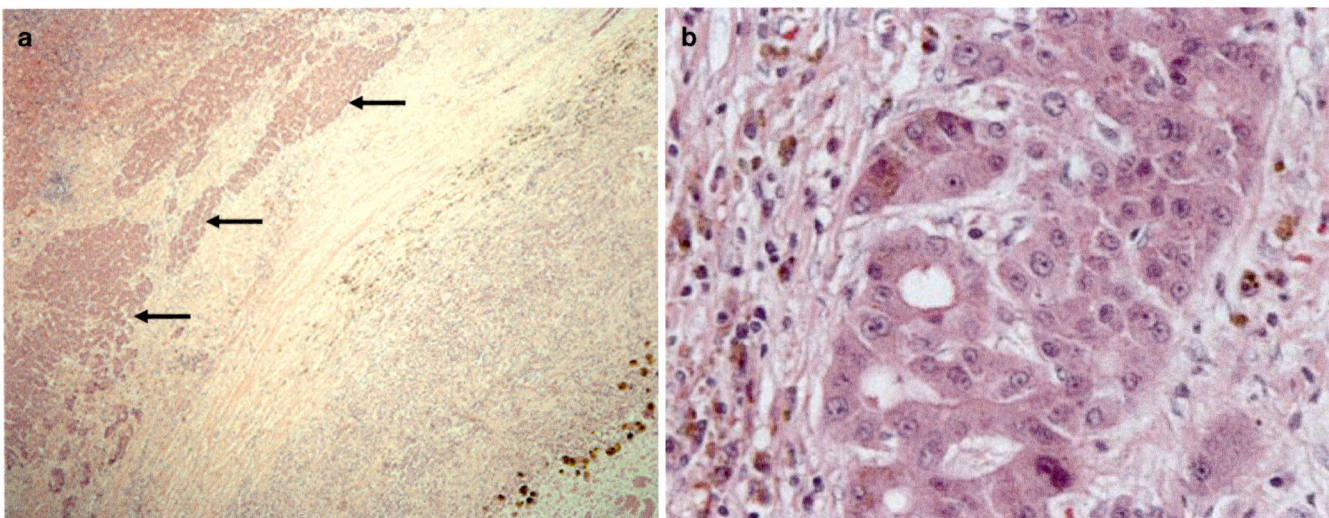

Fig. 17.11 Macro- or microscopic findings of hepatocellular carcinoma. Macroscopic findings of resected liver show a nodular tumor with a daughter nodule, and a necrotic area is seen in a main tumor (**a**). The main tumor shows trabecular type of hepatocellular carcinoma and a pseudoglandular structure is seen (**b**). Bile thrombus or cholestasis is seen in bile canaliculi and neoplastic cells (**c**) (Courtesy of Dr. T. Mori)

Fig. 17.12 Histological findings of hepatocellular carcinoma. A small tumor shows central necrosis with the presence of isolated tumor cells (arrow) in surrounding fibrosis (**a**). Neoplastic cells form trabecular and pseudoglandular structures (**b**) (Courtesy of Dr. T. Mori)

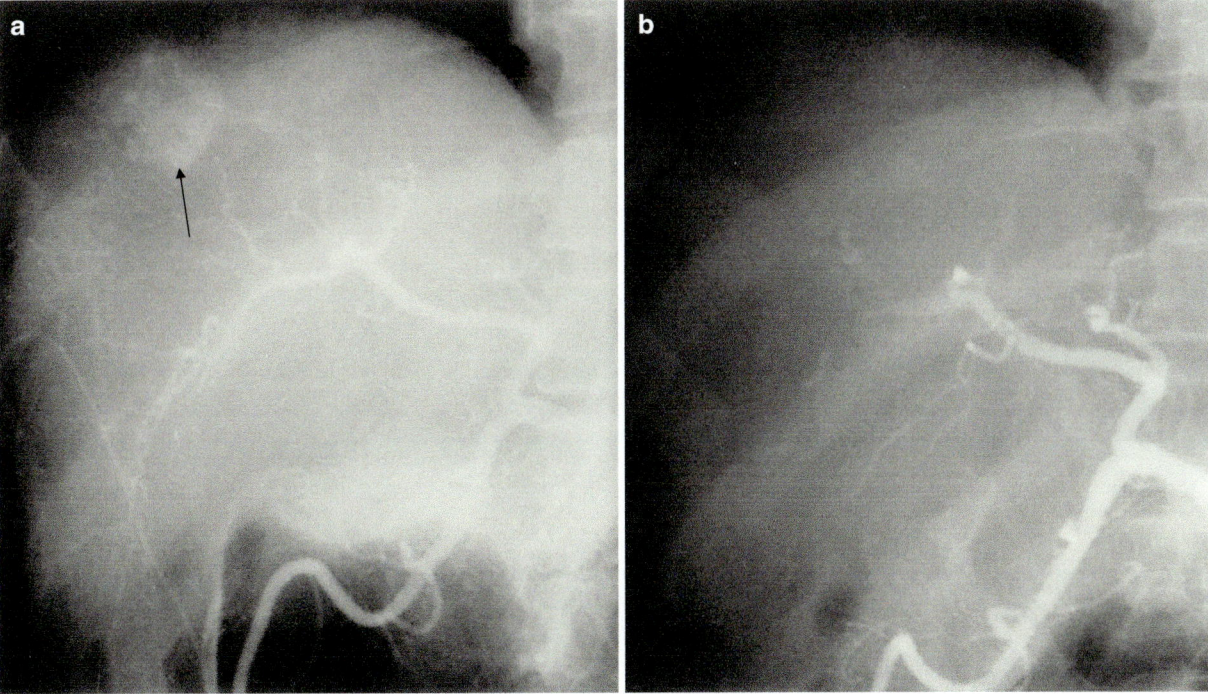

Fig. 17.13 Transarterial chemoembolization. The right hepatic angiography shows a hypervascular area (arrow) in S8 (anterosuperior subsegment of the right lobe) (**a**). Arteriography after TAE shows disappearance of arterial blood flow (**b**)

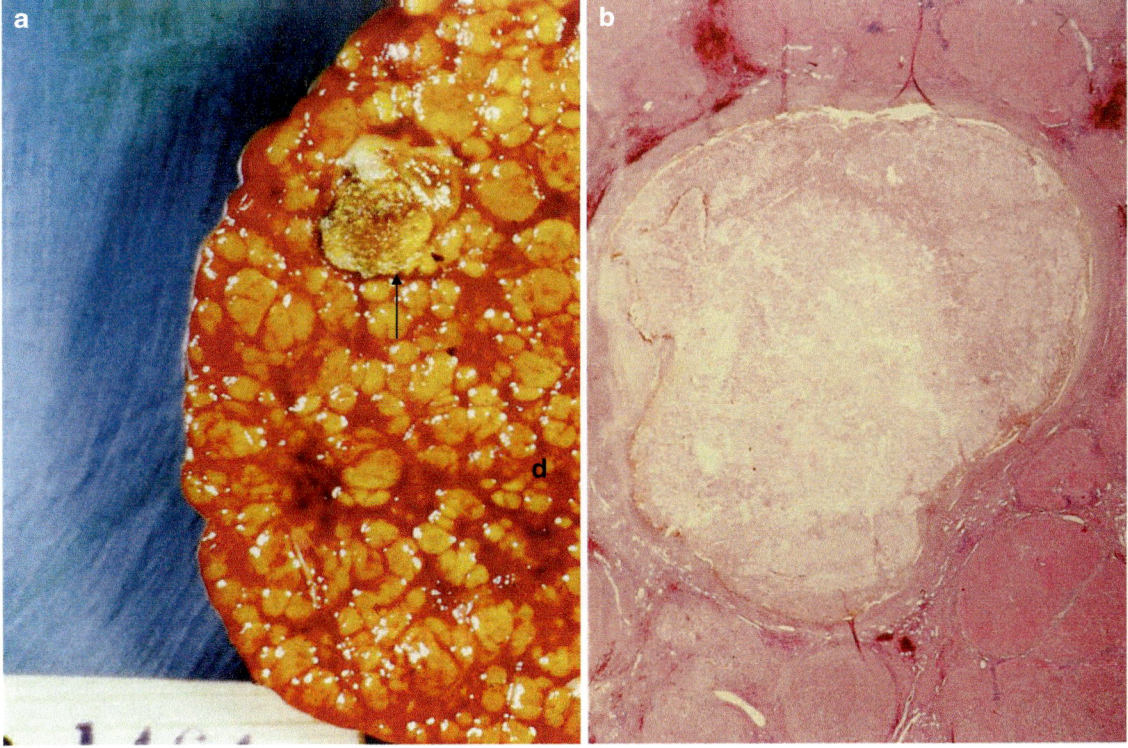

Fig. 17.14 Macro- and microscopic findings of the liver with hepatocellular carcinoma after transarterial embolization. Cut surface of the resected liver. The necrotic nodule (arrow) is surrounded by nonneoplastic regenerative nodules (**a**). Histology reveals an encapsulated tumor resulting in total necrosis. There is focal hemorrhage in the fibrous septa around the tumor (**b**)

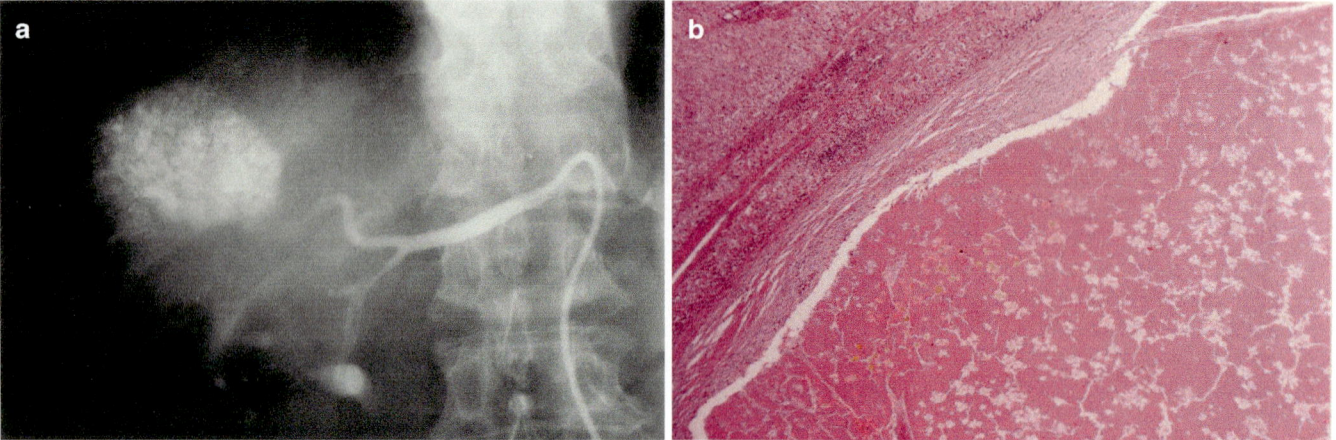

Fig. 17.15 Hepatic arterial infusion chemotherapy. Lipiodol is stained in the tumor area after infusion (**a**). The microscopic appearance confirms the complete necrosis of the tumor cells after hepatic arterial infusion chemotherapy (**b**)

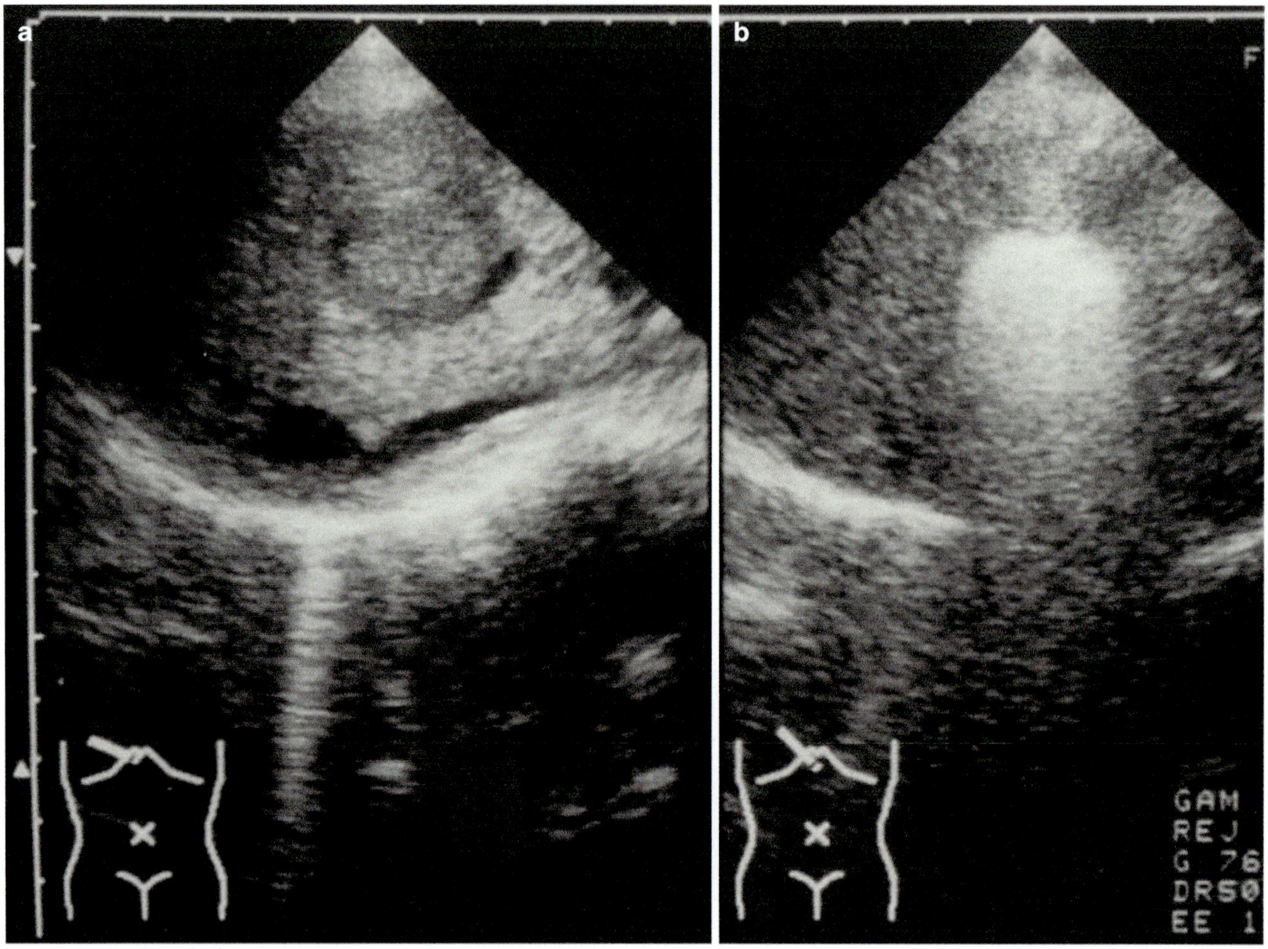

Fig. 17.16 Percutaneous ethanol injection. Ultrasonography shows an isoechoic space-occupying lesion (SOL) with halo (**a**). Ultrasonography shows hyperechoic SOL after PEI (**b**). The tumor (upper right) is totally necrotic. Nonneoplastic viable hepatocytes (lower left) are separated by fibrous connective tissue (**c**). The figures of this case are courtesy of Dr. Maki Iwai, Kyoto Prefectural University of Medicine

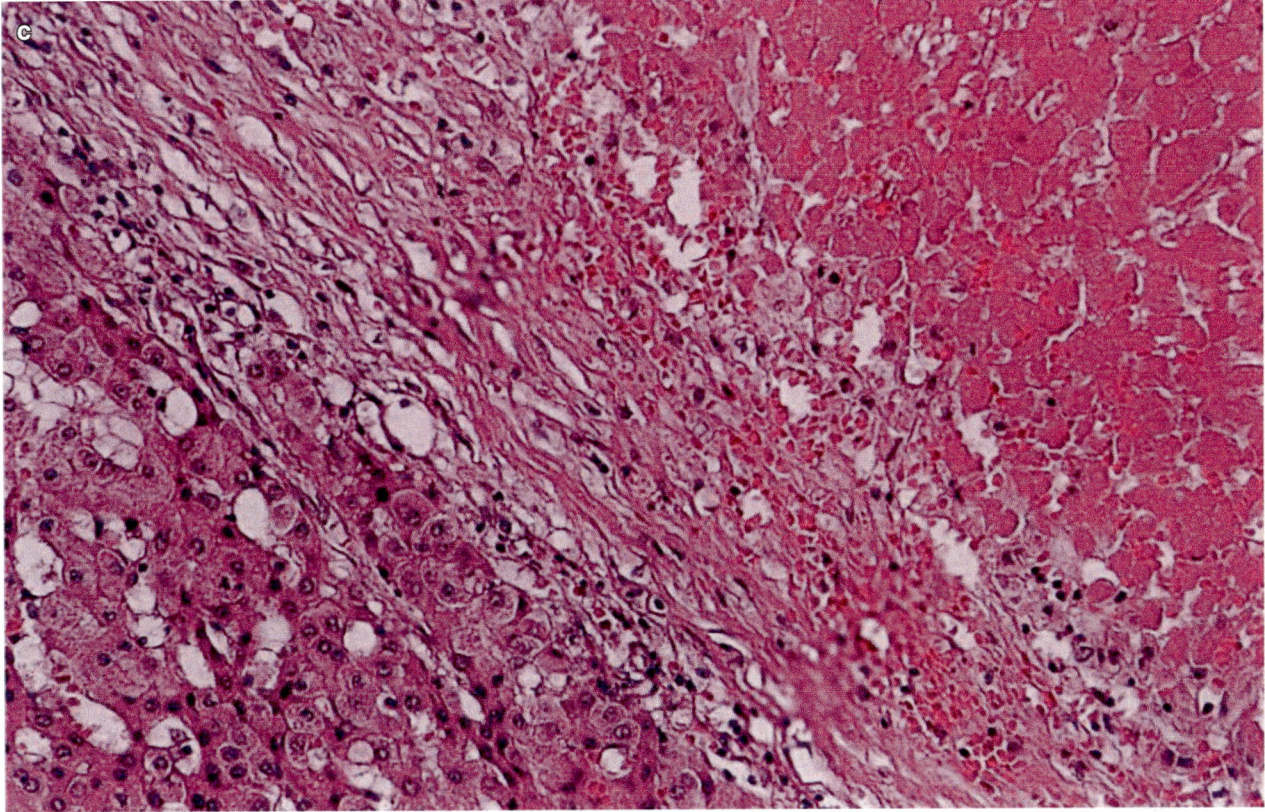

Fig. 17.16 (continued)

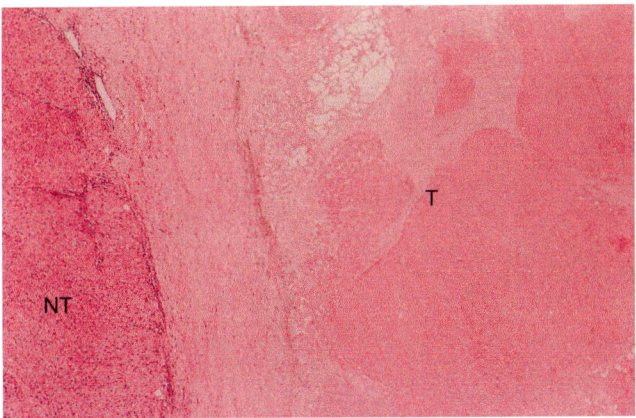

Fig. 17.17 Radiofrequency ablation. Massive necrosis of the encapsu-lated tumor (T) due to radiofrequency ablation NT, non-tumor

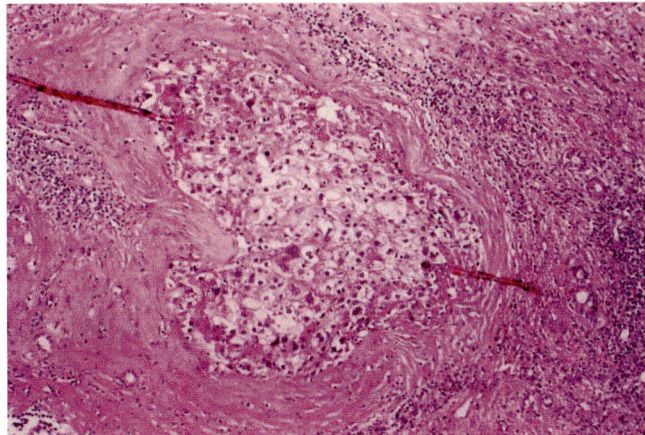

Fig. 17.18 Viable HCC cells after TACE. A small focus of viable neo-plastic cells is remained in the fibrous capsule after TACE

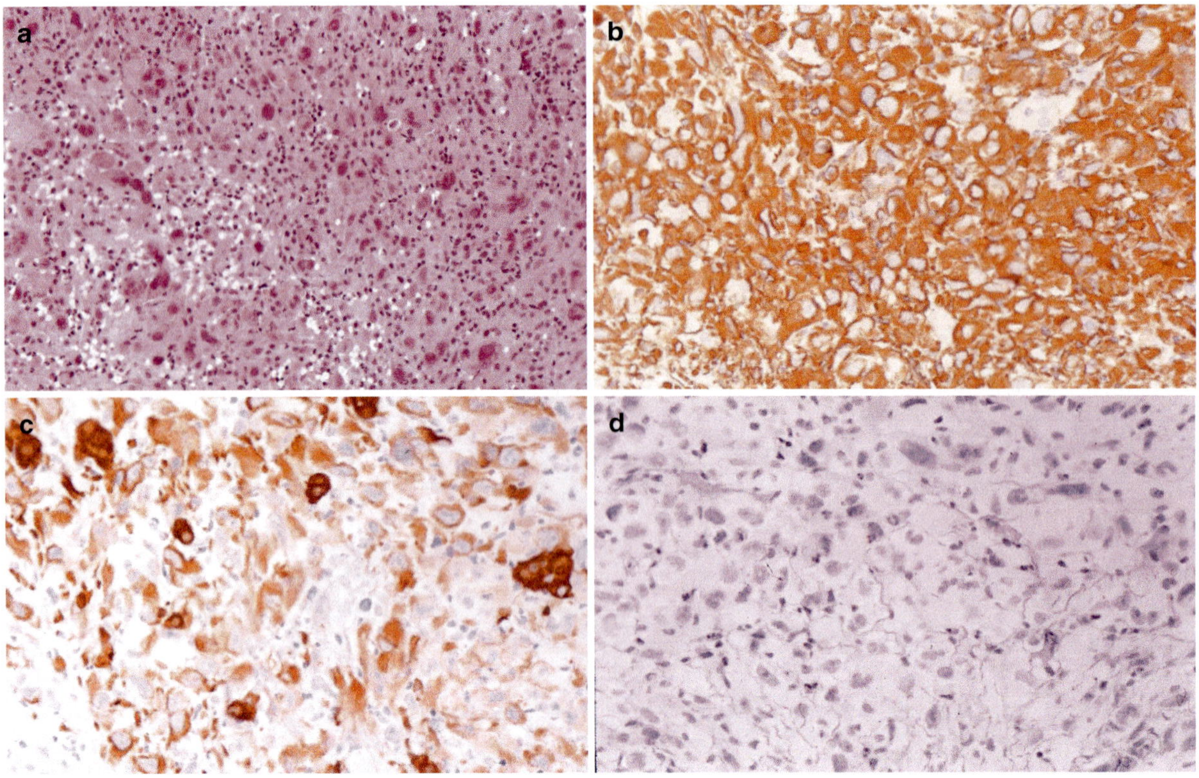

Fig. 17.19 Sarcomatous change in hepatocellular carcinoma. Multinucleated neoplastic cells are distributed with fibrous stroma cells (**a**). Expression of vimentin in neoplastic cells by immunohistochemis-try (**b**). Cytokeratin (CK) 19 is stained in neoplastic cells (**c**). CK20 immunoreactivity is not detected in neoplastic cells (**d**)

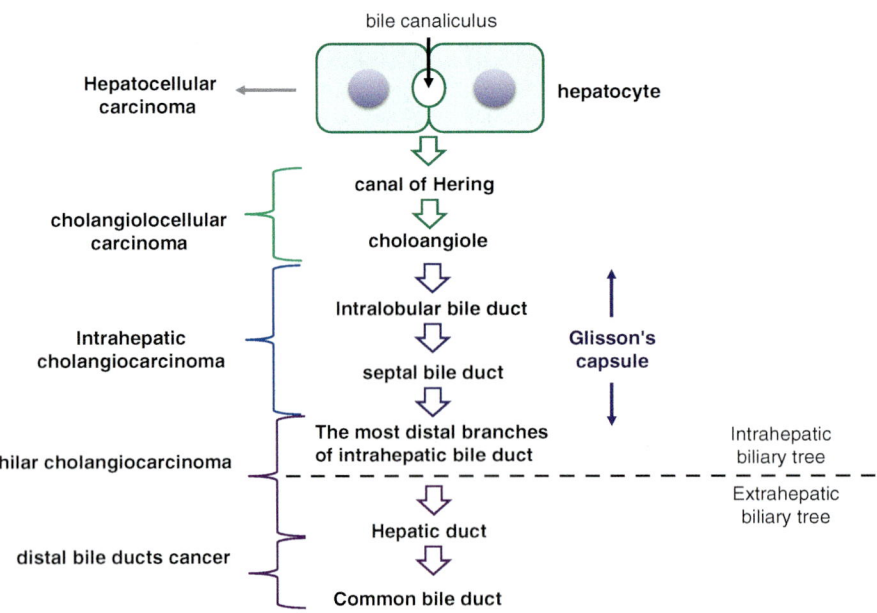

Fig. 17.20 Biliary tree and origin of cancer cell. Depending on whether they arise in the liver, near the hilum, or from the extrahepatic ducts, they are called carcinoma of the intrahepatic or peripheral bile duct, hilar cholangiocarcinoma (Klatskin tumor), or distal bile duct cancer, respectively. A subtype of CCC, morphologically similar to cholangioles, is known as cholangiolocellular carcinoma (CoCC), which is thought to be derived from Hering's canal. It is reported that Hering's canal might be composed of hepatic stem cells; CoCC sometimes contains HCC or CCC components within the tumor, suggesting that it could originate from hepatic stem cells

Fig. 17.21 Cholangiocellular carcinoma; US images. US shows an isoechoic tumor (arrow) in S4 and peripheral bile ducts (arrow head) are dilated around the tumor. The figures of this case are courtesy of Dr. Maki Iwai, Kyoto Prefectural University of Medicine

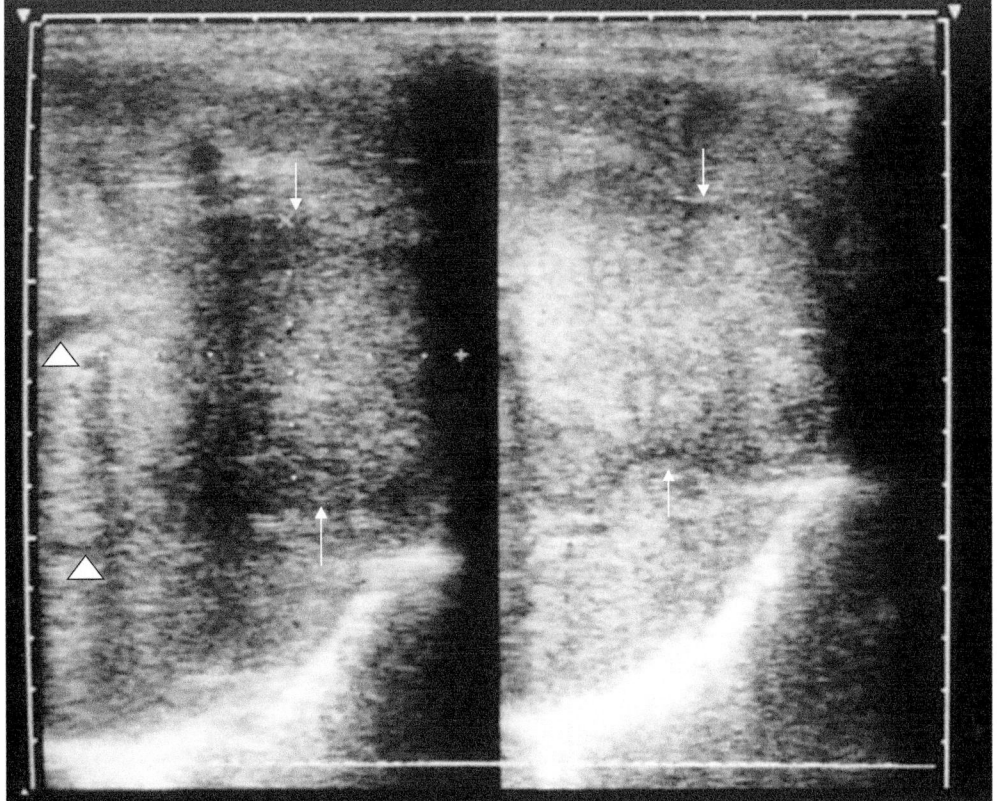

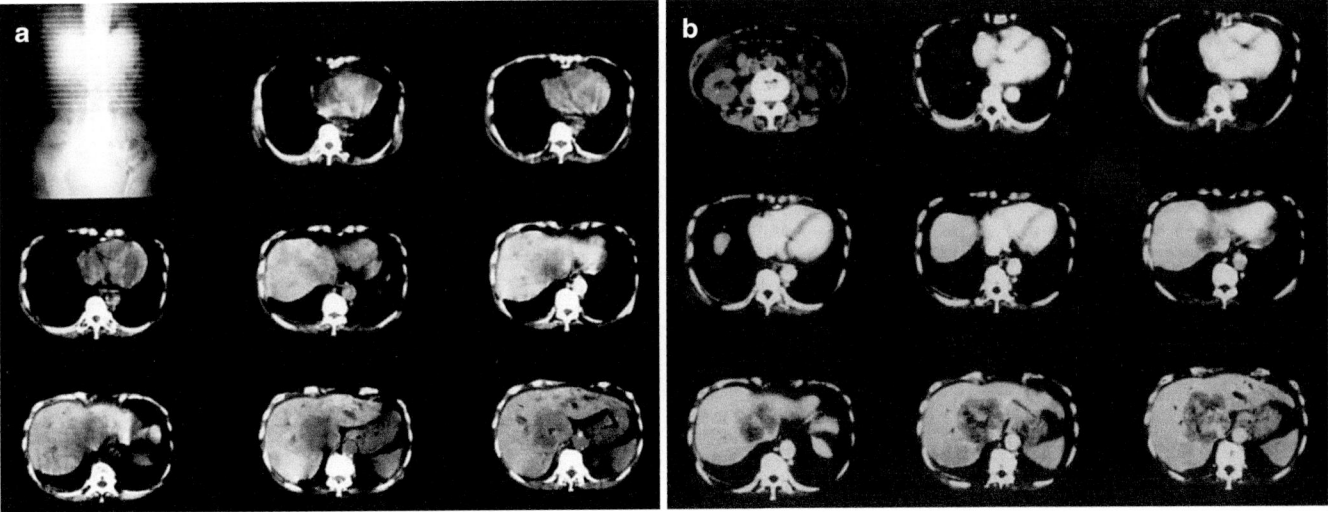

Fig. 17.22 Cholangiocellular carcinoma; CT images. CT shows a low-density area in S4 (**a**). A low-density area is partly enhanced by contrast medium (delayed enhancement); there is dilatation of the left intrahepatic bile duct and tumor invasion into the inferior vena cava (**b**)

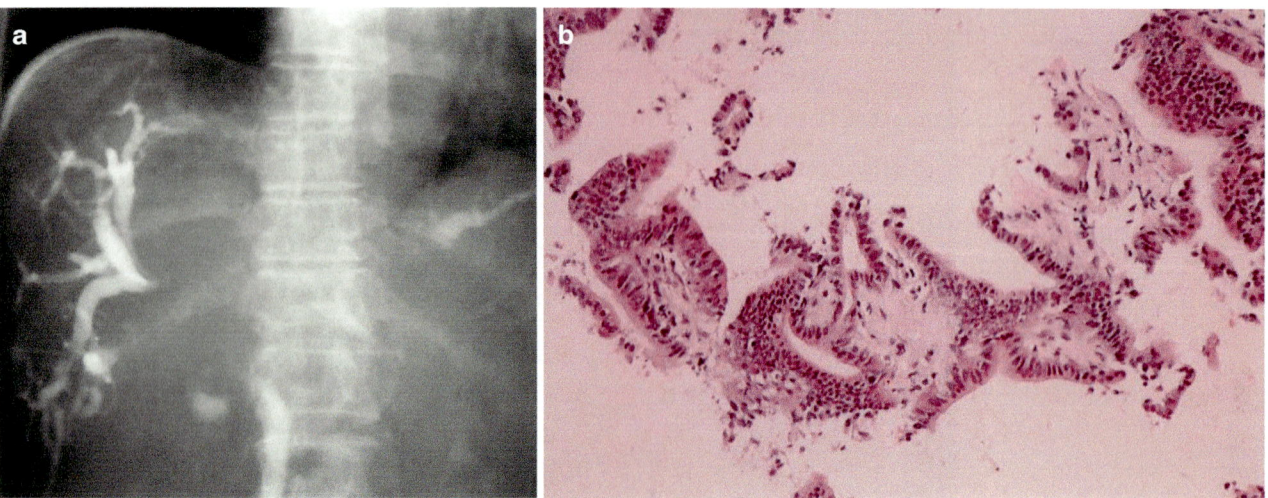

Fig. 17.23 Cholangiocellular carcinoma. Percutaneous transhepatic cholangiography (PTC) shows dilatation of the right and left intrahepatic bile ducts, and interruption of contrast medium is seen between the common and intrahepatic bile ducts (**a**). Needle biopsy of the tumor revealing neoplastic glands with focal loss of nuclear polarity and fibrous stroma (**b**)

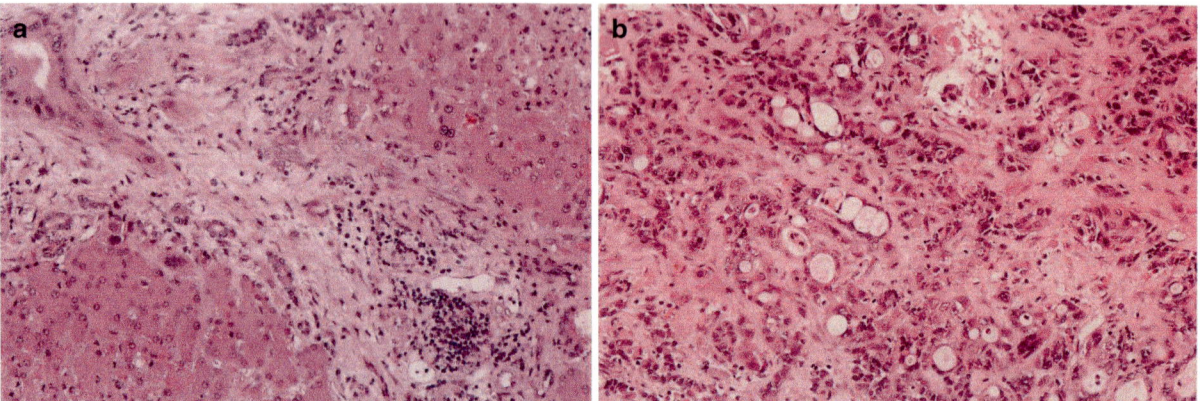

Fig. 17.24 Cholangiocellular carcinoma in the liver with infestation of *Clonorchis sinensis*. A neoplastic duct (upper left) is seen in the fibrous portal area with polymorphonuclear leukocyte infiltration, simulating a nonneoplastic interlobular bile duct (**a**). Poorly formed glands and cord-like structures are seen in the fibrous stroma (**b**)

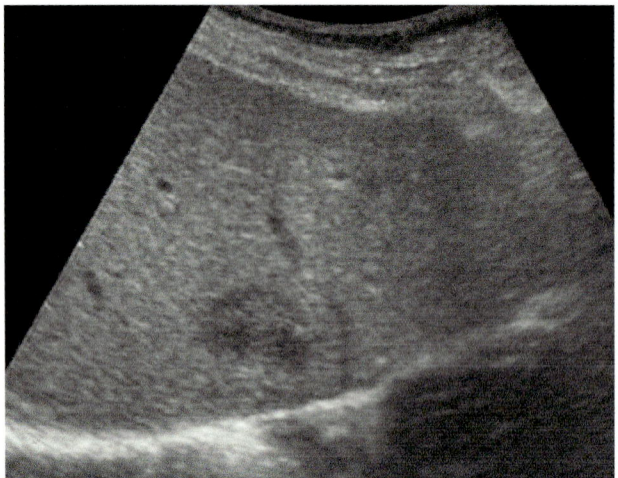

Fig. 17.25 Cholangiocellular carcinoma with the component of cholangiolocellular carcinoma; US images. The US showed a low-echoic nodule with heterogeneous isoechoic lesion inside

17.4 Mucinous Cystadenocarcinoma

Mucinous cystadenoma is regarded as a precursor or benign counterpart of mucinous cystadenocarcinoma [32]; the large majority occurs in middle-aged women and causes no symptoms or signs until the tumors are large. Metastasis is rare, and the tumor is considered as low-grade malignancy or carcinoma in situ when the neoplastic epithelium is contained within the cystic lesion. The operative results are good [34].

Case 17.8 (Mucinous Cystadenocarcinoma)

A 66-year-old male presented with an epigastric tumor, a high-echoic and papillary tumor with arterial flow (Fig. 17.30). CECT in the arterial phase revealed a low-density area with rim enhancement. In the delayed-phase image, the tumor is heterogeneous in density with prominent

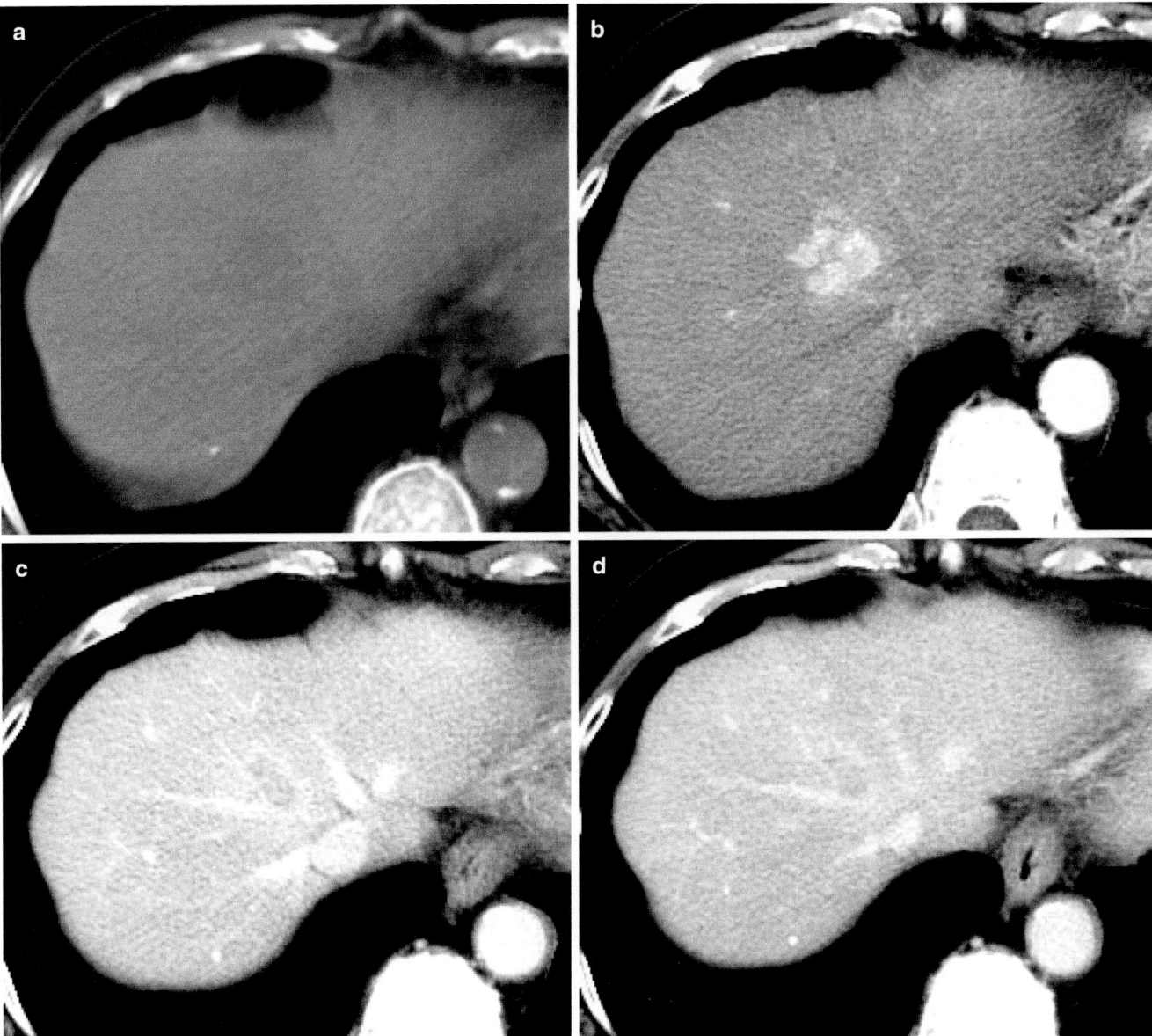

Fig. 17.26 Cholangiocellular carcinoma with the component of chol-angiolocellular carcinoma; CT images of the tumor. Plain CT image (**a**), arterial-phase image (**b**), portal-venous-phase image (**c**), and equilibrium-phase image (**d**) are shown. The nodule showed slightly low density in the pre-contrast, high density in the arterial, and partially low density in the central, accompanied with delayed enhancement in the peripheral region, in the portal-venous and equilibrium-phase image

rim enhancement pattern (Fig. 17.31). The T1-intensified image of MRI showed a mixture intensity in the tumor, and T2 image showed high intensity (Fig. 17.32). Angiography showed neovascularization and compression of the left hepatic artery. The resected tumor showed cystic structures surrounded by fibrous tissue and a cystic cavity lined by monolayer columnar epithelium. Much of the epithelium was desquamated. The remaining epithelium was basophilic and irregular in size, with displaced nuclei in the periphery. CA19-9 and carcinoembryonic antigen immunoreaction were seen in the cytoplasm, which contained mucinous material (Fig. 17.33).

Diagnosis of cystadenocarcinoma is made by both image analysis [35] and histological findings [32]. Resection leads to a high 5-year survival rate and good prognosis [36].

17.5 Hepatoblastoma

Hepatoblastoma is the most common liver tumor in childhood and is associated with congenital anomalies. The vast majority of cases are seen in children <5 years old, of which two-thirds are <2 years old. Boys are affected twice as frequently as girls. However, a few cases have been reported in middle-aged or

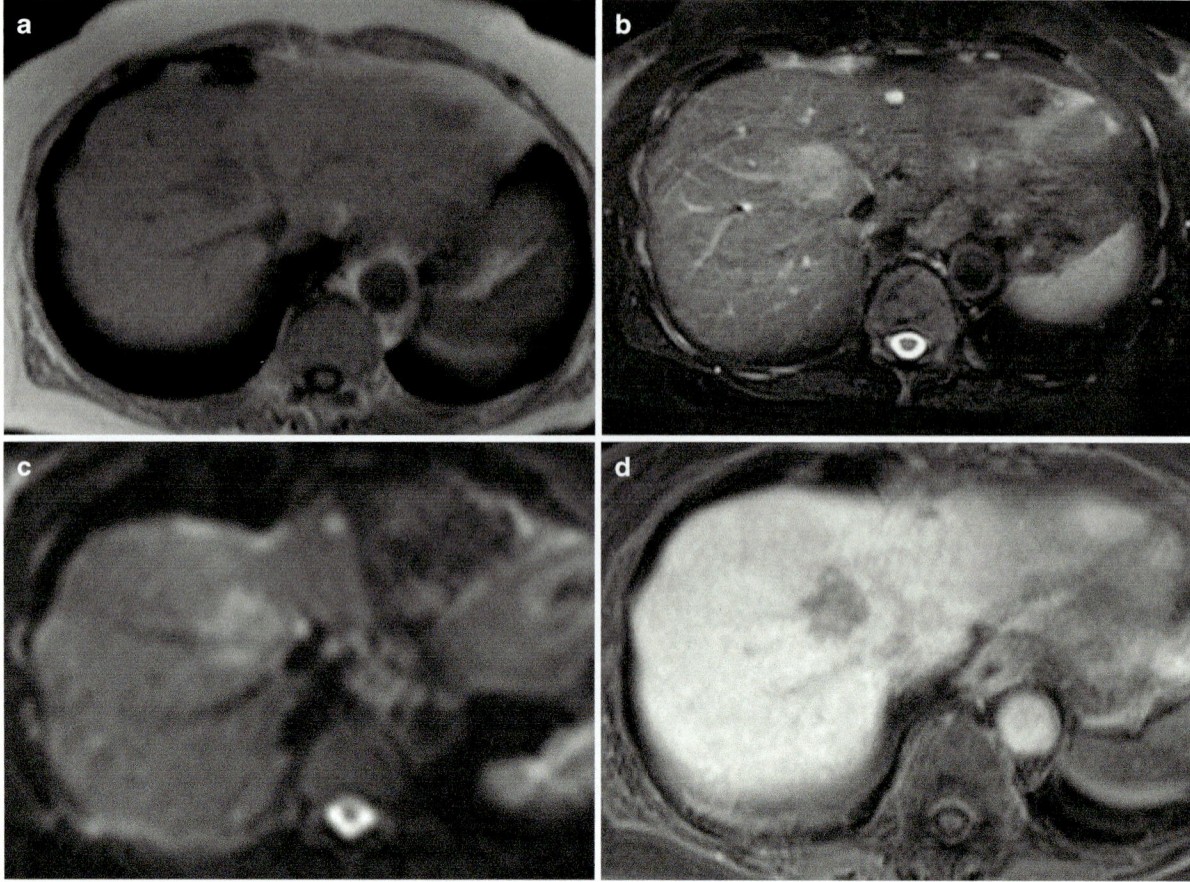

Fig. 17.27 Cholangiocellular carcinoma with the component of cholangiolocellular carcinoma; abdominal MRI images. The tumor revealed low intensity in the T1-weighted image (**a**) and high intensity in the T2-weighted and diffusion images (**b**, **c**). It was depicted as low-intensity nodule with irregular shape in the hepatobiliary phase of the Gd-EOB-DTPA-enhanced image (**d**)

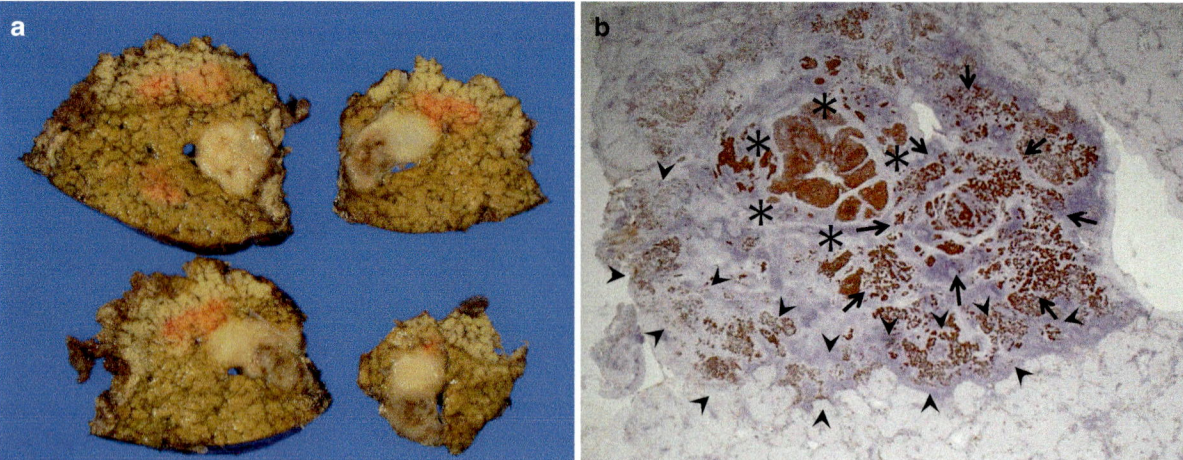

Fig. 17.28 Cholangiocellular carcinoma with the component of cholangiolocellular carcinoma; macroscopic view and loupe images. Macroscopic and loupe images of the tumor with CK7 immunostaining. Cross sections of the resected specimen (**a**). The tumor was whitish with an irregular boundary and without a capsule. Macroscopic view of the whole tumor with CK7 immunohistochemical staining (**b**). The tumor consisted of cholangiocellular carcinoma (CCC) components (arrow), cholangiolocellular carcinoma (CoCC) components (arrow head), and poorly differentiated CCC portion (asterisk)

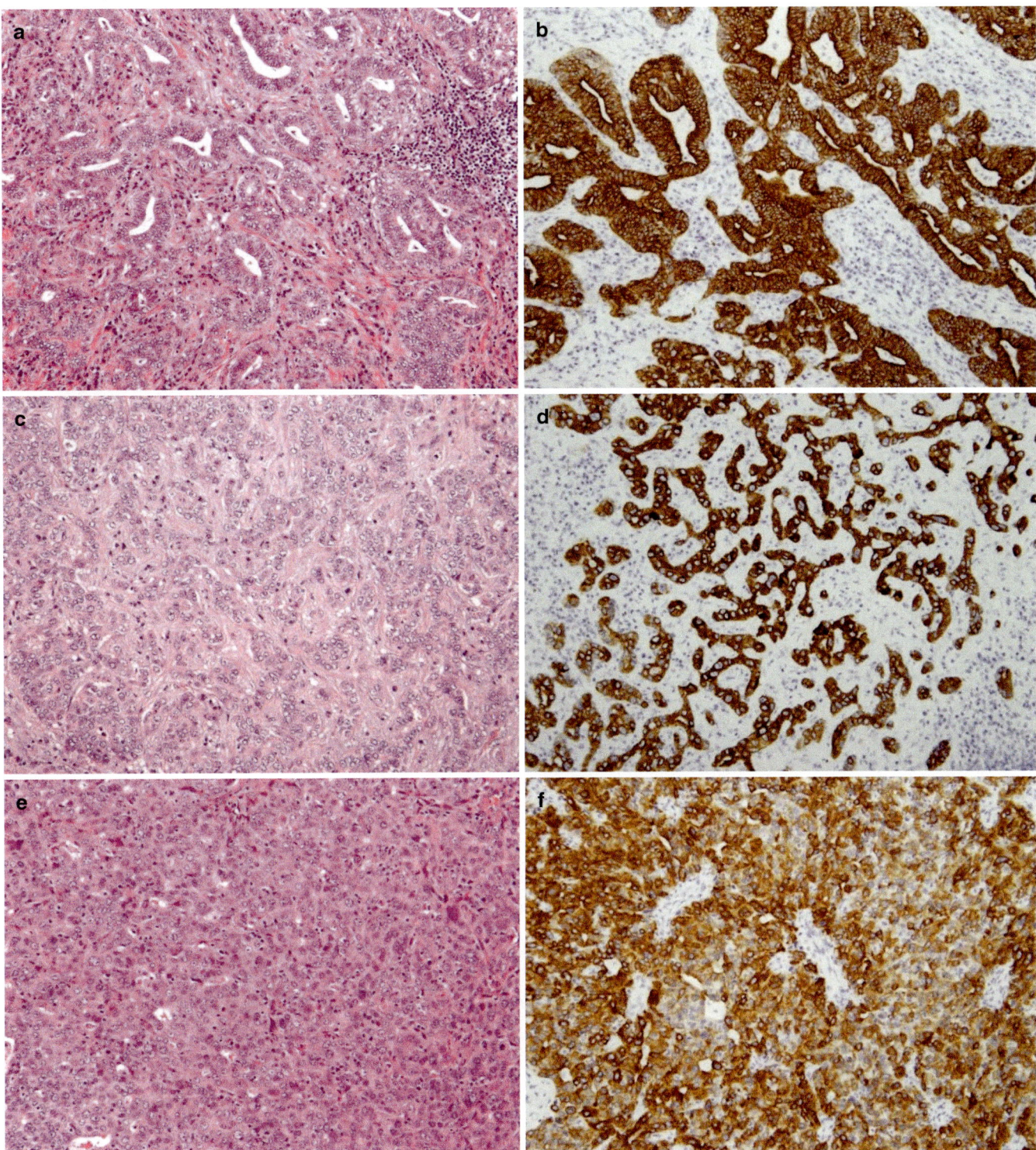

Fig. 17.29 Cholangiocellular carcinoma with the component of cholangiolocellular carcinoma; histologies and expression of CK7. Microscopic images of the tumor with HE and CK7 immunostaining. HE staining images of the CCC component (**a**), the CoCC component (**d**), and the poorly differentiated CCC component (**e**). Similarly, CK7 immunostainings of the CCC component (**b**), the CoCC component (**c**), and the poorly differentiated CCC component (**f**) are shown. In the CCC components of the tumor, cancer cells showed glandular duct-like structures, and lymphocytic infiltration was observed in fibrotic regions (**a**). Immunohistochemistry showed positivity for CK7 (**b**). In the CoCC component, smaller cancer cells resembling bile-ductular cells were observed, showing antler-like proliferation pattern (**c**). Immunohistochemistry also showed positivity for CK7 (**d**). In the poorly differentiated CCC component, pleomorphic cells showed severe cellular atypia with HCC-like compact proliferation with less fibrotic region (**e**). Immunohistochemical examination showed positive for CK7 (**f**)

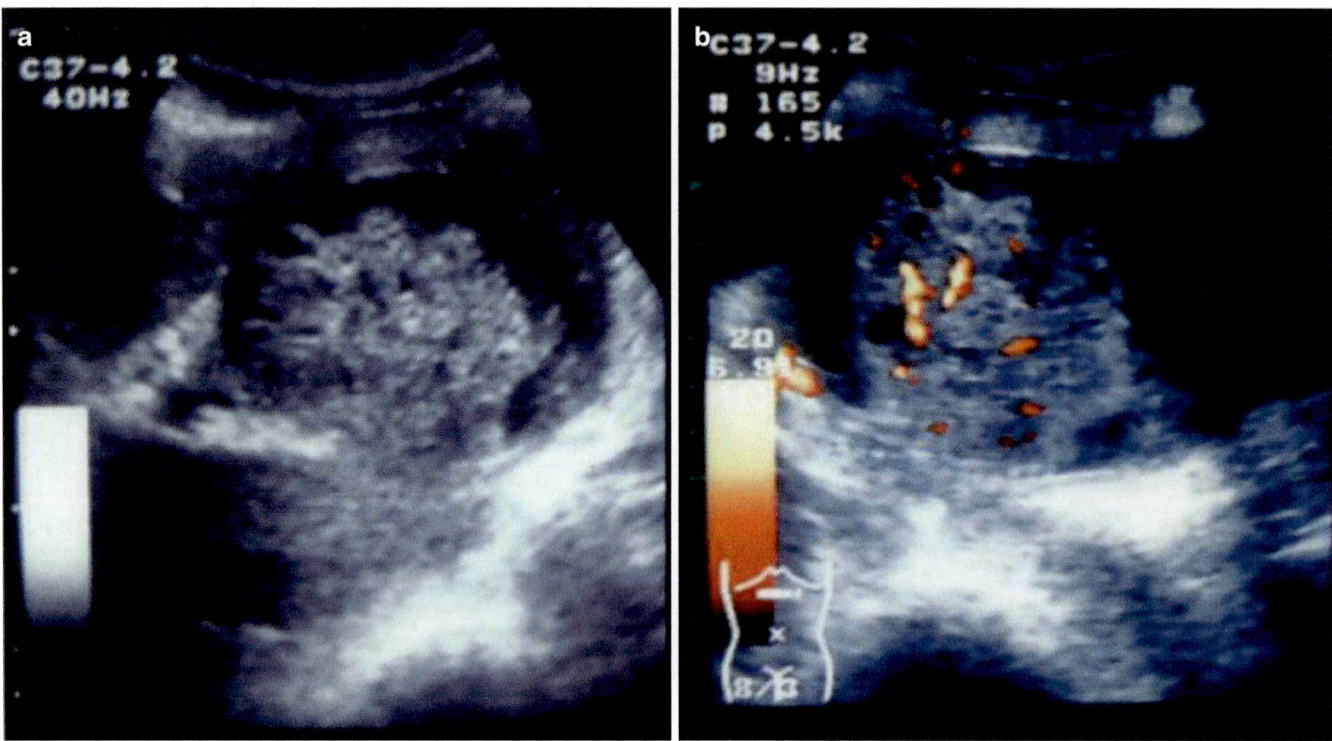

Fig. 17.30 Cystadenocarcinoma; US images. US shows a high-echoic tumor surrounded by a low-echoic area (**a**). Doppler US shows arterial flow in the tumor (**b**)

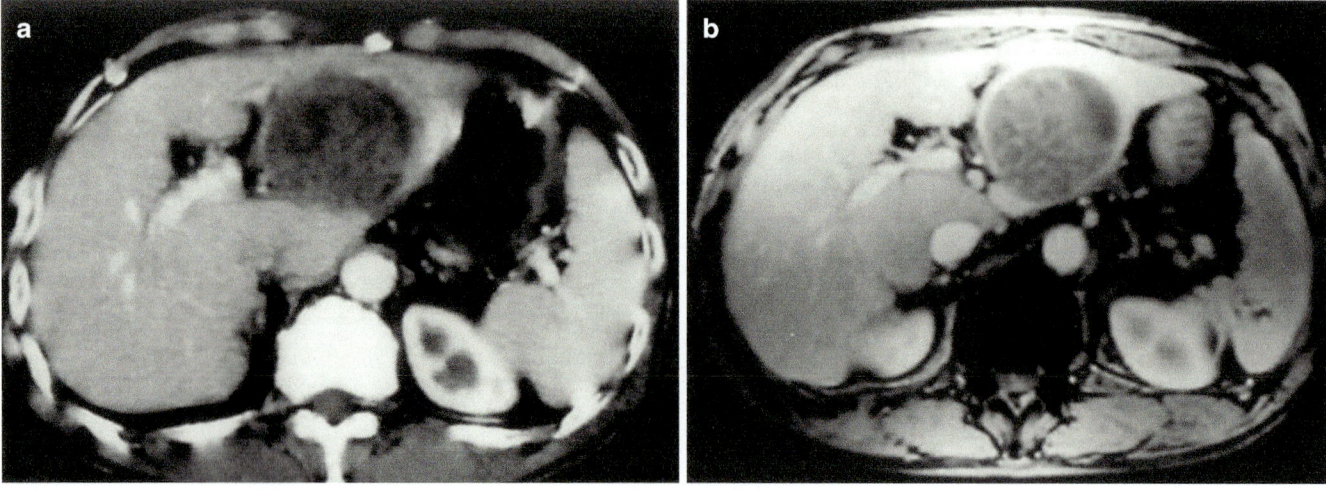

Fig. 17.31 Cystadenocarcinoma; CT images. CT in the early phase shows a low-density area in S4. There are arterial vessels in the tumor, and it is surrounded by arteries (**a**). CT in the late phase reveals low or heterogeneous density in the tumor, and there is a low-density area on edge (**b**)

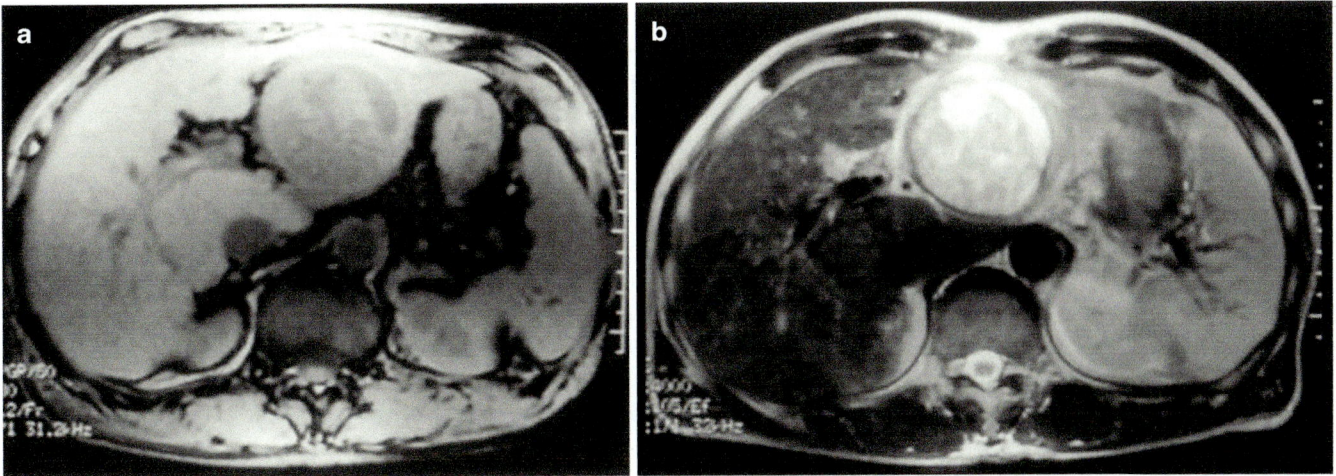

Fig. 17.32 Cystadenocarcinoma; MRI images. MRI with T1 intensification shows iso-intensity in the tumor with high intensity in its rim (**a**). MRI with T2 intensification shows high intensity in the tumor with low intensity in its rim (**b**)

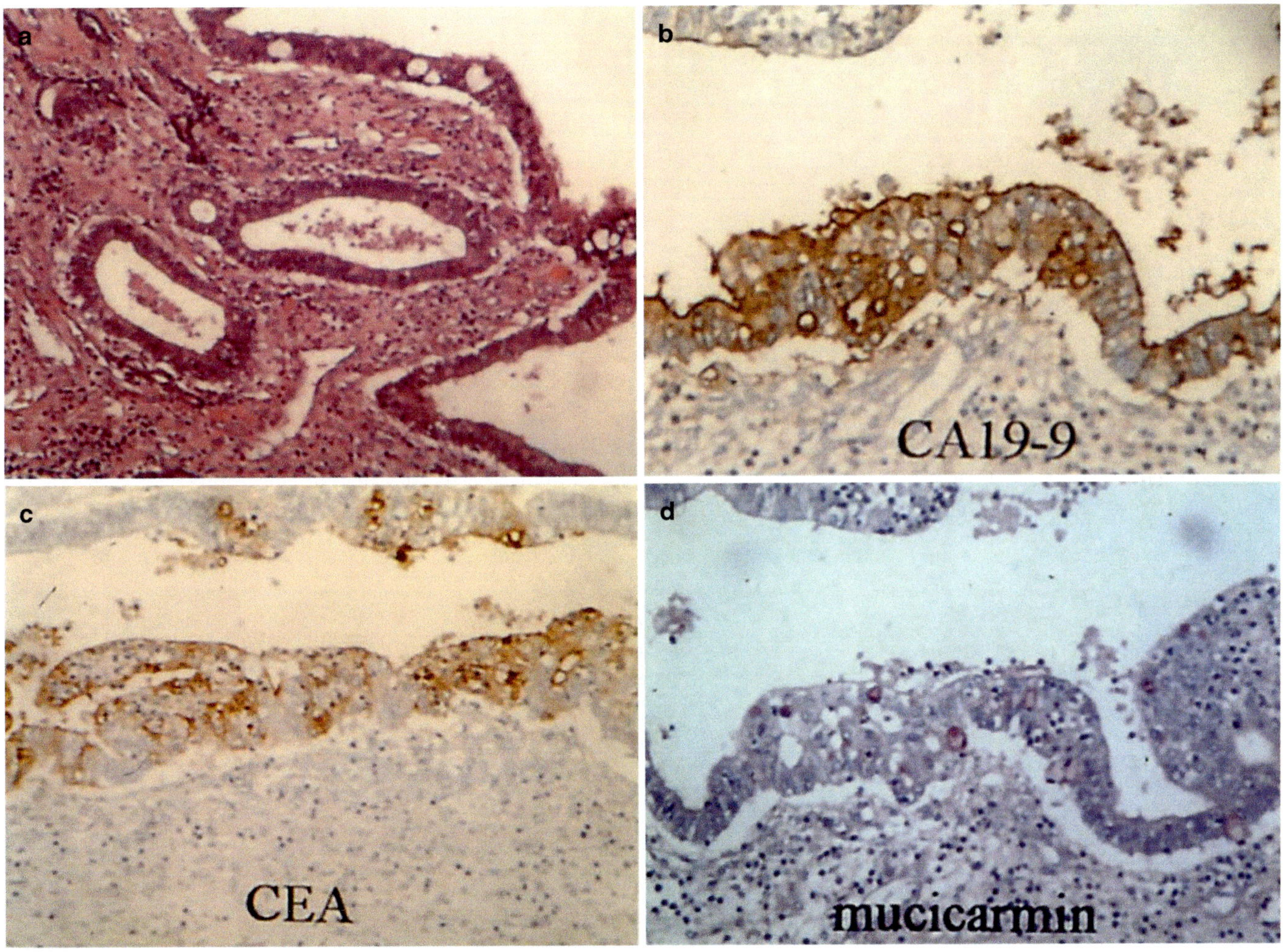

Fig. 17.33 Cystadenocarcinoma; microscopic views. Cystic areas lined by cuboidal to low columnar epithelium overlying cellular mesenchymal stroma (**a**). The tumor shows cytoplasmic and apical membranous staining for CA19-9 (**b**). Cystadenocarcinoma with membranous and cytoplasmic CEA staining. (**d**) Mucin in the epithelium of the cystadenocarcinoma is stained red with mucicarmine (**c**)

even in old-aged individuals [37]. The usual presentations are weight loss, large upper abdominal mass, and high serum AFP. Plain CT shows isodensity or low-density tumor with calcification on the periphery [38]. Histologically, there are three types of hepatoblastoma: epithelial, mixed epithelial-mesenchymal, and anaplastic [39]. Fetal hepatocytes contain more fat and glycogen than adult hepatocytes, and a pale appearance or light-and-dark pattern is seen in the fetal type of hepatoblastoma. Anaplastic type is characterized by high nuclear-cytoplasmic ratio, proliferative activity, poorly defined cellular margins, and squamous differentiation.

Case 17.9

A 5-month-old infant was admitted for an abdominal tumor. His serum AFP was as high as 61 × 10⁴ ng/mL, and CT showed a low-density area with calcification in S3 to S4 (Fig. 17.34). MRI revealed low intensity in S4 on T1-weighted image and high intensity on T2-weighted image (Fig. 17.35).

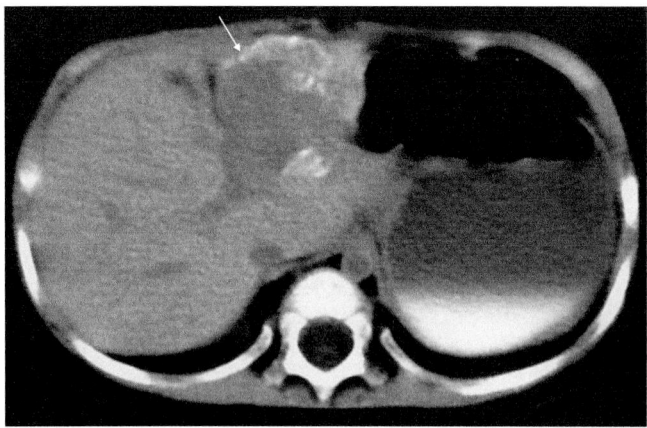

Fig. 17.34 Hepatoblastoma; CT images. A low-density tumor with calcification (arrow) is observed in S4 (medial segment) by CT

After diagnosis, the tumor was resected and showed cords of small hepatocytes (fetal epithelial type), tubular form in other areas (embryonal epithelial type), and focal keratinization (squamous differentiation) (Fig. 17.36).

Hepatomegaly and elevation of AFP in serum led to a working diagnosis of hepatoblastoma. Image analysis and liver biopsy confirm its diagnosis. Early detection may lead to curative resection. Preoperative chemotherapy reduces the size of the tumor. Surgical resection and liver transplantation need to be required [40].

17.6 Liver Sarcoma

Compared to carcinomas, sarcomas of the liver are very rare and should be differentiated from HCC.

17.7 Epithelioid Hemangioendothelioma

Endothelial tumor in the lung may present as primary liver tumor, and its prognosis varies widely. Some patients survive for decades, while others die within months. Its causes are unknown. A relationship to the use of oral contraceptive is postulated [41], and women are more often affected than men.

Case 17.10

A 44-year-old female with a history of oral contraceptive use presented with space-occupying lesions in the liver. CECT showed multiple tumors in the peripheral of S2, S4, S5, and S6 in the early phase (Fig. 17.37). Resected liver showed distribution of tumor cells and stroma in the periportal area, distribution of individual tumor cells in fibrous stroma, formation of vasculature from tumor cells, and

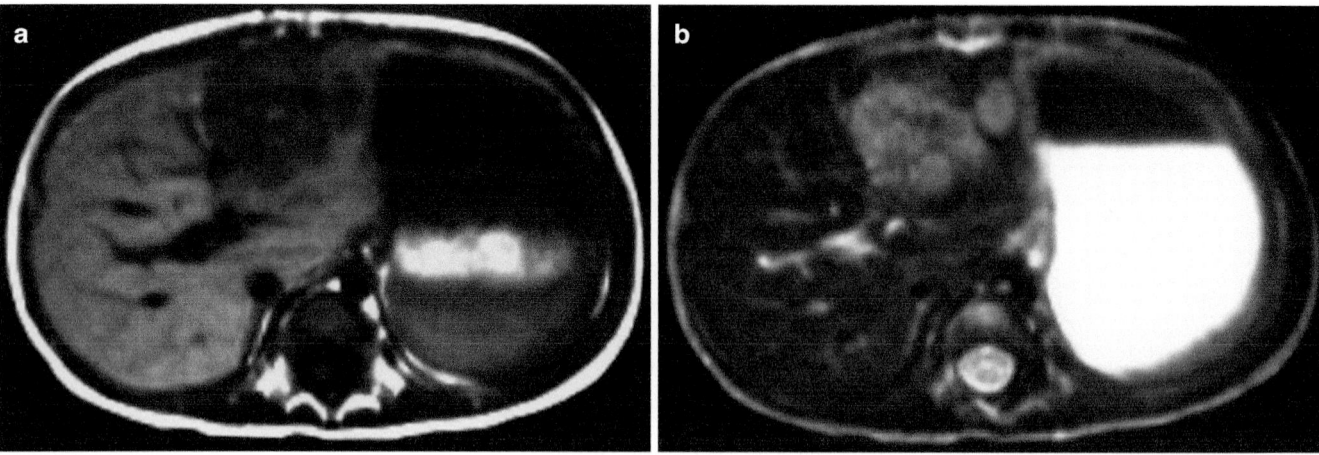

Fig. 17.35 Hepatoblastoma; MRI images. MRI shows low-intensity lesion with a calcified rim (**a**). MRI with T2 intensification reveals a high-intensity area in S4 (**b**)

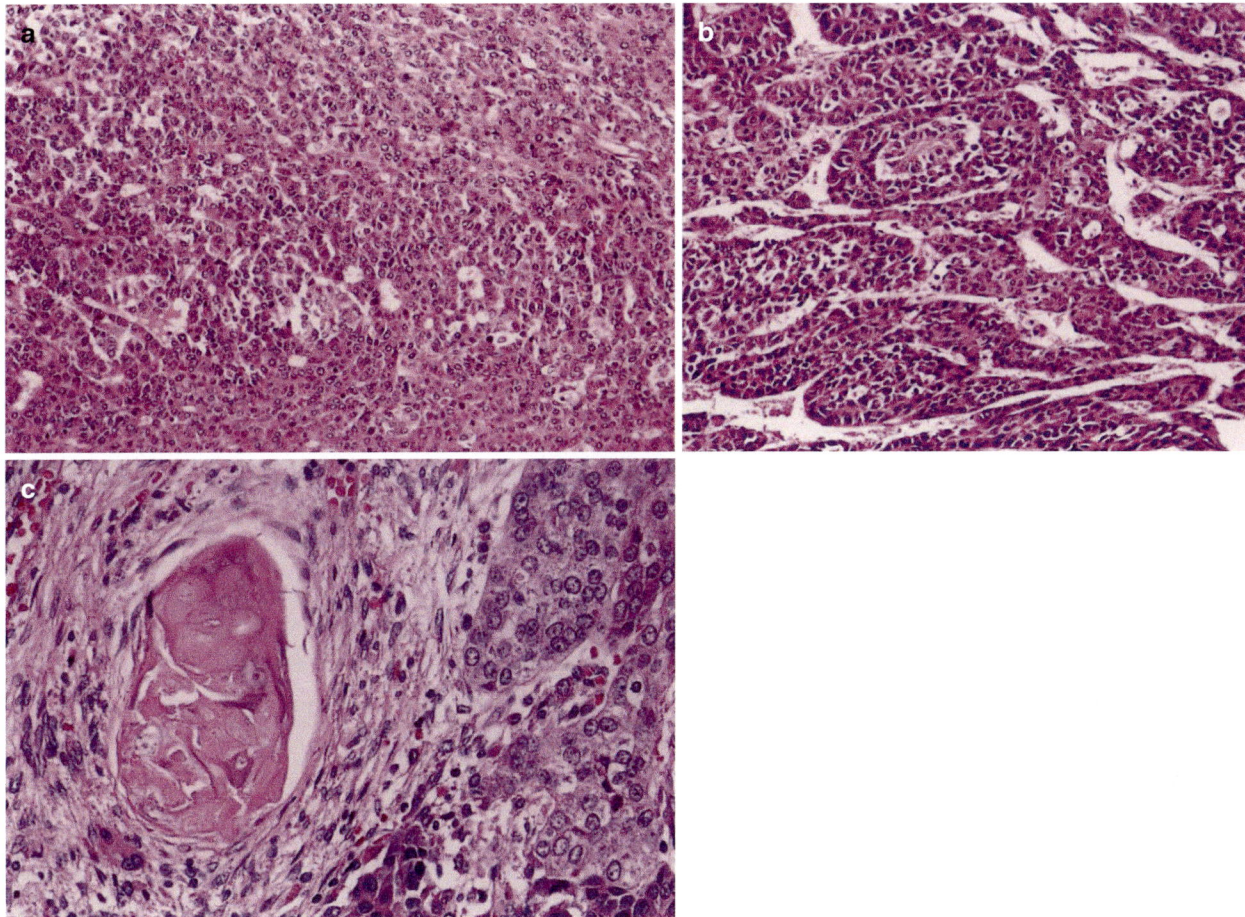

Fig. 17.36 Hepatoblastoma; histological view. (**a**) Hepatoblastoma, fetal epithelial type. The tumor is composed of sheets and thin trabeculae of small hepatocytes. (**b**) Hepatoblastoma, embryonal epithelial type. The tumor cells have a high nuclear-cytoplasmic ratio and are arranged in glandular pattern. (**c**) Hepatoblastoma. There is keratinization formation in hepatoblastoma

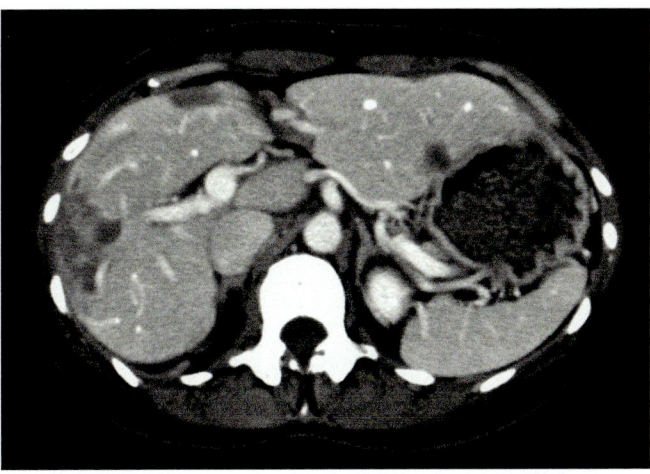

Fig. 17.37 Epithelioid hemangioendothelioma; CT images. CECT shows multiple low-density areas in the early phase, and these are localized mainly in the periphery of the liver. (Courtesy of Professor H Haga)

CD34 immunoreactivity in the tumor cells (Fig. 17.38). The tumor grows slowly but may metastasize [42]. Liver transplantation pertains to a favorable 5-year survival rate [43].

17.8 Angiosarcoma

Although it accounts for only 1–2% of primary hepatic malignancies, angiosarcoma is the most common sarcoma of the liver [44]. There are known predisposing factors, such as exposure to thorium (Thorotrast), vinyl chloride, and arsenic [44]. The incubation period is long from 15 to 25 years. Steroid hormones and urethane are also associated with the development of angiosarcoma [45, 46]. Symptoms and signs include pain, anemia, fever of unknown origin, weight loss, abdominal mass, and hemoperitoneum. The median survival is 6 months. Although imaging studies are helpful, they are inconclusive. Hence, liver biopsy is often required under peritoneoscopy.

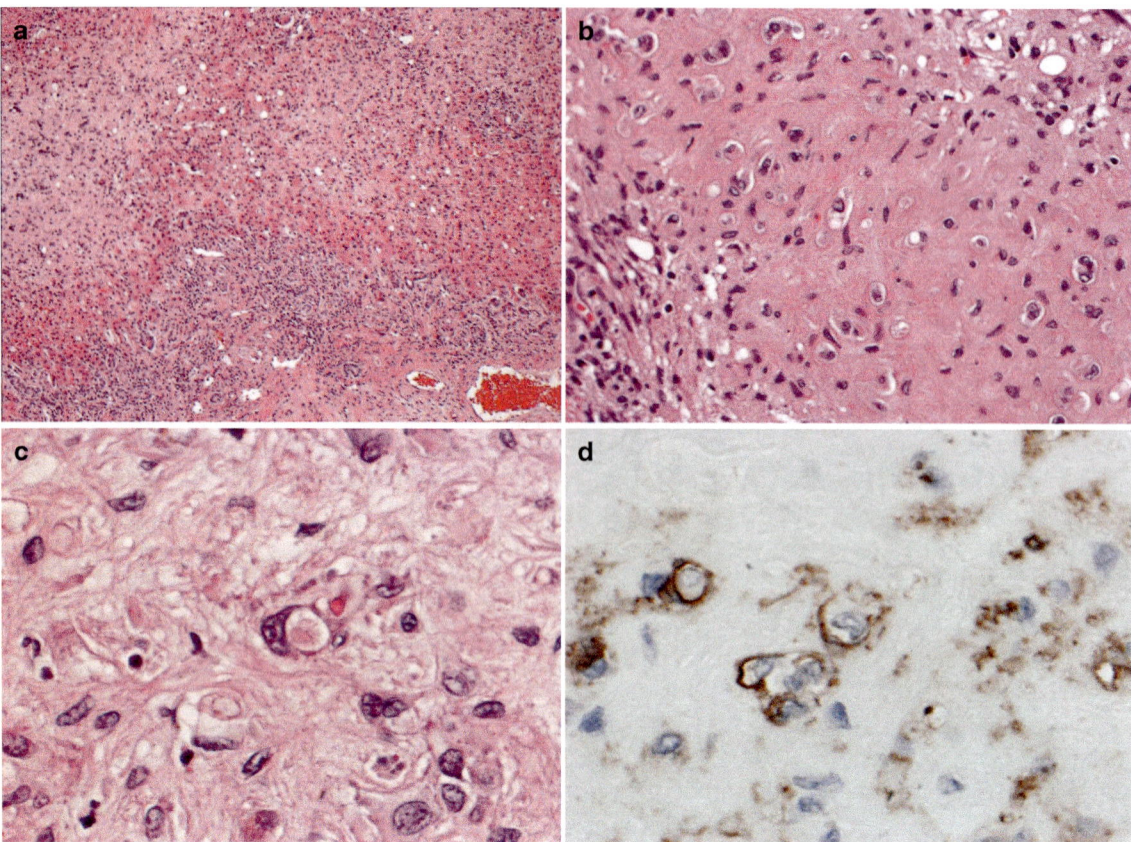

Fig. 17.38 Epithelioid hemangioendothelioma; microscopic views. Glandular structures of tumor cells are distributed in the periportal tract (**a**). Tumor cells are mixed with fibrosis (**b**). Tumor cells form a capil-lary structure (signet ringlike tumor cell) (**c**). CD34 immunoreactivity is seen in tumor cells (**d**). (Courtesy of Professor H Haga)

Case 17.11

A 47-year-old male presented with weight loss and a history of diabetes mellitus for 5 years. There were no predisposing factors, such as Thorotrast or vinyl chloride. His laboratory data showed T-BIL 1.9 mg/dL, AST 83 IU/L, ALT 111 IU/L, ALP 777 IU/L, LAP 1340 IU/L, GGT 3490 IU/L, FBS 191 mg/dL, AFP 2 ng/mL, $ICGR_{15}$ 56%, and PLT 9.6×10^4. US revealed many small tumors in the liver (Fig. 17.39). Plain CT presented heterogeneous tumor, and CECT did not reveal different densities (Fig. 17.40). Peritoneoscopy showed red nodules with prominence of the undersurface of the liver (Fig. 17.41). Angiography showed multiple staining with portal vein obstruction by a tumor thrombus (Fig. 17.42). He soon complained of epigastric pain and ascites and died of liver rupture.

Autopsy tissue revealed irregularly dilated sinusoids and congestion. The sinusoids were lined by atypical and multinucleated endothelial cells, which are in multiple layers, as well as compressed hepatocytes. Immunohistochemistry showed factor VIII in atypical endothelial cells (Fig. 17.43).

The tumor progresses quickly and grows multicentrically. Metastases occur in the lung, hilar lymph node, spleen, and bone. A sudden complication is rupture with hemoperitoneum; the course is progressive, and the prognosis is poor.

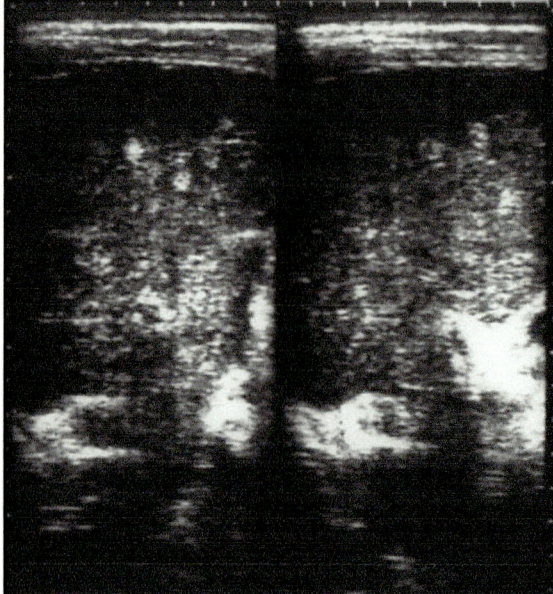

Fig. 17.39 Angiosarcoma; US images. US shows multiple high and small echogenic lesions in the liver. The figures of this case are courtesy of Dr. Maki Iwai, Kyoto Prefectural University of Medicine and (Reuse of Iwai M, et al. A case report of primary hepatic angiosarcoma. J Kyoto Pref Univ Med 1988; 97: 859–68, with permission of its chief editor)

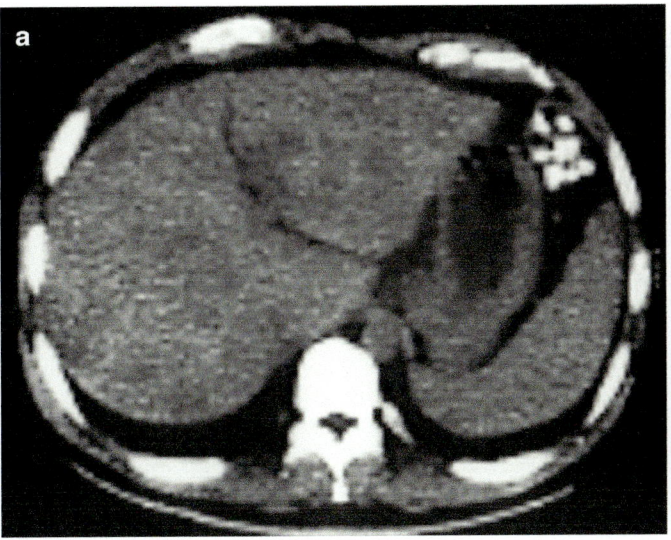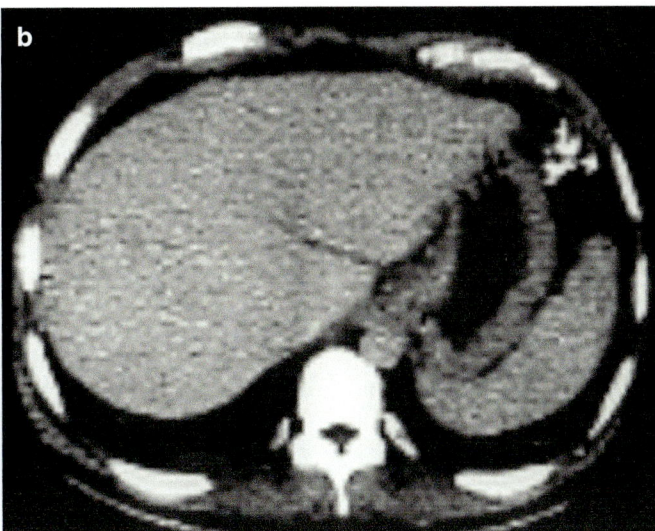

Fig. 17.40 Angiosarcoma; CT images. Plain CT shows heterogeneous density in the liver (**a**). CECT shows homogenous density in the liver (**b**). (Reuse of Iwai M, et al. A case report of primary hepatic angiosarcoma. J Kyoto Pref Univ Med 1988; 97: 859–68, with permission of its chief editor)

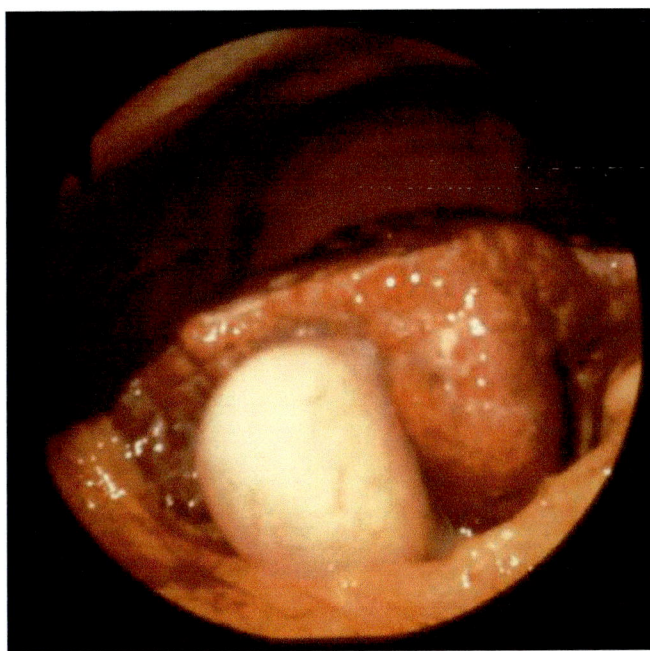

Fig. 17.41 Angiosarcoma; peritoneoscopy. Peritoneoscopy shows an irregular surface of the liver and protrusion of the undersurface in the inner area of the gallbladder. There is nodular formation on the surface, and the nodular surface is red in color and hypervascular. (Reuse of Iwai M, et al. A case report of primary hepatic angiosarcoma. J Kyoto Pref Univ Med 1988; 97: 859–68, with permission of its chief editor)

17.9 Primary Hepatic Neuroendocrine Tumor

A neuroendocrine neoplasm (NEN) derives from neuroendocrine cells which are present throughout the body in various organs such as the lungs and gastrointestinal tract. NEN is histologically classified based on morphology, Ki-67 index, and mitotic count. Neuroendocrine tumor (NET) G1 shows Ki-67 index ≤2%, NET G2 represents Ki-67 index = 3–20%, and neuroendocrine cancer (NEC) shows Ki-67 index >20%. NET is a slow-growing tumor; NEC is aggressive [47]. Primary hepatic neuroendocrine tumor is extremely rare.

Case 17.12

A 75-year-old female was pointed out approximately 20 mm hepatic tumor localized in S4 on CT. The results for blood routines, liver function, and tumor marker were within normal ranges. The tumor showed ring enhancement in the arterial phase (Fig. 17.44) and delayed enhancement on the central part of tumor. Similarly, CEUS also revealed ring enhancement accompanied by the delayed enhancement and defect in the post-vascular phase (Fig. 17.44). Resected liver tissues showed the distribution of tumor cells accompanied by fibrovascular stroma and pseudo-ductal structures (Fig. 17.45). The central part of the tumor was associated with hemorrhagic necrosis and edematous degeneration. Immunohistochemistry findings included chromogranin A (+), synaptophysin (+), CD56 (+), CDX2 (+), mucicarmine (−), CEA (−), cytokeratin7 (−), cytokeratin20 (−), and estrogen receptor (−) (Fig. 17.45). Ki-67 (MIB-1) index was less than 2%. Because no primary organ was found in postoperative examination, the tumor was considered as a primary neuroendocrine tumor of the liver (G1).

Acknowledgment We are grateful to Prof. Alex Y. Chang for constructive advice for first edition of this chapter.

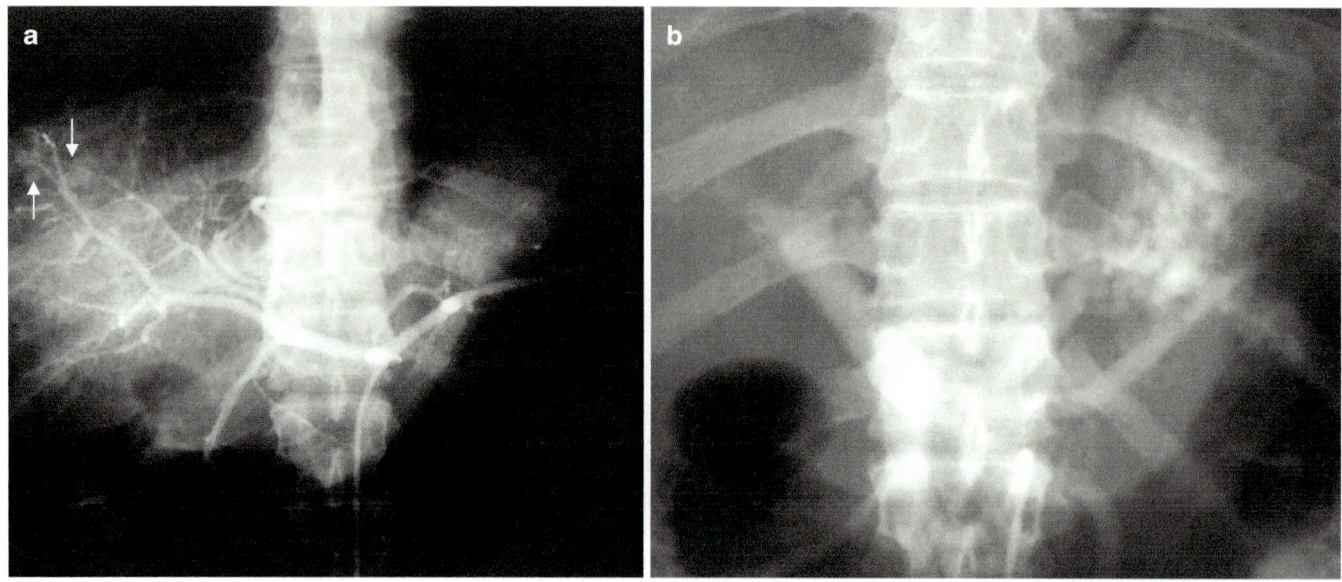

Fig. 17.42 Angiosarcoma; angiography. Angiography shows multiple small tumor staining (arrow) in the right lobe (**a**). Portography reveals tumor thrombus in portal trunk (**b**). (Reuse of Iwai M, et al. A case report of primary hepatic angiosarcoma. J Kyoto Pref Univ Med 1988; 97: 859–68, with permission of its chief editor)

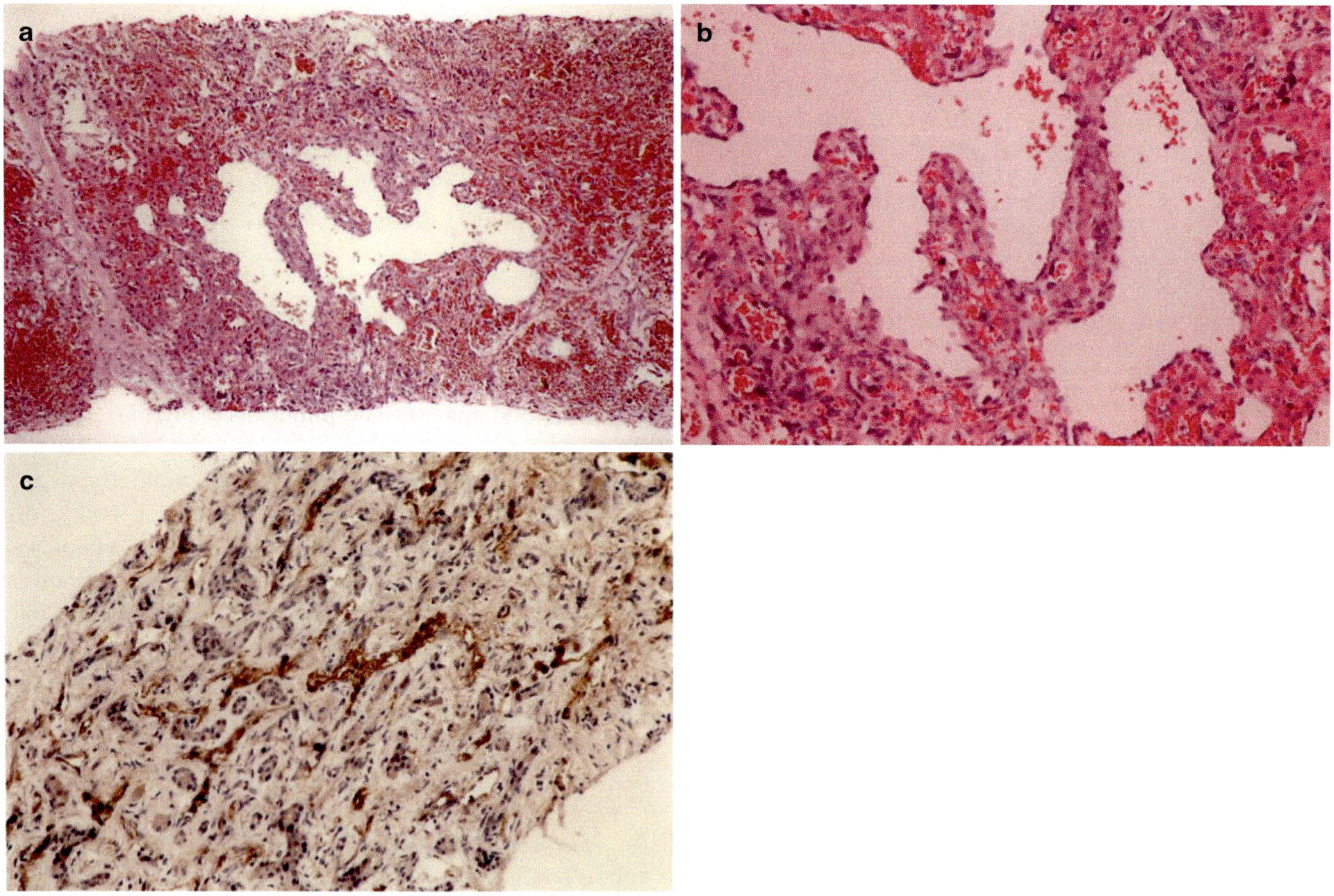

Fig. 17.43 Angiosarcoma; microscopic views. Irregularly dilated sinusoids and congestion are seen (**a**). The tumor shows cavernous sinusoids lined with pleomorphic and hyperchromatic endothelial cells. Hepatocytes are not seen (**b**). Immunostaining reveals that the tumor cells are focally positive for factor VIII (**c**). (Reuse of Iwai M, et al. A case report of primary hepatic angiosarcoma. J Kyoto Pref Univ Med 1988; 97: 859–68, with permission of its chief editor)

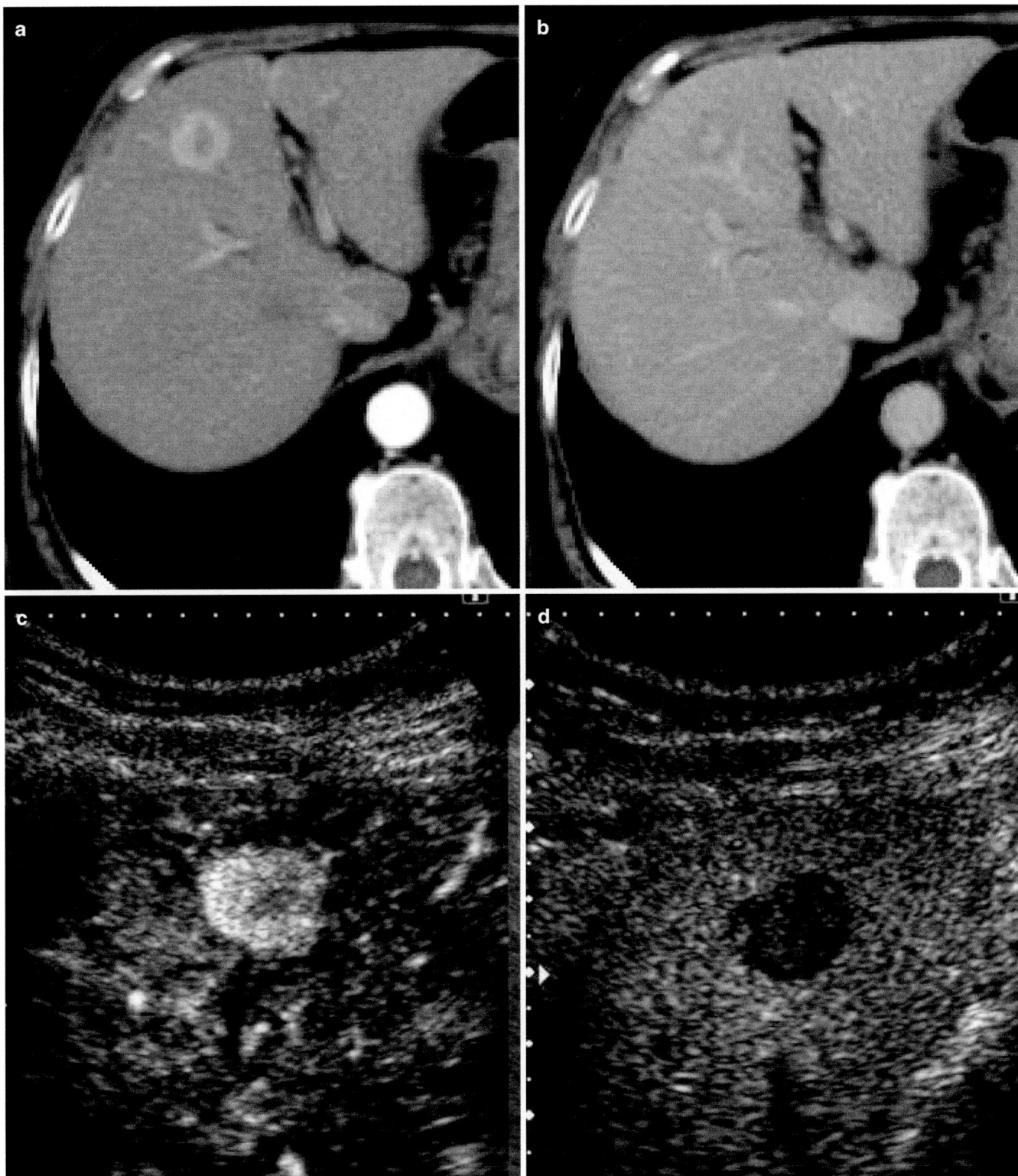

Fig. 17.44 Primary hepatic neuroendocrine tumor. CECT showed ring enhancement in the arterial phase (**a**) and delayed enhancement on the central part of tumor in the equilibrium phase (**b**). CEUS showed ring enhancement with delayed enhancement on the central part in the vascular phase (**c**) and complete defect in the post-vascular phase (**d**)

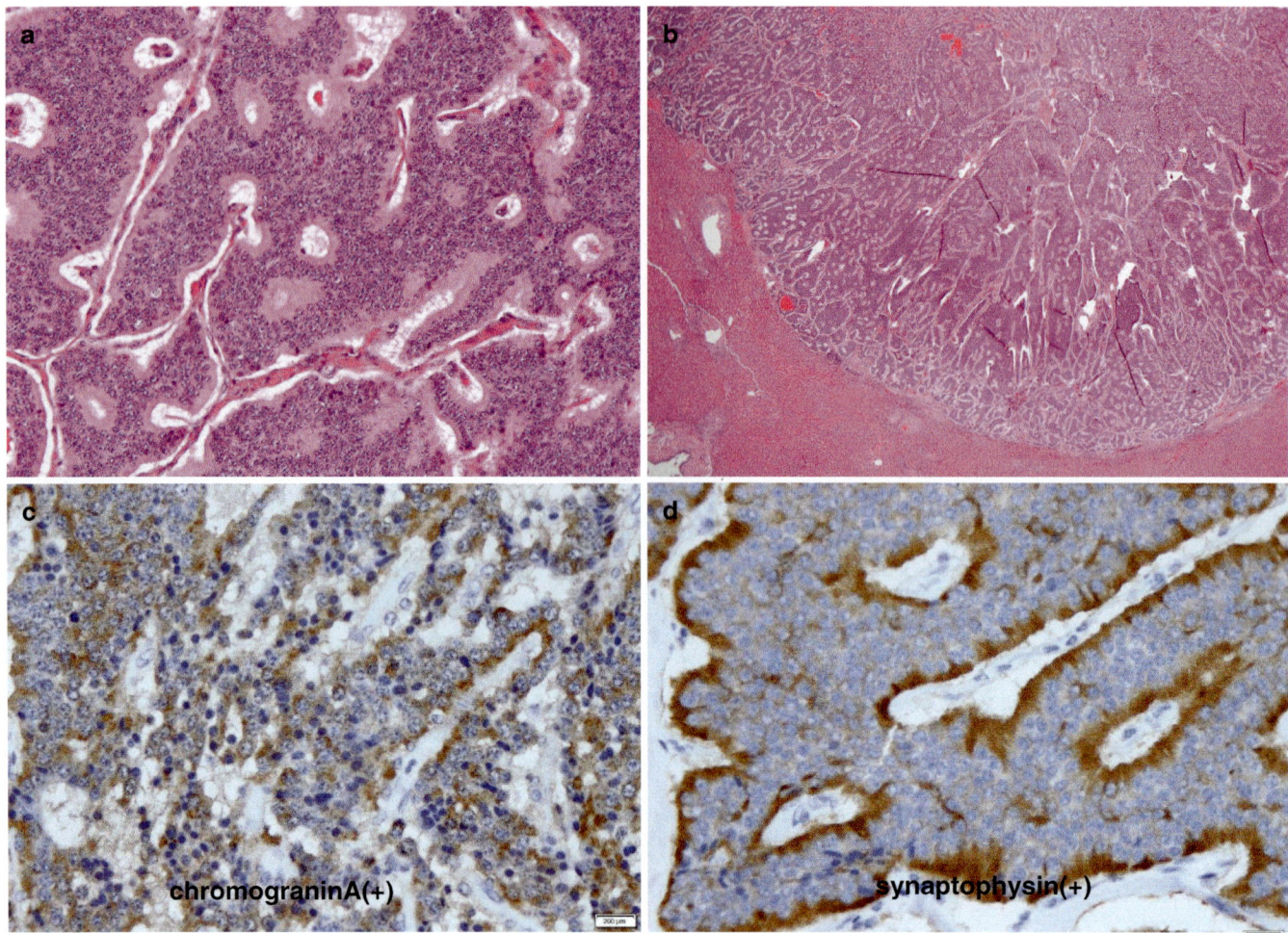

Fig. 17.45 Primary hepatic neuroendocrine tumor; microscopic views. Pathological findings showed the distribution of tumor cells accompanied by fibrovascular stroma and pseudo-ductal structures (**a**) and hem- orrhagic necrosis and edematous degeneration in the central part of the tumor (**b**). Immunostaining findings of chromogranin A (**c**) and synaptophysin (**d**) are shown

References

1. Lai CL, Yuen MF. Prevention of hepatitis B virus-related hepatocellular carcinoma with antiviral therapy. Hepatology. 2013;57:399–408.
2. Morgan RL, Baack B, Smith BD, Yartel A, Pitasi M, Falck-Ytter Y. Eradication of hepatitis C virus infection and the development of hepatocellular carcinoma: a meta-analysis of observational studies. Ann Intern Med. 2013;158:329–37.
3. Idilman R, De Maria N, Colantoni A, Van Thiel DH. Pathogenesis of hepatitis B and C-induced hepatocellular carcinoma. J Viral Hepat. 1998;5:285–99.
4. Wogan GN. Aflatoxins as risk factors for hepatocellular carcinoma in humans. Cancer Res. 1992;52:2114s–8s.
5. International Consensus Group for Hepatocellular Neoplasia. Pathologic diagnosis of early hepatocellular carcinoma: a report of the international consensus group for hepatocellular neoplasia. Hepatology. 2009;49:658–64.
6. Peng SY, Lai PL, Chu JS, Lee PH, Tsung PT, Chen DS, Hsu HC. Expression and hypomethylation of alpha-fetoprotein gene in unicentric and multicentric human hepatocellular carcinomas. Hepatology. 1993;17:35–41.
7. Aoyagi Y, Saitoh A, Suzuki Y, Igarashi K, Oguro M, Yokota T, Mori S, et al. Fucosylation index of alpha-fetoprotein, a possible aid in the early recognition of hepatocellular carcinoma in patients with cirrhosis. Hepatology. 1993;17:50–2.
8. Okuda H, Nakanishi T, Takatsu K, Saito A, Hayashi N, Takasaki K, Takenami K, et al. Serum levels of des-gamma-carboxy prothrombin measured using the revised enzyme immunoassay kit with increased sensitivity in relation to clinicopathologic features of solitary hepatocellular carcinoma. Cancer. 2000;88:544–9.
9. Bottelli R, Tibballs J, Hochhauser D, Watkinson A, Dick R, Burroughs AK. Ultrasound screening for hepatocellular carcinoma (HCC) in cirrhosis: the evidence for an established clinical practice. Clin Radiol. 1998;53:713–6.
10. Kim CK, Lim JH, Lee WJ. Detection of hepatocellular carcinomas and dysplastic nodules in cirrhotic liver: accuracy of ultrasonography in transplant patients. J Ultrasound Med. 2001;20: 99–104.
11. Kudo M. The 2008 Okuda lecture: management of hepatocellular carcinoma: from surveillance to molecular targeted therapy. J Gastroenterol Hepatol. 2010;25:439–52.
12. Kuszyk BS, Bluemke DA, Urban BA, Choti MA, Hruban RH, Sitzmann JV, Fishman EK. Portal-phase contrast-enhanced helical

CT for the detection of malignant hepatic tumors: sensitivity based on comparison with intraoperative and pathologic findings. AJR Am J Roentgenol. 1996;166:91–5.

13. Ward J, Guthrie JA, Scott DJ, Atchley J, Wilson D, Davies MH, Wyatt JI, et al. Hepatocellular carcinoma in the cirrhotic liver: double-contrast MR imaging for diagnosis. Radiology. 2000;216:154–62.

14. Forner A, Llovet JM, Bruix J. Hepatocellular carcinoma. Lancet. 2012;379:1245–55.

15. Vilgrain V, Van Beers BE, Pastor CM. Insights into the diagnosis of hepatocellular carcinomas with hepatobiliary MRI. J Hepatol. 2016;64:708–16.

16. Bruix J, Reig M, Sherman M. Evidence-based diagnosis, staging, and treatment of patients with hepatocellular carcinoma. Gastroenterology. 2016;150:835–53.

17. Llovet JM, Ricci S, Mazzaferro V, Hilgard P, Gane E, Blanc JF, de Oliveira AC, et al. Sorafenib in advanced hepatocellular carcinoma. N Engl J Med. 2008;359:378–90.

18. Bruix J, Qin S, Merle P, Granito A, Huang YH, Bodoky G, Pracht M, et al. Regorafenib for patients with hepatocellular carcinoma who progressed on sorafenib treatment (RESORCE): a randomised, double-blind, placebo-controlled, phase 3 trial. Lancet. 2017;389:56–66.

19. Kudo M, Finn RS, Qin S, Han KH, Ikeda K, Piscaglia F, Baron A, et al. Lenvatinib versus sorafenib in first-line treatment of patients with unresectable hepatocellular carcinoma: a randomised phase 3 non-inferiority trial. Lancet. 2018;391:1163–73.

20. Ishii H, Okada S, Okusaka T, Yoshimori M, Nakasuka H, Shimada K, Yamasaki S, et al. Needle tract implantation of hepatocellular carcinoma after percutaneous ethanol injection. Cancer. 1998;82:1638–42.

21. Kudo M. A new era of systemic therapy for hepatocellular carcinoma with regorafenib and lenvatinib. Liver Cancer. 2017;6:177–84.

22. Razumilava N, Gores GJ. Cholangiocarcinoma. Lancet. 2014;383:2168–79.

23. Shiota K, Taguchi J, Nakashima O, Nakashima M, Kojiro M. Clinicopathologic study on cholangiolocellular carcinoma. Oncol Rep. 2001;8:263–8.

24. Theise ND, Yao JL, Harada K, Hytiroglou P, Portmann B, Thung SN, Tsui W, et al. Hepatic 'stem cell' malignancies in adults: four cases. Histopathology. 2003;43:263–71.

25. Brunt E, Aishima S, Clavien PA, Fowler K, Goodman Z, Gores G, Gouw A, et al. cHCC-CCA: consensus terminology for primary liver carcinomas with both hepatocytic and cholangiocytic differentiation. Hepatology. 2018;68(1):113–26.

26. Okuda K, Nakanuma Y, Miyazaki M. Cholangiocarcinoma: recent progress. Part 1: epidemiology and etiology. J Gastroenterol Hepatol. 2002;17:1049–55.

27. Koga A, Ichimiya H, Yamaguchi K, Miyazaki K, Nakayama F. Hepatolithiasis associated with cholangiocarcinoma. Possible etiologic significance. Cancer. 1985;55:2826–9.

28. Bloustein PA. Association of carcinoma with congenital cystic conditions of the liver and bile ducts. Am J Gastroenterol. 1977;67:40–6.

29. Shaib Y, El-Serag HB. The epidemiology of cholangiocarcinoma. Semin Liver Dis. 2004;24:115–25.

30. Jusakul A, Cutcutache I, Yong CH, Lim JQ, Huang MN, Padmanabhan N, Nellore V, et al. Whole-genome and epigenomic landscapes of etiologically distinct subtypes of cholangiocarcinoma. Cancer Discov. 2017;7:1116–35.

31. Nakamura H, Arai Y, Totoki Y, Shirota T, Elzawahry A, Kato M, Hama N, et al. Genomic spectra of biliary tract cancer. Nat Genet. 2015;47:1003–10.

32. Nakanuma Y, Miyata T, Uchida T. Latest advances in the pathological understanding of cholangiocarcinomas. Expert Rev Gastroenterol Hepatol. 2016;10:113–27.

33. Bridgewater J, Galle PR, Khan SA, Llovet JM, Park JW, Patel T, Pawlik TM, et al. Guidelines for the diagnosis and management of intrahepatic cholangiocarcinoma. J Hepatol. 2014;60:1268–89.

34. Akwari OE, Tucker A, Seigler HF, Itani KM. Hepatobiliary cystadenoma with mesenchymal stroma. Ann Surg. 1990;211:18–27.

35. Vachha B, Sun MR, Siewert B, Eisenberg RL. Cystic lesions of the liver. AJR Am J Roentgenol. 2011;196:W355–66.

36. Shrikhande S, Kleeff J, Adyanthaya K, Zimmermann A, Shrikhande V. Management of hepatobiliary cystadenocarcinoma. Dig Surg. 2003;20:60–3.

37. Bortolasi L, Marchiori L, Dal Dosso I, Colombari R, Nicoli N. Hepatoblastoma in adult age: a report of two cases. Hepatogastroenterology. 1996;43:1073–8.

38. King SJ, Babyn PS, Greenberg ML, Phillips MJ, Filler RM. Value of CT in determining the resectability of hepatoblastoma before and after chemotherapy. AJR Am J Roentgenol. 1993;160:793–8.

39. Gonzalez-Crussi F, Upton MP, Maurer HS. Hepatoblastoma. Attempt at characterization of histologic subtypes. Am J Surg Pathol. 1982;6:599–612.

40. Kremer N, Walther AE, Tiao GM. Management of hepatoblastoma: an update. Curr Opin Pediatr. 2014;26:362–9.

41. Malamut G, Perlemuter G, Buffet C, Bedossa P, Joly JP, Colombat M, Kuoch V, et al. [Epithelioid hemangioendothelioma associated with nodular regenerative hyperplasia]. Gastroenterol Clin Biol. 2001;25:1105–7.

42. Demetris AJ, Minervini M, Raikow RB, Lee RG. Hepatic epithelioid hemangioendothelioma: biological questions based on pattern of recurrence in an allograft and tumor immunophenotype. Am J Surg Pathol. 1997;21:263–70.

43. Kayler LK, Merion RM, Arenas JD, Magee JC, Campbell DA, Rudich SM, Punch JD. Epithelioid hemangioendothelioma of the liver disseminated to the peritoneum treated with liver transplantation and interferon alpha-2B. Transplantation. 2002;74:128–30.

44. Chaudhary P, Bhadana U, Singh RA, Ahuja A. Primary hepatic angiosarcoma. Eur J Surg Oncol. 2015;41:1137–43.

45. Falk H, Thomas LB, Popper H, Ishak KG. Hepatic angiosarcoma associated with androgenic-anabolic steroids. Lancet. 1979;2:1120–3.

46. Cadranel JF, Legendre C, Desaint B, Delamarre N, Florent C, Levy VG. Liver disease from surreptitious administration of urethane. J Clin Gastroenterol. 1993;17:52–6.

47. Rindi G, Petrone G, Inzani F. The 2010 WHO classification of digestive neuroendocrine neoplasms: a critical appraisal four years after its introduction. Endocr Pathol. 2014;25:186–92.

Metastatic Liver Tumors

18

Louis J. Vaickus, Arief A. Suriawinata, and Masaki Iwai

Contents

Abbreviations

AFP	Alpha-fetoprotein
ALT	Alanine aminotransferase
AST	Aspartate aminotransferase
CK	Cytokeratin
CT	Computed tomography
GGT	Gamma-glutamyl transferase
LDH	Lactate dehydrogenase
TBIL	Total bilirubin

18.1 Introduction

Metastatic tumors are the most common type of malignancy in the liver, far exceeding primary tumors of the liver. The distinction between a primary tumor and a metastatic tumor in the liver has both therapeutic and prognostic significance. Knowledge of the primary tumor site and its morphology, if

L. J. Vaickus, MD, PhD · A. A. Suriawinata, MD (✉)
New Hampshire, USA
e-mail: Arief.A.Suriawinata@hitchcock.org

M. Iwai, MD, PhD
Gastroenterology, Hepatology and Internal Medicine,
Iwai Clinic, Kyoto, Japan

available, is important in evaluating and comparing it to its metastasis. Among tumor types, adenocarcinoma, neuroendocrine tumor, and lymphoma are the most common. Common primary sites include the colon (adenocarcinoma), pancreas (adenocarcinoma and pancreatic neuroendocrine tumor), stomach and small intestine (adenocarcinoma, neuroendocrine and gastrointestinal stromal tumor), lung (adenocarcinoma, small-cell and large-cell neuroendocrine carcinoma, and squamous cell carcinoma), breast, skin (melanoma), and kidney (renal cell carcinoma).

18.2 Clinical and Pathological Features

Besides the evaluation of morphologic features of the tumor, immunohistochemical stains or additional studies—such as flow cytometry or molecular studies—are often necessary in the diagnosis and treatment of metastatic tumors. For example, colonic adenocarcinomas, the most common type of metastasis of the liver, often demonstrate fairly well-formed glands with tall columnar cells and "dirty" necrotic debris in the glandular lumen. Further immunohistochemical stains, such as cytokeratin profile (CK7 negative and CK20 positive) or marker for enteric differentiation (CDX-2), are used to confirm or exclude other sites of origin with similar morphology. Molecular studies are often performed for identification of specific mutations and predicting response to antigrowth factor therapies. For the diagnosis of lymphoma,

© Springer Nature Singapore Pte Ltd. 2019
E. Hashimoto et al. (eds.), *Diagnosis of Liver Disease*, https://doi.org/10.1007/978-981-13-6806-6_18

flow cytometry can be performed in addition to immunohistochemical stains. Table 18.1 provides a list of immunohistochemical stains for various metastatic tumors.

Image analysis of metastatic tumors to the liver almost always shows hypovascularity, except for liver metastasis from carcinoids/neuroendocrine tumors which are hypervascular [1]. Diffuse metastatic lesions may not be detected by ultrasonography, computed tomography, or magnetic resonance imaging [2]. Therefore, laparoscopy with liver biopsy or, more commonly, radiology-guided fine needle aspiration (FNA) may be required for diagnosis, molecular pathology tissue procurement, and clinical trial/research protocol eligibility determination. Peritoneoscopy is helpful to visualize multiple metastatic nodules on the liver surface (Fig. 18.1), and central depression is often seen in metastatic nodules due to central necrosis as the result of insufficient blood supply.

Table 18.1 Common metastatic tumors in the liver and immunohistochemical stain profiles

Tumor type and origin	Immunohistochemical stain profile
Adenocarcinoma	• Coordinate CK7/CK20 staining is commonly used, and both are usually negative in hepatocellular carcinoma • Hepatocytes and hepatocellular carcinoma are positive for CK8, CK18, HepPar1, arginase and polyclonal carcinoembryonic antigen (canalicular staining). CK7 and CK19 are positive only in the presence of cholangiocellular differentiation • Cholangiocarcinoma is commonly CK7-positive, CK20-negative and HepPar1-negative and a diagnosis per exclusion from other metastatic tumors
Colon and rectum	• Mostly negative CK7 and positive CK20. Positive CDX-2 indicates intestinal differentiation
Stomach	• Stomach carcinomas show variable cytokeratin profiles • CK7 and CK20 can be positive or negative in any combination • Positive CDX-2 in tumors with intestinal differentiation
Pancreas	• CK7, CK19, and CK20 can be positive or negative in any combination • Positive CDX-2 in tumors with intestinal differentiation • 60% of tumors are negative for SMAD4
Lung	• Positive CK7, Napsin A, and nuclear TTF-1 • Negative CK20 except enteric subtype • Rare positive CDX-2 can be seen in mucinous type of bronchioalveolar carcinoma
Breast	• Positive CK7, mammaglobin, GATA3 • Negative CK20 • Estrogen and/or progesterone receptor can be positive or negative in any combination
Renal cell carcinoma	• Positive vimentin, CD10, RCC, CAIX, and CK7 • Negative CK20 • Renal cell carcinoma may resemble clear-cell variant of hepatocellular carcinoma
Transitional cell carcinoma	• Positive CK7, CK20, p63, p40, GATA3, uroplakin
Squamous cell carcinoma	• Positive broad cytokeratin, CK5, p40 and p63 • Negative CK7 and CK20
Serous carcinoma	• Positive PAX8, WT1, CK7, p53 • Negative CK20, Calretinin
Neuroendocrine tumors	
Pancreas neuroendocrine tumor	Positive chromogranin, synaptophysin, variable hormone (such as insulin, glucagon, and somatostatin), CD56, occasional PAX8
Carcinoid tumor	• Positive chromogranin, synaptophysin, and CD56 • Common primary sites are the stomach and small intestine
Large-cell neuroendocrine carcinoma	• Positive chromogranin, synaptophysin, and CD56 • MIB-1 shows high proliferation activity
Small-cell neuroendocrine carcinoma	• Positive chromogranin, synaptophysin, and CD56 • Positive nuclear TTF-1 can be seen in pulmonary and extrapulmonary (~50%) small-cell carcinoma
Mesenchymal tumors	
Gastrointestinal stromal tumor	• Positive vimentin, C-kit, DOG1, and CD34 • Negative desmin • Smooth muscle actin can be positive or negative in any combination • Treated tumors can be hypocellular and show reduced C-kit positivity
Leiomyosarcoma	• Positive vimentin, desmin, and smooth muscle actin • Negative C-kit
Melanoma	• Positive S-100 protein, SOX10, HMB45, Melan-A, and vimentin • Negative cytokeratin

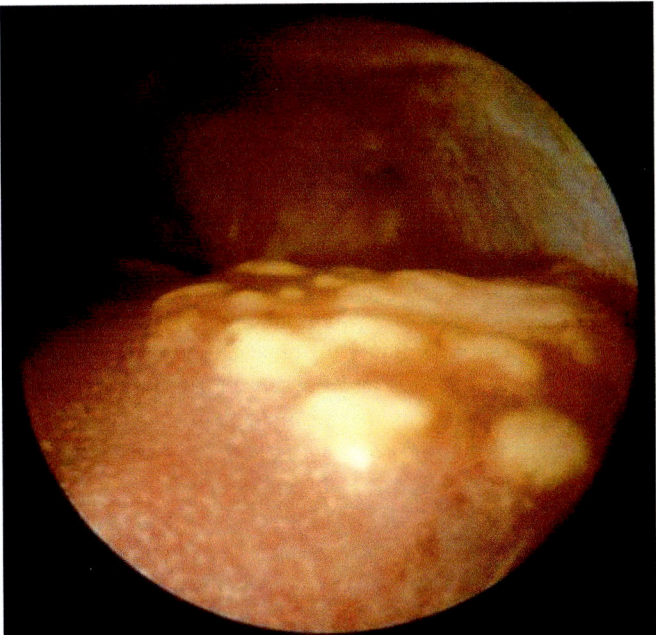

Fig. 18.1 Metastatic liver tumor. Peritoneoscopy shows multiple metastatic nodules with central excavation

On occasion, biopsy may miss the target metastatic lesion, yielding benign liver parenchyma with histological changes due to compression and local obstruction of bile duct and blood flow. In this case, histological changes show a triad, consisting of focal sinusoidal dilatation and congestion, ductular reaction, and neutrophils in edematous portal tracts [3].

18.3 Differentiation from Benign Liver Lesion

Benign liver lesions are frequently encountered during workups for metastatic lesions and should be in the differential diagnoses of these lesions. Simple biliary cyst, cavernous hemangioma, and focal fatty change can be distinguished from solid metastatic lesions with relative ease in imaging studies. Liver abscess can be difficult to differentiate from an extensively necrotic metastatic tumor but is usually accompanied by other constitutional symptoms such as fever. Inflammatory pseudotumor often requires biopsy to confirm the absence of malignant cells and the presence of chronic inflammation and storiform fibrosis.

Benign hepatocellular tumors, including focal nodular hyperplasia and hepatocellular adenoma, are not uncommon incidental findings. Focal nodular hyperplasia usually shows characteristic imaging features as a result of a prominent central scar containing large dystrophic vessels. The absence of an obvious central scar or the presence of steatosis in these

lesions may render an atypical appearance in imaging studies. Hepatocellular adenoma, usually encountered in young and middle-aged females with a history of oral contraceptive use or males with anabolic steroid use, requires complete resection because of its risk of bleeding and its slight risk of recurrence and malignant transformation.

Liver capsule or subcapsular nodules are often sampled during unrelated operations (gastric reduction surgery, pancreatoduodenectomy (whipple), etc.). Biliary hamartoma (von Meyenburg complex) is the most common nonmalignant cause of such nodules. On frozen section biliary hamartoma can be mistaken for well-differentiated adenocarcinoma but is usually readily apparent as a benign process. This lesion typically presents as a subcapsular cluster of angulated glands with surrounding fibrous reaction +/− neutrophilic inflammatory reaction. The epithelial cells themselves are typically bland with a low cuboidal morphology and smooth round-to-ovoid nuclei without nucleoli.

18.4 Case

Case 18.1
A patient presented with enlargement of the right submandibular gland and multiple small space-occupying lesions in the liver by ultrasonography. Computed tomography (CT) with contrast medium showed multiple low-density areas (Fig. 18.2). Peritoneoscopy showed small tumor nodules on the liver surface (Fig. 18.3). Echo-guided liver biopsy showed clusters of small neoplastic cells with hyperchromic nuclei, which were also positive for carcinoembryonic antigen. In this case, adenocarcinoma of the submandibular gland was diagnosed from metastatic lesions of the liver (Fig. 18.4).

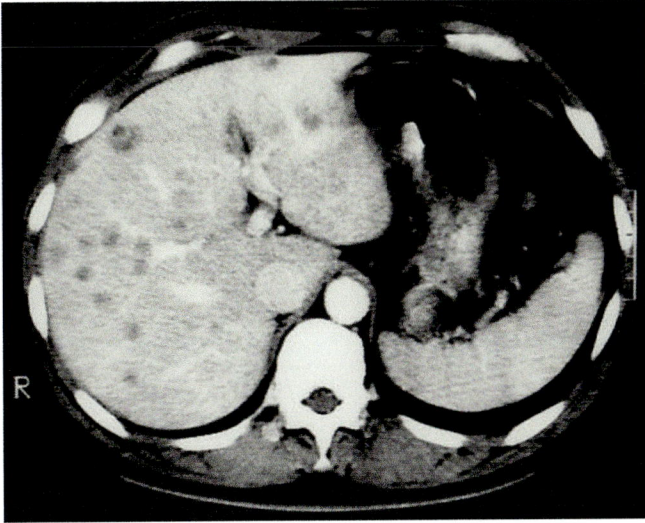

Fig. 18.2 Metastatic liver tumor. CT with contrast medium shows multiple low-density nodules

Case 18.2

A 55-year-old female complained of epigastric pain and diarrhea, and gastrointestinal fiberscope showed duodenal ulcers. Liver function tests revealed AST 136 IU/L, ALT 89 IU/L, LDH 336 IU/L, ALP 628 IU/L, GGT 189 IU/L, and AFP 570 ng/mL. The L3 fraction of AFP was 84.2% and serum gastrin was 6400 pg/mL. CT with contrast medium in the arterial phase showed multiple high-density areas in the liver and low density in the center. A low-density area in the pancreas was observed. High-density areas in the liver became low in the venous phase (Fig. 18.5). Biopsy of the liver tumor showed neoplastic cells with ani-

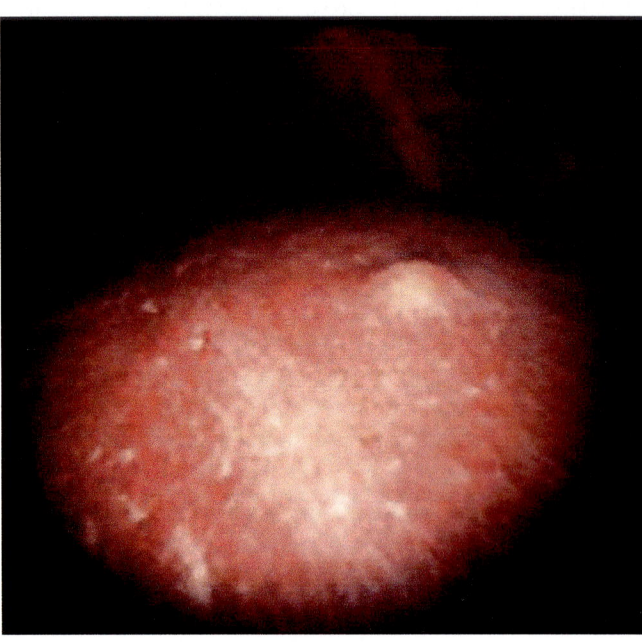

Fig. 18.3 Metastatic liver tumor. Peritoneoscopy shows nodular and granular liver surface

sonucleosis in comparison to normal hepatocytes; the neoplastic cells did not form a trabecular structure, and trabecular formation was preserved in non-tumoral area (Fig. 18.6). The tumor cells were positive for synaptophysin, CD56, chromogranin A, and AFP (Fig. 18.7). Serum test showed high values of gastrin and AFP. Image analysis revealed multiple hypervascular tumors in the liver and a hypovascular tumor of the pancreas. Histologically, neuroendocrine tumor was diagnosed from biopsy of liver metastasis. The pancreas was the suspected primary site. The tumor cells presumably produce gastrin and AFP. The elevation of serum AFP and human chorionic gonadotrophin-beta pertains to worse prognosis in patients with a neuroendocrine tumor [4].

Case 18.3

A 68-year-old female had a mastectomy for breast cancer, and a localized recurrence was found in the residual mammary gland 1 year later. General malaise and anorexia developed, and liver function tests showed TBIL 4.97 mg/dL, AST 219 IU/L, ALT 240 IU/L, ALP 1826 IU/L, and LDH 810 IU/L. CT by contrast medium showed heterogeneous enhancement in the liver at the arterial phase, but it decreased at the venous phase (Fig. 18.8). Peritoneoscopy showed enlarged liver with wavy surface and diffused white maculae (Fig. 18.9). Liver biopsy showed microthrombus of neoplastic cells in the portal veins and invasion beyond the portal tract, and the portal tract was edematous (Fig. 18.10). She was treated with systemic chemotherapy but died of acute liver failure due to diffuse invasion and proliferation of neoplastic cells. Breast cancer often metastasizes to the liver and produces multiple hypovascular tumors. In this patient, tumor cells invaded and proliferated diffusely in the peripheral portal veins. Hence, mass lesions were not detected in the liver, and heterogeneous density was seen on CT. The

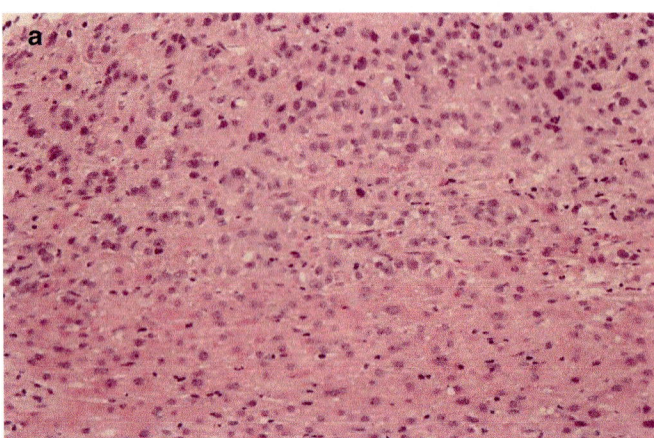

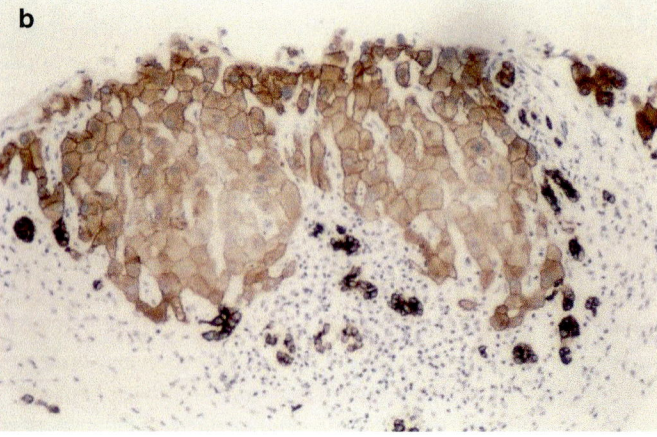

Fig. 18.4 Metastatic liver. (**a**) Small neoplastic cells at the upper two thirds of the picture are arranged in solid sheets with anisonucleosis and high nuclear cytoplasmic ratio. The lower third of the picture shows compressed non-tumoral hepatocytes in trabecular arrangement with low nuclear cytoplasmic ratio. (**b**) Carcinoembryonic antigen immunoreactivity is seen in neoplastic cells

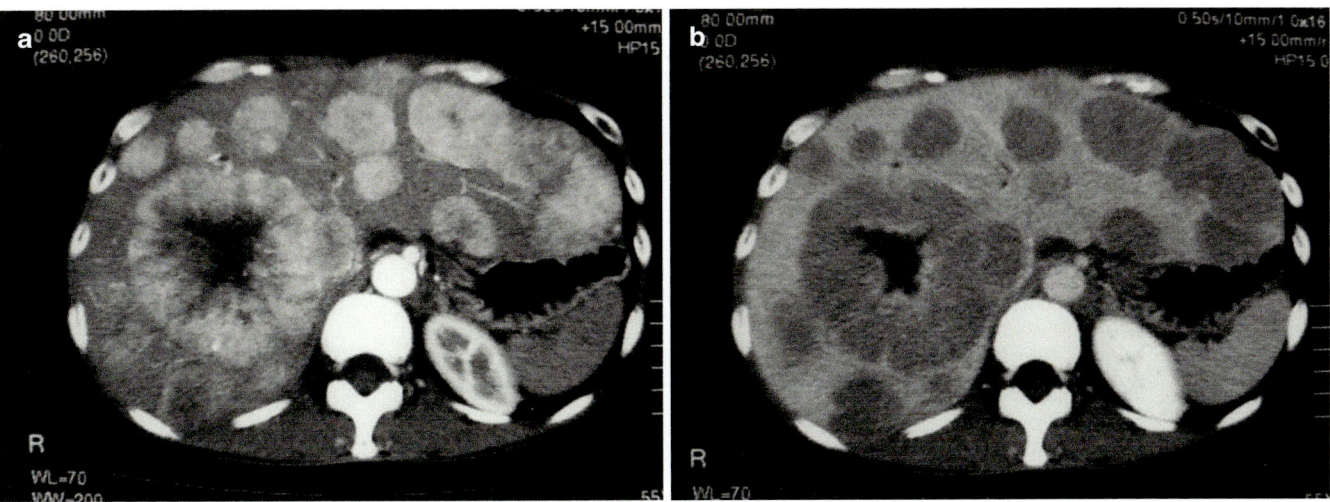

Fig. 18.5 Liver metastasis of neuroendocrine tumor. (**a**) CT with contrast medium shows multiple high-density areas with low density in the center at arterial phase. (**b**) CT shows low-density tumors at venous phase

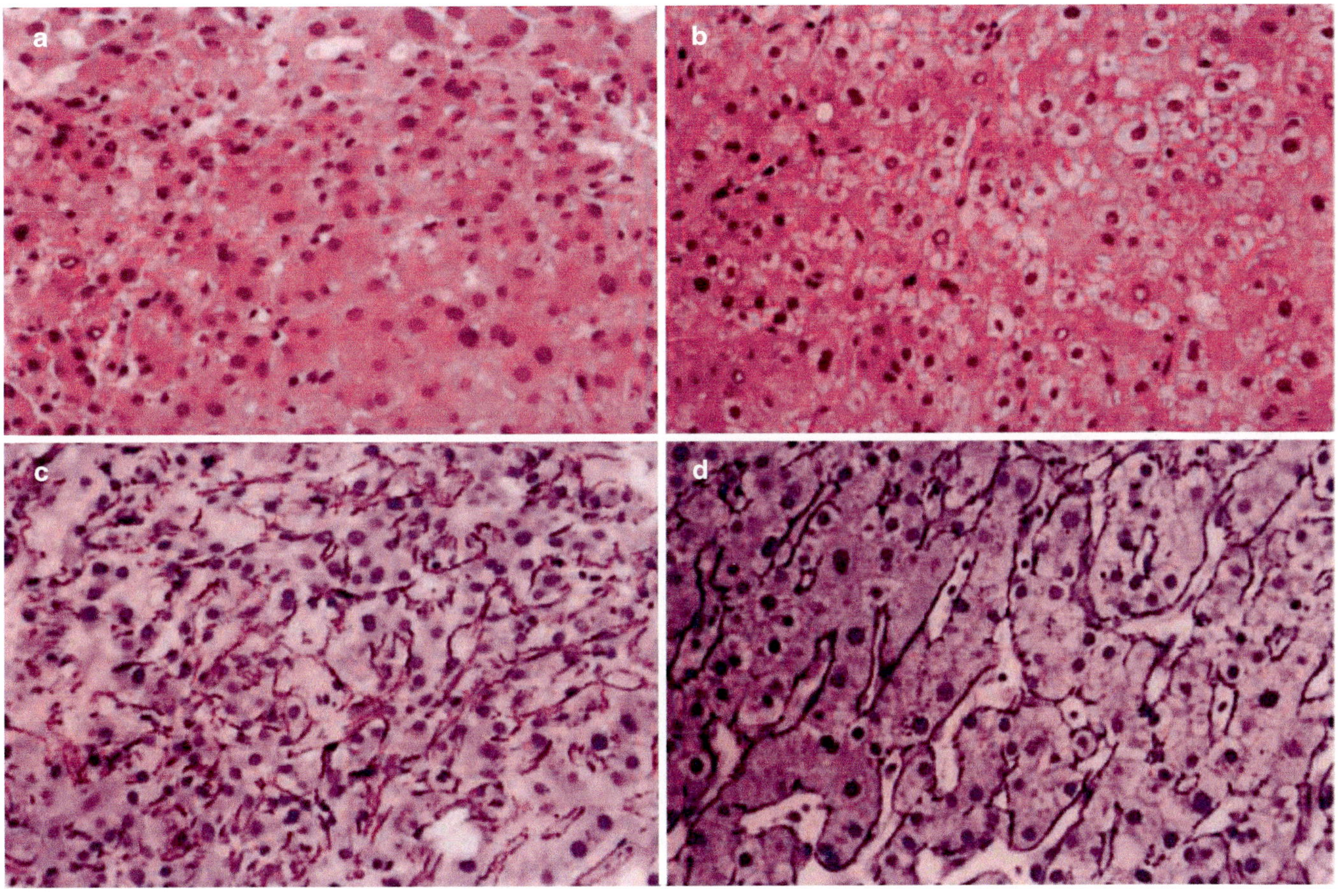

Fig. 18.6 Histological features of tumor area and non-tumor area. (**a**) Pleomorphic neoplastic cells in solid sheets. (**b**) Hepatocytes preserve the trabecular architecture in non-tumoral area. (**c**) Reticulin stain shows no trabecular arrangement of neoplastic cells. (**d**) Hepatocytes show trabecular arrangement

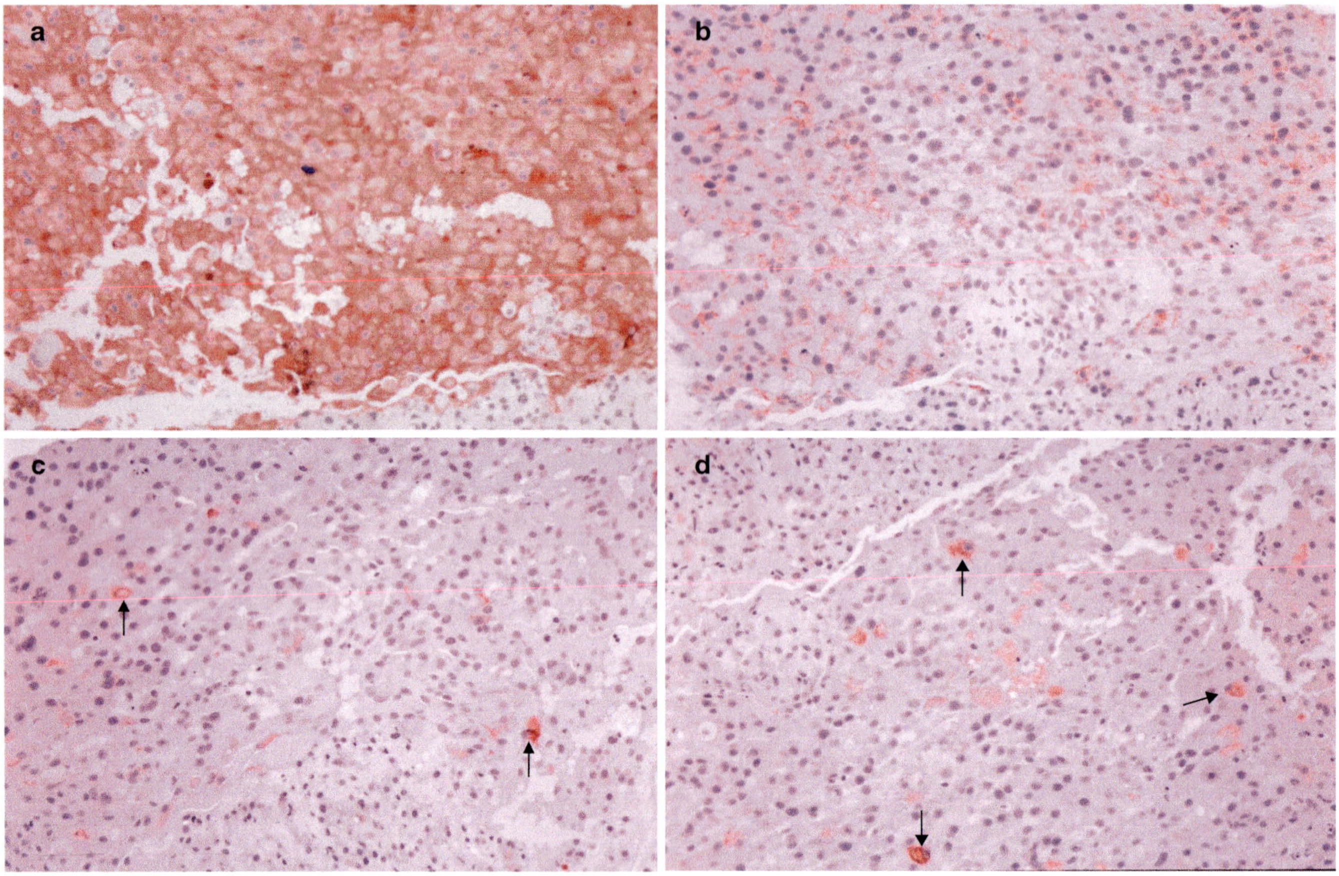

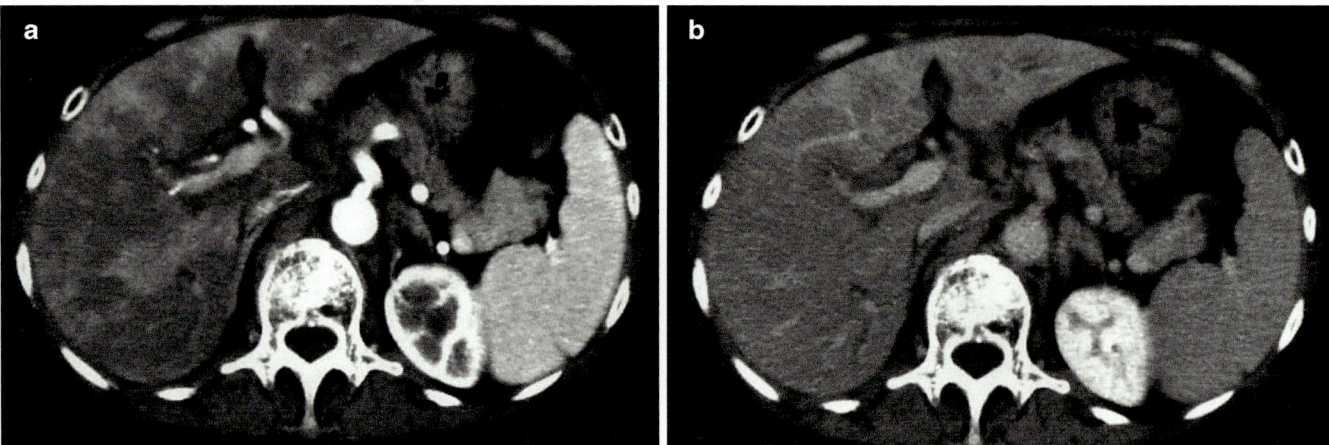

Fig. 18.7 Expression of synaptophysin, CD56, chromogranin A, and AFP immunoreactivity of the neoplastic cells. (**a**) Synaptophysin-immunoreactivity of the neoplastic cells. (**b**) CD56-immunoreactivity on the membrane of neoplastic cells. (**c**) Chromogranin A-immunoreactivity of some neoplastic cells (arrow). (**d**) Alpha-fetoprotein-immunoreactivity of some neoplastic cells (arrow)

Fig. 18.8 CT of metastatic liver. (**a**) Heterogeneous density at arterial phase with contrast medium. (**b**) Heterogeneous density is decreased at venous phase

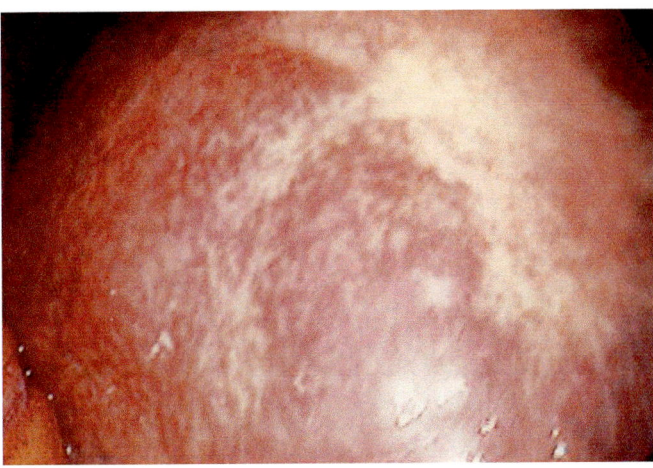

Fig. 18.9 Peritoneoscopic findings of metastatic liver. Large excavation and many white maculae are seen on liver surface

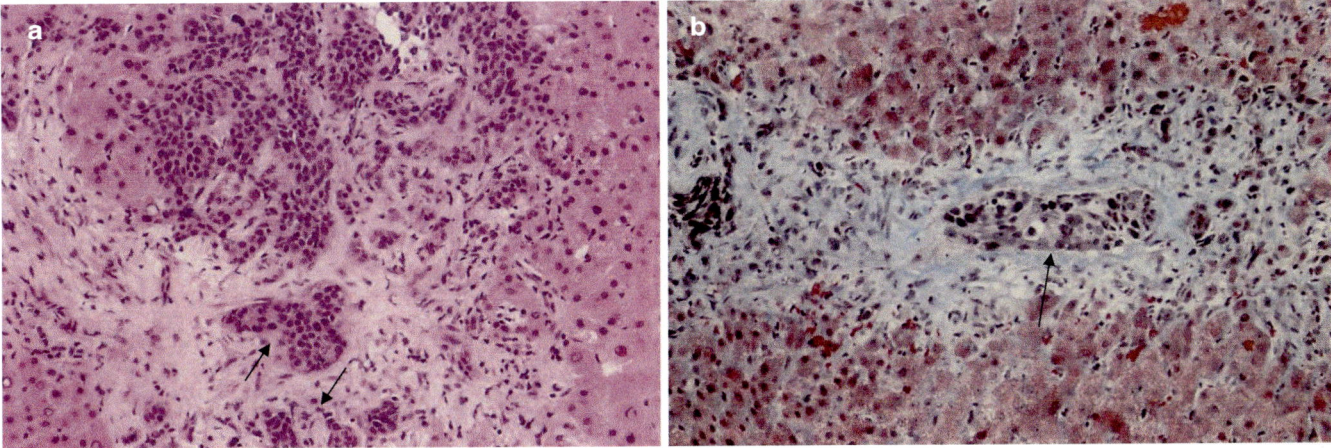

Fig. 18.10 Histological findings of metastatic liver. (**a**) Neoplastic cells proliferate in the portal tract with thrombi in the vessel (arrow) and invasion of the periportal area. (**b**) Portal tract is edematous with neoplastic thrombus (arrow) in the portal vein

development of diffuse metastasis and portal thrombus caused acute liver failure [5].

Acknowledgement Prof. Alex Y. Chang was a coauthor of the first edition of this chapter.

References

1. De Santis M, Santini D, Alborino S, Carubbi F, Romagnoli R. Liver metastasis from carcinoid: diagnostic imaging. Radiol Med. 1996;92:594–9.

2. Borja ER, Hori JM, Pugh RP. Metastatic carcinomatosis of the liver mimicking cirrhosis: case report and review of the literature. Cancer. 1975;35:445–9.

3. Gerber MA, Thung SN, Bodenheimer HC Jr, Kapelman B, Schaffner F. Characteristic histologic triad in liver adjacent to metastatic neoplasm. Liver. 1986;6:85–8.

4. Shah T, Srirajaskanthan R, Bhogal M, Toubanakis C, Meyer T, Noonan A, et al. Alpha-fetoprotein and human chorionic gonadotrophin-beta as prognostic markers in neuroendocrine tumour patients. Br J Cancer. 2008;99:72–7.

5. Athanasakis E, Mouloudi E, Prinianakis G, Kostaki M, Tzardi M, Georgopoulos D. Metastatic liver disease and fulminant failure: presentation of a case and review of the literature. Eur J Gastroenterol Hepatol. 2003;15:1235–40.

Liver Pathology in Transplantation

19

Hironori Haga

Contents

Abbreviations

ABMR	Antibody-mediated rejection
APC	Antigen-presenting cell
EBV	Epstein-Barr virus
GVHD	Graft-versus-host disease
H & E	Hematoxylin and eosin
HBV	Hepatitis B virus
HCV	Hepatitis C virus
HLA	Human leukocyte antigen
MHC	Major histocompatibility complex
NASH	Non-alcoholic steatohepatitis
PTLD	Posttransplant lymphoproliferative disorder
TCMR	T-cell-mediated rejection
Treg	Regulatory T cell

H. Haga, MD, PhD (✉)
Kyoto, Japan
e-mail: haga@kuhp.kyoto-u.ac.jp

19.1 Introduction

Liver transplantation is a treatment for almost all kinds of severe liver diseases that are otherwise incurable. More than 27,000 liver transplants were performed in 2015 worldwide, and about 20% of the donors were living donors [1]. In Japan, Southeast Asia, and Middle East, living donor liver transplantation is more common than transplantation from deceased donors due to problems with obtaining cadaveric organs. In cadaveric liver transplantation, the use of a whole allograft to replace the native diseased liver is the most common procedure. In live donor liver transplantation, the left lobe or left lateral segment of the live donor is usually used for pediatric patients. For neonates or very small children, use of a monosegment graft may be selected [2]. In some adult-to-adult living donor liver transplantation, the use of right lobe graft may be necessary to avoid small-for-size graft-associated liver dysfunction, but it might expose the live donor to considerable surgical risk. A cadaveric graft is also sometimes split into two grafts to save two recipients at a time. These partial grafts often need complicated surgical procedures and tend to have a greater risk of postoperative vascular and biliary anastomotic stricture or obstruction than livers resected for non-transplant settings.

© Springer Nature Singapore Pte Ltd. 2019
E. Hashimoto et al. (eds.), *Diagnosis of Liver Disease*, https://doi.org/10.1007/978-981-13-6806-6_19

Steady improvements in surgical techniques and immunosuppressive regimens to minimize postoperative complications have allowed lots of recipients (patients) to live decades after liver transplantation. Still, most patients experience various postoperative problems in the liver allograft. The main clinical practice of transplant pathology is to find the causes of graft dysfunction after transplantation. Major complications of liver allografts include (1) preservation/reperfusion injury, (2) postsurgical anastomotic complications, (3) allograft rejections, (4) complications related to immunosuppression, and (5) recurrence of the original liver disease.

Before discussing pathology of these complications, it would be useful to know that there is a time course of postoperative complications after liver transplantation. Most allograft complications were seen during specific posttransplant periods. In general, preservation/reperfusion injury manifests within the first week posttransplant period. Surgical complications are commonly seen in the first several weeks, except that biliary complications may also be seen months after transplantation. Typical acute allograft rejection is seen between 5 and 30 days posttransplantation [3]. Acute rejection can actually develop at any point thereafter especially when it is treatment-resistant or associated with nonadherence to immunosuppressive drugs. Incidence of recurrence of original liver diseases increases with time after transplantation. Recurrence of hepatotropic viral hepatitis may become evident within a few months after transplantation, while recurrence of autoimmune disease is usually noticed more than 6 months posttransplantation. In clinical practice, characteristic histological features may be found only focally or the findings may be subtle. Clinicopathological correlations are therefore imperative. The liver transplantation procedure, the timing of biopsy, the laboratory data, the types and dose of immunosuppressive drugs, and the findings of previous biopsy should all be considered before making a diagnosis of liver allograft biopsy.

19.2 Preservation/Reperfusion Injury

Preservation/reperfusion injury is associated with liver graft damage before implantation of the graft into the recipient's body. The main targets of the injury are hepatocytes and sinusoidal endothelial cells. Two types of ischemia are related to graft damage. Hepatocytes are sensitive to warm ischemia, which occurs before or during organ harvesting/procurement [4]. Cold ischemia, which is related to perfusion of hypothermic preservation solution and temporal storage of the graft in ice, causes sinusoidal endothelial damage [5]. After reperfusion, the formation and release of reactive oxygen species followed by Kupffer cell activation and other immune cell reaction worsen injury of both hepatocytes and endothelial cells.

Histologically, preservation/reperfusion injury is characterized by hepatocyte swelling (Fig. 19.1). Swelling of mitochondria and vacuoles in the hepatocytes is observed in electron microscopy [6]. Platelet adhesion occurs in the sinusoids but difficult to recognize in H&E stain [5]. Steatotic hepatocytes are more susceptible to preservation/reperfusion injury [7]. Most transplant surgeons will not use donor livers with severe fatty change (>60% of macrovesicular steatosis) because of poor patient outcome (Fig. 19.2) [8]. Primary graft non-function is a clinical term and is considered as the most severe form of preservation/reperfusion injury where the graft does not function at all after transplantation.

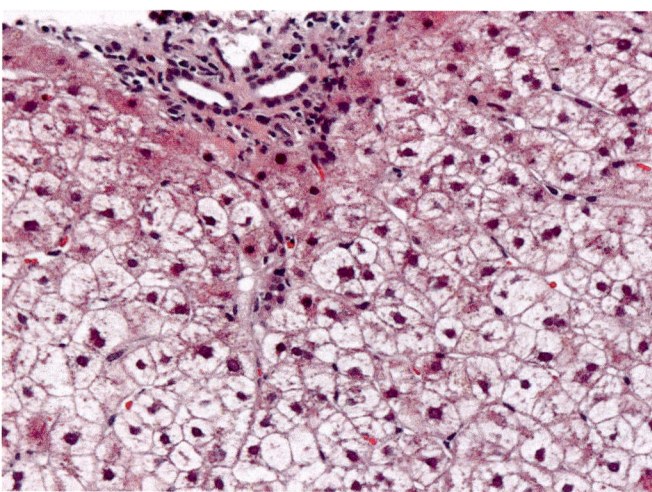

Fig. 19.1 Ischemia/reperfusion injury showing diffuse hepatocyte swelling without portal or lobular inflammation

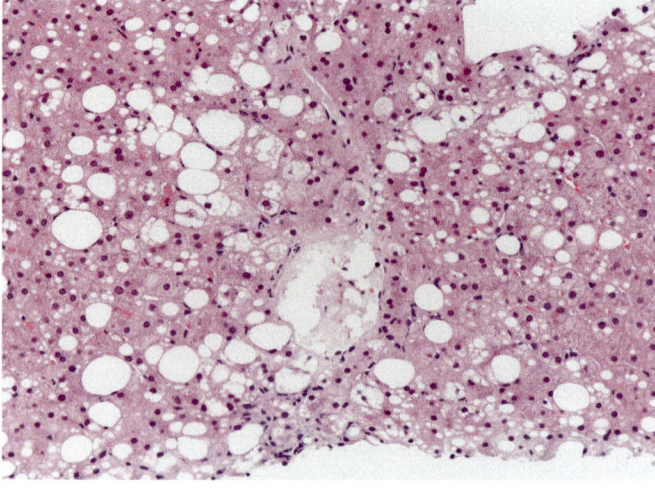

Fig. 19.2 Donor candidate with 60% of macrovesicular steatosis, which was not used for liver transplantation

19.3 Postsurgical Anastomotic Complications

Early complications of the vascular anastomoses can be associated with serious graft damage and can lead to graft failure if untreated. In principle, vascular anastomotic complications should be detected radiologically. Biopsy finding is relatively nonspecific, and it is often impossible to pinpoint affected vessels. Acute hepatic artery thrombosis, for example, can cause centrilobular hepatocyte coagulative necrosis (Fig. 19.3), but almost identical finding can be seen in grafts with acute portal vein thrombosis or severe venous outflow block. Hepatic vein stenosis, or outflow block, is usually associated with centrilobular congestion and hemorrhage (Fig. 19.4). Unlike hepatic artery thrombosis, the hepatocytes are atrophic and show thin cord-like arrangement. However, in partial graft, especially right lobe graft, focal congestion is sometimes seen without demonstrable large hepatic vein stenosis. Therefore, clinicopathological correlation is always necessary for interpretation of congestion of the allograft. Portal vein stenosis or obstruction found several months after transplantation tends to show more nonspecific findings, including periportal fibrosis, occlusion of small portal vein branches, focal sinusoidal dilatation, steatosis, or regenerative hyperplasia (Fig. 19.5) [9].

Biliary tract complication is more commonly seen than vascular complication after liver transplantation. Biliary reconstruction is usually performed by duct-to-duct anastomosis or hepaticojejunostomy and sometimes needs complicated procedures due to abnormal anatomy. Anastomotic biliary stricture usually occurs within the first several months posttransplantation, while non-anastomotic stricture tends to become apparent months or years after surgery. The large bile duct and surrounding peribiliary glands are supplied by a subepithelial layer of fine capillaries (peribiliary plexus) originated from the terminal branchings of the hepatic artery. Any insults associated with biliary tract ischemia can lead to disruption of bile flow. Major causes of biliary tract complication include preservation/reperfusion injury, hepatic artery thrombosis, antibody-mediated rejection, bacterial infection, cytomegalovirus infection, and recurrence of primary sclerosing cholangitis.

Biopsy is relatively sensitive to biliary complications. Portal and periportal edema, neutrophilic portal inflammation, ductular reaction, and hepatocanalicular cholestasis are the typical features of acute biliary complications (Fig. 19.6). Although neutrophils are most commonly seen in the periductal areas, there may be some intraductal inflammation

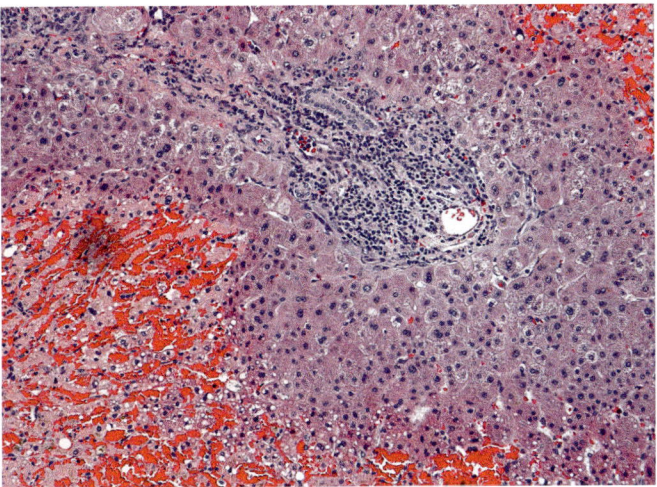

Fig. 19.3 Hepatic artery thrombosis. Centrilobular infarction is seen in the lower left corner. Portal inflammation suggests concurrent mild acute rejection

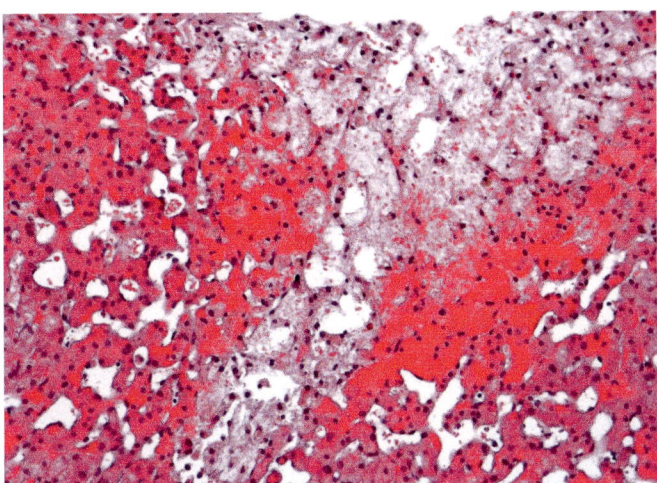

Fig. 19.4 Hepatic vein stenosis showing centrilobular congestion, dilatation of the sinusoids, and hepatocyte dropout

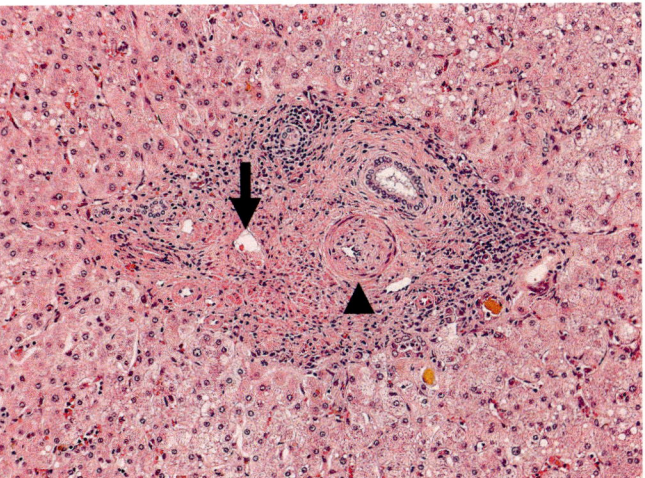

Fig. 19.5 Long-standing portal vein obstruction showing narrowing of the portal tract lumen (arrow) and intimal thickening of the hepatic artery (arrowhead)

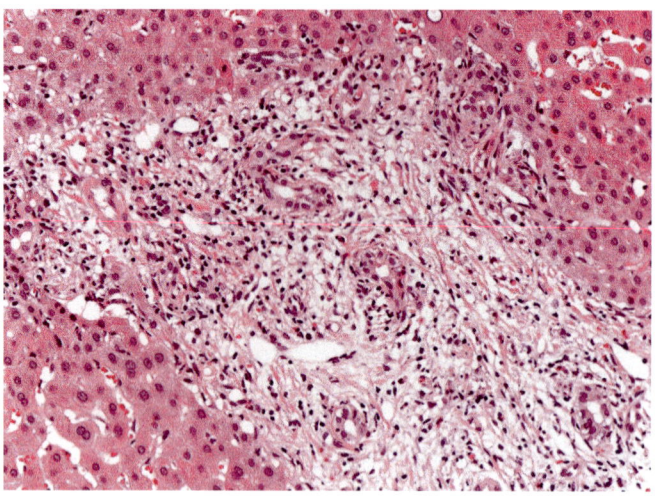

Fig. 19.6 Acute biliary obstruction showing portal edema and neutrophilic portal inflammatory cell infiltration

and neutrophil margination of the sinusoids. Prolonged biliary tract stricture is associated with mixed polymorphonuclear and mononuclear cell infiltration and periductal and periportal fibrosis, and these microscopic features appear similar to chronic hepatitis. Bile duct damage and cholestatic periportal hepatocytes can be the key to differentiate chronic biliary complications from chronic hepatitis. Loss of interlobular bile duct and ductules can occur in severe chronic biliary stenosis, and histology is sometimes indistinguishable from that of chronic ductopenic rejection. Both severe chronic biliary stenosis and late phase of chronic rejection are refractory to treatment and important causes of graft and patient loss.

19.4 Allograft Rejections

19.4.1 Mechanisms of Allograft Rejection

Allograft means a transplant graft from a genetically non-identical donor of the same species. Liver transplantation using xenograft (graft from other species/animals) has not been successful in human liver transplantation. Allograft rejection is an immunological reaction against allograft antigens. The main target of this reaction is major histocompatibility complex (MHC), a set of cell surface proteins which is related to peptide antigen presentation. The human MHC is also called the human leukocyte antigen (HLA). In transplant settings, MHC expressed by donor cells act as target of rejection unless the recipient has the same MHC. In the first several days or weeks after transplantation, the donor MHC antigens can be directly presented by donor antigen-presenting cells (APCs) (direct pathway). Direct pathway is believed to be related to acute rejection in early course of

transplantation. Subsequently recipient APCs start to engulf donor-derived antigens shed from the graft, and donor antigens were presented by the recipient APCs (indirect pathway). Because most of the donor APCs were killed by allograft rejection in early course of transplantation, indirect pathway is believed to be associated with late acute rejection and chronic rejection. It is also known that whole donor MHC-peptide complex can be transferred to recipient APCs through exosomes released from the graft cells and is used to cause immune reaction (semi-direct pathway) [10]. The role of semi-direct pathway in liver transplantation is not well understood.

19.4.2 Classification of Allograft Rejection

Rejection in liver transplantation can be classified into three main types based on the time course: hyperacute rejection, which starts from minutes after transplantation; acute rejection, which usually fully develop several days after transplantation; and chronic rejection, which may become apparent months or years after transplantation. However, there is no clear chronological definition for these immune reactions. Pathophysiologically, rejection is classified into two categories: antibody-mediated rejection (ABMR) and T-cell-mediated rejection (TCMR). This classification of rejection is well-recognized in kidney transplantation and other solid organ transplantations. In liver transplantation, however, histomorphological evaluation of liver allograft ABMR is often difficult, and there remains so much uncertainty about the role of ABMR. By contrast, histology of acute and chronic rejection is well-documented and has been widely used for management of liver allograft rejection. The terms of acute and chronic rejection are therefore mainly used in this chapter.

19.4.2.1 Hyperacute Rejection
Hyperacute rejection is a pure form of ABMR, mediated by preformed donor-specific anti-donor HLA antibodies (DSAs). Although recipients with high titers of DSA are at risk for ABMR, this type of rejection is rare in liver transplantation even the donor has DSAs. This relative resistance of liver allograft against ABMR, however, does not mean that hyperacute rejection does not occur at all. If hyperacute rejection develops, preformed DSAs bind donor endothelial cells and sinusoidal cells, and activation of complement causes thrombosis. Most of the vasculature within the graft is rapidly thrombosed, and massive necrosis of the liver parenchyma develops within hours after transplantation (Fig. 19.7a, b). Re-transplantation is the only way to save the recipient. Patients with high titers of DSA are therefore often precluded from cadaveric transplantation. In living donor liver transplantation, preoperative plasmapheresis and

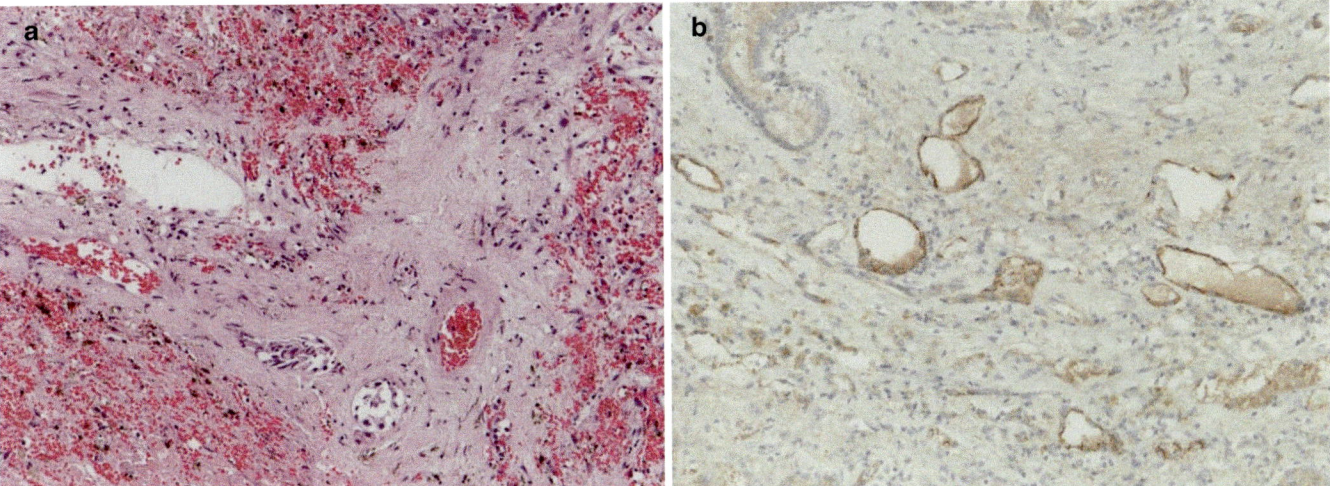

Fig. 19.7 (**a**) Hyperacute rejection showing massive hepatocyte necrosis. (**b**) Hyperacute rejection showing capillary C4d deposition, which suggests complement activation after antibody binding

administration of anti-CD20 antibody are performed to prevent ABMR for high-risk patients.

19.4.2.2 Acute Rejection

Acute cellular rejection (ACR) is often used as synonym for acute rejection because acute rejection is believed to be primarily caused by TCMR. This cellular process is supported by histological assessment. Acute rejection is characterized by (1) T-cell predominant but mixed portal and/or perivenular inflammation, (2) bile duct inflammation and damage, and (3) subendothelial inflammation of portal and/or terminal hepatic venules (Fig. 19.8a–d) [11]. To make the diagnosis of acute rejection, at least two of the above findings are required. Patients often show fever, abdominal pain, and reduced portal vein and bile flow. Blood test shows nonspecific liver injury (e.g., elevation of transaminase), and liver biopsy is necessary to confirm the diagnosis. Grading of acute rejection is proposed by the Banff Working Group on Liver Allograft Pathology, and acute rejection is graded as indeterminate, mild, moderate, and severe [11]. A basic concept of Banff grading is that grade is more than mild if more than half of the portal triads or perivenular areas are affected by inflammatory process. Most acute rejection is classified as mild or moderate and easily controlled by bolus of steroid and increased immunosuppression. More than mild acute rejection is often accompanied by eosinophilic infiltration and CD8+ cell-predominant infiltration and can be treatment-resistant [12, 13]. A diagnosis of severe acute rejection is made when parenchymal necroinflammation is observed in a majority of periportal and/or perivenular areas. Some therapy-resistant rejection may be treated by rabbit antihuman thymocyte immunoglobulin.

Involvement of ABMR in acute rejection of liver transplantation is thought to be uncommon. Patients with high-titer DSAs have a higher risk of developing ABMR. To make a definitive diagnosis of acute ABMR, positive serum DSA and microvascular deposition of C4d (degradation product of complement C4) are required in addition to histopathological pattern of injury consistent with acute ABMR such as endothelial swelling, capillary dilatation, and microvasculitis (Fig. 19.9a, b) [11]. ABMR can also be observed after ABO-incompatible transplantation if preoperative preventive management is inadequate (Fig. 19.10).

Late acute rejection, which is defined as acute rejection seen after 6 months posttransplantation, is likely attributable to indirect or semi-direct alloantigen presentation. Late acute rejection shows more monotonous lymphocytic infiltration and less bile duct and endothelial injury. In addition, lobular inflammation (periportal or perivenular) is more commonly seen even though clinical presentation does not suggest severe acute rejection. When there is marked plasma cell infiltration, the diagnosis of plasma cell-rich rejection (formerly known as "de novo autoimmune hepatitis") may be made (Fig. 19.11). Although patients with late acute rejection often initially have little or no symptoms, it is important to recognize and treat late acute rejection. Late acute rejection is a risk to patient and graft survival. Unlike typical (early) acute rejection, late acute rejection often recurs or persists and can cause liver cirrhosis or chronic rejection [14–16].

19.4.2.3 Chronic Rejection

Ductopenic rejection is a synonym of chronic rejection. Chronic rejection usually evolves from severe or persistent acute rejection. In some cases, it starts with intractable cholestasis with minimal inflammatory cell infiltrate. Owing to improvements of immunosuppression, this is a relatively uncommon problem in liver transplantation, but

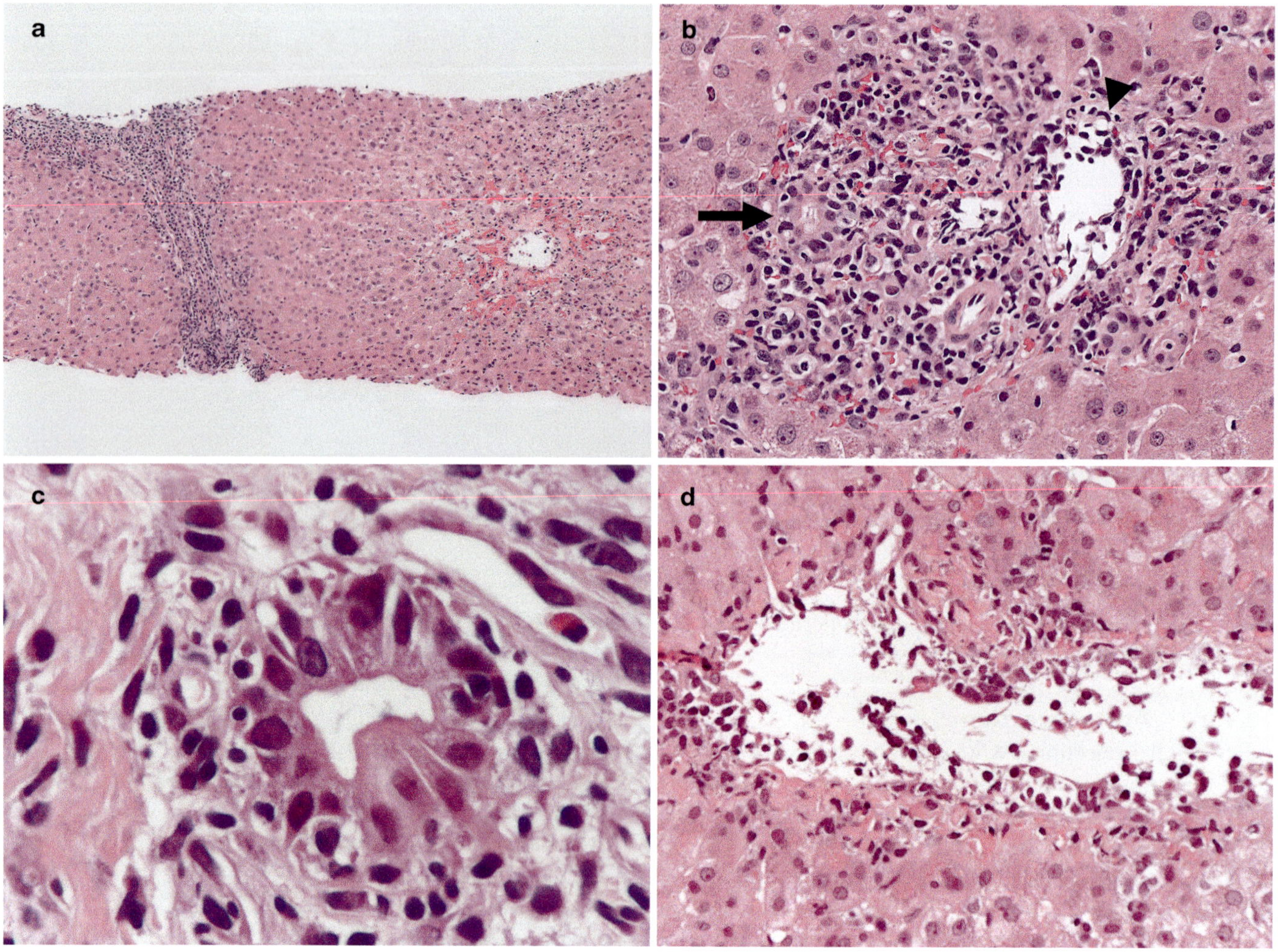

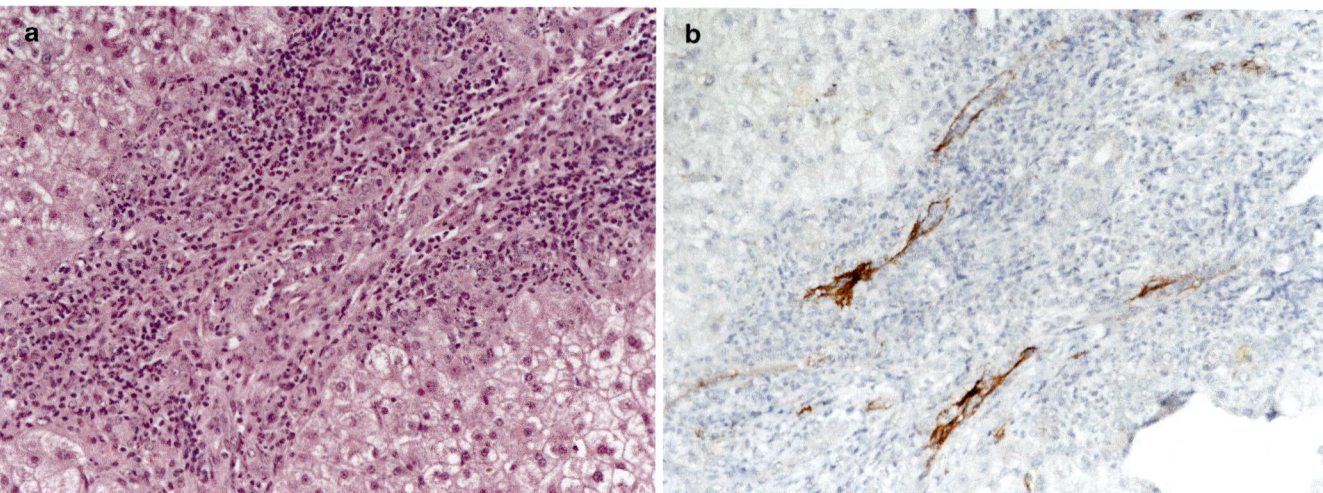

Fig. 19.8 (**a**) Low-power view of moderate acute rejection showing portal inflammation (left side) and perivenular inflammation (right side). Perivenular inflammation is accompanied by hemorrhage. (**b**) Acute rejection demonstrating bile duct inflammation damage (arrow, left side) and venous endothelial inflammation (arrow head, right). (**c**) Acute rejection showing degenerated biliary epithelium with inflammatory cell infiltration. (**d**) Acute rejection demonstrating endothelial detachment of the hepatic venule by subendothelial lymphocytic infiltration

Fig. 19.9 (**a**) Acute rejection with ABMR component. Mixed infiltrate is neutrophil predominant although neither biliary complication nor infection is not evident in this case. (**b**) Acute rejection with ABMR component showing C4d deposition in the sinusoids

it still consists of more than 10% of causes of pediatric retransplantation [17]. The most characteristic histological feature is interlobular bile duct loss and duct degeneration (atypia or senescence-like morphology) seen in more than half of the portal tracts (Fig. 19.12a, b). In typical cases, fibrous expansion of portal tracts is not conspicuous, and other portal structures such as arterioles often become atrophic and difficult to identify. Keratin 7 (cytokeratin 7) immunostaining is very useful to confirm the degeneration and loss of bile ducts and ductules (Figs. 19.12b and 19.13). Ductular reaction is usually absent, and there is aberrant expression of keratin 7 in the periportal and perivenular hepatocytes.

Unlike other solid organ allografts, the liver allograft with chronic rejection may response to rejection therapy and recovers its function to some extent. Staging of chronic rejection is therefore proposed by the Banff Working Group [11]. Early chronic rejection, which does not show severe cholestasis or bile duct loss in ≥50% of portal tracts, is potentially reversible or likely to response to potent immunosuppressive therapy. Late chronic rejection, in contrast, shows advanced histology with severe progressive cholestasis and is potentially irreversible. Venous obliteration is a feature of late chronic rejection (Fig. 19.14). Obliterative arteriopathy (Fig. 19.15) is another feature of late chronic rejection but usually dif-

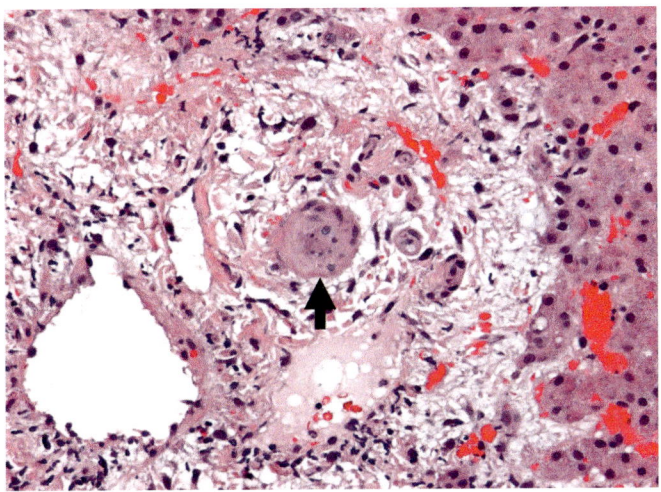

Fig. 19.10 ABO-incompatible acute ABMR showing portal edema, endothelial swelling (center, arrow) of the hepatic artery, and thromboses of the capillary (right side). There is not a component of TCMR

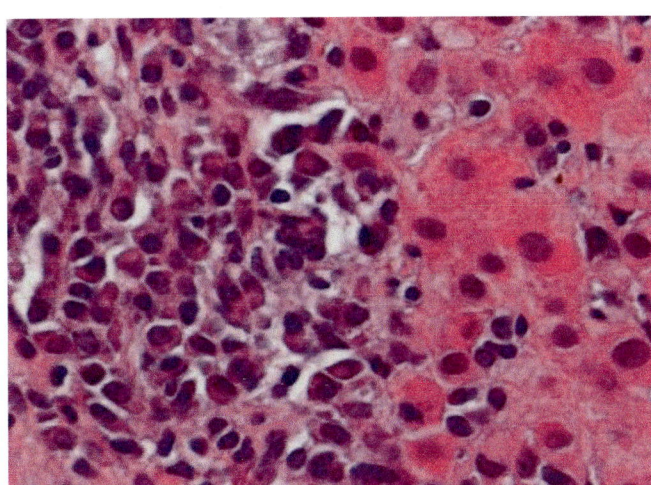

Fig. 19.11 Plasma cell-rich rejection (variant of late acute rejection) showing interface activity by lymphoplasmacytic infiltration

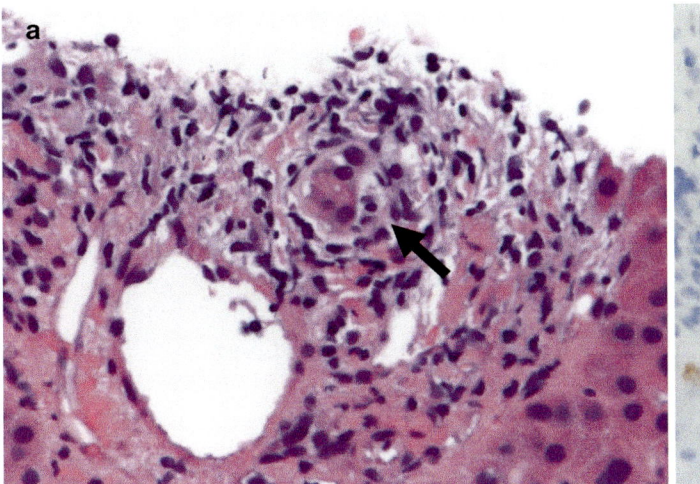

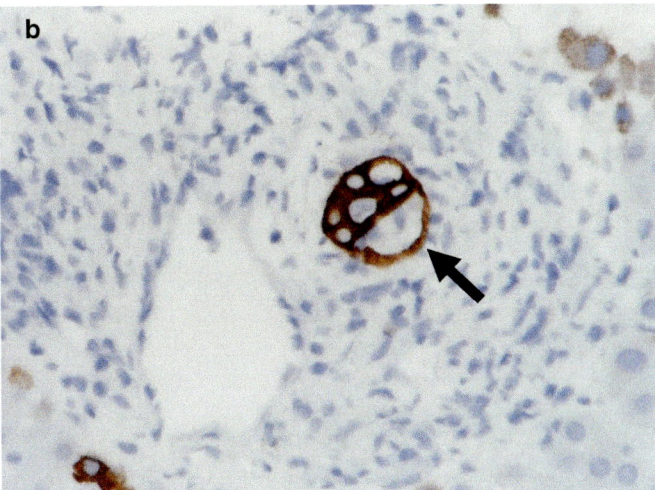

Fig. 19.12 (**a**) Early chronic rejection showing bile duct degeneration. (**b**) Early chronic rejection with keratin 7 immunostaining demonstrating luminal disruption and vacuolar changes of biliary epithelium

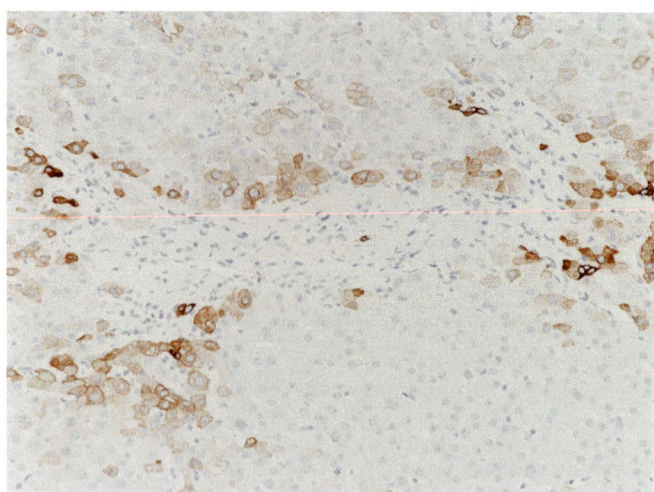

Fig. 19.13 Keratin 7 immunostaining confirms loss of bile ducts and bile ductules in late chronic rejection. Aberrant/compensatory keratin 7 expression is seen in some periportal hepatocytes

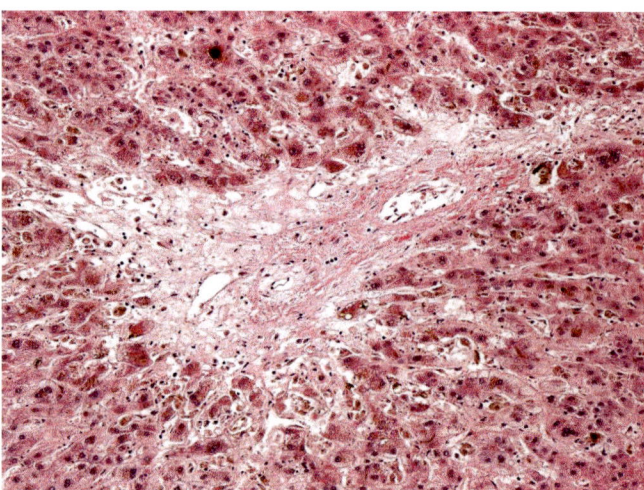

Fig. 19.14 Late chronic rejection showing fibrous obliteration of the terminal hepatic venule

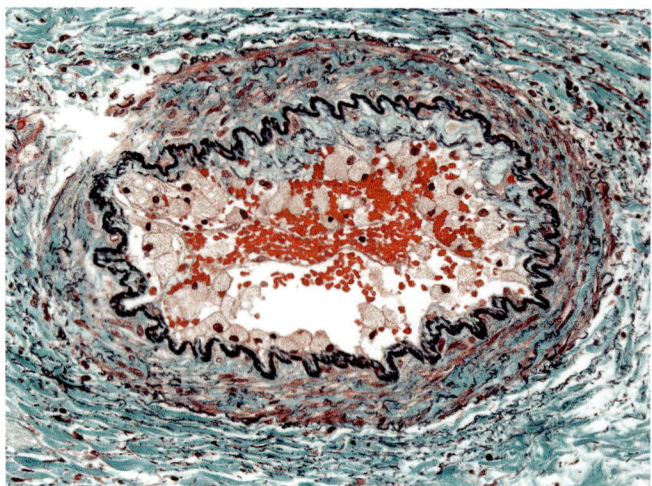

Fig. 19.15 Arterial lesion of late chronic rejection (Masson trichrome and Verhoeff elastic staining)

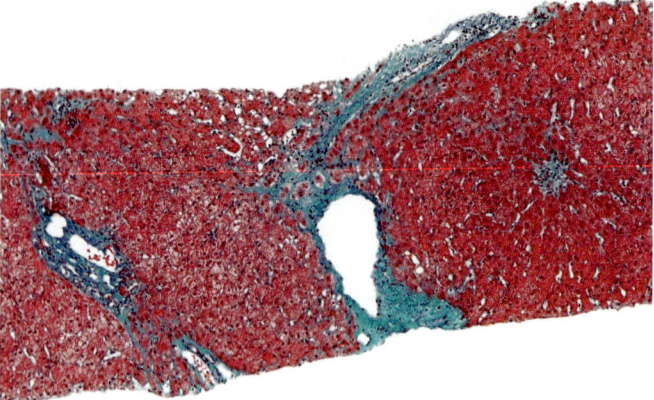

Fig. 19.16 Perivenular bridging fibrosis with minimal inflammation seen after complete withdrawal of immunosuppression

ficult to find in needle biopsy specimens. These features are usually associated with graft failure.

Graft-versus-host disease (GVHD) after hematopoietic stem cell transplantation shows similar histology to early chronic rejection; bile duct atypia and cholestasis are common, but portal inflammation tends to be mild, and endothelial inflammation is inconspicuous. Advanced GVHD shows similar histology and clinical course to late chronic rejection.

Chronic ABMR is an evolving concept. Some type of DSAs detected after months or years after transplantation is associated with chronic rejection and poor graft survival [18, 19]. Patients with DSAs often show portal and/or perivenular fibrosis, with minimal portal inflammation that does not fulfill the criteria of acute or chronic rejection [20, 21]. Such histology was initially reported in some pediatric recipients after complete cessation of immunosuppressive drugs (Fig. 19.16) [22]. These findings suggest that inadequate immunosuppression causes insidious progression of "nonspecific" allograft fibrosis, which would be a histological feature of chronic ABMR. To detect chronic ABMR, protocol biopsy (biopsy obtained in a patient with stable graft function) years after transplantation may be necessary. However, there is currently no defined treatment strategy for possible chronic ABMR.

19.4.3 Immune Tolerance in Liver Transplantation

It is known that some liver allograft recipients keep completely normal allograft histology and liver function after gradual weaning of immunosuppressive drugs and complete cessation of those drugs. This status is called "operational tolerance." Clinically this phenomenon is not uncommon, especially among pediatric liver transplantation. The mechanisms of "operational tolerance" are not clearly understood, but regulatory T cells (Tregs) seem to have an important role for liver allograft tolerance [23]. It is also true that majority of the patients cannot achieve operational tolerance due to overt rejection during weaning. Since progressive fibrosis with or without mild inflammation suggests subclinical rejection [22], weaning of immunosuppressive drugs should be carefully carried out with follow-up biopsy. A major goal in liver (and other solid organs) transplantation is to establish the ways to evaluate and induce graft tolerance.

19.5 Complications Related to Immunosuppression

Most serious infections associated with immunosuppressive status occur within the first 2 postoperative months. Various types of viral, fungal, and bacterial infection can occur. Bacterial infection of the allograft or systemic bacterial infection can cause sepsis (systemic inflammatory response syndrome in response to an infectious process) and sepsis-associated cholestasis. Histology of sepsis is characterized by canalicular and ductular cholestasis with bile plugs and periductular neutrophil infiltration (referred to as *cholangitis lenta*) (Fig. 19.17). Major opportunistic viral infections include cytomegalovirus and Epstein-Barr virus. The latter usually does not cause hepatitis but is associated with posttransplant lymphoproliferative disorder (PTLD) involving the allograft. PTLD seen the liver biopsy is mostly overt B-cell or T-cell lymphoma. Staining of EBV (EBER in situ hybridization) can be helpful to differentiate EBV-positive lymphoma from rejection, but EBV-negative T-cell lymphoma can mimic acute rejection.

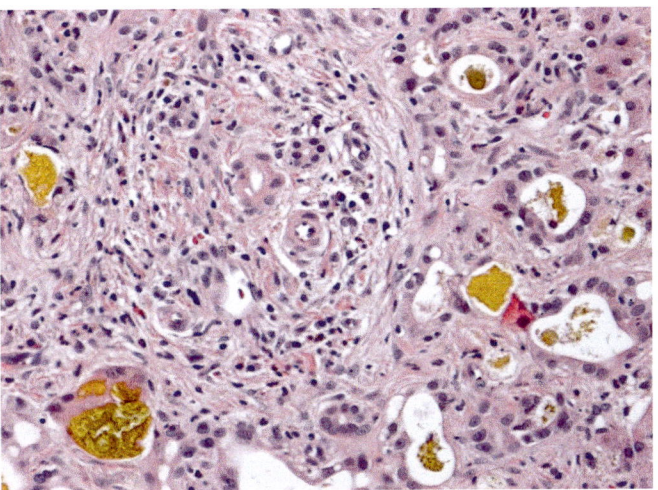

Fig. 19.17 Sepsis-related ductular cholestasis

19.6 Recurrence of the Original Liver Disease

Histology of recurrent disease is basically similar or identical to that of nontransplant settings. Timing of biopsy is an important factor for the diagnosis of recurrent disease. For example, recurrent alcoholic liver disease and recurrent NASH are usually seen in months or years after transplantation; graft steatosis in the first month posttransplantation is almost always attributed to donor-derived steatosis or parenteral nutrition.

Recurrence of hepatotropic virus infection (HBV and HCV) was once a common and serious complication after liver transplantation. Immunosuppression was often associated with accelerated course of recurrent hepatitis. After the introduction of effective and safe antiviral therapy, most cases of recurrent hepatitis can be treated without biopsy. Histology of recurrent hepatitis is rather nonspecific and can be similar to that of acute rejection. When acute rejection and recurrent HCV seem to coexist, antiviral therapy is recommended. Rejection therapy should be added only when acute rejection is graded as moderate or severe [24]. It is of note that late acute rejection can develop after treatment of recurrent HCV [25].

Autoimmune liver diseases, such as autoimmune hepatitis, primary biliary cholangitis, and primary sclerosing cholangitis, recur in about 10–50% of patients [26]. Histological findings are identical to those of nontransplant diseases. After more than a year after transplantation, biopsy from patients free from symptom and normal liver tests sometimes shows early stage of the recurrent disease. Graft and patient survival are generally good after liver transplantation for autoimmune liver disease except primary sclerosing cholangitis. Like other non-anastomotic late biliary complications, effective treatment for recurrent primary sclerosing cholangitis is not available. Compared to other autoimmune diseases, recurrent primary sclerosing cholangitis is associated with decreased graft and patient survival [26].

References

1. Global Observatory on Donation and Transplantation/World Health Organization. http://www.transplant-observatory.org/countliver [cited 1 Aug 2018].
2. Ogawa K, Kasahara M, Sakamoto S, et al. Living donor liver transplantation with reduced monosegments for neonates and small infants. Transplantation. 2007;83:1337–40.
3. An International Panel (Demetris AJ, Batts KP, Dhillon AP, et al.). Banff schema for grading liver allograft rejection: an international consensus document. Hepatology. 1997;25:658–63.
4. Teoh NC, Farrell GC. Hepatic ischemia reperfusion injury: pathogenic mechanisms and basis for hepatoprotection. J Gastroenterol Hepatol. 2003;18:891–902.

5. Cywes R, Mullen JB, Stratis MA, et al. Prediction of the outcome of transplantation in man by platelet adherence in donor liver allografts. Evidence of the importance of preservation injury. Transplantation. 1993;56:316–23.

6. Bochimoto H, Matsuno N, Ishihara Y, et al. The ultrastructural characteristics of porcine hepatocytes donated after cardiac death and preserved with warm machine perfusion preservation. PLoS One. 2017;12:e0186352.

7. Chu MJ, Premkumar R, Hickey AJ, et al. Steatotic livers are susceptible to normothermic ischemia-reperfusion injury from mitochondrial Complex-I dysfunction. World J Gastroenterol. 2016;22:4673–84.

8. Feng S, Lai JC. Expanded criteria donors. Clin Liver Dis. 2014;18:633–49.

9. Ueda M, Oike F, Kasahara M, et al. Portal vein complications in pediatric living donor liver transplantation using left-side grafts. Am J Transplant. 2008;8:2097–105.

10. Marino J, Paster J, Benichou G. Allorecognition by T lymphocytes and allograft rejection. Front Immunol. 2016;7:582.

11. Demetris AJ, Bellamy C, Hübscher SG, et al. 2016 comprehensive update of the Banff Working Group on liver allograft pathology: introduction of antibody-mediated rejection. Am J Transplant. 2016;16:2816–35.

12. Kubota N, Sugitani M, Takano S, et al. Correlation between acute rejection severity and CD8-positive T cells in living related liver transplantation. Transpl Immunol. 2006;16:60–4.

13. Kishi Y, Sugawara Y, Tamura S, et al. Histological eosinophilia as an aid to diagnose acute cellular rejection after living donor liver transplantation. Clin Transpl. 2007;21:214–8.

14. Miyagawa-Hayashino A, Haga H, Egawa H, et al. Outcome and risk factors of de novo autoimmune hepatitis in living-donor liver transplantation. Transplantation. 2004;78:128–35.

15. Uemura T, Ikegami T, Sanchez EQ, et al. Late acute rejection after liver transplantation impacts patient survival. Clin Transpl. 2008;22:316–23.

16. Thurairajah PH, Carbone M, Bridgestock H, et al. Late acute liver allograft rejection; a study of its natural history and graft survival in the current era. Transplantation. 2013;95:955–9.

17. Neves Souza L, de Martino RB, Sanchez-Fueyo A, et al. Histopathology of 460 liver allografts removed at retransplantation: a shift in disease patterns over 27 years. Clin Transpl. 2018;32:e13227.

18. Kaneku H, O'Leary JG, Taniguchi M, et al. Donor-specific human leukocyte antigen antibodies of the immunoglobulin G3 subclass are associated with chronic rejection and graft loss after liver transplantation. Liver Transpl. 2012;18:984–92.

19. Couchonnal E, Rivet C, Ducreux S, et al. Deleterious impact of C3d-binding donor-specific anti-HLA antibodies after pediatric liver transplantation. Transpl Immunol. 2017;45:8–14.

20. Minagawa-Hayashino A, Yoshizawa A, Uchida Y, et al. Progressive graft fibrosis and donor-specific human leukocyte antigen antibodies in pediatric late liver allografts. Liver Transpl. 2012;18:1333–42.

21. Dao M, Habès D, Taupin JL, et al. Morphological characterization of chronic antibody-mediated rejection in ABO-identical or ABO-compatible pediatric liver graft recipients. Liver Transpl. 2018;24:897–907.

22. Yoshitomi M, Koshiba T, Haga H, et al. Requirement of protocol biopsy before and after complete cessation of immunosuppression after liver transplantation. Transplantation. 2009;87:606–14.

23. Todo S, Yamashita K, Goto R, et al. A pilot study of operational tolerance with a regulatory T-cell-based cell therapy in living donor liver transplantation. Hepatology. 2016;64:632–43.

24. Demetris AJ, Eghtesad B, Marcos A, et al. Recurrent hepatitis C in liver allografts: prospective assessment of diagnostic accuracy, identification of pitfalls, and observations about pathogenesis. Am J Surg Pathol. 2004;28:658–69.

25. Chan C, Schiano T, Agudelo E, et al. Immune-mediated graft dysfunction in liver transplant recipients with hepatitis C virus treated with direct-acting antiviral therapy. Am J Transplant. 2018;18(10):2506–12.

26. Montano-Loza AJ, Bhanji RA, Wasilenko S, et al. Systematic review: recurrent autoimmune liver diseases after liver transplantation. Aliment Pharmacol Ther. 2017;45:485–500.

Peritoneal Diseases

20

Masaki Iwai, Yosuke Kunishi, and Arief A. Suriawinata

Contents

Abbreviations

BAP1	Breast cancer-associated protein 1
CA125	Carcinogenic antigen-125
CA19-9	Carcinogenic antigen 19-9
FDG-PET	18F-fluorodeoxyglucose positron emission tomography
SEP	Sclerosing encapsulating peritonitis
TNF	Tumor necrosis factor
TS-1	Combination capsule of tegafur, gimeracil, and oteracil potassium

The peritoneum is an organ of serosa with combined epithelial and mesenchymal features. It consists mainly of mesothelial cells arranged in a monolayer. Peritoneal disorders include primary or secondary tumors, benign or malignant tumors, and inflammatory disorders. Hence, they are not only of tuberculosis and sarcoidosis but also mesothelioma

and carcinomatosis which can impair physiological functions [1] and produce massive ascites. Sclerosing encapsulating peritonitis leads to peritoneal fibrosis and obstruction of small intestine which mimics liver cirrhosis.

20.1 Peritoneal Tuberculosis

Ascites always occur in peritoneal tuberculosis, besides constitutional symptoms such as weight loss, abdominal discomfort, anorexia, night sweat [2], fever, and general malaise. The ascitic fluid is exudative and rich in albumin and lymphocytes [3]. Abdominal US and CT scanning is useful for the diagnosis of peritoneal tuberculosis [4, 5]. FDG-PET is crucial in the differential diagnosis from peritoneal carcinomatosis [6]. An accurate diagnosis can be made based on the value of adenosine deaminase in the fluid [7] and by laparoscopy [8] with selective biopsy of peritoneal granulomas [9]. Positive staining for acid-fast bacilli in granulomatous tissue confirms the diagnosis, while positive culture of tissue biopsied from the peritoneum is regarded as the gold standard test [2]. Furthermore, polymerase chain reaction (PCR) for mycobacterial tuberculosis is used to confirm tubercle bacilli [2]. In some cases, examination cannot prove the presence of the mycobacteria. Hence, first-line antituberculous drugs such as isoniazid, rifampicin, ethambutol, and pyrazinamide are administered [3] for definite or probable tuberculosis.

M. Iwai, MD, PhD (✉)
Kyoto, Japan
e-mail: masaiwai@koto.kpu-m.ac.jp

Y. Kunishi, MD, PhD
Tochigi, Japan

A. A. Suriawinata, MD
New Hampshire, USA

© Springer Nature Singapore Pte Ltd. 2019
E. Hashimoto et al. (eds.), *Diagnosis of Liver Disease*, https://doi.org/10.1007/978-981-13-6806-6_20

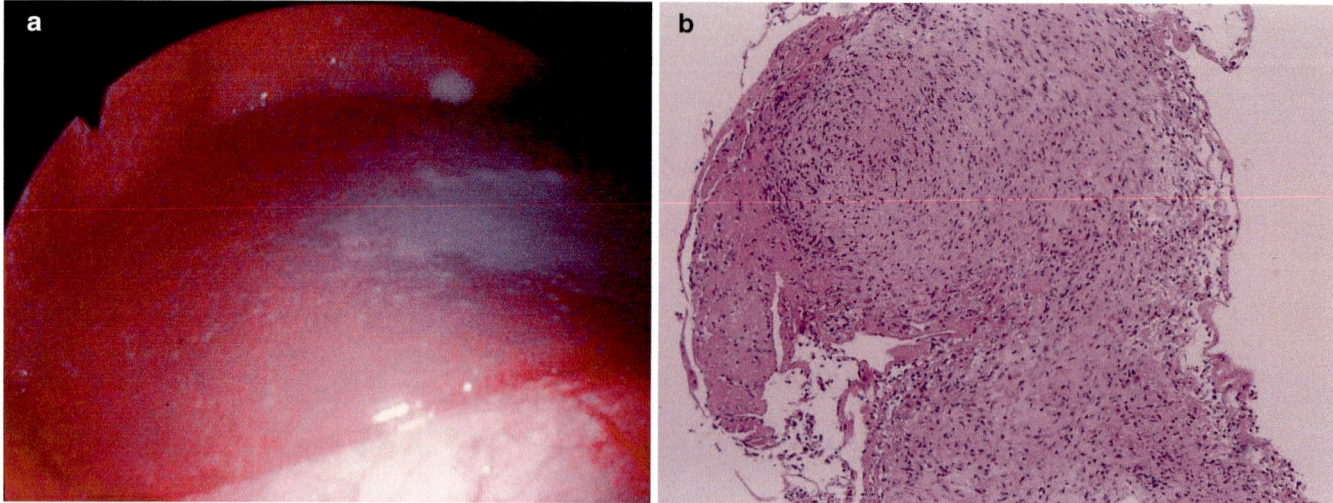

Fig. 20.1 Peritoneal tuberculosis. (**a**) Laparoscopy showing white maculae on the peritoneum and thick white plaque with small granules on the liver capsule. (**b**) Biopsy from white maculae on the peritoneum showing formation of granuloma

Case 20.1

A 51-year-old patient complained of epigastric pain and low-grade fever. Liver function test was normal. Ascites were detected by ultrasonography. Examination of ascitic fluid showed increased lymphocytes, but PCR was negative for *Mycobacterium tuberculosis*. Peritoneoscopy revealed a white-coated capsule and small nodules or maculae on liver surface. White nodules or granulomas were also seen in the peritoneum. Biopsy from a white nodule on the peritoneum showed necrotizing epithelioid granuloma (Fig. 20.1). Six months of empirical treatment with first-line antituberculous drugs resulted in reduced ascites and abdominal pain and no fever. Peritoneoscopic findings in another patient with tuberculosis showed an adhesive membrane between the peritoneum and liver. Granulomas were not visible on the peritoneum or liver surface (Fig. 20.2), a finding that is suggestive of cured or old tuberculosis in the peritoneum [8, 10].

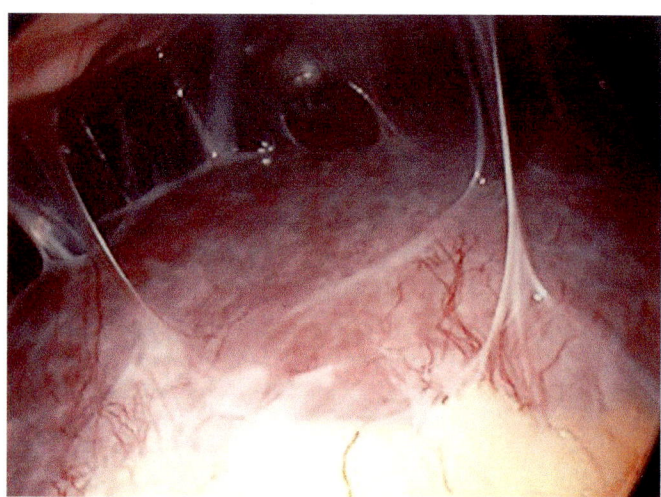

Fig. 20.2 Peritoneal tuberculosis. Laparoscopy showing adhesion between the diaphragm or abdominal wall and the thickened liver capsule with prominent vascularization

20.2 Peritoneal Sarcoidosis

Sarcoidosis is a multisystemic idiopathic granulomatous disease with lung and lymphoid system being the most commonly involved sites. The abdomen is the most common extra-thoracic site, but peritoneum involvement is extremely rare and is not always isolated [11]. CT scan is an excellent means of detecting ascites and soft tissue infiltration of the peritoneal ligaments and mesenteries but hardly distinguishes peritoneal sarcoidosis from tuberculosis, mesothelioma, malignant lymphoma, or carcinomatosis. Gallium scintigram is a useful tool for diagnosis of sarcoidosis in cases involving lacrimal and parotid glands [12]. An accurate diagnosis can be made by laparoscopic-guided biopsy of peritoneal lesions. Multiple small white granulomas are observed on the peritoneum, and the biopsy revealed non-caseating granulomas [13]. Enlarged lymph nodes are also observed in peritoneal sarcoidosis. Lymph nodes are often seen in porta hepatis, para-aortic region, and the celiac axis [14]. The lymph nodes are generally smaller than 2 cm in diameter and are more discrete rather than confluent [11], and these features distinguish sarcoidosis from malignant lymphoma [15]. Most cases of peritoneal sarcoidosis have a benign course, evolving spontaneously. Corticosteroid therapy should be considered for reducing ascites or improving functional impairment of gastrointestinal tract. Methotrexate, azathioprine, or TNF-alpha antagonists may potentially be a second-line treatment in the future [16, 17].

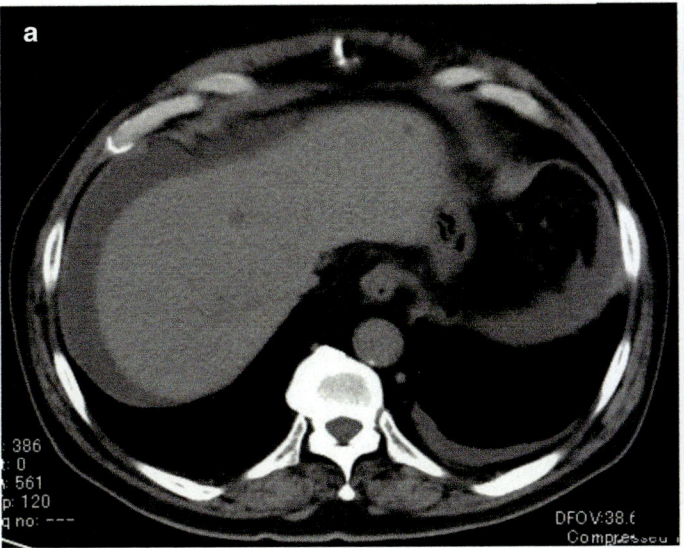

Fig. 20.3 Peritoneal sarcoidosis. (**a**) CT showing ascites around the liver. (**b**) Heterogeneous hyper-density of the omentum (arrow heads). Reprinted from Nihon Shokakibyo Gakkai Zasshi. 2016;113. Kunishi Y, Yoshie K, Ota M, et al. Peritoneal sarcoidosis: an unusual cause of ascites. pp. 143–151. Copyright 2016 with permission from Nihon Shokakibyo Gakkai

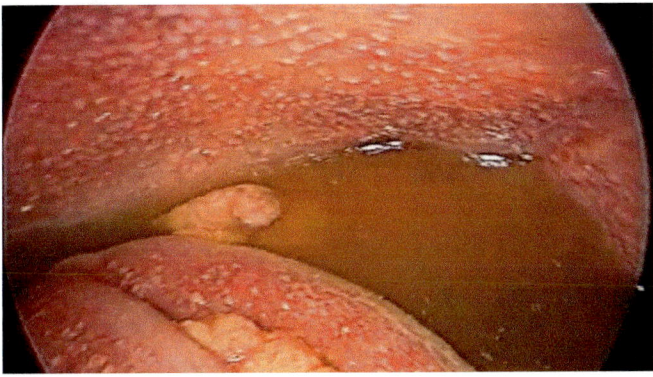

Fig. 20.4 Peritoneal sarcoidosis. Laparoscopy showing multiple white small nodules on the peritoneum. Reprinted from Nihon Shokakibyo Gakkai Zasshi. 2016;113. Kunishi Y, Yoshie K, Ota M, et al. Peritoneal sarcoidosis: an unusual cause of ascites. pp. 143–151. Copyright 2016 with permission from Nihon Shokakibyo Gakkai

Case 20.2

An 83-year-old man presented with abdominal fullness. A computed tomography demonstrated pleural effusion, ascites, peritoneal thickness, and panniculitis (Fig. 20.3). Multiple small white nodules on the peritoneum were observed during laparoscopy (Fig. 20.4), and biopsy revealed non-caseating granulomas (Fig. 20.5). A gallium scintigram demonstrated accumulation in the peritoneum with a characteristic "panda sign" that has been reported to indicate sarcoidosis [12] (Fig. 20.6). The patient was treated with steroid (40 mg/day of prednisolone), resulting in the resolution of ascites and negative gallium scintigram. He was then placed on low-dose steroid therapy and maintained a complete response.

20.3 Sclerosing Encapsulating Peritonitis

Sclerosing encapsulating peritonitis (SEP) is a chronic inflammatory process in which the small intestines are encased by a dense fibro-collagenous membrane [18, 19]. SEP is divided into primary (idiopathic) and secondary forms according to the underlying etiological cause [19, 20]. Idiopathic form is also known as abdominal cocoon [18]. The secondary form is associated with continuous peritoneal dialysis and other rare causes including abdominal surgery, recurrent peritonitis, beta-blocker treatment, peritoneovenous shunting, abdominal tuberculosis, sarcoidosis, intraperitoneal chemotherapy, cirrhosis, liver transplantation, gastrointestinal malignancy, and endometriosis [19]. The early clinical features of SEP are often unrecognized. Clinical manifestation of SEP includes ascites and recurrent acute, subacute, or chronic episodes of intestinal obstruction [21] which are sometimes complicated by life-threatening enterocutaneous fistula, small intestinal necrosis, and malnutrition. Preoperative diagnosis of SEP has become possible with technological advances in image analysis of computed tomography [22], but most cases are diagnosed incidentally at laparotomy. Laparotomy reveals ascites and characteristic gross thickening of the peritoneum, which encloses some or all small intestine and other organs (e.g., appendix, cecum, ascending colon, liver, ovary, etc.). Histologically, the peritoneum shows sheets of dense collagenous tissue with the presence of a mononuclear inflammatory infiltrate [23]. Surgery is the most effective management option for SEP [21], although controversy surrounds the indication, optimal timing, and mode of surgical

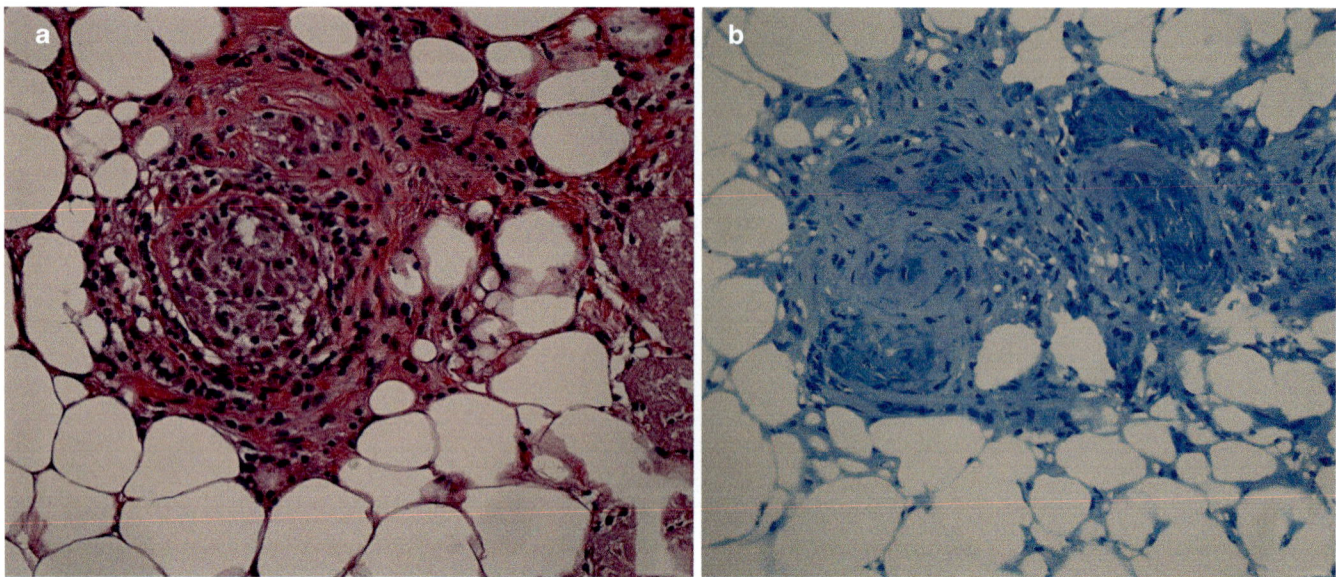

Fig. 20.5 Peritoneal sarcoidosis. (**a**) Hematoxylin and eosin-stained biopsy revealed non-caseating granulomas. (**b**) Ziehl-Neelsen-stained biopsy was negative. Reprinted from Nihon Shokakibyo Gakkai Zasshi. 2016;113. Kunishi Y, Yoshie K, Ota M, et al. Peritoneal sarcoidosis: an unusual cause of ascites. pp. 143–151. Copyright 2016 with permission from Nihon Shokakibyo Gakkai

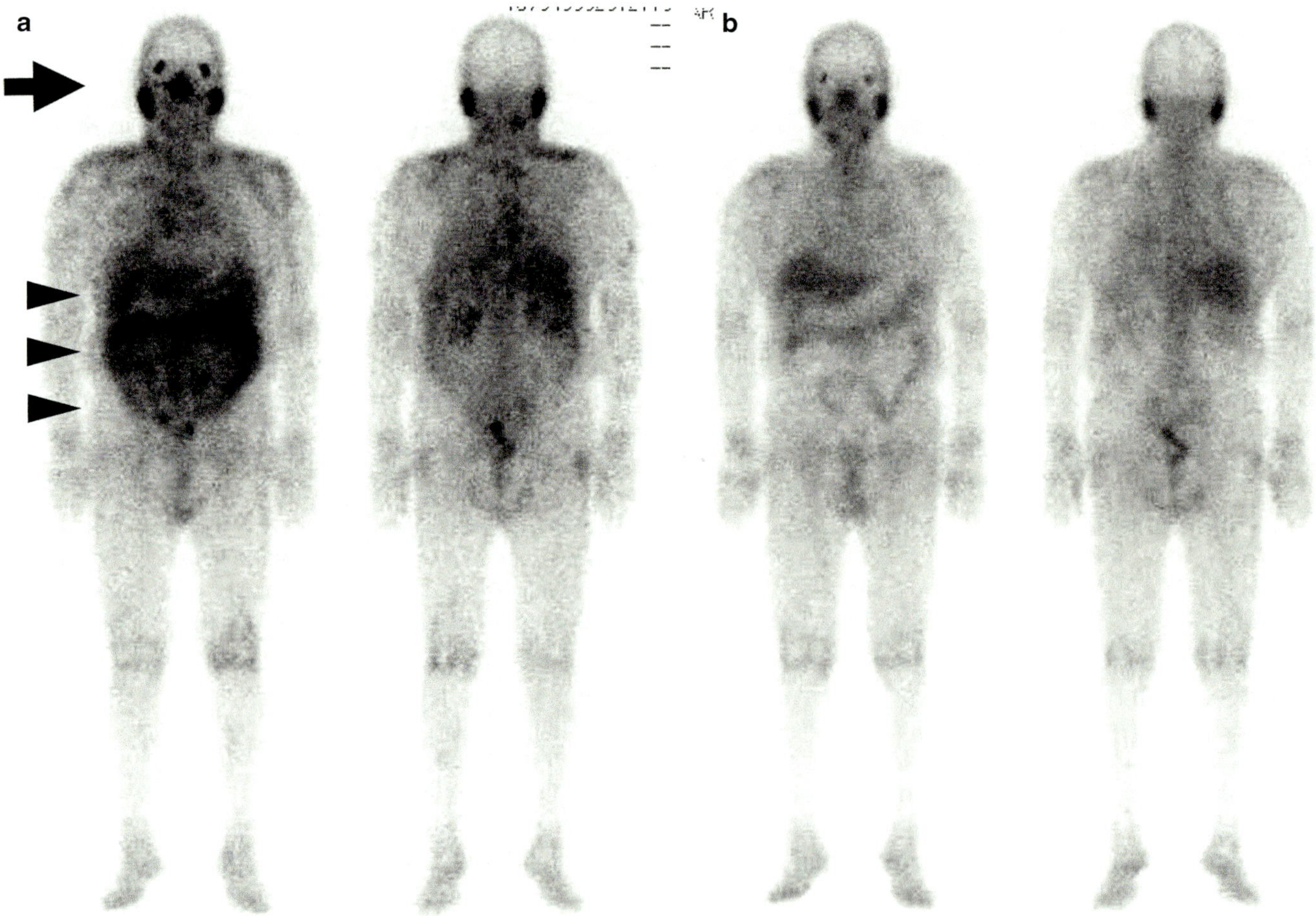

Fig. 20.6 Peritoneal sarcoidosis. (**a**) Gallium scintigram demonstrated an accumulation in the peritoneum (arrow heads). These accumulations were also observed in the lacrimal and parotid glands (arrow), the so-called panda sign. (**b**) Gallium scintigram demonstrating reduced accumulation (improvement) after 2 weeks of treatment with steroids. Reprinted from Nihon Shokakibyo Gakkai Zasshi. 2016;113. Kunishi Y, Yoshie K, Ota M, et al. Peritoneal sarcoidosis: an unusual cause of ascites. pp. 143–151. Copyright 2016 with permission from Nihon Shokakibyo Gakkai

operation. Steroid, tamoxifen, and immunosuppressants are effective in alleviating incomplete obstruction of the small intestine [24].

Case 20.3

A 66-year-old male had suffered from ascites due to alcoholic liver cirrhosis. CT with contrast showed dilated small intestines, thickening of peritoneum, and massive ascites (Fig. 20.7), which was exudative, and neither malignant cell nor bacterium was detected, and ADA was negative. Laparoscopic findings showed sheets of thick, firm, and white-colored membrane on the surface of the liver, stomach, small intestine, and colon (Fig. 20.8a, b). Biopsy of the membrane revealed fibro-collagenous tissue with many inflammatory cells (Fig. 20.8c, d). IgG- and IgG4-positive plasma cells were dominantly present (Fig. 20.9). With the diagnosis of SEP, prednisolone was administered. Ascites disappeared, and repeat CT found reduced thickness of peritoneal wall after treatment. Secondary form of SEP in liver cirrhosis is associated with prolong ascites and sporadic bacterial infection if a patient has neither peritoneal dialysis nor peritoneal-venous shunting [25]. Infiltration of mononuclear cells is seen in fibro-collagenous tissues [23]. The role of IgG- and IgG4-positive plasma cells should further be studied in the pathogenesis of SEP.

20.4 Peritoneal Mesothelioma

Peritoneal mesothelioma is a very rare but a serious and often fatal primary tumor. It has been linked to toxic exposure to industrial pollutants, especially asbestos as well as pleural mesothelioma. Massive and exudative ascites is usually present [26] with an increase in lymphocytes and a high level of hyaluronic acid [27]. Features of peritoneal mesothelioma on computed tomography (CT) range from a "dry" appearance, comprised of peritoneum-based nodular masses, to a "wet" appearance comprised of ascites and peritoneum thickening, which may be nodular or diffuse [28, 29]. Mesothelial tumors are classified into well-differentiated papillary, multicystic, and malignant mesotheliomas. Histologically, malignant mesothelioma is further classified into epithelial, fibrous (sarcomatoid), and mixed types. The prognosis of multicystic mesothelioma is good [30]. Mutations in the BAP1 tumor suppressor gene are associated with malignancy as well as somatic loss of other tumor suppressor genes [31, 32]. The prognosis of epithelial malignant mesothelioma is better than sarcomatoid type. Most patients are not a surgical candidate and are often offered palliative chemotherapy and supportive medical management. Active chemotherapeutic agents include cisplatin, pemetrexed, or a

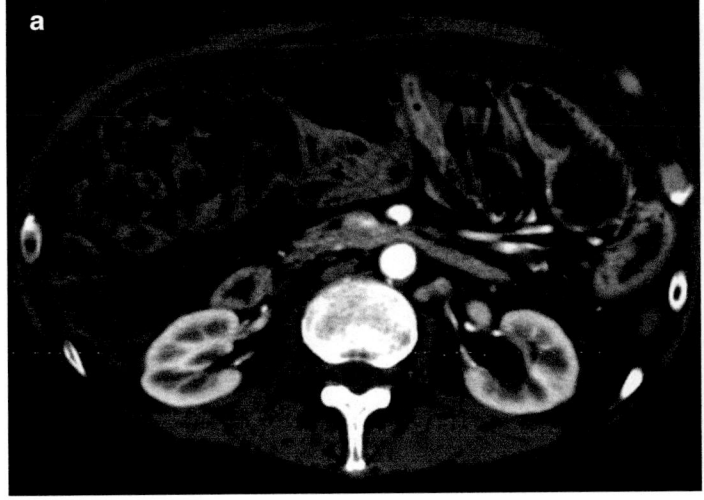
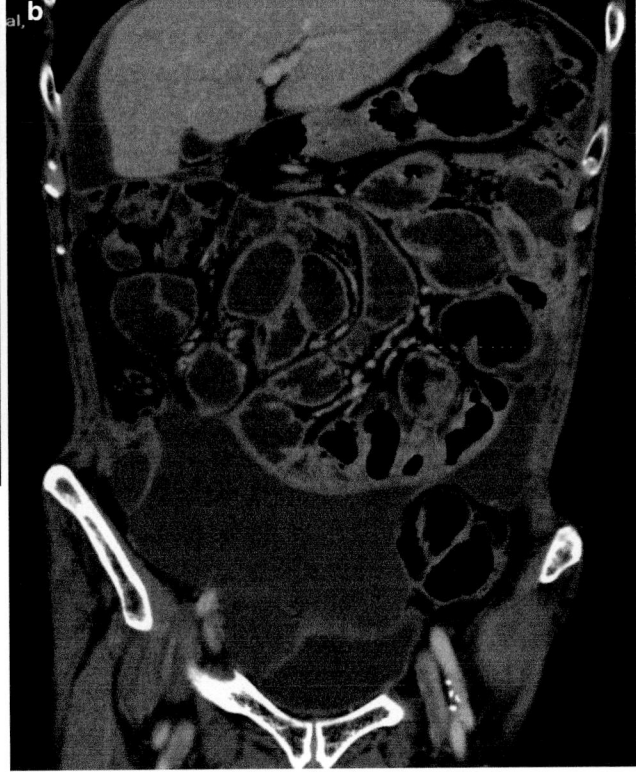

Fig. 20.7 Sclerosing encapsulating peritonitis. (**a**) Abdominal CT with contrast shows mass of dilated and thickened small intestine and ascites. (**b**) Sagittal section of CT shows mass of dilated small intestine and massive ascites. The peritoneum and wall of small intestines are thickened. The lumen of dilated small intestine is filled by fluid

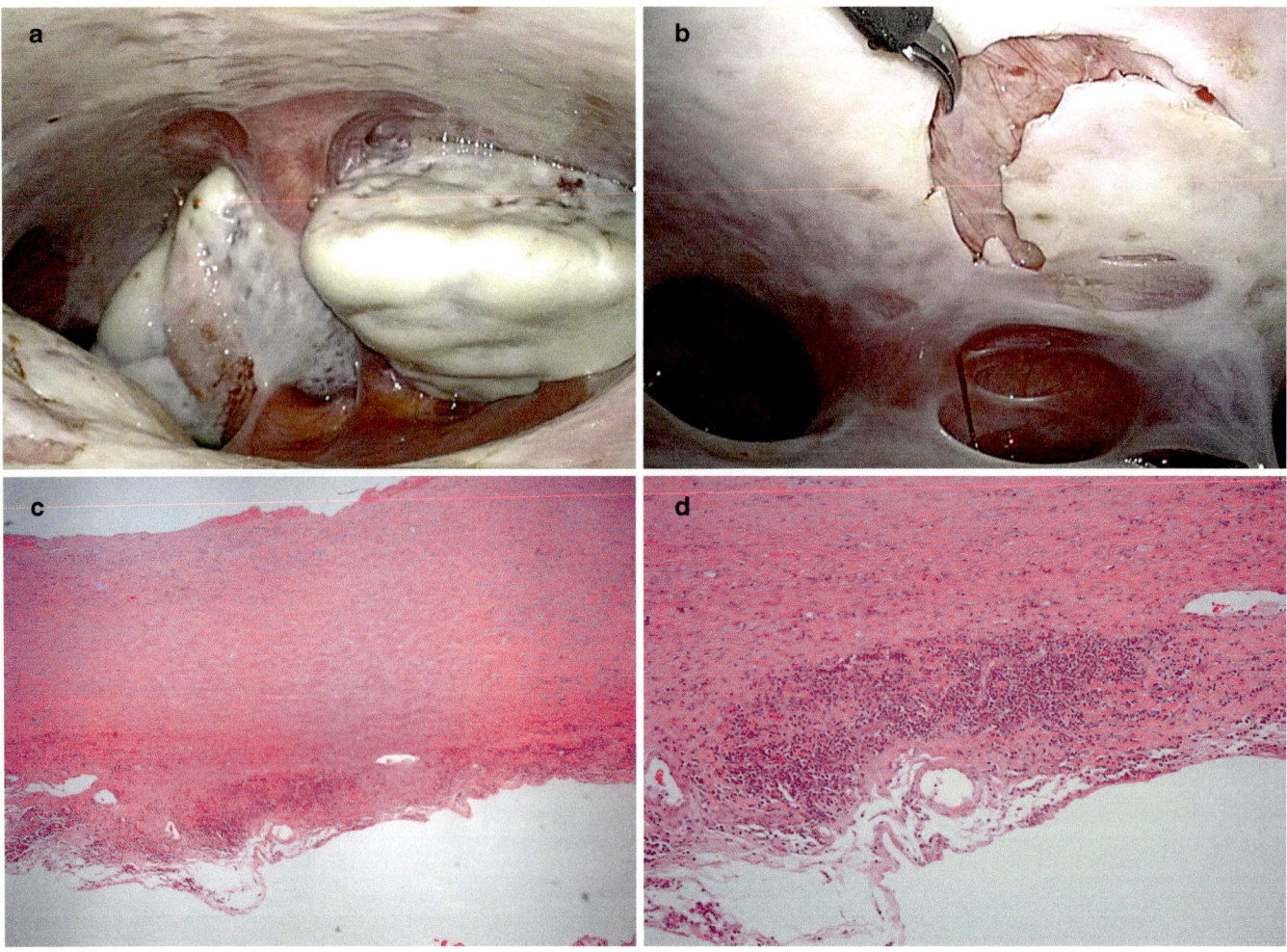

Fig. 20.8 Sclerosing encapsulating peritonitis. (**a**) Peritoneoscopy shows thick-white membrane covering the surface of the liver and peritoneum with adhesion of the peritoneum to the liver. (**b**) Thick-white membrane with adhesion between the peritoneum and omentum. (**c**) Biopsy of thick-white membrane shows fibro-collagenous structure. (**d**) Lower portion of fibro-collagenous membrane is infiltrated by many inflammatory cells

combination of both [33]. Gemcitabine, mitomycin C, inter-leukin-2, and interferon also have modest therapeutic activity [34]. Intraperitoneal chemotherapy has been used to control and relieve symptoms of ascites [35]. Cytoreduction followed by hyperthermal intraperitoneal chemotherapy is now the recommended treatment [36, 37].

Case 20.4

A 42-year-old male presented with yellowish ascites on paracentesis. Lymphocytes and neutrophils were seen microscopically, but there were no neoplastic cells. The serum value of hyaluronic acid was 322 ng/mL, but it was 442,000 ng/mL in the ascitic fluid. CA125 in serum was 43 ng/mL. CT with contrast showing ascites and an irregular peritoneal surface (Fig. 20.10). Mesothelioma of the peritoneum was suspected. Peritoneoscopy showed numerous cystic formations in the abdominal wall and omentum, and solid nodules were seen in the subdiaphragmatic peritoneum (Fig. 20.11). Biopsy of a peritoneal cystic lesion showed mesothelial cells (Fig. 20.12). Cisplatin was administered intraperitoneally, and ascites subsided. The mesothelioma gradually became resistant to cisplatin, while hyaluronic acid increased in the serum and ascitic fluid. The patient died of renal failure 3.5 years later.

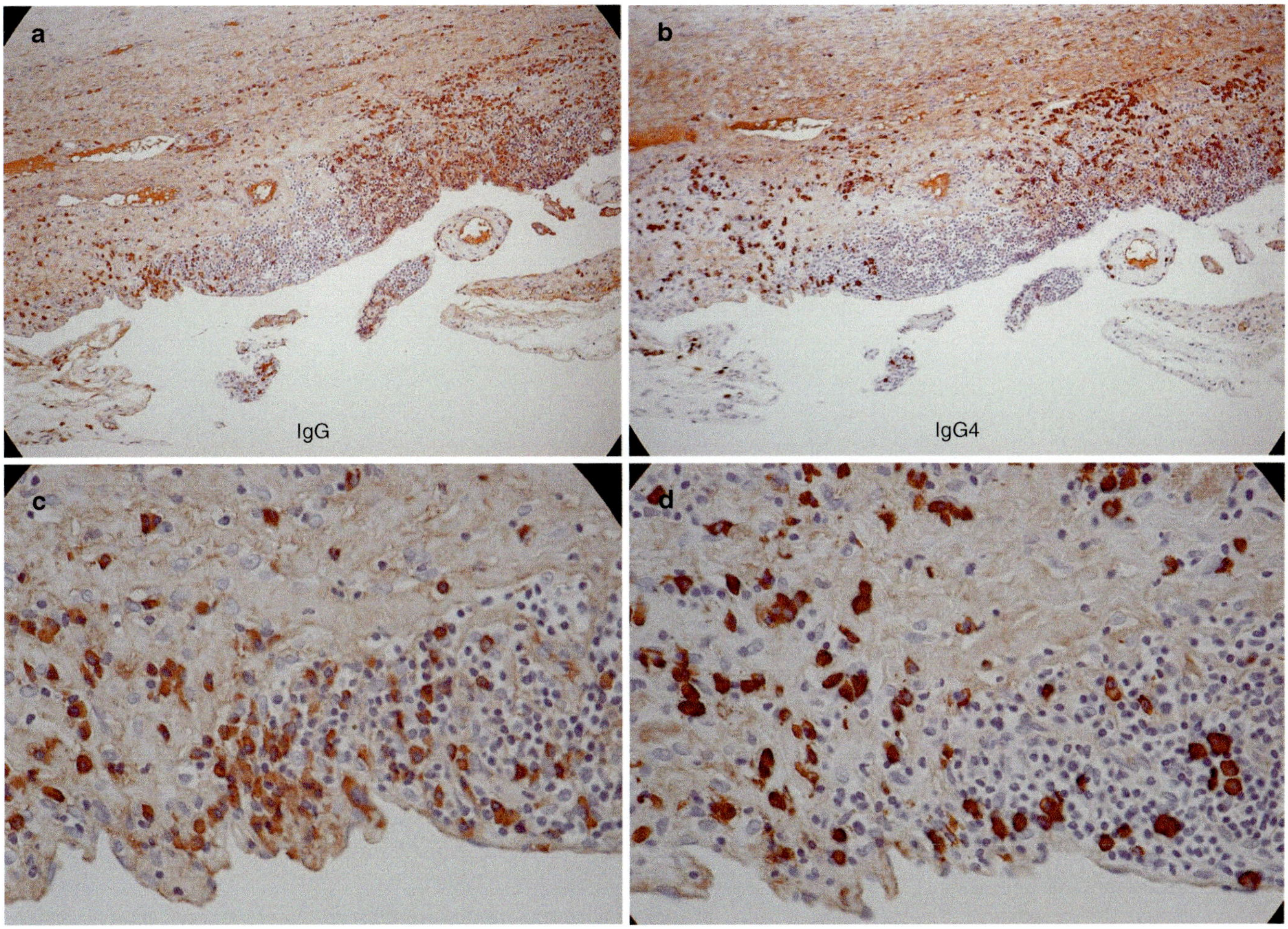

Fig. 20.9 Sclerosing encapsulating peritonitis. (**a, b**) Immunohistochemistry shows presence of IgG-positive inflammatory cells. (**c, d**) Serial sections show the presence of IgG4-positive cells simultaneously in area of IgG-positive cells

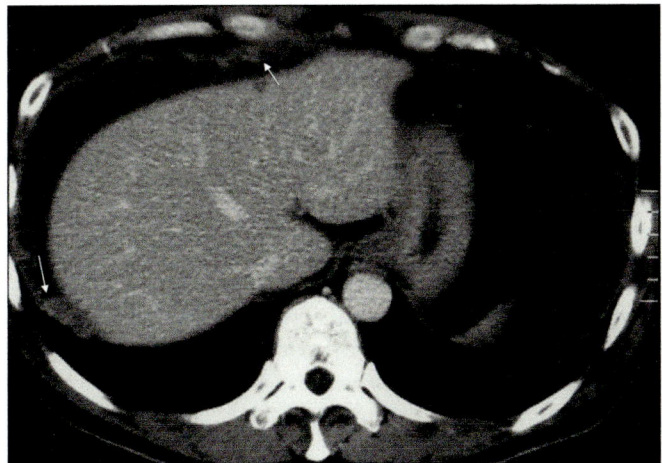

Fig. 20.10 Peritoneal mesothelioma. CT with contrast showing ascites and an irregular and enhanced surface of peritoneum (arrows)

Case 20.5

A 73-year-old male with a history of exposure to asbestos was referred for persistent and massive ascites. Serum hyaluronic acid level was 26,100 ng/mL, and its level was extremely high in the ascitic fluid. Lymphocytes were seen microscopically, but no neoplastic cells were detected. Peritoneoscopy revealed small cystic lesions and nodules on the omentum or peritoneum (Fig. 20.13). Biopsy of a small cystic lesion in the peritoneum showed a sheet of neoplastic cells admixed with fibrosis. Immunohistochemistry showed positivity for cytokeratin 5 and 6, calretinin, and epithelial membrane antigen (Fig. 20.14), consistent with malignant mesothelioma. Cisplatin was administered intravenously, and the patient survived for 1 year.

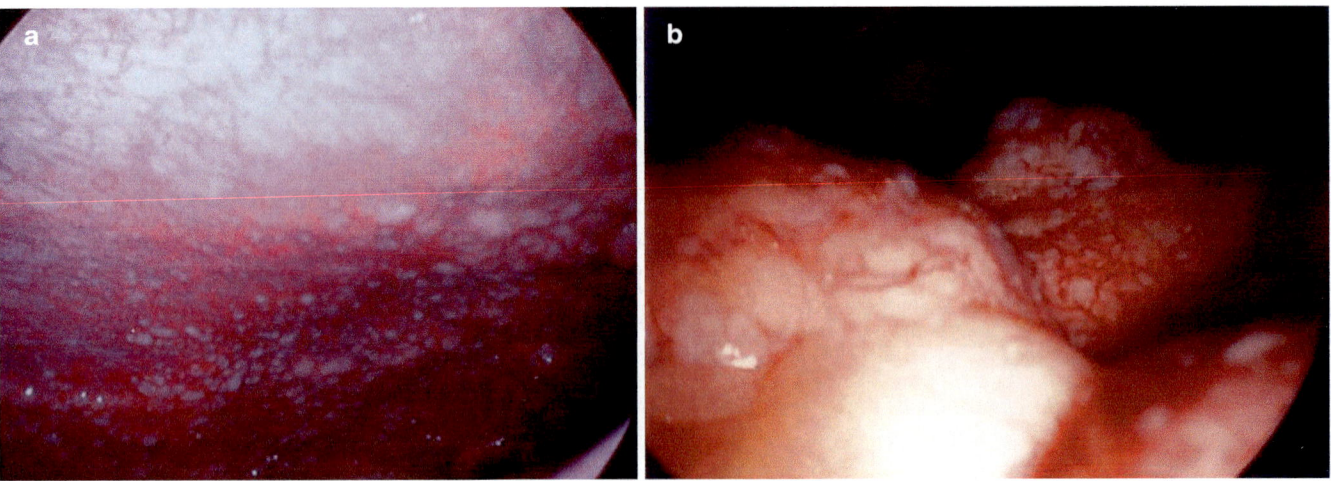

Fig. 20.11 Peritoneal mesothelioma. (**a**) Laparoscopic findings include cystic or nodular lesions in the peritoneum, subdiaphragmatic surface, or abdominal wall. (**b**) Cystic lesions are seen diffusely on the omentum

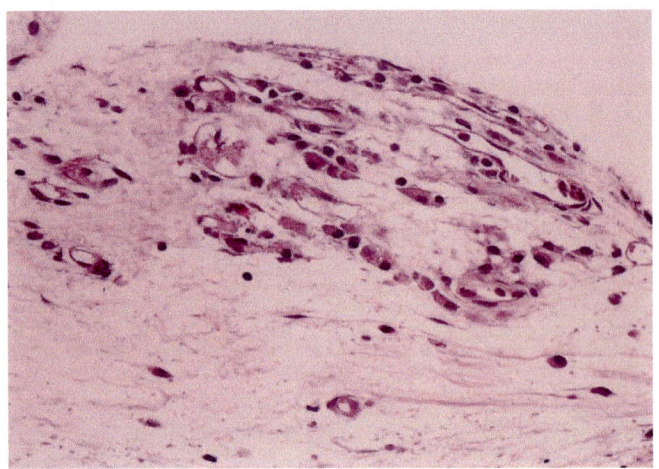

Fig. 20.12 Peritoneal mesothelioma. Biopsy from cyst shows scattered mesothelial cells in coarse mesenchyme

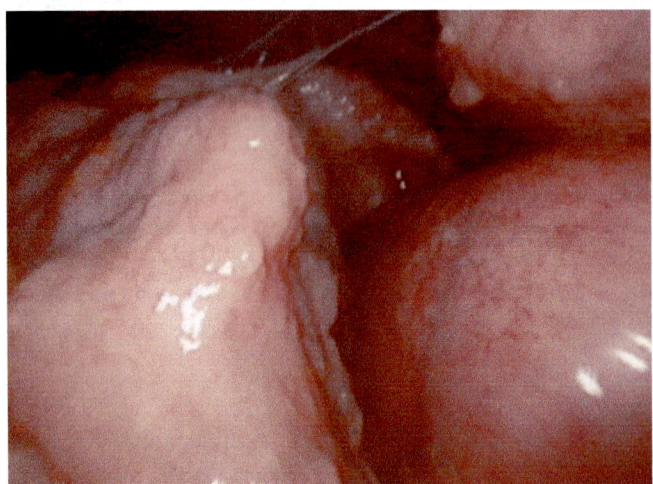

Fig. 20.13 Peritoneal mesothelioma. Diffuse cystic lesions on the omentum and peritoneum with adhesion between the omentum and liver surface

20.5   Peritoneal Carcinomatosis

The peritoneum is the site of metastatic lesions from primary cancer of the gastrointestinal tract [38], pancreas [39], and ovary [40]. Massive ascites often follows peritoneal carcinomatosis. It is important to discriminate carcinomatosis from tuberculosis involvement and mesothelioma and lymphoma involvement. CT or positron emission tomography, laparoscopy with biopsy, and endoscopic ultrasound-guided fine-needle aspiration are used to determine the stage of malignancy for surgical treatment of primary and peritoneal lesions [41–43]. TS-1 with cisplatin chemotherapy is currently the most commonly used first-line chemotherapeutic regimen in patients with advanced gastric cancer [44].

Case 20.6

A 53-year-old female complained of epigastralgia for 1 year, and her serum chemistry showed CRP 1.41 mg/dL, LDH 269 IU/L, ChE 163 IU/L, TP 5.7 g/dL, albumin 2.8 g/dL, and CA19-9 1514 U/mL. Upper gastrointestinal fiberscope revealed giant folds at the greater curvature of the stomach. The stomach extension was poor, but no malignant cells are detected in the biopsy. Upper abdominal CT showed thick stomach wall and swelling of several lymph nodes around the lesser and greater curvature of the stomach. Peritoneoscopy showed a white patch and maculae on the subdiaphragmatic peritoneum, and biopsy showed neoplastic cells admixed with fibrosis, some formed glandular structures (Fig. 20.15). Repeat gastrointestinal fiberscope with biopsy showed poorly differentiated adenocarcinoma of the stomach (Bormann IV and scirrhous type). TS-1 with cisplatin chemotherapy was administered for 6 months, but she died of anasarca within a year.

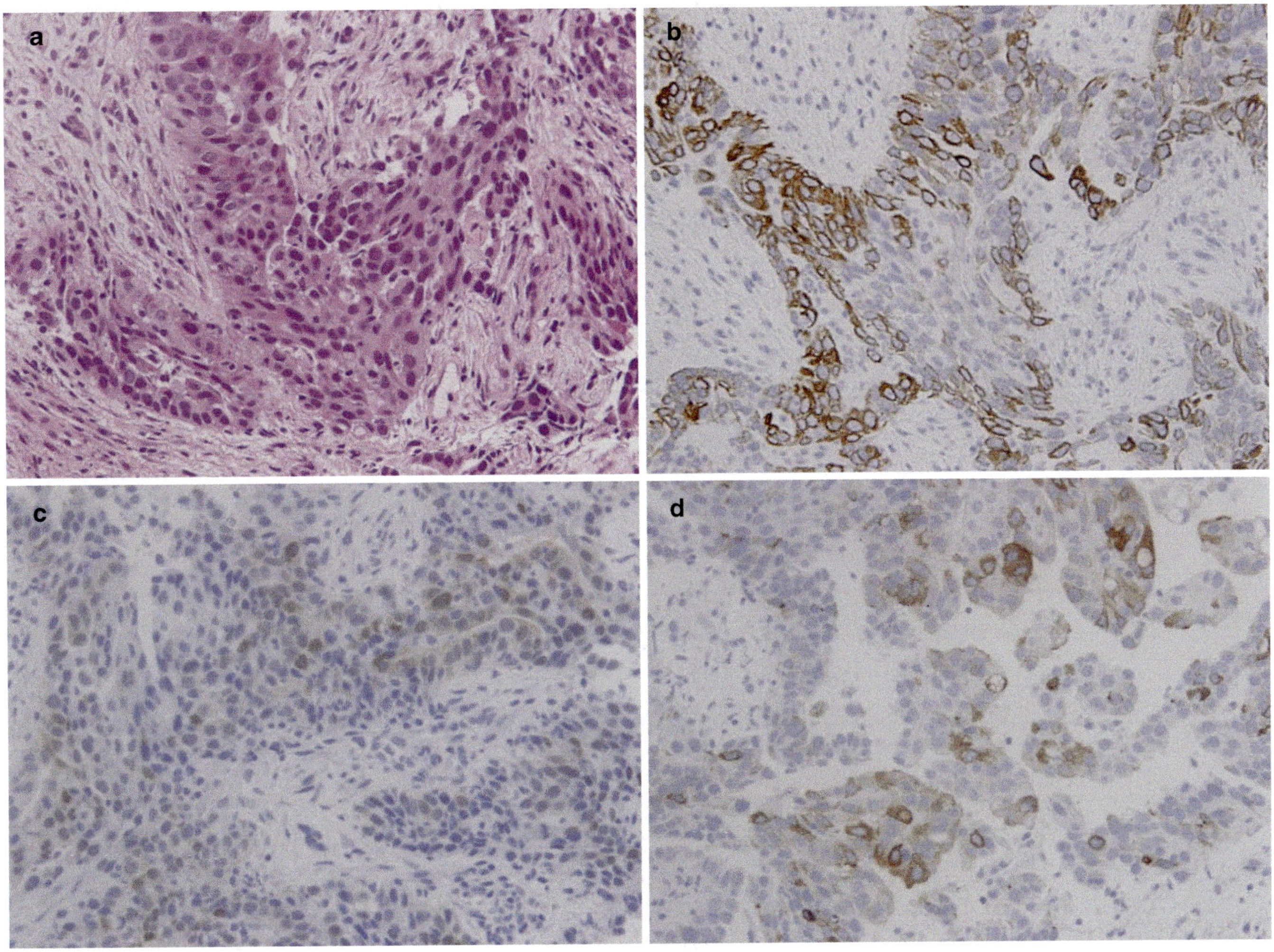

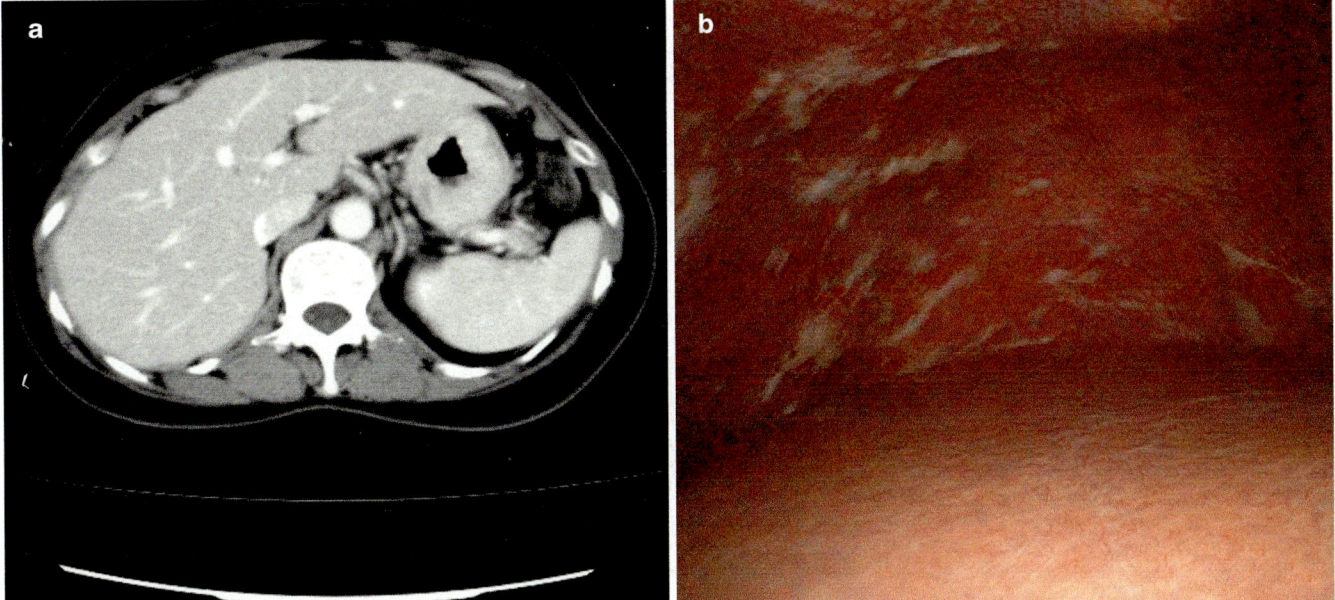

Fig. 20.14 Mesothelioma. (**a**) Neoplastic cells are in sheets and admixed with fibrosis. (**b**) Neoplastic cells are positive for cytokeratin 5 and 6. (**c**) Calretinin-immunoreactivity is seen in the nuclei and cyto-plasm of neoplastic cells. (**d**) Epithelial membrane antigen-immunoreactivity is seen in the cytoplasm of some neoplastic cells

Fig. 20.15 Peritoneal carcinomatosis. (**a**) CT with contrast shows enhanced and thick wall of the stomach, slight presence of ascites, and swelling of small lymph nodes. (**b**) Laparoscopy shows white patches and maculae on the subdiaphragmatic peritoneum. (**c**) Hematoxylin and eosin-stained liver tissue shows mixed neoplastic cells with fibrosis

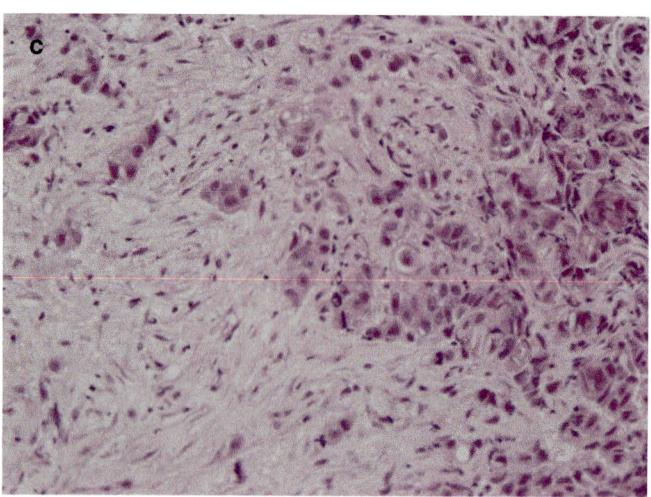

Fig. 20.15 (continued)

References

1. van Baal JOAM, Van de Vijver KK, Nieuwland R, van Noorden CJF, van Driel WJ, Sturk A, Kenter GG, Rikkert LG, Lok CAR. The histophysiology and pathophysiology of the peritoneum. Tissue Cell. 2017;49:95–105.
2. Uzunkoy A, Harma M, Harma M. Diagnosis of abdominal tuberculosis: experience from 11 cases and review of the literature. World J Gastroenterol. 2004;10:3647–9.
3. Sanai FM, Bzeizi KI. Systematic review: tuberculous peritonitis—presenting features, diagnostic strategies and treatment. Aliment Pharmacol Ther. 2005;22:685–700.
4. Malik A, Saxena NC. Ultrasound in abdominal tuberculosis. Abdom Imaging. 2003;28:574–9.
5. Sinan T, Sheikh M, Ramadan S, Sahwney S, Behbehani A. CT features in abdominal tuberculosis: 20 years-experience. BMC Med Imaging. 2002;2:3–16.
6. Shimamoto H, Hamada K, Higuchi I, et al. Abdominal tuberculosis: peritoneal involvement shown by F-18 FDG PET. Clin Nucl Med. 2007;32:716–8.
7. Riquelme A, Calvo M, Salech F, Valderrama S, Pattillo A, Arellano M, et al. Value of adenosine deaminase (ADA) in ascitic fluid for the diagnosis of tuberculous peritonitis: a meta-analysis. J Clin Gastroenterol. 2006;40:705–10.
8. Henning H, Lightdale CJ, Look D. Color atlas of diagnostic laparoscopy. New York: Thieme Medical Publishers; 1994. p. 199–200.
9. Milingos S, Protopapas A, Papadimitriou C, Rodolakis A, Kallipolitis G, Skartados N, et al. Laparoscopy in the evaluation of women with unexplained ascites: an invaluable diagnostic tool. J Minim Invasive Gynecol. 2007;14:43–8.
10. Jorge AD. Peritoneal tuberculosis. Endoscopy. 1984;16:10–2.
11. Gezer NS, Başara I, Altay C, Harman M, Rocher L, Karabulut N, et al. Abdominal sarcoidosis: cross-sectional imaging findings. Diagn Interv Radiol. 2015;21:111–7.
12. Kurdziel KA. The panda sign. Radiology. 2000;215:884–5.
13. Kunishi Y, Yoshie K, Ota M, Kuboi Y, Kanno M, Tanaka S, et al. Peritoneal sarcoidosis: an unusual cause of ascites. Nihon Shokakibyo Gakkai Zasshi. 2016;113:143–51.
14. Warshauer DM, Molina PL, Hamman SM, Koehler RE, Paulson EK, Bechtold RE, et al. Nodular sarcoidosis of the liver and spleen: analysis of 32 cases. Radiology. 1995;195:757–62.
15. Warshauer DM, Lee JKT. Imaging manifestations of abdominal sarcoidosis. Am J Roentgenol. 2004;182:15–28.
16. Judson MA. Advances in the diagnosis and treatment of sarcoidosis. F1000Prime Rep. 2014;6:89–65.
17. Dasilva V, Breuil V, Chevallier P, Euller-Ziegler L. Relapse of severe sarcoidosis with uncommon peritoneal location after TNF-alpha blockade. Efficacy of rituximab: report of a single case. Joint Bone Spine. 2010;77:82–3.
18. Foo KT, Ng KC, Rauff A, Foong WC, Sinniah R. Unusual small intestinal obstruction in adolescent girls: the abdominal cocoon. Br J Surg. 1978;65:427–30.
19. Akbulut S. Accurate definition and management of idiopathic sclerosing encapsulating peritonitis. World J Gastroenterol. 2015;21:675–87.
20. Tannoury JN, Abboud BN. Idiopathic sclerosing encapsulating peritonitis: abdominal cocoon. World J Gastroenterol. 2012;18:1999–2004.
21. Li N, Zhu W, Li Y, Gong J, Gu L, Li M, Cao L, Li J. Surgical treatment and perioperative management of idiopathic abdominal cocoon: single-center review of 65 cases. World J Surg. 2014;38:1860–7.
22. George C, Al-Zwae K, Nair S, Cast JE. Computed tomography appearances of sclerosing encapsulating peritonitis. Clin Radiol. 2007;62:732–7.
23. Honda K, Oda H. Pathology of encapsulating peritoneal sclerosis. Perit Dial Int. 2005;25(Suppl 4):S19–29.
24. Habib SM, Betjes MG, Fieren MW, Boeschoten EW, Abrahams AC, Boer WH, et al. Management of encapsulating peritoneal sclerosis: a guideline on optimal and uniform treatment. Neth J Med. 2011;69:500–7.
25. Yamamoto S, Sato Y, Takahashi T, Kobayashi T, Hatakeyama K. Sclerosing encapsulating peritonitis in two patients with liver cirrhosis. J Gastroenterol. 2004;39:172–5.
26. Averbach AM, Sugarbaker PH. Peritoneal mesothelioma: treatment approach based on natural history. Cancer Treat Res. 1996;81:193–211.
27. Friedman MT, Gentile P, Tarectecan A, Fuchs A. Malignant mesothelioma: immunohistochemistry and DNA ploidy analysis as methods to differentiate mesothelioma from benign reactive mesothelial cell proliferation and adenocarcinoma in pleural and peritoneal effusions. Arch Pathol Lab Med. 1996;120:959–66.
28. Pickhardt PJ, Bhalla S. Primary neoplasms of peritoneal and subperitoneal origin: CT findings. Radiographics. 2005;25:983–95.
29. Park JY, Kim KW, Kwon HJ, Park MS, Kwon GY, Jun SY, et al. Peritoneal mesotheliomas: clinicopathologic features, CT findings, and differential diagnosis. AJR Am J Roentgenol. 2008;191:814–25.
30. Søreide JA, Søreide K, Körner H, Søiland H, Greve OJ, GudLaugsson E. Benign peritoneal cystic mesothelioma. World J Surg. 2006;30:560–6.
31. Nasu M, Emi M, Pastorino S, et al. High incidence of somatic BAP1 alterations in sporadic malignant mesothelioma. J Thorac Oncol. 2015;10(2):565–76.
32. Cercek A, Zaderer M, Rimner A, et al. Confirmation of high prevalence of BAP1 inactivation in mesothelioma. J Clin Oncol. 2015;33(Suppl):Abstract 7564.
33. Vogelzang NJ, Rusthoven JJ, Symanowski J, Denham C, Kaukel E, Ruffie P, et al. Phase III study of pemetrexed in combination with cisplatin versus cisplatin alone in patients with malignant pleural mesothelioma. J Clin Oncol. 2003;21:2636–44.
34. Hassan R, Alexander R, Antman K, Boffetta P, Churg A, Coit D, et al. Current treatment options and biology of peritoneal mesothelioma: meeting summary of the first NIH peritoneal mesothelioma conference. Ann Oncol. 2006;17:1615–9.
35. Mohamed F, Sugarbaker PH. Peritoneal mesothelioma. Curr Treat Options Oncol. 2002;3:375–86.

36. Baratti D, Kusamura S, Cabras AD, Dileo P, Laterza B, Deraco M. Diffuse malignant peritoneal mesothelioma: failure analysis following cytoreduction and hyperthermic intraperitoneal chemotherapy (HIPEC). Ann Surg Oncol. 2009;16:463–72.

37. Kim J, Bhagwandin S, Labow DM. Malignant peritoneal mesothelioma: a review. Ann Transl Med. 2017;5:236–46.

38. Muntean V, Mihailov A, Iancu C, Toganel R, Fabian O, Domsa I, et al. Staging laparoscopy in gastric cancer. Accuracy and impact on therapy. J Gastrointestin Liver Dis. 2009;18:189–95.

39. del Castillo CF, Warshaw L. Peritoneal metastases in pancreatic carcinoma. Hepatogastroenterology. 1993;40:430–2.

40. Groutz A, Carmon E, Gat A. Peritoneal tuberculosis versus advanced ovarian cancer: a diagnostic dilemma. Obstet Gynecol. 1998;91:868.

41. Suzuki A, Kawano T, Takahashi N, Lee J, Nakagami Y, Miyagi E, et al. Value of 18F-FDG PET in the detection of peritoneal carcinomatosis. Eur J Nucl Med Mol Imaging. 2004;31:1413–20.

42. Pomel C, Provencher D, Dauplat J, Gauthier P, Le Bouedec G, Drouin P, et al. Laparoscopic staging of early ovarian cancer. Gynecol Oncol. 1995;58:301–6.

43. Sharma V, Rana SS, Ahmed SU, Guleria S, Sharma R, Gupta R. Endoscopic ultrasound fine-needle aspiration from ascites and peritoneal nodules: a scoping review. Endosc Ultrasound. 2017;6:382–8.

44. Koizumi W, Tanabe S, Saigenji K, Ohtsu A, Boku N, Nagashima F, et al. Phase I/II study of S-1 combined with cisplatin in patients with advanced gastric cancer. Br J Cancer. 2003;89: 2207–12.

Index

© Springer Nature Singapore Pte Ltd. 2019
E. Hashimoto et al. (eds.), *Diagnosis of Liver Disease*, https://doi.org/10.1007/978-981-13-6806-6

Printed by Printforce, the Netherlands